MOLECULAR BIOLOGY OF
PSEUDOMONADS

MOLECULAR BIOLOGY OF
PSEUDOMONADS

Edited by

Teruko Nakazawa
Department of Microbiology
Yamaguchi University School of Medicine
Ube, Yamaguchi, Japan

Kensuke Furukawa
Department of Agricultural Chemistry
Kyushu University
Fukuoka, Japan

Dieter Haas
Laboratoire de Biologie Microbienne
Université de Lausanne
Lausanne, Switzerland

Simon Silver
Department of Microbiology and Immunology
University of Illinois
Chicago, Illinois

ASM PRESS, Washington, D.C.

1325 Massachusetts Ave., NW
Washington, DC 20005

Library of Congress Cataloging-in-Publication Data

International Symposium on Pseudomonads: Molecular Biology and Biotechnology (5th : 1995 : Tsukuba-shi, Japan)
Molecular biology of pseudomonads / edited by Teruko Nakazawa . . . [et al.]
p cm.
Proceeding of the Fifth International Symposium on Pseudomonads: Molecular Biology and Biotechnology, in Tsukuba, Japan, August 1995.
Includes bibliographical references and index.
ISBN 1-55581-104-3
1. Pseudomonad—Molecular aspects—Congresses. I. Nakazawa, Teruko. II. Title.
QR82.P78I58 1995
589.9′5—dc20 96-18032
CIP

Printed in the United States of America

Cover photo: The view of an octameric BphC molecule along the fourfold axis (see Senda and Mitsui, chapter 27, this volume) (photo courtesy T. Senda)

CONTENTS

IV. DYNAMIC FEATURES OF PSEUDOMONADS

V. ENVIRONMENTAL AND INDUSTRIAL MICROBIOLOGY

VI. PROTEIN STRUCTURE AND ENGINEERING

VII. CELL ENVELOPE, TRANSPORT, AND RESISTANCES

VIII. MEDICAL ASPECTS AND PATHOGENESIS

IX. PLANT-BACTERIAL INTERACTIONS

CONTRIBUTORS†

Mitsuko Abe (40) • Department of Microbiology, Yamaguchi University School of Medicine, Ube, Yamaguchi 755, Japan

Hiroyuki Arai (26) • Laboratory of Microbiology, The Institute of Physical and Chemical Research (RIKEN), 2-1 Hirosawa, Wako, Saitama 351-01, Japan

Marc Bally (37) • Laboratoire d'Ingénierie et Dynamique des Systèmes Membranaires, Centre National de la Recherche Scientifique UPR 9027, 31 Chemin Joseph Aiguier, B.P. 71, 13402 Marseille Cedex 20, France

Paola Barbieri (5) • Dipartimento di Genetica e di Biologia dei Microrganismi, via Celoria 26, 20133 Milan, Italy

Fabrizio Beltrametti (5) • Dipartimento di Genetica e di Biologia dei Microrganismi, via Celoria 26, 20133 Milan, Italy

Bernard Berger (20) • Laboratoire de Biologie Microbienne, Université de Lausanne, CH-1015 Lausanne, Switzerland

Hélène Bergeron (14) • Biotechnology Research Institute, National Research Council Canada, 6100 Royalmount Avenue, Montreal, Quebec H4P 2R2, Canada

Giovanni Bertoni (5) • Centro Nacional de Biotecnologia, Campus de Cantoblanco, UAM 28049 Madrid, Spain

Giuseppina Bestetti (5) • Dipartimento di Genetica e di Biologia dei Microrganismi, via Celoria 26, 20133 Milan, Italy

Rafael Blasco (10) • Departamento de Bioquimica y Biologia Molecular, Universidad de Cordoba, Avenida S. Alberto Magno S/N, 14071 Cordoba, Spain

Sophie Bléves (37) • Laboratoire d'Ingénierie et Dynamique des Systèmes Membranaires, Centre National de la Recherche Scientifique UPR 9027, 31 Chemin Joseph Aiguier, B.P. 71, 13402 Marseille Cedex 20, France

Fabrizio Bolognese (5) • Dipartimento di Genetica e di Biologia dei Microrganismi, via Celoria 26, 20133 Milan, Italy

John C. Boucher (34) • Department of Microbiology and Immunology, 5641 Medical Science Building II, University of Michigan Medical School, Ann Arbor, Michigan 48109-0620

Melissa Brown (38) • Department of Microbiology and Immunology, University of British Columbia, Vancouver, B.C. V6T 1Z3, Canada

Barrie W. Bycroft (16) • Department of Pharmaceutical Sciences, University of Nottingham, Nottingham NG7 2RD, United Kingdom

M. Callanan (44) • Department of Microbiology, University College Cork, Cork, Ireland

Miguel Camara (16) • Department of Pharmaceutical Sciences, University of Nottingham, Nottingham NG7 2RD, United Kingdom

† Numbers in parentheses indicate chapter number.

Carlos Cervantes (35) • Instituto de Investigaciones Químico-Biológicas, Universidad Michoacana, Edificio B-1, Cd. Universitaria, 58240 Morelia, Mich., Mexico

Ananda M. Chakrabarty (11) • Department of Microbiology and Immunology, University of Illinois at Chicago, Chicago, Illinois 60612

Virginie Chapon (37) • Laboratoire d'Ingénierie et Dynamique des Systèmes Membranaires, Centre National de la Recherche Scientifique UPR 9027, 31 Chemin Joseph Aiguier, B.P. 71, 13402 Marseille Cedex 20, France

Qi Chen (4) • Institute of Biotechnology, Swiss Federal Institute of Technology, ETH-Hoenggerberg, 8093 Zürich, Switzerland

Heather L. Currie (39) • Department of Microbiology, University of Guelph, Guelph, Ontario N1G 2W1, Canada

Charles Dean (33) • Department of Microbiology and Immunology, Queen's University, Kingston, Ontario K7L 3N6, Canada

Teresa R. de Kievit (39) • Department of Microbiology, University of Guelph, Guelph, Ontario N1G 2W1, Canada

I. Delany (44) • Department of Microbiology, University College Cork, Cork, Ireland

Asunción Delgado (17) • Department of Biochemistry, Molecular and Cellular Biology of Plants, Consejo Superior de Investigaciones Científicas, Apdo 419, E-18008 Granada, Spain

Víctor de Lorenzo (13) • Department of Microbial Biotechnology, Centro Nacional de Biotecnología, Campus de Cantoblanco, 28049 Madrid, Spain

V. Deretic (34) • Department of Microbiology and Immunology, 5641 Medical Science Building II, University of Michigan Medical School, Ann Arbor, Michigan 48109-0620

Caroline A. DeVries (41) • Department of Microbiology and Immunology, University of Tennessee and VA Medical Center, Memphis, Tennessee 38163

Patrizia Di Gennaro (5) • Dipartimento di Genetica e di Biologia dei Microrganismi, via Celoria 26, 20133 Milan, Italy

Bauke W. Dijkstra (28) • Laboratory of Biophysical Chemistry, NL-9747 AG Groningen, The Netherlands

D. N. Dowling (44) • Department of Microbiology, University College Cork, Cork, Ireland

Robert Drew (29) • Department of Biochemistry and Molecular Biology, University College London, Gower Street, London WC1E 6BT, United Kingdom

Tim Falla (38) • Department of Microbiology and Immunology, University of British Columbia, Vancouver, B.C. V6T 1Z3, Canada

S. Fedi (44) • Department of Microbiology, University College Cork, Cork, Ireland

A. Fenton (44) • Department of Microbiology, University College Cork, Cork, Ireland

Silvia Fernández (13) • Department of Microbial Biotechnology, Centro Nacional de Biotecnología, Campus de Cantoblanco, 28049 Madrid, Spain

Shafique Fidai (38) • Department of Microbiology and Immunology, University of British Columbia, Vancouver, B.C. V6T 1Z3, Canada

Alain Filloux (37) • Laboratoire d'Ingénierie et Dynamique des Systèmes Membranaires, Centre National de la Recherche Scientifique UPR 9027, 31 Chemin Joseph Aiguier, B.P. 71, 13402 Marseille Cedex 20, France

Dennis D. Focht (7) • Department of Soil and Environmental Sciences, University of California, Riverside, California 92521

Maryline Foglino (37) • Laboratoire d'Ingénierie et Dynamique des Systèmes Membranaires, Centre National de la Recherche Scientifique UPR 9027, 31 Chemin Joseph Aiguier, B.P. 71, 13402 Marseille Cedex 20, France

Michael J. Franklin (41) • Department of Microbiology and Immunology, University of Tennessee and VA Medical Center, Memphis, Tennessee 38163

Masao Fukuda (6) • Department of Bioengineering, Nagaoka University of Technology, Kamitomioka, Nagaoka, Niigata 940-21, Japan

Jun Fukushima (42) • Department of Bacteriology, Yokohama City University School of Medicine, 3-9 Fukuura, Kanazawa-ku, Yokohama 236, Japan

Kensuke Furukawa (8) • Department of Agricultural Chemistry, Kyushu University, Hakozaki, Fukuoka 812-81, Japan

Maria-Trinidad Gallegos (17) • Department of Biochemistry, Molecular and Cellular Biology of Plants, Consejo Superior de Investigaciones Científicas, Apdo 419, E-18008 Granada, Spain

Enrica Galli (5) • Dipartimento di Genetica e di Biologia dei Microrganismi, via Celoria 26, 20133 Milan, Italy

James Garnon (14) • Biotechnology Research Institute, National Research Council Canada, 6100 Royalmount Avenue, Montreal, Quebec H4P 2R2, Canada

Gijs Gerritse (28) • Genencor, NL-2600 MA Delft, The Netherlands

Monisha Gough (38) • Department of Microbiology and Immunology, University of British Columbia, Vancouver, B.C. V6T 1Z3, Canada

Irwin C. Gunsalus (2) • Gulf Ecology Division, U.S. Environmental Protection Agency, 1 Sabine Island Drive, Gulf Breeze, Florida 32561-5299

Dieter Haas (20, 28) • Laboratoire de Biologie Microbienne, Université de Lausanne, CH-1015 Lausanne, Switzerland

Robert E. W. Hancock (38) • Department of Microbiology and Immunology, University of British Columbia, Vancouver, B.C. V6T 1Z3, Canada

Shigeaki Harayama (21) • Marine Biotechnology Institute, Kamaishi Laboratories, 3-75-1 Heita, Kamaishi City, 026 Iwate, Japan

Jürgen Havel (9) • Bergische Universität, Gesamthochschule Wuppertal, Chemische Mikrobiologie, Gaußstraße 20, D-42097 Wuppertal, Germany

Osamu Hayaishi (1) • Osaka Bioscience Institute, 6-2-4 Furuedai, Suita, Osaka 565, Japan

David Heinrichs (33) • Department of Microbiology and Immunology, Queen's University, Kingston, Ontario K7L 3N6, Canada

William Hendrickson (22) • Department of Microbiology and Immunology, University of Illinois, Chicago, Illinois 60612

Sunggi Heu (45) • Plant Molecular Biology Laboratory, Agricultural Research Service, U.S. Department of Agriculture, Beltsville, Maryland 20705

Tung Hoang (19) • Department of Microbiology and Infectious Diseases, University of Calgary, Calgary, Alberta T2N 4N1, Canada

Bernd Hofer (10) • Division of Microbiology, National Research Centre for Biotechnology, Mascheroder Weg 1, 38124 Braunschweig, Germany

Bruce W. Holloway (3) • Department of Genetics and Developmental Biology, Monash University, Clayton, Victoria, 3168 Australia

Anette Hübner (22) • Department of Microbiology and Immunology, University of Illinois, Chicago, Illinois 60612

Steven W. Hutcheson (45) • Department of Plant Biology, University of Maryland at College Park, College Park, Maryland 20742; joint appointment with the Center of Agricultural Biotechnology of the University of Maryland Biotechnology Institute

Yasuo Igarashi (26) • Department of Biotechnology, University of Tokyo, Yayoi 1-1-1, Bunkyo-ku, Tokyo 113, Japan

Tadayuki Imanaka (25) • Department of Biotechnology, Graduate School of Engineering, Osaka University, 2-1 Yamadaoka, Suita, Osaka 565, Japan

Junko Ishii (32) • The Department of Molecular Life Science, Tokai University School of Medicine, Isehara 259-11, Japan

Ryo Iwakiri (8) • Department of Agricultural Chemistry, Kyushu University, Hakozaki, Fukuoka 812-81, Japan

Karl-Erich Jaeger (28) • Lehrstuhl Biologie der Mikroorganismen, Ruhr-Universität, D-44780 Bochum, Germany

Deokjin Jahng (24) • Department of Chemical and Biochemical Engineering, University of California, Irvine, Irvine, California 92717-2575

Songmu Jin (45) • Department of Plant Biology, University of Maryland at College Park, College Park, Maryland 20742

Thomas Kasberg (9) • Bergische Universität, Gesamthochschule Wuppertal, Chemische Mikrobiologie, Gaußstraße 20, D-42097 Wuppertal, Germany

Stefan R. Kaschabek (9) • Bergische Universität, Gesamthochschule Wuppertal, Chemische Mikrobiologie, Gaußstraße 20, D-42097 Wuppertal, Germany

Junichi Kato (15) • Department of Fermentation Technology, Hiroshima University, Higashi-Hiroshima, Hiroshima 739, Japan

Andrew Kavanaugh-Black (22) • Department of Microbiology and Immunology, University of Illinois, Chicago, Illinois 60612

Susumu Kawamoto (42) • Department of Bacteriology, Yokohama City University School of Medicine, 3-9 Fukuura, Kanazawa-ku, Yokohama 236, Japan

Shinji Kawasaki (26) • Department of Biotechnology, University of Tokyo, Yayoi 1-1-1, Bunkyo-ku, Tokyo 113, Japan

Laurie Kilburn (33) • Department of Microbiology and Immunology, Queen's University, Kingston, Ontario K7L 3N6, Canada

Craig S. Kim (24) • Department of Chemical and Biochemical Engineering, University of California, Irvine, Irvine, California 92717-2575

Nobutada Kimura (8) • Department of Agricultural Chemistry, Kyushu University, Hakozaki, Fukuoka 812-81, Japan

Tanya Klassen (19) • Department of Microbiology and Infectious Diseases, University of Calgary, Calgary, Alberta T2N 4N1, Canada

Tohru Kodama (26) • Department of Biotechnology, University of Tokyo, Yayoi 1-1-1, Bunkyo-ku, Tokyo 113, Japan

Kathleen Krebes (33) • Department of Microbiology and Immunology, Queen's University, Kingston, Ontario K7L 3N6, Canada

Minoru Kurata (42) • Department of Bacteriology, Yokohama City University School of Medicine, 3-9 Fukuura, Kanazawa-ku, Yokohama 236, Japan

Akio Kuroda (15) • Department of Fermentation Technology, Hiroshima University, Higashi-Hiroshima, Hiroshima 739, Japan

Diane Labbé (14) • Biotechnology Research Institute, National Research Council Canada, 6100 Royalmount Avenue, Montreal, Quebec H4P 2R2, Canada

Joseph S. Lam (39) • Department of Microbiology, University of Guelph, Guelph, Ontario N1G 2W1, Canada

Amel Latifi (37) • Laboratoire d'Ingénierie et Dynamique des Systèmes Membranaires, Centre National de la Recherche Scientifique UPR 9027, 31 Chemin Joseph Aiguier, B.P. 71, 13402 Marseille Cedex 20, France

Peter C. K. Lau (14) • Biotechnology Research Institute, National Research Council Canada, 6100 Royalmount Avenue, Montreal, Quebec H4P 2R2, Canada

Andrée Lazdunski (37) • Laboratoire d'Ingénierie et Dynamique des Systèmes Membranaires, Centre National de la Recherche Scientifique UPR 9027, 31 Chemin Joseph Aiguier, B.P. 71, 13402 Marseille Cedex 20, France

Xian-Zhi Li (31) • Department of Microbiology, University of Saskatchewan, Saskatoon, Saskatchewan, Canada S7N 0W0

Michael C. Lidell (45) • Department of Plant Biology, University of Maryland at College Park, College Park, Maryland 20742

Klaus Liebeton (28) • Lehrstuhl Biologie der Mikroorganismen, Ruhr-Universität, D-44780 Bochum, Germany

Steven E. Lindow (43) • Department of Environmental Science, Policy, and Management, University of California, Berkeley, California 94720-3110

Paul J. Loida (30) • Abbott Laboratories, Abbott Park, Illinois 60064

Stephen Lory (36) • Department of Microbiology, Box 357242, University of Washington, Seattle, Washington 98195

Hong-Mei Lu (36) • Department of Microbiology, Box 357242, University of Washington, Seattle, Washington 98195

Dzwokai Ma (31) • Department of Physiology, University of California, San Francisco, California 94143

Sheng Ma (41) • Department of Microbiology and Immunology, University of Tennessee and VA Medical Center, Memphis, Tennessee 38163

Maximino Manzanera (17) • Department of Biochemistry, Molecular and Cellular Biology of Plants, Consejo Superior de Investigaciones Científicas, Apdo 419, E-18008 Granada, Spain

Silvia Marqués (17) • Department of Biochemistry, Molecular and Cellular Biology of Plants, Consejo Superior de Investigaciones Científicas, Apdo 419, E-18008 Granada, Spain

Daniel W. Martin (34) • Department of Microbiology and Immunology, Stanford University School of Medicine, D052 Fairchild Building, Stanford, California 94305

Jaime M. Martinez-Salazar (34) • Depto. de Genetica Molecular, Centro de Investigacion sobre Fijacion de Nitrogeno, UNAM, Av. Universidad s/n Col Chamilpa, Cuernavaca, Morelos, Mexico 62100

Kalai Mathee (41) • Department of Microbiology and Immunology, University of Tennessee and VA Medical Center, Memphis, Tennessee 38163

Sally M. McFall (11) • Department of Microbiology and Immunology, University of Illinois at Chicago, Chicago, Illinois 60612

B. McHugh (44) • Department of Microbiology, University College Cork, Cork, Ireland

David McKay (10) • Division of Microbiology, National Research Centre for Biotechnology, Mascheroder Weg l, 38124 Braunschweig, Germany

Craig J. McPherson (41) • Department of Microbiology and Immunology, University of Tennessee and VA Medical Center, Memphis, Tennessee 38163

Mallavarapu Megharaj (10) • Department of Microbiology, University of Otago, POB 56, Dunedin, New Zealand

Gérard Michel (37) • Laboratoire d'Ingénierie et Dynamique des Systèmes Membranaires, Centre National de la Recherche Scientifique UPR 9027, 31 Chemin Joseph Aiguier, B.P. 71, 13402 Marseille Cedex 20, France

Yukio Mitsui (27) • Department of BioEngineering, Nagaoka University of Technology, Nagaoka, Niigata 940-21, Japan

Keisuke Miyauchi (6) • Department of Biotechnology, The University of Tokyo, Bunkyo-ku, Tokyo 113, Japan

Y. Moenne-Loccoz (44) • Department of Microbiology, University College Cork, Cork, Ireland

Heiner Mokroß (9) • Bergische Universität, Gesamthochschule Wuppertal, Chemische Mikrobiologie, Gaußstraße 20, D-42097 Wuppertal, Germany

Masaaki Morikawa (25) • Department of Material and Life Sciences, Graduate School of Engineering, Osaka University, 2-1 Yamadaoka, Suita, Osaka 565, Japan

Ernest J. Mueller (30) • Sigma Chemical Company, 3500 DeKalb Street, St. Louis, Missouri 63178

Detlef Müller (9) • Bergische Universität, Gesamthochschule Wuppertal, Chemische Mikrobiologie, Gaußstraße 20, D-42097 Wuppertal, Germany

Maryse Murgier (37) • Laboratoire d'Ingénierie et Dynamique des Systèmes Membranaires, Centre National de la Recherche Scientifique UPR 9027, 31 Chemin Joseph Aiguier, B.P. 71, 13402 Marseille Cedex 20, France

Yuji Nagata (6) • Department of Biotechnology, The University of Tokyo, Bunkyo-ku, Tokyo 113, Japan

Taiji Nakae (32) • The Department of Molecular Life Science, Tokai University School of Medicine, Isehara 259-11, Japan

Teruko Nakazawa (40) • Department of Microbiology, Yamaguchi University School of Medicine, Ube, Yamaguchi 755, Japan

Seiji Negoro (23) • Department of Biotechnology, Faculty of Engineering, Osaka University, 2-1 Yamada-oka, Suita, Osaka 565, Japan

Shadi Neshat (33) • Department of Microbiology and Immunology, Queen's University, Kingston, Ontario K7L 3N6, Canada

Maarten Nieboer (4) • Institute of Biotechnology, Swiss Federal Institute of Technology, ETH-Hoenggerberg, 8093 Zürich, Switzerland

Hiroshi Nikaido (31) • Department of Molecular and Cell Biology, University of California, Berkeley, California 94720

Akito Nishi (8) • Department of Agricultural Chemistry, Kyushu University, Hakozaki, Fukuoka 812-81, Japan

F. O'Gara (44) • Department of Microbiology, University College Cork, Cork, Ireland

Bernard O'Hara (29) • Department of Biochemistry and Molecular Biology, University College London, Gower Street, London WClE 6BT, United Kingdom

Dennis E. Ohman (41) • Department of Microbiology and Immunology, University of Tennessee and VA Medical Center, Memphis, Tennessee 38163

Hisao Ohtake (15) • Department of Fermentation Technology, Hiroshima University, Higashi-Hiroshima, Hiroshima 739, Japan

Kenji Okuda (42) • Department of Bacteriology, Yokohama City University School of Medicine, 3-9 Fukuura, Kanazawa-ku, Yokohama 236, Japan

Haruko Okusu (31) • Department of Molecular and Cell Biology, University of California, Berkeley, California 94720

Matthew R. Parsek (11) • Department of Microbiology, University of Iowa, Iowa City, Iowa 52242

Jeffrey C. Pepe (36) • Department of Microbiology, Box 357242, University of Washington, Seattle, Washington 98195

José Pérez-Martín (13) • Department of Microbial Biotechnology, Centro Nacional de Biotecnología, Campus de Cantoblanco, 28049 Madrid, Spain

Statis Philippou (28) • Institut für Pathologie, Ruhr-Universität, DD-44780 Bochum, Germany

Dietmar H. Pieper (10) • Division of Microbiology, National Research Centre for Biotechnology, Mascheroder Weg 1, 38124 Braunschweig, Germany

Kevin Piers (38) • Department of Microbiology and Immunology, University of British Columbia, Vancouver, B.C. V6T 1Z3, Canada

Minna U. Pirhonen (45) • Department of Molecular Genetics, Swedish University of Agricultural Sciences, Box 7010, 75007 Uppsala, Sweden

Keith Poole (33) • Department of Microbiology and Immunology, Queen's University, Kingston, Ontario K7L 3N6, Canada

Irfan D. Prijambada (23) • Department of Biotechnology, Faculty of Engineering, Osaka University, 2-1 Yamada-oka, Suita, Osaka 565, Japan

Siri Ram Chhabra (16) • Department of Pharmaceutical Sciences, University of Nottingham, Nottingham NG7 2RD, United Kingdom

Juan L. Ramos (17) • Department of Biochemistry, Molecular and Cellular Biology of Plants, Consejo Superior de Investigaciones Científicas, Apdo 419, E-18008 Granada, Spain

Stéphane Ransac (28) • Laboratory of Biophysical Chemistry, NL-9747 AG Groningen, The Netherlands

Manfred T. Reetz (28) • Max-Planck-Institut für Kohlenforschung, D-45470 Mülheim, Germany

Cornelia Reimmann (20) • Laboratoire de Biologie Microbienne, Université de Lausanne, CH-1015 Lausanne, Switzerland

Walter Reineke (9) • Bergische Universität, Gesamthochschule Wuppertal, Chemische Mikrobiologie, Gaußstraße 20, D-42097 Wuppertal, Germany

Daniel L. Rowley (45) • Department of Plant Biology, University of Maryland at College Park, College Park, Maryland 20742

Yukihiro Sakai (15) • Department of Fermentation Technology, Hiroshima University, Higashi-Hiroshima, Hiroshima 739, Japan

George P. C. Salmond (16) • Department of Biological Sciences, University of Warwick, Coventry CV4 7AL, United Kingdom

Rafael Salto (17) • Department of Biochemistry, Molecular and Cellular Biology of Plants, Consejo Superior de Investigaciones Científicas, Apdo 419, E-18008 Granada, Spain

Sergio Schmid (20) • Ingenieurschule Wallis, CH-1950 Sion, Switzerland

Bernd Schneidinger (28) • Lehrstuhl Biologie der Mikroorganismen, Ruhr-Universität, D-44780 Bochum, Germany

Michael J. Schurr (34) • Department of Microbiology and Immunology, 5641 Medical Science Building II, University of Michigan Medical School, Ann Arbor, Michigan 48109-0620

Herbert P. Schweizer (19) • Department of Microbiology and Infectious Diseases, University of Calgary, Calgary, Alberta T2N 4N1, Canada, and Department of Microbiology, Colorado State University, Fort Collins, Colorado 80523

Michael Seeger (10) • Division of Microbiology, National Research Centre for Biotechnology, Mascheroder Weg 1, 38124 Braunschweig, Germany

Thomas Seitz (20) • Laboratoire de Biologie Microbienne, Université de Lausanne, CH-1015 Lausanne, Switzerland

Toshiya Senda (27) • Department of BioEngineering, Nagaoka University of Technology, Nagaoka, Niigata 940-21, Japan

R. Sexton (44) • Department of Microbiology, University College Cork, Cork, Ireland

Takashi Shigematsu (42) • Department of Bacteriology, Yokohama City University School of Medicine, 3-9 Fukuura, Kanazawa-ku, Yokohama 236, Japan

Victoria Shingler (12) • Department of Cell and Molecular Biology, Umeå University, 901 87 Umeå, Sweden

Simon Silver (35) • Department of Microbiology and Immunology, University of Illinois College of Medicine, M/C 790, Room 703, 835 South Wolcott Avenue, Chicago, Illinois 60612-7344

Stephen G. Sligar (30) • Beckman Institute for Advanced Science and Technology, University of Illinois, Urbana, Illinois 61801

Gordon S. A. B. Stewart (16) • Department of Applied Biochemistry and Food Science, University of Nottingham, Sutton Bonington Campus, Loughborough LE12 5RD, United Kingdom

Adam K. Sun (24) • Department of Chemical and Biochemical Engineering, University of California, Irvine, Irvine, California 92717-2575

Akiko Suyama (8) • Department of Agricultural Chemistry, Kyushu University, Hakozaki, Fukuoka 812-81, Japan

Kazunori Taguchi (15) • Department of Fermentation Technology, Hiroshima University, Higashi-Hiroshima, Hiroshima 739, Japan

Masamichi Takagi (6) • Department of Biotechnology, The University of Tokyo, Bunkyo-ku, Tokyo 113, Japan

Kenneth N. Timmis (10) • Division of Microbiology, National Research Centre for Biotechnology, Mascheroder Weg 1, 38124 Braunschweig, Germany

Masataka Tsuda (18) • Department of Biology, Faculty of Science, Okayama University, Okayama 700, Japan

Itaru Urabe (23) • Department of Biotechnology, Faculty of Engineering, Osaka University, 2-1 Yamada-oka, Suita, Osaka 565, Japan

Jan B. van Beilen (4) • Institute of Biotechnology, Swiss Federal Institute of Technology, ETH-Hoenggerberg, 8093 Zürich, Switzerland

Ying Wang (14) • Biotechnology Research Institute, National Research Council Canada, 6100 Royalmount Avenue, Montreal, Quebec H4P 2R2, Canada

Paul Williams (16) • Department of Pharmaceutical Sciences, University of Nottingham, Nottingham NG7 2RD, United Kingdom

Rachel Williams (29) • Department of Biochemistry and Molecular Biology, University College London, Gower Street, London WC1E 6BT, United Kingdom

Michael K. Winson (16) • Department of Applied Biochemistry and Food Science, University of Nottingham, Sutton Bonington Campus, Loughborough LE12 5RD, United Kingdom

Bernard Witholt (4) • Institute of Biotechnology, Swiss Federal Institute of Technology, ETH-Hoenggerberg, 8093 Zürich, Switzerland

Rolf-Michael Wittich (10) • Division of Microbiology, National Research Centre for Biotechnology, Mascheroder Weg 1, 38124 Braunschweig, Germany

Thomas K. Wood (24) • Department of Chemical and Biochemical Engineering, University of California, Irvine, Irvine, California 92717-2575

Daniel J. Wozniak (41) • Department of Microbiology and Immunology, Wake Forest University, Bowman Gray School of Medicine, Winston-Salem, North Carolina 27157-1064

Manhong Wu (38) • Department of Microbiology and Immunology, University of British Columbia, Vancouver, B.C. V6T 1Z3, Canada

Marcel Wubbolts (4) • Institute of Biotechnology, Swiss Federal Institute of Technology, ETH-Hoenggerberg, 8093 Zürich, Switzerland

Satoshi Yamamoto (21) • Marine Biotechnology Institute, Kamaishi Laboratories, 3-75-1 Heita, Kamaishi City, 026 Iwate, Japan

Hiroshi Yoneyama (32) • The Department of Molecular Life Science, Tokai University School of Medicine, Isehara 259-11, Japan

Eisaku Yoshihara (32) • The Department of Molecular Life Science, Tokai University School of Medicine, Isehara 259-11, Japan

Zhiying You (42) • Department of Bacteriology, Yokohama City University School of Medicine, 3-9 Fukuura, Kanazawa-ku, Yokohama 236, Japan

Lisa Young (33) • Department of Microbiology and Immunology, Queen's University, Kingston, Ontario K7L 3N6, Canada

Hongwei Yu (34) • Department of Microbiology and Immunology, 5641 Medical Science Building II, University of Michigan Medical School, Ann Arbor, Michigan 48109-0620

Elisabetta Zennaro (5) • Dipartimento di Biologia Cellulare e dello Sviluppo, p.le A. Moro 5, 00185 Rome, Italy

INTRODUCTION

These reports, which are from the Fifth International Symposium on Pseudomonads: Molecular Biology and Biotechnology, offer an overview of the evolving molecular biological and biotechnological aspects of pseudomonad bacteria, which are important to basic science, medical science, and the biosphere as a whole.

The introductory chapter offers a historical review of pseudomonad catabolism and the discovery of oxygenase, showing us the pseudomonad's world before the era of molecular biology. "*Pseudomonas:* a Century of Biodiversity" outlines the history and some of the personalities involved with *Pseudomonas* research from the Delft School to the merging disciplines of the present. "*Pseudomonas* Genetics and Taxonomy" describes how the formal genetic analysis of earlier days has been replaced in the context of molecular genetics, and introduces modern pseudomonad taxonomy with new views on arrangements of species and genera.

Pseudomonads are well known for their nutritional and metabolic versatility and for their wide distribution in the biosphere. Metabolism of hydrocarbons and chlorinated hydrocarbons by soil pseudomonads is important for production of chemicals and for biodegradation of environmental pollutants. Bacteria with novel genetic systems as well as engineered strains carrying hybrid pathways or operons are reviewed. These efforts will eventually allow expanded and enhanced degradability of these pollutants.

Transcriptional regulatory systems in pseudomonads have been very extensively studied. Analyses of the structure-function relationships of regulatory proteins and their target DNA sequences provide basic understanding of how the systems sense and respond to the presence of hydrocarbons in the environment, leading to the expression of catabolic genes. Chemotactic signal transduction and signal transduction through "quorum sensing" enable bacteria to respond to their environment and to mount appropriate adaptive strategies.

One dynamic feature of pseudomonads is "catabolic transposons," which frequently undergo genetic rearrangements. Another interesting and novel feature is the multiple chromosomes in the genus *Burkholderia,* which introduces a new concept for the evolution of degradative pathways. New tools for biotechnology such as broad-host-range general-purpose cloning vectors, new gene cassettes, and linker insertion mutagenesis are described.

In the field of environmental microbiology, the assessment of bioremediation effectiveness by engineered bacteria is important. An alternative method for detection and identification of pseudomonad strains is presented that overcomes some difficulties of 16S rDNA-sequence-based identification of closely related bacteria. The pseudomonads are host bacteria for a wide variety of enzyme systems that participate in degradation of various hydrocarbons. The three-dimensional structure of one of the *meta*-cleavage dioxygenases is presented (see Senda and Mitsui, chapter 27, and the cover of this book). It has a barrel-shaped central cavity for the iron molecule and a putative binding cavity for the O_2 molecule. Such protein structural analysis is essential for the future development of protein engineering.

The biotechnology of pseudomonads started with the construction of new bacterial strains which have useful abilities such as production of chemicals and biodegradation of pollutants. Great advances have been made, as reviewed in this monograph. Applications to industry, agriculture, and medicine require further improvements, and for these purposes we must work toward new directions in the molecular biology of pseudomonads, not only studying biochemical pathways of interest but also viewing pseudomonads as living organisms in the ecosystem.

All living cells are separated from their environments by the cell envelope. Recent findings on the structure-function relationships of the bacterial cell envelope are remarkable and are reviewed in several important papers in this monograph. Much of the intrinsic resistance of *Pseudomonas aeruginosa* and related bacteria is due to an active efflux system that exports various antibiotics. The efflux machinery consists of an inner membrane pump, a linker protein between the inner and outer membranes, and an outer membrane channel. Resistance to toxic heavy metal ions is also due to a related efflux system in pseudomonads. The acquisition of iron is facilitated by siderophores which bind ferric ion and deliver it to the bacterium via cell surface receptors specific for the ferric siderophore complex. Expression of these receptors is inducible by the specific siderophore, and such induction is mediated by two-component regulators which include a sensor and a regulator-activator component. *P. aeruginosa* and *Burkholderia* (formerly *Pseudomonas) cepacia* secrete a number of extracellular enzymes via a specialized mechanism, the general secretion pathway, located in the bacterial cell envelope. This pathway allows precursor proteins to be translocated across the inner membrane and allows the periplasmic intermediate to specifically cross the outer membrane. The key components of this pathway share sequence similarities with the type IV pilin of *P. aeruginosa.*

Infections caused by *P. aeruginosa* and its related bacteria are a major problem in the medical field. Several antipseudomonal drugs have been produced, but soon after their introduction, bacteria acquire resistance against the new drugs. Cationic peptides that show synergy with classical antibiotic activity can be applied to combat multidrug-resistant pseudomonads. The mucoid phenotype of *P. aeroginosa* associated with chronic pulmonary cystic fibrosis patients is due to the overproduction of the exopolysaccharide alginate, which also confers increased resistance to the host animal's immune response. AlgU-dependent stress-responsive systems are involved in regulation of this process. The bacterial strategies of colonization in mammalian hosts, escape from host defense, and survival are being more understood and yet seem more complex, year by year. Such basic understanding of host-bacterial interactions is very important for prevention and therapy of infectious diseases due to pseudomonads.

Interactions between plant host cells and pseudomonads are the last topic in this volume. Ice nucleation by phytopathogenic bacterial cells is a stress-induced phenotype. Similarly, synthesis of siderophores and several antifungal metabolites is under the control of environmental signals. The recent discovery of *hrp* genes of phytopathogenic pseudomonads is reviewed. These findings opened a new era of host-bacterial interactions: bacteria utilize similar strategies to interact with hosts, whether plants or animals. A plant response elicitor is secreted by the *hrp*-independent translocation system, which is controlled by a response regulatory system. Coregulated with the *hrp* genes are a set of host range determinants which are postulated to produce specific plant defense response elicitors.

All living things, humans, animals, plants, and microorganisms, live together on this planet and socially and ecologically interact with each other, constituting one large community. A number of means for communication between pseudomonads and host organisms have evolved and developed, but from the view of molecular biology, the ways of communication appear to be more or less the same. By responding to environmental signals, cells excrete signal molecules that affect other cells. Interaction between bacteria and hosts is well organized so that both can survive. Signal transduction systems of both organisms operate within the cells to support such intimate communication. The editors of this monograph believe that pseudomonads, among the most ubiquitously distributed microorganisms in nature, provide vital information on signal transduction, cell-to-cell communication, and above all the communication of all living things on this planet.

The Fifth International Symposium on Pseudomonads: Molecular Biology and Biotechnology was held at the AIST Conference Hall, Tsukuba, Japan, in August 1995. Over 250 participants from 22 countries attended. The organizing committee consisted of T. Nakazawa (chair), K. Furukawa (co-chair), S. Harayama (co-chair), M. Fukuda (secretary), K. Kimbara (secretary), Y. Kudo, E. Mikami, K. Nakamura, K. Nakamura, and H. Ohtake. The international advisory committee consisted of A. M. Chakrabarty, V. de Lorenzo, E. Galli, D. Haas, R. Hancock, B. Iglewski, S. Silver, K. N. Timmis, and B. Witholt. The success of the symposium was demonstrated by the planning for the next pseudomonad meeting, expected to be held in Madrid, Spain, in 1997.

Teruko Nakazawa

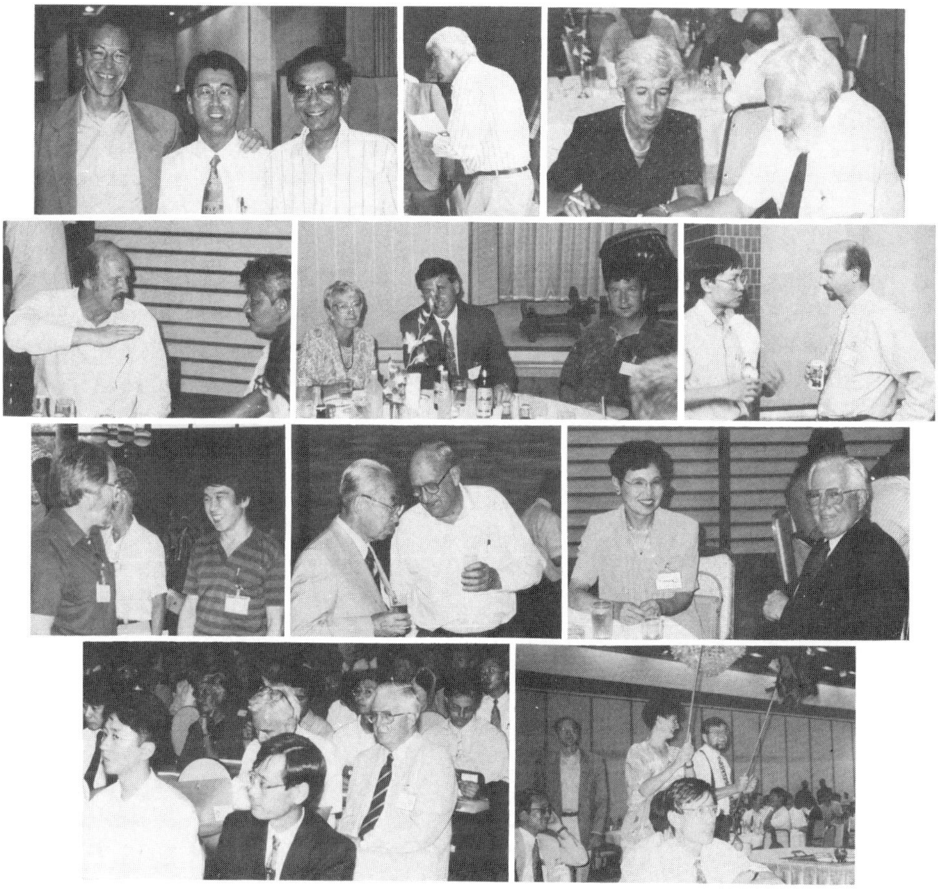

Row 1: Witholt, Fukuda, Chakrabarty; Haas; Galli, Silver. **Row 2:** Hancock, ?; Iglewski, O'Gara, Deretic; ?, de Lorenzo. **Row 3:** ?, Harayama; Hayaishi, Gunsalus; Nakazawa, Holloway. **Row 4:** ?, Galli, Furukawa (foreground), Silver, Holloway, others; Furukawa (foreground), others.

Section I

GLOBAL PROSPECTS

Molecular Biology of Pseudomonads
Edited by T. Nakazawa et al.

Chapter 1

Discovery of Oxygenases in Pseudomonads

Osamu Hayaishi

In 1945, almost exactly 50 years ago, I started my career in basic medical science, or should I say that I attempted or struggled to start my career in biomedical research. With the end of the second World War, I returned to my hometown, Osaka, from military service and found that the entire city had been almost completely demolished by bombing. The home of my parents and family had completely vanished. Food was scarce, and supplies of most commodities—gas, electricity, and even water—were extremely limited. There were no research funds. Research facilities were poor, chemicals were scarce, and we had no laboratory animals. To overcome these difficulties, I decided to use microorganisms for my research. So I went to the backyard of the university, took some soil samples from the ruins, mixed them with a small amount of tryptophan and water in a test tube, and waited. It was a very simple and inexpensive experiment. After a few days, I observed some cloudiness in the supernatant. Thus, by this enrichment culture technique, I was able to isolate several strains of soil bacteria that could grow on tryptophan as their sole source of carbon and nitrogen. These soil bacteria were subsequently identified as pseudomonads. For me, the pseudomonads found in the ruins turned out to be a gold mine of information.

About that time, it was already known, mainly through the efforts of Kotake and associates, that in mammals, tryptophan is degraded through kynurenine to the end metabolites kynurenic acid, anthranilic acid, and xanthurenic acid (Fig. 1). However, I was able to show that, in this soil microorganism, anthranilate was further metabolized to catechol and then to muconic acid and was ultimately oxidized to CO_2, ammonia, and H_2O.

Encouraged by these unexpected findings, we proceeded to isolate and purify the enzymes involved in this pathway. However, at that time, isolating enzymes in a cell-free form from bacterial cells was technically impossible except for the enzyme that catalyzed the oxidative cleavage of catechol to produce *cis,cis*-muconic acid as the reaction product (Fig. 2). This enzyme was a nonheme iron protein and had a molecular weight of approximately 90,000. Because two atoms of oxygen were consumed, I took it for granted that oxygen atoms had been incorporated into the substrate. I named this enzyme "pyrocatechase" (Hayaishi and Hashimoto, 1950) instead of catechol oxidase because

Osamu Hayaishi • Osaka Bioscience Institute, Suita, Osaka 565, Japan.

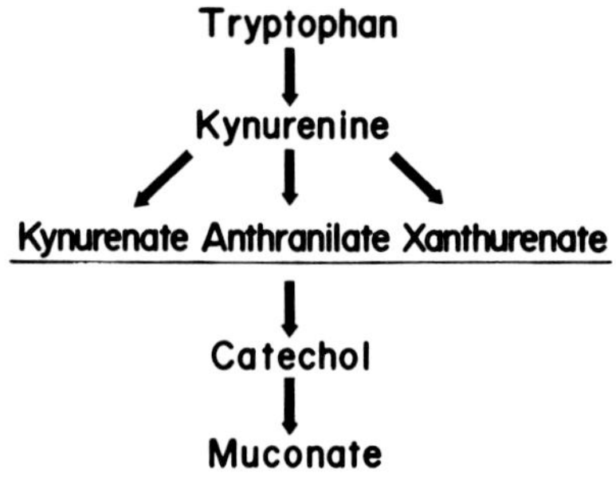

Figure 1. Major metabolic pathways of tryptophan as understood around 1950.

although a number of catechol oxidases had already been reported by that time, these enzymes seemed to be very different from pyrocatechase because they did not cleave the aromatic structure of catechol. Furthermore, they were copper proteins rather than nonheme iron proteins. Thus the catalytic mechanism of this newly found pyrocatechase remained unclarified for some years.

Being a very naive and inexperienced biochemist, I assumed that the oxygen consumed must have been incorporated into catechol, as depicted by Lavoisier in the 18th century. According to Lavoisier, the principle of biological oxidation was the addition of oxygen atoms to a substrate, and the opposite process, that of reduction, was the removal of oxygen atoms from an oxide.

$$X + O_2 \underset{\text{reduction}}{\overset{\text{oxidation}}{\rightleftharpoons}} XO_2$$

I was startled to learn, however, that at the beginning of the present century, the enzymatic incorporation of molecular oxygen into substrates had been completely ruled out by Professor Heinrich Wieland, German Nobel laureate.

According to "the dehydrogenation theory" proposed by Wieland, the principle of biological oxidation processes is the transfer of hydrogen atoms, or its equivalent, from the substrate molecule XH_2 to an appropriate acceptor A, such as coenzymes and various dyes. Oxygen molecules may, in some instances, serve as the immediate electron acceptor (Wieland, 1932). In these instances, the enzymes are termed oxidases.

$$XH_2 + A \underset{\text{reduction}}{\overset{\text{oxidation}}{\rightleftharpoons}} X + AH_2$$

Thus, according to Professor Wieland, molecular oxygen accepts hydrogen atoms and is reduced to water or hydrogen peroxide. However, the oxygen is never incorporated into the substrate, as was originally proposed by Lavoisier and his contemporaries some 200 years ago.

According to the dehydrogenation theory of Wieland, when the overall reaction is envisaged as the addition of oxygen, the oxygen atoms are always derived from the water molecule rather than from atmospheric oxygen (Wieland, 1932). For example,

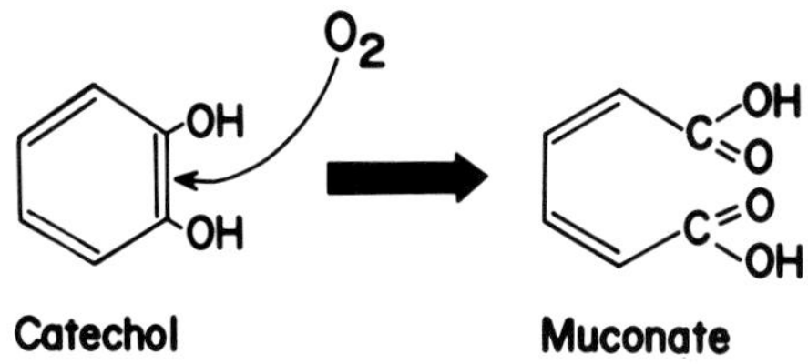

Figure 2. Pyrocatechase-catalyzed reaction.

when aldehydes are converted to acids, aldehydes are first hydrated and then dehydrogenated, so the sum is the addition of oxygen to substrate X to form XO, but this oxygen atom is derived from water rather than from molecular oxygen. Therefore, according to Professor Wieland, the direct addition of molecular oxygen to a substrate was completely irrelevant to biological oxidation.

Nevertheless, we considered the possibility that pyrocatechase may incorporate molecular oxygen into the substrate rather than dehydrogenate catechol because, first, oxygen could not be replaced by known coenzymes or electron acceptor dyes, and second, orthobenzoquinone, the dehydrogenation product of catechol, was not the intermediate of the overall reaction. In 1955, while working at the National Institutes of Health in Bethesda, Md., I decided to explore this possibility. I performed a set of experiments in which a heavy oxygen isotope, ^{18}O, was used in air in one flask and in the form of water in another. The product, muconic acid, was isolated and analyzed by mass spectrometry for its ^{18}O content. If pyrocatechase is a dehydrogenase or an oxidase, the incorporated oxygen atoms should have been derived from water, according to the theory of Professor Wieland. However, contrary to the then generally held belief, our results clearly demonstrated that oxygen atoms incorporated into product molecules were derived almost exclusively from molecular oxygen and not from the oxygen of the water molecule (Hayaishi et al., 1955). Despite our clear-cut results, our data at first met with skepticism and were brushed off by our peers. Concurrently and independently, Mason and associates demonstrated that the phenolase complex of the mushroom incorporated one atom of molecular oxygen into a substrate, 3,4-dimethylphenol, to form 4,5-dimethylcatechol (Mason et al., 1955). These findings, together with subsequent work by Bloch, Gunsalus, and others, established that oxygen fixation does indeed occur in biological systems, and thus the new concept of biological oxygenation was introduced. In essence, this was a revival of the old concept of Lavoisier.

In 1956, the first symposium on oxygenases was held in Atlantic City, N.J., as part of an American Chemical Society meeting. There, we proposed that the enzymes responsible for these reactions, that is, pyrocatechase and phenolase, be termed "dioxygenase"and "monooxygenase," respectively; Mason used the term "mixed function oxidase" for monooxygenase. At first, these reactions were generally thought to be rather unusual and limited to only primitive living organisms such as soil bacteria or mushrooms. Several years passed before the ubiquity of oxygenases was confirmed in many laboratories.

Figure 3 shows the metabolic map of tryptophan. The black arrows in this chart denote oxygenase reactions, and the oxygen atoms indicated by heavy black O's have been incorporated into substrates by the actions of various oxygenases. You can see that a

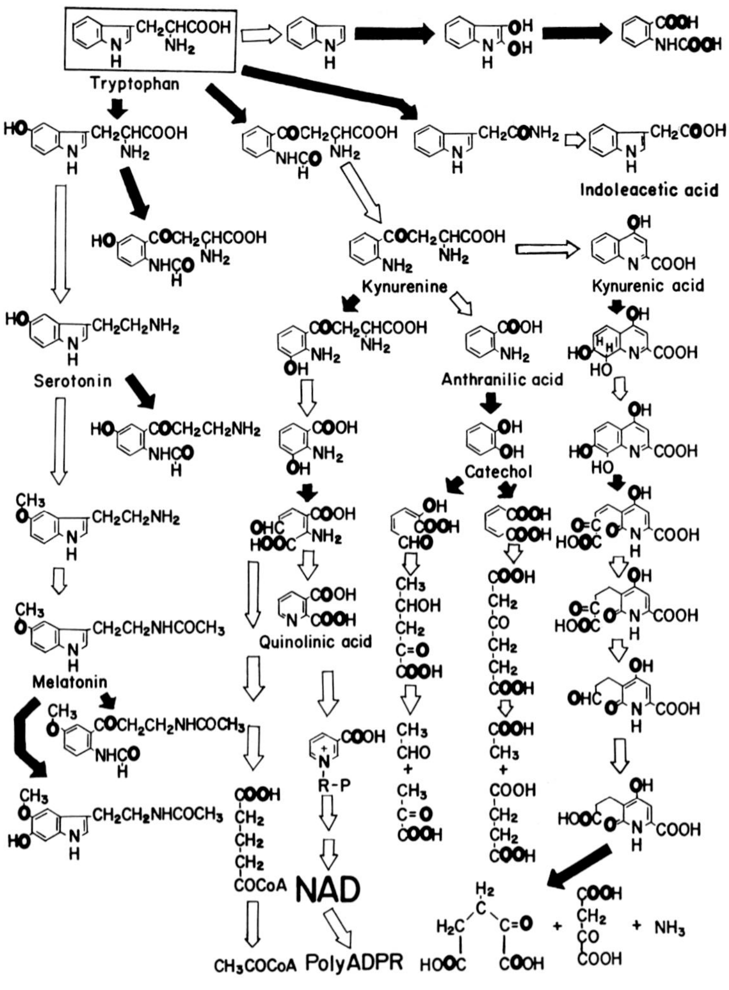

Figure 3. Tryptophan metabolism. CoA, coenzyme A; polyADPR, poly(ADP-ribose).

large number of oxygenases are involved in these important metabolic pathways. In fact, the two most important metabolic pathways of tryptophan in mammals, those leading to the formation of pyridine nucleotide coenzymes and ultimately to poly(ADP-ribose) in one case and to various indoleamines in the other, are initiated by the well-known oxygenases tryptophan 2,3-dioxygenase and tryptophan 5-monooxygenase, respectively.

During the next decade, a number of oxygenases were isolated from animals, plants, and microorganisms, and some were highly purified and crystallized. In 1958, I returned to Japan, and soon afterwards, Dr. Nozaki in my department purified metapyrochatechase from a pseudomonad and succeeded in producing the first crystalline dioxygenase preparation. Encouraged by his success, my colleagues in the Kyoto laboratory crystallized several other oxygenases, including protocatechuate dioxygenase, imidazoleacetate monooxygenase, and lysine monooxygenase. With the use of these highly purified oxygenase preparations, studies of their structures, properties, and mechanisms of action as well as of the nature of the active form of oxygen were initiated in many laboratories worldwide.

It is now clear that the enzymes involved in biological oxidation processes can be classified into two major categories. Dehydrogenases and oxidases transfer electrons and are involved mainly, if not exclusively, in ATP synthesis. Oxygenases, on the other hand, transfer molecular oxygen and play important roles in the metabolism of essential nutrients and foreign compounds.

It has been nearly 20 years since I left the field of pseudomonads. Today, molecular biology dominates the world of biomedical science, yet not all of biochemistry deserves to be relegated to history. It is a great pleasure to look back on the good old days and also to acquaint young molecular biologists with subjects not widely known or taught today.

REFERENCES

Hayaishi, O., and Z. Hashimoto. 1950. Pyrocatechase. A new enzyme catalyzing oxidative breakdown of pyrocatechin. *J. Biochem.* **37:**317–374.

Hayaishi, O., M. Katagiri, and S. Rothberg. 1955. Mechanism of the pyrocatechase reaction *J. Am. Chem. Soc.* **77:**5450–5451.

Mason, H. S., W. L. Fowlks, and E. Peterson. 1955. Oxygen transfer and electron transport by the phenolase complex. *J. Am. Chem. Soc.* **77:**2914–2915.

Wieland, H. 1932. *On the Mechanism of Oxidation.* Yale University Press, New Haven, Conn.

Molecular Biology of Pseudomonads
Edited by T. Nakazawa et al.

Chapter 2

Pseudomonas: a Century of Biodiversity

Irwin C. Gunsalus

When Coleridge tried to define beauty, he returned always to one deep thought; beauty, he said, is 'unity in variety.' Science is nothing else than the search to discover unity in the wild variety of nature—or more exactly, in the variety of our experience.

(Kluyver, 1959, p. 68)

The Fifth International *Pseudomonas* Symposium in Tsukuba brought a welcome opportunity to offer tribute to a century of versatility, to recall the gracious contribution from Ken Timmis of the first Symposium of this series in Geneva nearly a decade ago, and to share recent discoveries. It was a pleasure to find myself on a program with Professor Osamu Hayaishi, whose exquisite experiments, two oxygenase volumes (Hayaishi, 1962, 1974), many students with whom we still interact today, and friendship are fundamental monuments. His $^{18}O_2$ experiments in 1955 validated our pursuit of enzyme systems active on "inert" structures.

This chapter has a dual purpose: first, a reminder of the gifts from *Pseudomonas* research to the present day, with the route traveled. Selected references to original publications are supplemented with recent reviews giving a view of current findings and literature. A more important question, however, is how these talents can, and will, affect the plethora of insults to world ecology, especially those we call anthropogenic. What is appropriate given the surge in human population with its insatiable energy demands, especially for fossil fuels, and the risks and errors in the transport of such fuels?

The beginnings of our science are clear and still pertinent. In mid-20th century, genes and enzymes became known in chemical terms. They are now part dogma and part methods and have rapidly expanded into near universal use. To engage the question of how, within the world pool of knowledge, microbes can be applied in curbing the current human impact on nature, one must turn to the early fundamentals, reinforced with the new molecular tools available to biology and the new attention from chemistry and physics. The extensive use of pseudomonad systems to determine gene and enzyme, structure and

Irwin C. Gunsalus • Gulf Ecology Division, U.S. Environmental Protection Agency, 1 Sabine Island Drive, Gulf Breeze, Florida 32561-5299.

function, is abundantly documented, and the extension of these findings to crucial applications is equally clear (Sokatch,1986; Gunsalus,1973).

To consider the essential role of microbes in today's urgent challenges, let me outline the time frame. For the late 19th century (Gest, 1987) and much of the first half of the 20th, we relied largely on European science (Kluyver, 1959; Kluyver et al., 1956; Pfennig, 1993). I shall mention later a few notable exceptions. In the explosive growth during the two decades bridging the mid-20th century, America and Asia also contributed to the lore and, more importantly, to the fundamentals. Now the Fifth Symposium brings us to the present. But is the current status of *Pseudomonas* research excellent enough for the tasks facing our societies and populations, now and in the future? How many of us use these fundamental bases for decision, and how well? Is the future opaque or only, a bit annoyingly, like frosted glass?

History can be frail: it consists of perceptions of events, rather than what actually happened. Life continues as it must, rather than as it ought. In discussions while we worked together, Wayne Umbreit cautioned often, quoting Kant: "It takes a long neck to view the firmament from a single window." Future predictions are even more risky. Janus, the patron god of beginnings and endings in Roman myth, looked both forward and aft; though the look back may be familiar, the forward view remains unclear.

EARLY 20TH CENTURY FUNDAMENTALS: ECOLOGY, ENRICHMENT, AND BIOCHEMICAL UNITY

Under the genus *Pseudomonas,* coined by Migula in 1895, a wide range of creatures have been gathered over the past century, now chopped into several taxonomic bits by innovators in search of natural relationships. Understanding their character and roles truly began with the 1895 appointment of Martinus Beijerinck to the Chair of General and Applied Microbiology at the Technical University of Delft, Holland, and construction of a laboratory to his specifications there. After his quarter century of leadership the "Delft School" was superbly amplified beyond mid-century by his successor A. J. Kluyver, 1922–1956 (Kluyver, 1959).

Beijerinck, a fierce, dominant, intuitive botanist in an engineering school, introduced enrichment culture techniques. His approach to microbiology was through microbial ecology—the relation between environmental conditions and the corresponding special life forms (Woese, 1994). As evidence of Beijerinck's keen, persistent observations, notebooks from the turn of the century are still available in the Delft Laboratory that include sketches of cells dividing under his microscope during a single observation period running well past midnight. The magnificent original data from Beijerinck's studies earned broad respect and frequent consultation by his successor and many others.

S. N. Winogradsky, a Russian scientist and contemporary of Beijerinck, was also a major contributor to the general microbial ecology of soil organisms, populations, and activities. Norbert Pfennig (Pfennig,1993, Epilogue, p. 23) provides a charming vignette:

> S. N. Winogradsky's and L. Pasteur's studies more than a hundred years ago mark the beginning of microbial ecology. Both were aware that the real nature of a microbe cannot truly be understood if it is not considered in the context of the biogeochemical processes on earth. For a lecture on "the role

> of the microbes in the general cycle of life" in 1896 in St. Petersburg, Winogradsky chose as a motto a quotation of Pasteur: ". . .the role of the infinitely small appears to me infinitely large. . ."

Pfennig's view of the scientific debt due to the collected works of Winogradsky enjoys a broad accord. Winogradsky was indeed a major leader, equal to, if not exceeding, contemporaries. He left many marks for later work.

A. J. Kluyver, a Delft graduate, chemist, and engineer, was recalled from the Dutch East Indies in 1922 as second appointee to the Delft Chair, succeeding Beijerinck, and held that position until his death in 1956. Kluyver was an inspiring lecturer and leader as well as a sensitive, considerate mentor, gentle listener, and friend. On accepting the Delft Chair, he became intent on learning everything about microbiology. The laboratory soon filled with students, visitors, and new developments. Delft became a microbiological Mecca. His concept of "unity in biochemistry" soon dominated an age, and was used to bridge the Wieland-Warburg dehydrogenase-oxidase controversy (Kluyver and van Niel, 1956; Kluyver, 1959, p. 114). Kluyver also traveled and lectured extensively in the United States in the mid-1930s—at Ames, Iowa, he observed two groups of graduate students, those who read Dutch and a few who did not. (Publications from the Delft School from the 1920s required purchasing many Dutch dictionaries. The publication *Bacterial Metabolism* by Marjorie Stephenson [Cambridge, U.K.] significantly increased awareness of the rich European literature, especially that from the Delft laboratory [Stephenson, 1939].) After 1945, Kluyver's U.S. travel resumed; occasionally he lectured with van Niel (Kluyver et al., 1956).

C. B. (Kees) van Niel, the third master to arise from the Delft School, presented himself as student candidate at Delft the day after Kluyver's inaugural address and followed L. E. Den Dooren de Jong as Assistant from 1923 to 1925. In 1928 he was recruited to the Hopkins Marine Station of Stanford University, in Pacific Grove, California, and markedly enriched the American landscape thereafter. His summer courses at the Marine Station attracted students of all levels, as well as domestic and international research colleagues, throughout his lifelong tenure.

MID-20TH CENTURY: ORGANISMS AND TOOLS, BIOLOGY, CHEMISTRY, AND SERVICES

Norbert Pfennig sensed fully his generation's debt to earlier leaders and contributed actively himself in the transition from the first to the second half of the 20th century, including to the present. Born in the year of van Niel's thesis in Delft, from a different line of youth and scientific ancestry, he brought meritorious original work of astonishing breadth to international science. His "Reflections of a Microbiologist, or How To Learn from the Microbes" (Pfennig, 1993) summarizes a rich insight and the best in human values. The section "Microbial Ecology and Limnology in Konstanz,1980–1990" in that paper is especially pertinent to the present endeavor. With Ralph Wolfe (Wolfe, 1991) and a few others, Pfennig followed the naturalist approach, bringing advances to biology per se from fundamental microbiology. From a more biochemical prospect, the 1937 finding by Harland Wood that CO_2 is an essential cell metabolite for microbes—in fact, for all living cells—is an important landmark in a remarkable life work (Wood, 1985).

These advances to general biology through the study of microbes and the metabolism part of microbial physiology, in many ways remarkable, did not come out of the blue. Rather they came from gradual accumulations; in Wood's case, of redox balances in fermentation calculations that were lacking earlier when Sherman and van Niel worked with the same propionic acid bacteria. In fact, the latter reported succinate yields, which Wood accounted for as CO_2 from the added calcium carbonate.

Other pivotal gifts from the United States before 1940 include an Otto Rahn volume on qualitative bacterial physiology (Rahn,1926; also Rahn,1945), discovery of changes in cell morphology during growth of a microbial culture (Henrici,1928), and observation of increased metabolic activity in the earlier growth phases (Hershey, 1939).

Rahn made very specific remarks on the separation of growth rate and endpoint, clearly differentiated growth from fermentation, and made precise distinction between observations and theories: all concepts much appreciated and incorporated into the Delft thinking (Kluyver, 1959).

The Henrici volume (Henrici, 1928) contains drawings of cells of a variety of bacterial species to illustrate the size differences in the various portions of the growth curve, the cells being larger in the late lag and early logarithmic phases, and decreasing until the smallest cells are found at the endpoint of growth. More recently, these properties have been exploited in experiments to introduce cell mass into porous media, for example into deep well borings, among others.

The notion of "physiological youth," a much higher metabolic activity per unit cell mass an hour or so after initiation of growth on inoculation into new medium, decreasing with advance through the logarithmic phase to the endpoint, was documented in a series of elegant papers (Hershey, 1939). This Hershey insight was again evident in the 1952 Hershey-Chase experiments showing that phage inject DNA rather than protein into cells (Cairns et al., 1966, p. 100–109).

A. T. Henrici also introduced an advance over the enrichment technique in assaying natural microbial communities, a technique later used by Tom Brock in discovery of the photosynthetic and other flora in the thermal pools of the Yellowstone and elsewhere (Brock, 1995). Henrici, an inveterate fisherman of the Minnesota Lakes, had suspended microscope slides at various depths from small floats, which he visited over time, very much in the fashion of monitoring lobster traps. By this device he discovered a wide variety of stock bacteria in natural habitats.

These concepts, while applying to pseudomonads, are more general; they are universal. But, unless we use them every day in experimental planning and interpretation, folklore and fuzziness prevail.

In the period shortly following mid-century, microbiology moved from Lamarckian concepts to developments in genetics: Josh Lederberg's two-factor crosses with *Escherichia coli,* and later replicate plating, with indirect selection of bacterial mutants (Lederberg, 1947; Lederberg and Lederberg,1952); Max Delbruck's phage group studies (see Cairns et al., 1966, p. 9); the critical Hershey-Chase experiments mentioned above; and the work of Salva Luria and his students at Indiana University with Renato Dulbecco, Jim Watson as a graduate student, and others. These, but samples of the rich innovations dating from mid-century, soon altered the landscape toward molecular biology with the infusion of chemistry, and physics via genetics, to hasten the transfer of new concepts in precision, physical theory, and experimental technique.

CHEMISTRY OF PERSISTENCE AND METABOLISM, AN AMERICAN *PSEUDOMONAS* HERITAGE

The fundamental microbiology from Western Europe before 1940 included Marjorie Stephenson and her students in the Cambridge biochemical school of Gowen Hopkins. The growth of microbiology as a chemical metabolic science in the U.K. bloomed with groups at Bristol, Leeds, Oxford, Sheffield, Stratford upon Tyne, and other places. The intellectual mix within Europe was extensive. New fundamentals came especially from the Medical Research Council in Cambridge and the Pasteur Institute in Paris, extending the great Delft initiative. The influx of world youth (American postdocs partially fueled European laboratories) provided an exponential growth to biology with a major component in fundamental microbiology. In the United States, this developed from the grassroots level, with European enrichment (Gunsalus, 1992; Kluyver and van Niel, 1956; Wood, 1985; Wolfe, 1991).

Microbiology in American universities was enriched and distributed broadly by graduate students in the decade of the 1930 Depression, and again after the war. The attraction of students to land grant colleges and public universities added numbers and a refreshing naiveté which was most significant to growth. In the Midwest at Wisconsin, a major center for most of this century, at Iowa State University in Ames, and further west at the University of California at Berkeley, strong nuclei in general microbiology were based on the land grant college agriculture of crop and livestock production. Similarly, Alex Wood and J. J. R. Campbell attended the Cornell-land grant hybrid, sent by Blythe Eagles from the University of British Columbia, and later Roberts Smith and Willard Razzell went to Illinois on Jack Campbell's initiative.

Shortly before 1950, University of Illinois President George Stoddard, "encouraged" by E. B. Fred, then President of the University of Wisconsin, ignited a major microbiological effort at Urbana, now of eminence throughout a half century. A fruitful blending was soon established with excellent chemistry (and also biochemistry) and the quality science personnel from the now "applied life sciences" of the land grant genius. Genetics and biophysics were also growing. (The first age of Illinois quality in bacteriology was before the 1900s, with T. J. Burrill's studies on the fire-blight bacterium and the early teaching of bacteriology in the laboratory with student microscopes. The second blossoming was also set off by Burrill, who as University President recruited Otto Rahn in 1912.)

As they did for Professor Hayaishi, pseudomonads came to my attention in the mid-1940s. Meeting Roger Stanier as he left the van Niel laboratory to return to his native Canada at the beginning of the war was instrumental, an effect that intensified into a lifelong friendship. Professor Hayaishi's major research interests and contributions broadened materially beyond his early studies in Osaka, and his subsequent experiments on tryptophan and aromatic fission with Stanier benefited them both (Hayaishi, this volume). After I followed Stanier at Indiana in 1947, the superb genetics there, and interactions with Salva Luria, built a firm base, extended as Luria and I moved together to Illinois in 1950. There I focused on new enzymes, reactions, and structures, and in this warm collegial atmosphere shared in the strong input of chemistry and, later, physics (Bradshaw et al., 1959; Gunsalus, 1988). The first year at Indiana included a break to spend the summer of 1948 with Kees van Niel at the Hopkins Marine Station. We had first been introduced in 1939 by Otto Rahn following a microbiology congress in New

York. My first strong impression had endured through a decade, enhanced by the van Niel intellect, knowledge, and personality. As I discovered for myself the Delft School, from val Niel there developed a lasting gift of support and friendship. The Delft School influence was extended the following summer, in 1949, as I taught at Berkeley, worked with Roger Stanier's laboratory students, and shared lunch conversations with Stanier, Mike Doudoroff, Nook Barker, and Severo Ochoa, who was also lecturing there.

A fortuitous focus of common research by Stanley Dagley (at Leeds, U.K.) and Jack Campbell with Roberts Smith (at the University of British Columbia) on isocitratase led in the 1960s to additional blending of European enrichment with the emerging microbial strengths in the Urbana Incubator. Roberts Smith had brought the isocitrate problem to Illinois as his Ph.D. thesis topic. Stanley Dagley, on 1963–64 leave from Leeds at Illinois, where four of his Ph.D. students became postdoctorates, generated a new relationship, now best characterized as the Dagley-Gibson initiative. (The "persistence and metabolism" in the title of this section derives from an early National Academy effort to assess the effects on the environment of food production for an increasing population, to which Dagley contributed after taking up a Professorship at Minnesota [Gunsalus, 1973].)

In 1963, my students and I were working in a laboratory at Cold Spring Harbor, on the floor below Al Hershey, who served as consultant. Luria worked sometimes at the bench to aid us, and his son Daniel served as the summer media cook. The Cold Spring Harbor laboratory experience, with courses and learning, continued through the following three summers.

Other figures from those early years come readily to mind, reaching back to the 1920 Delft days with Den Dooren de Jong. They include, in addition to Roger Stanier and Mike Doudoroff, their students, several of whom worked later for a time in Urbana; the British groups mentioned previously; and those of Australia and elsewhere. The chief player in *Pseudomonas* genetics is Bruce Holloway, to whom, among others, I owe a lasting debt. Even as I worked in the Cold Spring Harbor Laboratory in the summer of 1963 with *Pseudomonas putida* PpGl and cam (for camphor) to add a genetic tool to our enzyme research, Holloway, on sabbatical from Australia at the Massachusetts Institute of Technology with Luria, visited Cold Spring Harbor and shared freely his advice and knowledge, and later sent strains and students. I add homage to Irving Crawford, to whom the first *Pseudomonas* volume was dedicated, who brought me through early scoring with tryptophan auxotrophs, and to Al Chakrabarty, who provided transduction phage and, as a colleague, the extra refinement of a keen and generous mind through several years of memorable interactions, in part shared with Nick Ornston, Mark Wheelis, and others. And I hasten to add a warm tribute to Ryo Sato of P-450 for many kindnesses and precious bits of information and learning.

TO THE PRESENT: MANDELATE RACEMASE; THE ENOLASE SUPERFAMILY

Roger Stanier had three goals for his 1953 sabbatical in Urbana: to learn to make cell extracts, enzyme separations, and assays. Within a few months, the Stanier *P. putida* strain ATCC 12366 (Stanier et al., 1966, culture #90) provided mandelate racemase, dehydrogenase, decarboxylase, and dehydrogenases to benzoate (C. F. Gunsalus et al., 1953; I. C. Gunsalus et al., 1953; Stanier et al., 1953). The methods developed at Cornell in the 1940s, with the humanoid nutritive requirements of lactic acid bacteria, lyophilized cell reagents, extracts, deficient nutrient detection of function, and new factors, were transferred to the self-sufficient pseudomonads (C. F. Gunsalus et al., 1953; I. C. Gunsalus et al., 1953; Stanier et al., 1953; Gunsalus, 1992).

Studies by Stanier (with Bill Sistrom, Nick Ornston, George Hageman, and others over more than a decade) identified the enzymes and pathways for mineralization of D- and L-mandelate. The anapleurotic intermediate products essential to cellular metabolism were identified. An array of papers published in biochemical and microbiological journals fully document this early advance in aromatic metabolic patterns (Ornston et al., 1990). Hageman and G. L. Kenyon pursued with solid progress the properties of the unique aromatic hydroxy acid racemase.

A beautifully detailed series of recent studies in the laboratories of Gerlt, Kenyon, and Petsko (Babbit et al.,1995; Kenyon et al.,1995) has provided detailed structures and summarized the metals and amino acids of the catalytic center and the reversible reaction mechanism (Fig.1; the analogous MLE [mucono-lactonizing enzyme] and GalD [galactose dehydratase] are also shown). These authors provided tertiary structures and associated the mechanism with a superfamily of alpha-hydroxyl acid enzyme catalysts,

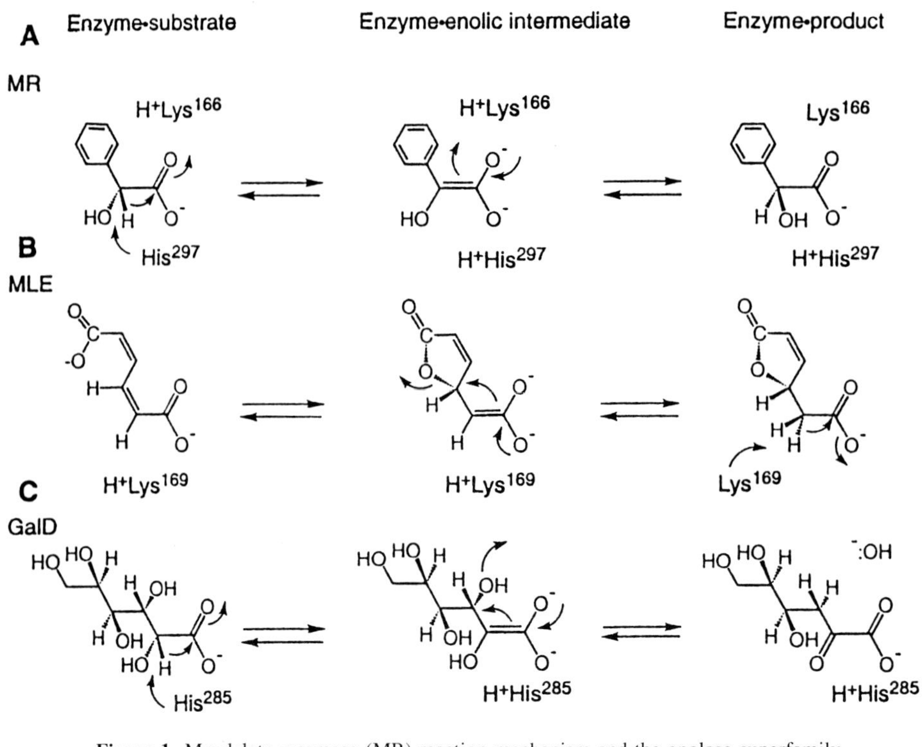

Figure 1. Mandelate racemase (MR) reaction mechanism and the enolase superfamily (Babbit et al., 1995). The analogous MLE (mucono-lactonizing enzyme) and GalD (galactose dehydratase) are also shown.

so far about a dozen, under the term "enolase superfamily" (P. C. Babbit and J. Gerlt, personal communication). New insights continue to be added on hydrogen biocatalysis.

OXYGENASES, METABOLIC PLASMIDS, HEME AND SULFUR IRON, STRUCTURE, AND DYNAMICS: P-450cam

These examples of *Pseudomonas* biological, chemical, and physical services are brought forward in summary of detailed analysis of the preferred heme model, P-450cam. The biology (Unger et al., 1986), structure (Sharrock et al., 1973; Sligar et al., 1974; Poulos et al., 1985), dynamics (Austin et al., 1973; Lipscomb et al., 1973; Martinis et al., 1991), and physical characterization (Gunsalus, 1988; Sligar et al., this volume) have been thoroughly documented. Many terpene oxygenase-positive pseudomonads were isolated and characterized by Bhattacharyya and colleagues (at the Indian Institute of Science, Bangalore) as graduate theses, and these are widely used (Madyastha and Bhattacharyya, 1968; Madyastha et al., 1977). The chemical structures of mineralization intermediates have been identified and metabolic pathways have been suggested. In several cases, the substrate specificity has been systematically explored (Madyastha et al., 1977; Gunsalus et al., 1985; Ropp et al., 1993). Recent and continuing advances appear from the Sligar laboratory (Sligar et al., this volume). The metabolic plasmids encoding genes for Cam, Oct, and Nah, discovered and characterized in Urbana in the early 1970s (Chou et al., 1974), are also widely distributed and under intensive analysis.

We asked in the early 1950s how enzymes initiate reactions on "inert hydrocarbons." Terpenes were chosen, enrichment cultures were started, and a dozen or so pure cultures were isolated that grew on a variety of mono-terpenes in mineral media. W. H. Bradshaw, a postdoctoral student from H. A. Barker, provided a pseudomonad now termed PpG1 from camphor enrichments, and Robert Baum, a graduate student, isolated from an alpha-terpineol culture the gram-positive, orange-pigmented strain T2. Both PpG1 and T2 grow on D,L-camphor (the oxygenated, biocyclic 2-bornanone) and accumulate neutral and acidic compounds in fermentation broth.

Bradshaw's fluorescent pseudomonad PpG1 was later assigned to *P. putida* biotype A by Stanier (Stanier et al.,1966, culture #77). It was found to initiate camphor metabolism by either of two aerobic reactions, formation of a 1,2-lactone (campholide) or an exhydroxylation on carbon 5 (Bradshaw et al., 1959). The gram-positive strain T2 was assigned to the *Rhodobacterium rhodochrous* group by Peter Chapman (Chapman et al., 1965). It had been found to initiate a 6-endo-hydroxylation on D,L-camphor. Several intermediates and enzymes were identified; then concentration followed on the pseudomonad.

At the enzyme level the PpG1 strain was found to contain two mono-oxygenases, an iron sulfur "keto-lactonase-1" (Conrad et al., 1965) and a (cytochrome) P-450 5-exo-hydroxylase. Each was driven by reduced pyridine nucleotide and an individual flavoprotein, coupled to the substrate-reactive oxygen activation reaction center of the iron sulfide redox transfer system. Peter Trudgill, later revisiting camphor metabolism, found that the second ring fission (keto-lactonase-2), though similar to the first, requires an acylcoenzyme A derivative to open the remaining carbocyclic ring (Fig. 2) (Trudgill, 1986).

The P-450 superfamily now exceeds 200 members (Nelson et al., 1996). The majority are associated with hepatic microsomal detoxification. A small number are involved in

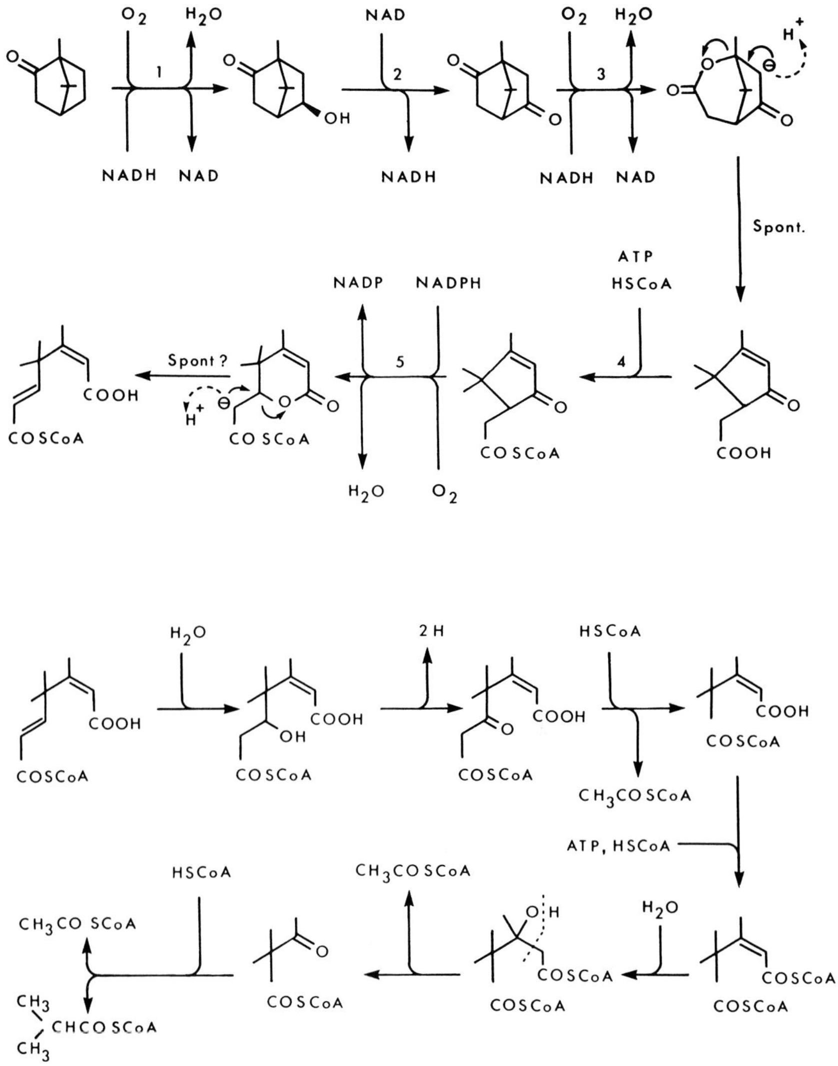

Figure 2. (+)-Camphor mono-oxygenases; terpene mineralization (from Trudgill et al., 1986, p. 509, Fig. 17 and 18, with permission).

synthesis of mammalian regulators, prostaglandin, steroid hormones, and bile acid intermediates. About a dozen microbial isolates with P-450 mono-oxygenases have been identified (Nelson et al., 1996). Several of the best studied catalyze the initial steps in hydrocarbon oxidation, while others are synthetic, for example, *eryF* in erythromycin synthesis (Andersen et al., 1993).

The tertiary structure of P-450cam, as published in 1985, is shown in Fig. 3. The structure was completed in J. Kraut's laboratory at the University of California-San Diego from a crystalline form prepared by Gerry Wagner in our Urbana laboratory (Poulos et al., 1985). Yu et al. (1974) had prepared the first P-450cam crystals from which early

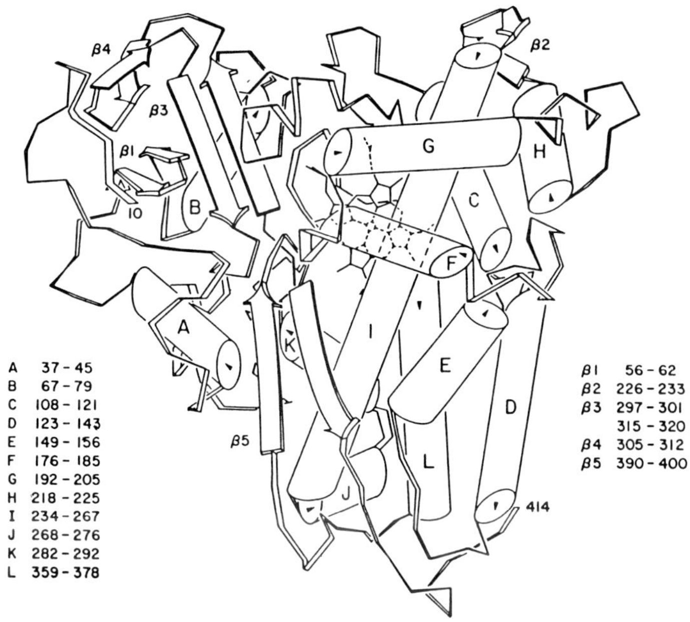

Figure 3. Crystal structure of substrate-bound P-450cam (from Poulos et al., 1985, with permission).

data were taken, but the thinness of the crystals precluded resolution. Now three additional microbial P-450 protein structures have become available. They have been compared, and they confirm the validity of the original P-450cam model (Cupp-Vickery and Poulos, 1995; Hasemann et al., 1995). The general folding patterns and catalytic site residues are retained, but the primary amino acid structures are far less so. As expected, the substrate pockets vary to accommodate structural differences in carbon substrate. More differences arise from the stringent or relaxed specificity of binding and activities.

To date, the more polar microsomal and mitochondrial P-450 proteins have resisted crystallization. Many amino acid sequences have been deduced from DNA gene sequences, and other primary protein structures have been obtained by direct amino acid sequencing. With the three new P-450 structures, from *Bacillus megaterium* BM-3, from a second pseudomonad, *ter,* and from a specific group *of Streptomyces, eryF*, the presumed difference between microsomal and microbial redox proteins has been clarified. The *B. megaterium* BM-3 enzyme resembles the animal P-450 in redox couple and more nearly in primary structure size, but it still retains the common folding pattern of its bacterial counterparts (Poulos et al., 1985; Cupp-Vickery and Poulos, 1995; Hasemann et al., 1995).

The early terpene product studies were markedly favored by the generosity of the University of Illinois Organic Chemistry Division, especially the advice and experimental participation of E. J. Corey and his students. The first physical (EPR) data on the pure two-iron, two-sulfide, four-cysteineyl protein ligand redoxin (Fe_2S_2*Cys_4) center were obtained with Helmut Beinert and William Orme-Johnson at Wisconsin, and, as mentioned, the P-450cam folding was described by Poulos and Kraut at the University of

California-San Diego. A primary driving force was a new generation of physical-biological scientists that emerged from the free flow, in both directions, of students, ideas, and information with Peter Debrunner and Hans Frauenfelder in the University of Illinois Physics Department.

The diversity of pseudomonads has attracted to biology many science talents, concepts, and experimental developments in fruitful multidisciplinary efforts. These have afforded the P-450cam system and its two energy-coupling proteins a major role in providing current structural and dynamic knowledge. This large family of proteins and systems, important in protective and synthetic roles throughout biology, is now open to interpretation.

The camphor hydroxylase system (particularly its P-450cam model) has given us a "hydrogen atom" for the fundamental principles of molecular recognition and of catalysis in a full spectrum of biochemical transformations. Commercial goals such as bioremediation that are important to society require precise understanding of the underlying chemical and physical principles. Movement on a path to rationally engineered P-450 for xenobiotic and natural product mineralization has revealed the importance of protein structure in control of regiospecific oxidation/reduction and redox coupling, as described by Sligar and his colleagues in this volume.

SUMMARY

With the influx of an increased variety and level of chemicals to the environment, bacterial strains, particularly pseudomonads, are being isolated in increasing number and kind. Snapshots are being assembled of oxidative fermentations on substrates ranging from natural biogenic materials, including fossil fuels, to synthetic chemicals of agricultural and industrial commerce. To a lesser extent, process dynamics, gene distributions, structural homologies, and correlations of activities in hetero-oligomer recombinations have been documented. However, of the few microbial strains that are studied in detail, still fewer are compared, nor are the implications thoughtfully considered. Thus the fundamentals of microbial characters, populations, changes, and control could well use more coherence. Researchers who enter the fray now find themselves facing culture numbers with scant designations, nearly all, save the mammalian synergist *E. coli,* simply designated "odd bugs." To those in need of the basic biology and a microbiological update beyond the scope of Pfennig's 1993 vignette, attention is directed to the perceptive insights of Nicholas Ornston in Editorial prefaces to *Annual Reviews of Microbiology,* for example, volumes 47–49 (1993, 1994, 1995), and the extended content by the authors selected therein. Several general population aspects are considered, though not in molecular terms, in the contemporary and historical perspective of Wilson's *Environmental Ethic* (Wilson, 1992, chapters 10, 12, and 15).

Fundamental advances in physical chemistry and materials science have enabled applications of sophisticated imaging and manipulation methods, such as atomic force microscopy and monolayer membrane film technology. The protein aggregate structures found in *Pseudomonas* metabolic processing in particular are within working parameters. Thus, merging the research paths of chemists in catalytic mechanisms with physicists in electronic structure and redox transport and biochemists in genetic engineering brings synergistic applications of technology to the resolution of problems in cellular biology.

A succinct encapsulation of the benefits of directing many disciplines toward one set of problems may be found in Frauenfelder's "Complexity in Proteins" (Frauenfelder,1995):

> The four concepts (structure, energy landscape, dynamics, function) provide a framework, but the new concepts and laws only emerge when experiments are performed and theories are being built to explain the facts.
>
> The approach and tools. . . are not different from any other field of physics. We must combine essentially every tool available in atomic, chemical, and condensed matter physics. Two aspects, however, are different from conventional physics. First, without close collaboration with biochemists and biologists, it is easy to encounter unnecessary difficulties such as spoiled samples. Such a collaboration requires that the physicist learns a new language, but the effort is fun and the result can be exciting. Second, in pure physics it is usually useless to ask for instance "Why are atoms the way they are?" In biological physics, however, the question of "why" for instance an enzyme works the way it does is legitimate and useful.

The use of bacteria for studies of structure and dynamic biochemistry is important in the ecology of a varied and safe biosphere. Hazards to flora and fauna are major concerns. The environment is captive to a cost-intensive, information-poor struggle. The need is to achieve safety, health, esthetics, and to maintain, yes to enhance, the food chain in wholesome abundance. The reward of interdisciplinary communication and transfer, the gift of free flow of information, brings increased optimism for Janus, looking forward.

REFERENCES

Andersen, J. F., K. Tatsuta, H. Gunji, T. Ishiyama, and C. R. Hutchinson. 1993. Substrate specificity of 6-deoxyerythronolide B hydroxylase, a bacteria cytochrome P450 of erythromycin A biosynthesis. *Biochemistry* **32:**1905–1913.

Austin, R. H., K. Beeson, L. Eisenstein, H. Frauenfelder, I. C. Gunsalus, and V. P. Marshall. 1973. Dynamics of carbon monoxide binding by heme proteins. *Science* **181:**541–543.

Babbit, P. C., G. T. Mrachko, M. Hasson, G. W. Huisman, R. Kolter, D. Ringe, G. A. Petsko, G. L. Kenyon, and J. A. Gerlt. 1995. A functionally diverse enzyme superfamily that abstracts the α-protons of carboxylic acids. *Science* **267:**1159–1161.

Bradshaw, W. H., E. H. Conrad, E. J. Corey, and I. C. Gunsalus. 1959. Microbiological degradation of (+)-camphor. *J. Am. Chem. Soc.* **81:**5507.

Brock, T. D. 1995. The road to Yellowstone—and beyond. *Annu. Rev. Microbiol.* **49:**2–24.

Cairns, J., G. S. Stent, and J. D. Watson. 1966. *Phage and the Origins of Molecular Biology*. Cold Spring Harbor Laboratory, Cold Spring Harbor, N.Y.

Chapman, P. J., G. Meerman, and I. C. Gunsalus. 1965. The microbiological transformation of fenchone. *Biochem. Biophys. Res. Commun.* **20:**104–108.

Chou, G. I. N., D. Katz, and I. C. Gunsalus. 1974. Fusion and compatibility of camphor and octane plasmids in *Pseudomonas*. *Proc. Natl. Acad. Sci. USA* **71:**2675–2678.

Conrad, H. E., K. Lieb, and I. C. Gunsalus. 1965. Mixed function oxidation. III. An electron transport complex in camphor ketolactonization. *J. Biol. Chem.* **240:**4029–4037.

Cupp-Vickery, J. R., and T. L. Poulos. 1995. Structure of cytochrome P450eryF involved in erythromycin biosynthesis. *Nature Struct. Biol.* **2:**144–153.

Frauenfelder, H. 1995. Complexity in proteins. *Nature Struct. Biol.* **2:**821–823.

Gest, H. 1987. Three giants in infectious disease research, Pasteur, Koch, Jenner, p. 153–160. *In The World of Microbes*. Science Tech Publishers, Inc., Madison, Wis.

Gunsalus, C. F., R. Y. Stanier, and I. C. Gunsalus. 1953. The enzymatic conversion of mandelic acid to benzoic acid. III. Fractionation and properties of the soluble enzymes. *J. Bacteriol.* **66:**548–553.

Gunsalus, I. C. 1973. *Productive Agriculture and a Quality Environment.* National Academy of Sciences, Washington, D.C.

Gunsalus, I. C. 1988. Learning with Hans from iron and oxygen. Proceedings of the International Symposium on Frontiers in Science, Urbana, Ill. *Am. Inst. Physics Proc.* **180:**1–24.

Gunsalus, I. C. 1992. Molecules and microbes of merit: 50 years ago and now. *FASEB J.* **6:**3423–3425.

Gunsalus, I. C., P. K. Bhattacharyya, and K. Suhara. 1985. Bioregulation of binding and dynamics: the cytochrome P-450_{cam} model. *Curr. Top. Cell. Regul.* **26:**295–309.

Gunsalus, I. C., C. F. Gunsalus, and R Y. Stanier. 1953. The enzymatic conversion of mandelic acid to benzoic acid. I. Gross fractionation of the system into soluble and particulate components. *J. Bacteriol.* **66:**538–542.

Hasemann, C. A., R. G. Curumbail, S. S. Boddupally, J. A. Peterson, and J. Deisenhofer. 1995. Structure and function of cytochromes P450: a comparative analysis of three crystal structures. *Structure* **3:**41–62.

Hayaishi, O. (ed.). 1962. *Oxygenases.* Academic Press Inc., New York.

Hayaishi, O. 1974. *Molecular Mechanisms of Oxygen Activation.* Academic Press Inc., New York.

Henrici, A. T. 1928. Morphologic variation and the rate of growth of bacteria, p.1–194. *In Microbiology Monographs,* vol. 1. Bailliere, Tindall, and Cox, London.

Hershey, A. D. 1939. Factors limiting bacterial growth. VII. Respiration and growth properties *of Escherichia coli* surviving sublethal temperatures. *J. Bacteriol.* **38:**563–578.

Kenyon, G. L., J. A. Gerlt, G. A. Petsko, and J. W. Kozarich. 1995. Mandelate racemase: structure-function studies of a pseudosymmetric enzyme. *Accts. Chem. Res.* **8:**178–186.

Kluyver, A. J. 1959. *Contributions to Microbiology and Biochemistry. His Life and Work.* North Holland Publishing Co., Amsterdam.

Kluyver, A. J., and C. B. van Niel. 1956. Microbial metabolism; further evidence of life's unity, p. 31–72, 130–154. *In The Microbe's Contribution to Biology,* vol. 5. Harvard University Press, Cambridge, Mass.

Lederberg, J. 1947. Gene recombination and linked segregation in *E. coli. Genetics* **32:**505–525.

Lederberg, J., and E. M. Lederberg. 1952. Replica plating and indirect selection of bacterial mutants. *J. Bacteriol.* **63:**399–406.

Lipscomb, J. D., C. A. Tyson, and I. C. Gunsalus. 1973. Cytochrome P-450 reduction and oxygenation, p. 583–603. *In* T. E. King, H. S. Mason, and M. Morrison (ed.), *Oxidases and Related Redox Systems.* University Park Press, Baltimore.

Madyastha, K. M., and P. K. Bhattacharyya. 1968. Microbiological transformations of terpenes. XII. Fermentation of p-cymene by a soil pseudomonad (PL-strain). *Indian J. Biochem.* **5:**102–111.

Madyastha, K. M., P. K. Bhattacharyya, and C. S. Vaidyanathan. 1977. Metabolism of a monoterpene alcohol, linalool, by a soil pseudomonad (lin-strain). *Can. J. Microbiol.* **23:**230–239.

Martinis, S. A., J. D. Ropp, S. G. Sligar, and I. C. Gunsalus. 1991. Molecular recognition by cytochrome P450cam: substrate specificity, catalysis and electron transfer. *Frontiers Biotransformation* **4:**54–86.

Nelson, D. R., L. Koymans, T. Kamataki, J. J. Stegeman, R. Feyereisen, D. J. Wazman, M. R Waterman, O. Gotoh, M. J. Coon, R W. Estabrook, I. C. Gunsalus, and D. W. Nebert. 1996. P450 superfamily: update on new sequences, gene mapping, accession numbers, and nomenclature. *DNA Cell Biol.* **15:**1–60.

Ornston, L. N., J. Houghton, E. L. Neidle, and L. A. Gregg. 1990. Subtle selection and novel mutation during evolutionary divergence of the β-ketoadipate pathway, p. 207–225. *In* S. Silver, A. M. Chakrabarty, B. Iglewski, and S. Kaplan (ed.), *Pseudomonas: Biotransformations, Pathogenesis, and Evolving Biotechnology.* American Society for Microbiology, Washington, D.C.

Pfennig, N. 1993. Reflections of a microbiologist, or how to learn from the microbes. *Annu. Rev. Microbiol.* **47:**1–29.

Poulos, T. L., B. C. Finzel, I. C. Gunsalus, G. C. Wagner, and J. Kraut. 1985. The 2.6Å crystal structure of *Pseudomonas putida* cytochrome *P*-450. *J. Biol. Chem.* **260:**16122–16130.

Rahn, O. 1926. Growth, p. 162–269. *In Physiology of Bacteria.* Blakiston's Son & Co., Philadelphia.

Rahn, O. 1945. *Microbes of Merit.* C C Thomas & Co., Springfield, Ill.

Ropp, J. D., I. C. Gunsalus, and S. G. Sligar. 1993. Cloning and expression of a new cytochrome P-450 family: cytochrome P-450lin from *Pseudomonas putida (incognita). J. Bacteriol.* **175:**6028–6037.

Sharrock, M., E. Munck, P. G. Debrunner, V. Marshall, J. D. Lipscomb, and I. C. Gunsalus. 1973. Mossbauer studies of cytochrome P450cam. *Biochemistry* **12:**258–265.

Sligar, S. G., P. G. Debrunner, J. D. Lipscomb, M. J. Namtvedt, and I. C. Gunsalus. 1974. A role of the putidaredoxin COOH-terminus in P450cam (cytochrome m) hydroxylations. *Proc. Natl. Acad. Sci. USA* **71:**3906–3910.

Sokatch, J. R. (ed.). 1986. *The Bacteria*, vol. 10: *The Biology of Pseudomonas*. Academic Press, Inc., Orlando, Fla.

Stanier, R. Y., I. C. Gunsalus, and C. F. Gunsalus. 1953. The enzymatic conversion of mandelic acid to benzoic acid. II. Properties of the particulate fractions. *J. Bacteriol.* **66:**543–547.

Stanier, R. Y., N. J. Palleroni, and M. Doudoroff. 1966. The aerobic pseudomonads: a taxonomic study. *J. Gen. Microbiol.* **43:**159–271.

Stephenson, M. 1939. *Bacterial Metabolism*. Longmans, Green and Co., London.

Trudgill, P. W. 1986. Terpenoid metabolism by *Pseudomonas*, p. 483–485. *In* J. R. Sokatch (ed.), *The Bacteria*, vol. 10: *The Biology of Pseudomonas*. Academic Press, Inc., Orlando, Fla.

Unger, B. P., I. C. Gunsalus, and S. G. Sligar. 1986. The biology *of Pseudomonas* cytochrome P450, p. 557–589. *In* J. R. Sokatch (ed.), *The Bacteria*, vol. 10: *The Biology of Pseudomonas*. Academic Press, Inc., Orlando, Fla.

Wilson E. O. 1992. *Environmental Ethic*, p. 182–211, 243–280, 343–351. Harvard University Press, Cambridge, Mass.

Wolfe, R S. 1991. My kind of biology. *Annu. Rev. Microbiol.* **45:**1–35.

Woese, C. R. 1994. There must be a prokaryote somewhere: microbiology's search for itself. *Microbiol. Rev.* **58:**1–9.

Wood, H. G. 1985. Then and now. *Annu. Rev. Microbiol.* **54:**1–41.

Yu, C.-A., I. C. Gunsalus, M. Katagiri, K. Suhara, and S. Takemori. 1974. Cytochrome P450cam. I. Crystallization and properties. *J. Biol. Chem.* **249:**94–101.

Molecular Biology of Pseudomonads
Edited by T. Nakazawa et al.

Chapter 3

Pseudomonas Genetics and Taxonomy

Bruce W. Holloway

The last 5 years have seen a complete change in the way that genetic information is obtained with bacteria. The classical techniques of conjugation, transduction, and transformation are used only in special circumstances. In their place, techniques for constructing different types of genetic maps and gaining an understanding of whole genomic structures are used. This change has particular importance for those genera of bacteria formerly grouped into the genus *Pseudomonas*. The miscellany of names used is shown in Table 1. The common occurrence of plasmids in naturally occurring isolates of these organisms and the recent demonstration of multiple chromosomes in *Burkholderia cepacia* (Cheng and Lessie, 1994) attest to the genomic complexity of these bacteria.

THE NEW TECHNIQUES

The basis of the new techniques of genomic analysis is fragmentation of the physical structures of the bacterial genome, that is, the chromosome(s) and plasmids, into smaller, manageable pieces. These fragments can be individually analyzed, and their individual former relative positions in the whole genome can be determined, a top-down approach that is in contrast to the more traditional bottom-up method. For bacteria, the genome can be fragmented by using infrequently cutting enzymes, and the resultant segments can be separated by pulsed-field gel electrophoresis (PFGE). A variety of techniques, including linking clones (Ratnaningsih et al., 1990), two-dimensional PFGE (Römling and Tümmler, 1991), and end labeling (Römling and Tümmler, 1991), are used to establish the original arrangement. The last two techniques overcome the problems created by repetitive DNA. When retention of the fragment is desirable, a variety of cloning vehicles is available, including phage lambda, numerous plasmids, and, for cloning of larger fragments, cosmids. Cosmids derived from wide-host-range plasmids have the advantage of transferring the cloned fragment between different species, which is a benefit when gene identification by complementation is required (Simon et al., 1983; Holloway et al., 1992).

Bruce W. Holloway • Department of Genetics and Developmental Biology, Monash University, Clayton, Victoria, 3168 Australia.

Table 1. New generic assignments for pseudomonads

rRNA homology group	Organism(s)	Reference
I (γ-proteobacteria)	*P. aeruginosa*, "true pseudomonads"	Palleroni, 1992
II and III (β-proteobacteria)	*Acidovorax, Burkholderia, Ralstonia*	Willems et al., 1990
		Willems et al., 1992
		Yabuuchi et al., 1995
IV (α-proteobacteria)	*Brevundimonas*	Segers et al., 1994
V (γ-proteobacteria)	*Stenotrophomonas*	Palleroni and Bradbury, 1993

The increased availability of and access to sequence data for bacterial genes has created opportunities for generating probes from cloned genes either from the same or similar species or from quite different species of bacteria. In the latter case, a degree of sequence similarity is assumed, and optimally, a region of sequence homology that will give unequivocal probing results is identified (Mohr et al., 1994).

All of the techniques named above have the advantage of being applicable to any isolate of any bacterial species, so that investigators are not confined to using only one isolate of a given species (Holloway, 1993). This flexibility is clearly advantageous in studies involving isolates from diseased animals, plants, or humans; for isolates from natural sources that may have biochemical characteristics of interest; and for environmental investigations.

GENOME ANALYSIS OF PSEUDOMONADS

Pseudomonas aeruginosa

The best-characterized species with respect to genome structure is *P. aeruginosa*, which has the benefit of more than 30 years of classical genetic investigation (Holloway and Morgan, 1986). The availability of effective chromosome-mobilizing plasmids made possible the construction of a circular genetic chromosome map (Royle et al., 1981; O'Hoy and Krishnapillai, 1987). Techniques for combined physical mapping and genetic mapping were developed (Ratnaningsih et al., 1990; Römling et al., 1989; Römling and Tümmler, 1991; Römling et al., 1992), and this work has developed to the point that we now have a combined physical and genetic map for *P. aeruginosa* that is circular and has in excess of 180 genes mapped. Most of the genes were mapped by using the enzyme *Spe*I, but some genes were mapped by using *Dpn*I as well (Holloway et al., 1994b). The genome size for strain PAO is 5.9 Mbp, but this number has been shown to vary with other strains (Schmidt et al., 1996). The genome is contained in one circular chromosome, and in strain PAO, there is no evidence of any plasmid components in the genome. Partial *Dra*I (Shortridge et al., 1991) and *Hpa*I (Ronald et al., 1992) maps are available. The current physical and genetic maps or *P. aeruginosa* PAO are shown in Fig. 1 and 2.

Though it has been an advantage to have a common strain, PAO, for the accumulation of these data, the techniques that have resulted in the combined genetic and molecular map are applicable to any *P. aeruginosa* strain. This applicability is important for clinical research, both for identifying genes important for pathogenesis and for providing a new type of epidemiological data. As the number and range of mapped genes increase, it

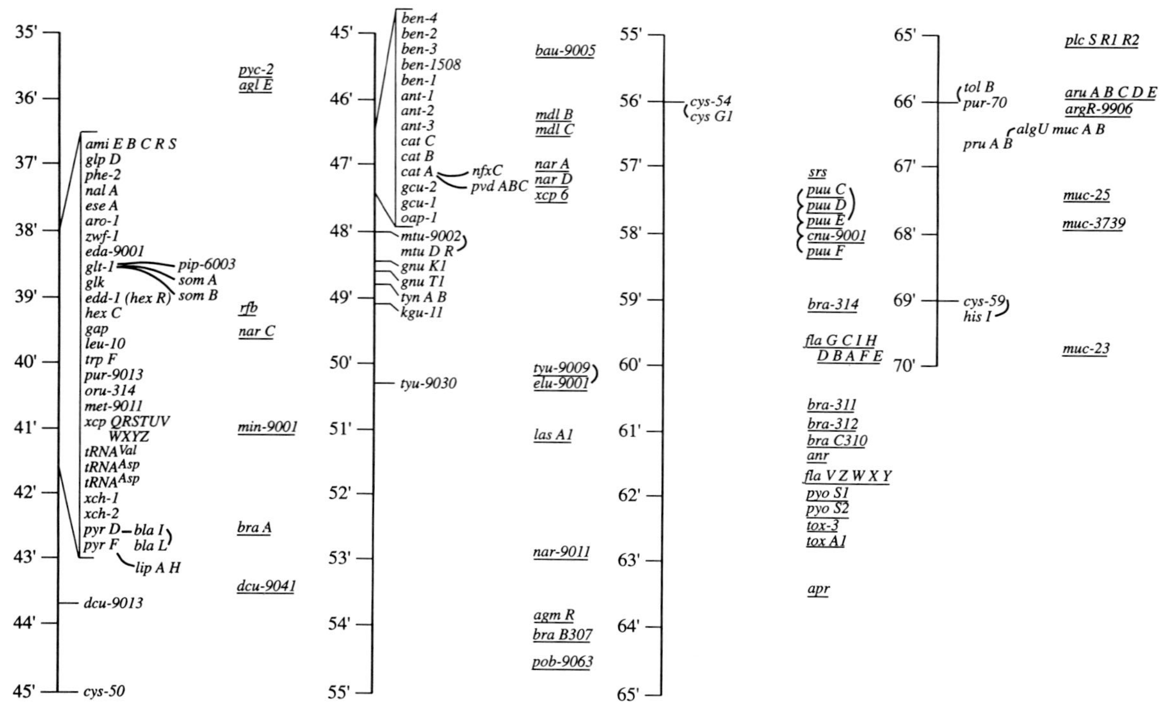

Figure 1. Genetic map of *P. aeruginosa* PAO (from Holloway et al., 1994b, with permission). The 0-min or origin site has been arbitrarily located at the *ilvB/C* locus. A description of the markers mapped is given by Holloway et al. (1994b). Markers whose locations are indicated by straight lines joining locus designations to the map were located by interrupted matings using FP2, FP5, pMO514, or IncP-1 insert donor strains. A square bracket surrounding a group of markers indicates that the gene order of those markers has been established. Curved lines joining a marker to the chromosome indicate that the markers so joined are contransducible using one or more of the bacteriophages F116, F116L, G101, and E79*tv-2*. Markers that are underlined have not been precisely mapped, but there is evidence to locate the marker in the area where the symbol has been placed, and in most such cases, the relationships to flanking markers have not been determined.

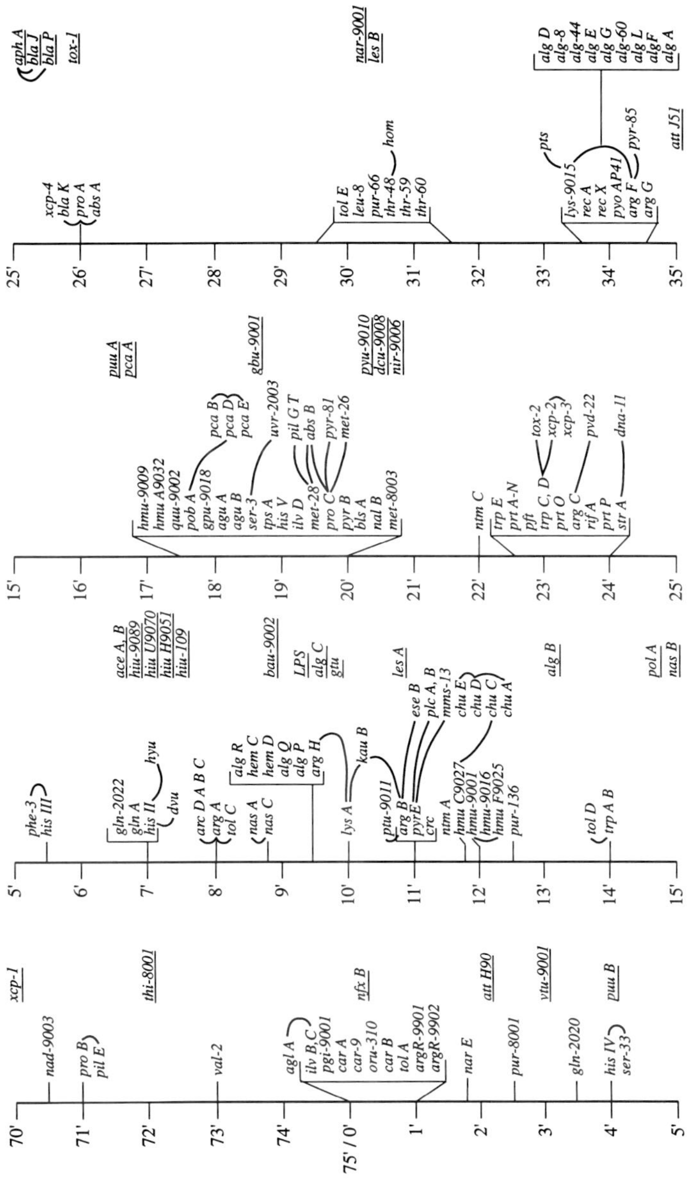

Figure 1. *Continued*

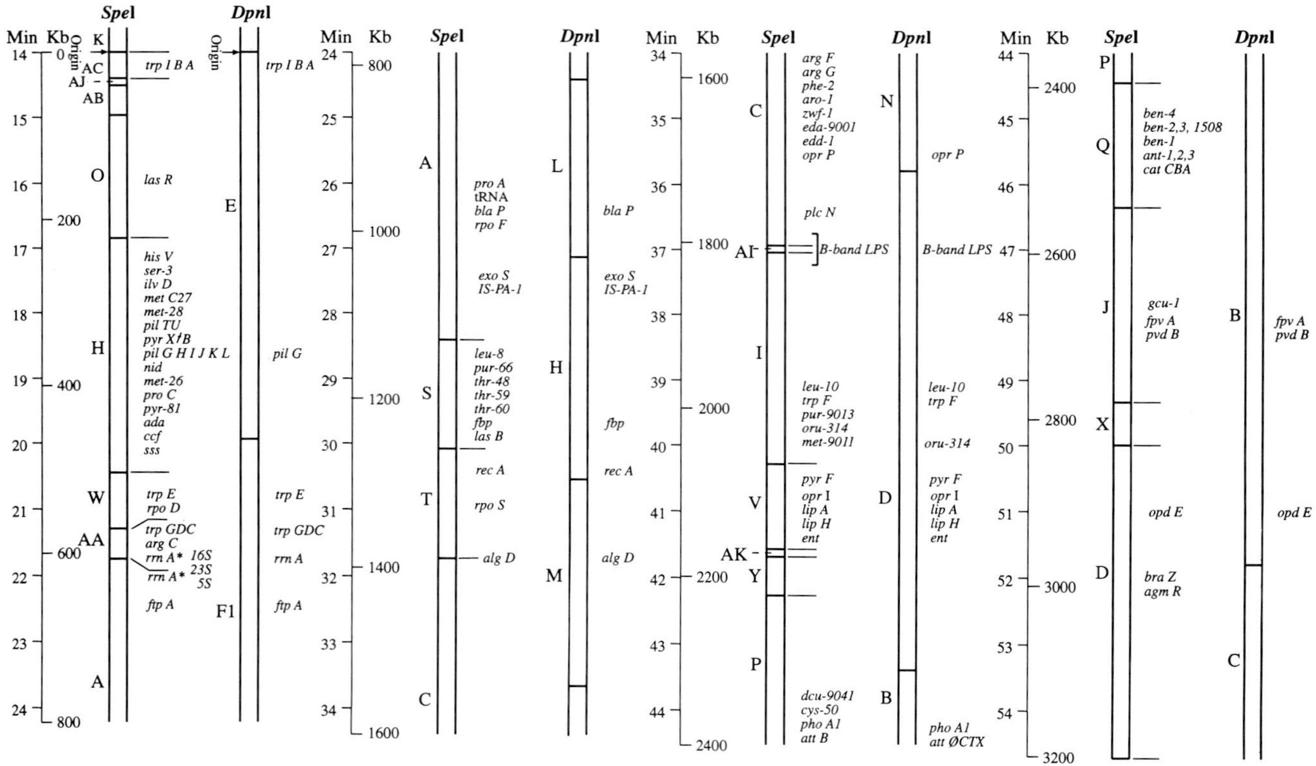

Figure 2. Physical map of *P. aeruginosa* PAO. The *oriC* site has been nominated as the origin of the physical map. The physical and genetic maps have been aligned by locating the 14-min site of the genetic map at one end of the *Spe*I AC fragment. Markers identified only from sequence data are indicated by daggers (†). An asterisk indicates that the probe hybridizes with the adjacent fragments. No conclusions can be drawn from the data with respect to the relative arrangement of markers on any individual *Spe*I fragment. From Holloway et al. (1994b), with permission.

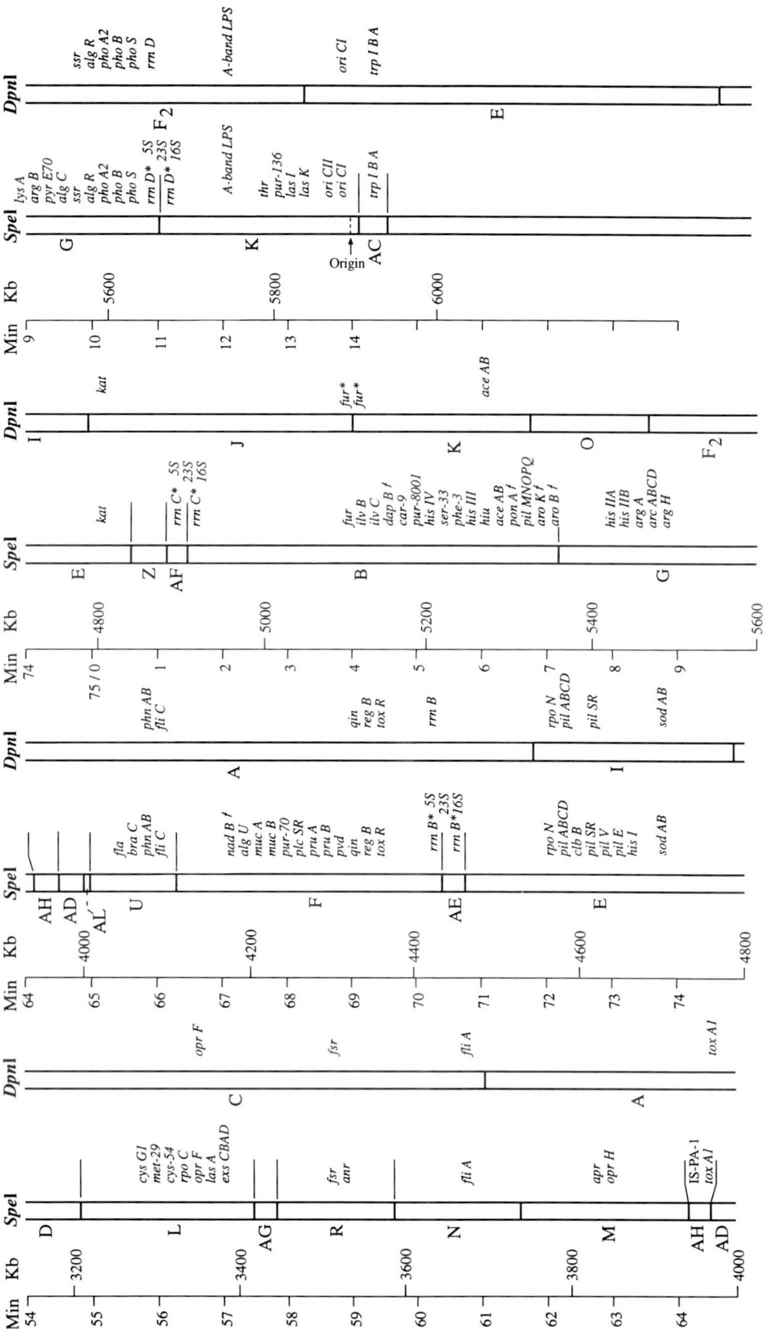

Figure 2. *Continued*

will be possible to draw conclusions about genomic architecture and the evolution and function of specific gene arrangements. Holloway and Morgan (1986) have already identified auxotropic marker-rich regions in *P. aeruginosa* and *P. putida* and have proposed mechanisms by which these and other genes may have acquired their present arrangements. The availability of an extensive physical and genetic map and a characterized cosmid library for this organism will be of considerable benefit should the sequencing of the entire genome of *P. aeruginosa* be undertaken. New approaches to genome sequencing may minimize the value of existing data, as shown by the recent whole-genome sequencing of *Haemophilus influenzae* (Fleischmann et al., 1995).

P. fluorescens

A low-resolution physical and genetic map of *P. fluorescens* SBW25 was made (Rainey and Bailey, 1996). The circular map has 15 *Pac*I fragments, 52 *Spe*I fragments, and a genome size of 6.65 Mbp, with 30 markers located, including *oriC* and rRNA operons (*rrnA* through *rrnE*). *P. fluorescens* and *P. aeruginosa* show similarities in their chromosomal gene arrangements.

Burkholderia solanacearum

A physical and genetic map of *B. solanacearum* was constructed by using the techniques established with *P. aeruginosa.* Strain PS1000, a biovar 3, race 1 strain isolated from diseased eggplant, was used to construct an *Spe*I map that shows a minimum of 30 fragments arranged in six contigs. The genome size is at least 5.5 Mbp. Nearly 50 genes have been located on these fragments, including some involved in the disease processes of bacterial wilt (Holloway et al., 1994a). Assembling a more comprehensive physical map has been made difficult by the presence of repetitive DNA, but this is being overcome by the use of two-dimensional PFGE.

Burkholderia cepacia

Using the same techniques as were found to be effective in *P. aeruginosa*, Cheng and Lessie (1994) showed that *B. cepacia* has three large circular replicons of 3.4, 2.5, and 0.9 Mbp. Inclusion of the already identified 170-kbp cryptic plasmid thus gives a genome size of 7 Mbp for this organism. Each of the three large replicons carries rRNA genes, indicating that they possess essential genetic information and thus identifying them as chromosomes rather than plasmids. A number of genes and insertion sequences have been mapped on these replicons, thus providing the first physical and genetic map of this organism. This organism is the first example of a beta-group proteobacterium with multiple chromosomes, although this situation was also demonstrated with three members of the alpha group of proteobacteria: *Rhodobacter sphaeroides* (Suwanto and Kaplan, 1989), *Agrobacterium tumefaciens* (Allard-Servent et al., 1993), and *Brucella melitensis* (Michaux et al., 1993). Additional studies of the genomes of *B. cepacia* and *B. solanacearum* demonstrating that isolates of the genus *Burkholderia* commonly have a multireplicon genomic structure are described by Rodley et al. (1995). In such organisms, it is now more difficult to distinguish between what is a chromosome and what is a plasmid.

MODERN TAXONOMY OF PSEUDOMONADS

Rationalization and greater precision in the taxonomy of pseudomonads have resulted from the increasing use of genetic techniques (Table 2). The aims of such work include defining organismal diversity and interrelationships and providing a logical and orderly arrangement of the component organisms. Palleroni (1992) gave a historical account that noted the importance of DNA hybridization and of the identification of the value of conserved regions of the genome, particularly the rRNA genes, which led to identification of five major groups. Indeed, molecular phylogeny is now the major basis of bacterial systematics, with the comparative sequence analysis of rRNAs (or rather, their corresponding genes) providing the major input of new data. The 16S rRNAs are the major phylogenetic marker molecules, and the 23S rRNAs provide additional information. However, the work of Harayama and Yamamoto (this volume) demonstrates the value to molecular taxonomy of genes coding for proteins such as *gyrB* and *rpoD*. The 16S RNA sequences of more than 1,500 bacteria are now available. In pseudomonads, these sequences have about 2,900 bases (Ludwig and Schleifer, 1994).

The relative importance of the role of a single molecule in bacterial systematics has been widely debated (Olsen and Woese, 1993), and for the pseudomonads, a solution to the heterogeneity of the genus has been to use a variety of criteria. In this process, the original genus has been modified by the introduction of new generic descriptions of species that were formerly included in the genus *Pseudomonas*. These modifications are based on the identification of five rRNA groups in this genus (Palleroni et al., 1973; De Vos and De Ley, 1983). rRNA homology group I continues to be referred to as the "true pseudomonads," and the other groups have been reassigned to new genera. The rRNA homology groups II and III (β-proteobacteria) now include the new genera *Acidovorax* (Willems et al., 1990, 1992) and *Burkholderia* (Yabuuchi et al., 1992; Urakami et al., 1994). As a result, the former *P. cepacia, P. mallei, P. pseudomallei, P. carophyllii, P. gladioli, P. pickettii, P. plantarii,* and *P. glumae* are now assigned to the genus *Burkholderia*. Some species of rRNA group IV (α-proteobacteria) have been included in the new genus *Brevundimonas*, for example, *B. diminuta* and *B. vesicularis* (Segers et al., 1994). *P. maltophilia* of rRNA homology group V (γ-proteobacteria) has been renamed *Stenotrophomonas maltophilia* (Palleroni and Bradbury, 1993).

As we use these new taxonomic criteria and accumulate new data, additional changes may have to be made. For example, Gillis et al. (1995) proposed emendments to the description of the genus *Burkholderia*. They described a new species, *B. vietnamiensis*,

Table 2. Taxonomic criteria important for pseudomonads

Taxonomic criterion	Reference
16S rRNA gene sequences	Li et al., 1993
23S rRNA Gene sequences	Ludwig et al., 1995
gyrB gene sequences	Yamamoto and Harayama, 1995
rpoD gene sequences	Harayama and Yamamoto (this volume)
rRNA-DNA hybridization	Palleroni et al., 1973
DNA-DNA homology values	Johnson and Palleroni, 1989
Cellular lipid and fatty acid compositions	Stead, 1992

that includes nitrogen-fixing isolates from rice in Vietnam. Yabuuchi et al. (1995) suggested that *B. pickettii, B. solanacearum*, and *Alcaligenes eutrophus* be transferred to a new genus, *Ralstonia*. In addition to 16S rRNA, other regions of the genome are being tested for higher specificity for taxonomic purposes than the rRNA-based probes have. One possible candidate is *gyrB*, which encodes the subunit B protein of DNA gyrase (topoisomerase type II). This gene is effective in the detection and taxonomic analysis of *P. putida* strains (Yamamoto and Harayama, 1995; and this volume).

MOLECULAR GENETIC TECHNIQUES FOR THE IDENTIFICATION OF FIELD STRAINS OF PSEUDOMONADS

In a conjunction of genetics and taxonomy in agriculture and medical microbiology, the identification of specific strains of a given species or genus can contribute to the solution of practical problems. One example of such a solution involves bacterial wilt of crop plants, a disease caused by *Burkholderia solanacearum*. It is important to classify field isolates of this organism in terms of their host range and infectious ability, and former methods of doing this were not sufficiently precise. By using 16S rRNA sequences (Taghavi et al., 1996) and random amplified polymorphic DNA approaches (Opina et al., submitted), procedures have been developed that make possible the precise differentiation of *B. solanacearum* from other bacteria and that also differentiate between isolates with similar cultural characteristics that could not otherwise be distinguished by current techniques.

Acknowledgments. Work in my laboratory is supported by the Australian Centre for International Agricultural Research. I thank Jeremy Timmis, Chris Hayward, Viji Krishnapillai, and Paul Rainey for permission to quote unpublished data and for suggestions about the manuscript.

REFERENCES

Allard-Servent, A., S. Micheaux-Charachon, E. Jumas-Bilak, L. Karayan, and M. Ramuz. 1993. Presence of one linear and one circular chromosome in the *Agrobacterium tumefaciens* C58 genome. *J. Bacteriol.* **175:**7869–7874.

Cheng, H.-P., and T. G. Lessie. 1994. Multiple replicons constituting the genome of *Pseudomonas cepacia* 17616. *J. Bacteriol.* **176:**4034–4042.

De Vos, P., and J. De Ley. 1983. Intra- and intergeneric similarities of *Pseudomonas* and *Xanthomonas* ribosomal ribonucleic acid cistrons. *Int. J. Syst. Bacteriol.* **33:**487–509.

Fleischmann, R. D., M. D. Adams, O. White, R. A. Clayton, E. F. Kirkness, A. R. Kerlavage, C. J. Bult, J.-F. Tomb, B. A. Dougherty, J. M. Merrick, K. McKenney, G. Sutton, W. Fitzhugh, C. Fields, J. D. Gocayne, J. Scott, R. Shirley, L.-I. Lie, A. Glodek, J. M. Kelley, J. F. Weidman, C. A. Philipps, T. Spriggs, E. Hedblom, M. D. Cotton, T. R. Utterback, M. C. Hanna, D. T. Nguyen, D. M. Saudek, R. C. Brandon, L. D. Fine, J. L. Fritchman, J. L. Fuhrmann, N. S. M. Geoghagen, C. L. Gnehm, L. A. McDonald, K. V. Small, C. M. Fraser, H. O. Smith, and J. C. Venter. 1995. Whole-genome random sequencing and assembly of *Haemophilus influenzae* Rd. *Science* **269:**496–512.

Gillis, M., T. V. Van, R. Bardin, M. Goor, P. Hebbar, A. Willems, P. Segers, K. Kersters, T. Heulin, and M. P. Fernandez. 1995. Polyphasic taxonomy in the genus *Burkholderia* leading to an emended description of the genus and proposition of *Burkholderia vietnamiensis* sp. nov. for N_2-fixing isolates from rice in Vietnam. *Int. J. Syst. Bacteriol.* **45:**274–289.

Holloway, B. W. 1993. Genetics for all bacteria. *Annu. Rev. Microbiol.* **47:**659–684.

Holloway, B. W., M. D. Escuadra, A. F. Morgan, R. Saffery, and V. Krishnapillai. 1992. The new approaches to whole genome analysis of bacteria. *FEMS Microbiol. Lett.* **100:**101–106.

Holloway, B. W., V. Krishnapillai, and M. D. Escuadra. 1994a. Whole genome analysis of pseudomonads and its application to *Pseudomonas solanacearum*, p. 59–76. *In* A. C. Hayward and G. L. Hartman (ed.), *Bacterial Wilt: the Disease and Its Causative Agent, Pseudomonas solanacearum*. C.A.B. International, Wallingford, United Kingdom.

Holloway, B. W., and A. M. Morgan. 1986. Genome organization in *Pseudomonas*. *Annu. Rev. Microbiol.* **40:**79–105.

Holloway, B. W., U. Römling, and B. Tümmler. 1994b. Genomic mapping of *Pseudomonas aeruginosa*. *Microbiology* **140:**2907–2929.

Johnson, J. L., and N. J. Palleroni. 1989. Deoxyribonucleic acid similarities among *Pseudomonas* species. *Int. J. Syst. Bacteriol.* **39:**230–235.

Li, X., M. Dorsch, T. Del Dot, L. Sly, E. Stackebrandt, and A. C. Hayward. 1993. Phylogenetic studies of the rRNA group II pseudomonads based on 16S rRNA gene sequences. *J. Appl. Bacteriol.* **74:**324–329.

Ludwig, W., R. Rosselló-Mora, R. Aznar, S. Klugbauer, S. Spring, K. Reetz, C. Beimfohr, E. Brockmann, G. Kirchhof, S. Dorn, M. Bachleitner, N. Klugbauer, N. Springer, D. Lane, R. Nietupsky, M. Weizenegger, and K.-H. Schleifer. 1995. Comparative sequence analysis of 23S rRNA from *Proteobacteria*. *Syst. Appl. Microbiol.* **18:**164–188.

Ludwig, W., and K. H. Schleifer. 1994. Bacterial phylogeny based on 16S and 23S rRNA sequence analysis. *FEMS Microbiol. Rev.* **15:**155–173.

Michaux, S., J. Paillisoon, M. J. Carles-Nurit, G. Bourg, A. Allardet-Servent, and M. Ramuz. 1993. Presence of two independent chromosomes in the *Brucella melitensis* 16M genome. *J. Bacteriol.* **175:**701–705.

Mohr, C. D., S. K. Sonsteby, and V. Deretic. 1994. The *Pseudomonas aeruginosa* homologs of *hemC* and *hemD* are linked to the gene encoding the regulator of mucoidy *algR*. *Mol. Gen. Genet.* **242:**177–184.

O'Hoy, K., and V. Krishnapillai. 1987. Recalibration of the *Pseudomonas aeruginosa PAO* chromosome map in time units using high-frequency-of-recombination donors. *Genetics* **115:**611–618.

Olsen, G. J., and C. R. Woese. 1993. Ribosomal RNA: a key to phylogeny. *FASEB J.* **7:**113–123.

Opina, N., F. Tavner, G. Hollway, J.-F. Wang, S. Li, R. Maghirang, M. Fegan, C. Hayward, V. Krishnapillai, W. F. Hong, B. W. Holloway, and J. Timmis. DNA probes for *Pseudomonas solanacearum*: PCR detection, specificity and sensitivity. Submitted for publication.

Palleroni, N. J. 1992. Present situation of the taxonomy of aerobic Pseudomonads, p. 105–115. *In* E. Galli, S. Silver, and B. Witholt (ed.), *Pseudomonas: Molecular Biology and Biotechnology*. American Society for Microbiology, Washington, D.C.

Palleroni, N. J., and J. F. Bradbury. 1993. *Stenotrophomonas*, a new bacterial genus for *Xanthomonas maltophilia* (Hugh 1980) Swings et al. 1982. *Int. J. Syst. Bacteriol.* **43:**606–609.

Palleroni, N. J., R. Kunisawa, R. Contopoulou, and M. Doudoroff. 1973. Nucleic acid homologies in the genus *Pseudomonas*. *Int. J. Syst. Bacteriol.* **23:**333–339.

Rainey, P. B., and M. J. Bailey. 1996. Physical and genetic map of the *Pseudomonas fluorescens* SBW25 chromosome. *Mol. Microbiol.* **19:**521–534.

Ratnaningsih, E., S. Dharmsthiti, V. Krishnapillai, A. Morgan, M. Sinclair, and B. W. Holloway. 1990. A combined physical and genetic map of *Pseudomonas aeruginosa* PAO. *J. Gen. Microbiol.* **136:**2351–2357.

Rodley, P. D., U. Römling, and B. Tümmler. 1995. A physical genome map of the *Burkholderia cepacia* type strain. *Mol. Microbiol.* **17:**57–67.

Römling, U., M. Duchênne, D. W. Essar, D. Galloway, C. Guidi-Rontani, D. Hill, A. Lazdunski, R. V. Miller, K. H. Schleifer, D. W. Smith, H. Y. Toschka, and B. Tümmler. 1992. Localization of *alg, opr, phn, phoR*, 5S RNA, 6S RNA, *tox, trp*, and *xcp* genes, *rrn* operons, and the chromosomal origin on the physical genome map of *Pseudomonas aeruginosa* PAO. *J. Bacteriol.* **174:**327–330.

Römling, U., D. Grothues, W. Bautsch, and B. Tümmler. 1989. A physical genome map of *Pseudomonas aeruginosa* PAO. *EMBO J.* **8:**4081–4089.

Römling, U., and B. Tümmler. 1991. The impact of two-dimensional pulsed-field gel electrophoresis techniques for the consistent and complete mapping of bacterial genomes: refined physical map of *Pseudomonas aeruginosa* PAO. *Nucleic Acids Res.* **19:**3199–3206.

Ronald, S., M. A. Farinha, B. J. Allan, and A. M. Kropinski. 1992. Cloning and physical mapping of transcriptional regulatory (sigma) factors from *Pseudomonas aeruginosa*, p. 249–257. *In* E. Galli, S. Silver, and B. Witholt (ed.), *Pseudomonas: Molecular Biology and Biotechnology*. American Society for Microbiology, Washington, D.C.

Royle, P., H. Matsumoto, and B. W. Holloway. 1981. Genetic circularity of the *Pseudomonas aeruginosa* chromosome. *J. Bacteriol.* **145:**145–155.

Schmidt, K. D., B. Tümmler, and U. Römling. 1996. Comparative mapping of *Pseudomonas aeruginosa* PAO with *P. aeruginosa* C, which belongs to a major clone in cystic fibrosis patients and aquatic habitats. *J. Bacteriol.* **178:**85–93.

Segers, P., M. Vancanneyt, B. Pot, V. Torck, B. Hoste, D. Dewettingck, E. Falsen, K. Kersters, and P. de Vos. 1994. Classification of *Pseudomonas diminuta* Leifson and Hugh 1954 and *Pseudomonas vesicularis* Büsing, Döll, and Freytag 1953 in *Brevundimonas* gen. nov. as *Brevundimonas diminuta* comb. nov. and *Brevundimonas vesicularis* comb. nov., respectively. *Int. J. Syst. Bacteriol.* **44:**499–510.

Shortridge, V. D., M. L. Pato, A. I. Vasil, and M. L. Vasil. 1991. Physical mapping of virulence-associated genes in *Pseudomonas aeruginosa* transverse alternating-field electrophoresis. *Infect. Immun.* **59:**3596–3603.

Simon, R., U. Priefer, and A. Pühler. 1983. A broad host range mobilization system for in vivo genetic engineering transposon mutagenesis in gram negative bacteria. *Bio/Technology* **1:**784–791.

Stead, D. E. 1992. Grouping of plant-pathogenic and some other *Pseudomonas* spp. by using cellular fatty acid profiles. *Int. J. Syst. Bacteriol.* **42:**281–295.

Suwanto, A., and S. Kaplan. 1989. Physical and genetic mapping of the *Rhodobacter sphaeroides* 2.4.1 genome: genome size, fragment identification and gene localization. *J. Bacteriol.* **171:**5840–5849.

Taghavi, M., C. Hayward, L. I. Sly, and M. Fegan. 1996. Analysis of the phylogenetic relationships of strains of *Burkholderia solanacearum, Pseudomonas syzygii*, and the blood disease bacterium of banana based on sequencing of the 16S rRNA gene sequences. *Int. J. Syst. Bacteriol.* **46:**10–15.

Urakami, T., C. Ito-Yoshida, H. Araki, T. Kijima, K. I. Suzuki, and K. Komagata. 1994. Transfer of *Pseudomonas plantarii* and *Pseudomonas glumae* to *Burkholderia* as *Burkholderia* spp. and description of *Burkholderia vandii* sp. nov. *Int. J. Syst. Bacteriol.* **44:**235–245.

Willems, A., E. Falsen, B. Pot, E. Jantzen, B. Hoste, P. Vandamme, M. Gillis, K. Kersters, and J. De Ley. 1990. *Acidovorax*, a new genus for *Pseudomonas facilis*, *Pseudomonas delafieldii* E. Falsen (EFO group 13, EF group 16) and several clinical isolates, with the species *Acidovorax facilis* comb. nov., *Acidovorax delafieldii* comb. nov., and *Acidovorax temperans* sp. nov. *Int. J. Syst. Bacteriol.* **40:**384–398.

Willems, A., M. Goor, S. Thielemans, M. Gillis, and K. Kersters. 1992. Transfer of several phytopathogenic *Pseudomonas* species to *Acidovorax* as *Acidovorax avenae* subsp. *avenae* subsp. nov. comb. nov., *Acidovorax avenae* subsp. *citrulli*, *Acidovorax avenae* subsp. *cattleyae*, and *Acidovorax konjaci*. *Int. J. Syst. Bacteriol.* **42:**107–119.

Yabuuchi, E., Y. Kosako, I. Yano, H. Hotta, and Y. Nishiuchi. 1995. Transfer of two *Burkholderia* and an *Alcaligenes* species to *Ralstonia* gen nov—proposal of *Ralstonia pickettii* (Ralston, Palleroni and Doudoroff 1973) comb nov *Ralstonia solanacearum* (Smith 1896) comb nov and *Ralstonia eutropha* (Davis 1969) comb nov. *Microbiol. Immunol.* **39:**897–904.

Yabuuchi, E., K. Yoshimasa, H. Oyaizu, I. Yano, H. Hotta, Y. Hashimoto, T. Ezaki, and M. Arakawa. 1992. Proposal of *Burkholderia* gen. nov. and transfer of seven species of the genus *Pseudomonas* homology group II to the new genus, with the type species *Burkholderia cepacia* (Palleroni and Holmes 1981) comb. nov. *Microbiol. Immunol.* **36:**1251–1275.

Yamamoto, S., and S. Harayama. 1995. PCR amplification and direct sequencing of *gyrB* genes with universal primers and their application to the detection and taxonomic analysis of *Pseudomonas putida* strains. *Appl. Environ. Microbiol.* **61:**1104–1109.

Section II

METABOLISM OF HYDROCARBONS AND CHLORINATED HYDROCARBONS

Molecular Biology of Pseudomonads
Edited by T. Nakazawa et al.

Chapter 4

Effects of Two-Liquid-Phase Systems and Expression of *alk* Genes on the Physiology of Alkane-Oxidizing Strains

Jan B. van Beilen, Marcel Wubbolts, Qi Chen, Maarten Nieboer, and Bernard Witholt

Bacterial oxygenases involved in the biotransformation of apolar compounds have industrial potential because they catalyze the regio- and stereoselective introduction of oxygen into unactivated organic substrates, a reaction that by classical synthetic chemistry remains difficult.

Pseudomonas oleovorans GPo1 (TF4-1L, ATCC 29347) (Schwartz and McCoy, 1973) is able to grow on medium-chain-length *n*-alkanes by virtue of the alkane hydroxylase system. Modification of the alkane oxidation pathway allows us to develop practical biosynthetic pathways for the synthesis of potentially interesting industrial synthons such as alkanols, aldehydes, carboxylic acids, and epoxides. This approach is beginning to be explored by several industries for the production of aromatic alcohols and other fine chemicals by using the *P. oleovorans* alkane-oxidizing system or the related xylene monooxygenase of *Pseudomonas putida* mt-2, as illustrated by Table 1.

To be able to apply such enzyme systems, it is necessary to develop appropriate bioconversion systems, suitable host strains, bioreactor systems, and downstream processing. Because the substrates for these enzyme systems are very hydrophobic and toxic, two-liquid-phase media are an interesting option for protecting cells from substrate-educt or for continuously extracting educt. This option does, however, produce new challenges in reactor design, operation, and safety, while the interaction of microorganisms with a second organic phase is largely unknown territory and warrants the study of cell physiology in two-liquid-phase systems.

THE *P. OLEOVORANS* ALKANE OXIDATION SYSTEM

Baptist et al. (1963) reported the isolation of a *P. oleovorans* strain able to grow directly on *n*-hexane. The strain was later classified as *P. putida* biotype A (Stanier et al.,

Jan B. van Beilen, Marcel Wubbolts, Qi Chen, Maarten Nieboer, and Bernard Witholt • Institute of Biotechnology, Swiss Federal Institute of Technology, ETH-Hoenggerberg, 8093 Zürich, Switzerland.

Table 1. Patented bioconversion routes that make use of *P. oleovorans, P. putida* mt-2, or recombinants thereof

Product or process	Company	Reference[a]
4-(2-Methoxyethyl)phenylglycidyl ethers	Gist-brocades/Shell	1
1-Amino-3-aryloxy-2-propanol beta blockers	Gist-brocades/Shell	2
4-Epoxypropoxy-phenylacetate esters	Gist-brocades/Shell	3
Terminal hydroxyl or epoxy group formation	Groningen University	4
α-Aryl and α-alkyl sulfoxide production	Idemitsu	5
Resolution of optically active *sec* alcohols	Idemitsu	6
Methyl group oxidation on aromatic heterocycles	Lonza A.G.	7
Ethyl group oxidation on aromatic heterocycles	Lonza A.G.	8

[a] 1, European patent 193 228, September, 1986; 2, European patent 193 227, September, 1986; 3, European patent 256 586, February, 1988; 4, European patent 277 674, August, 1988, and U.S. patent 5,173,428, August, 1992; 5, Japanese patent J61195694, August, 1986; 6, Japanese patent J01257484, October, 1989; 7, European patent 477 828, April, 1992; 8, European patent 466 115, January, 1992, and European patent 502 524, September, 1992.

1966) but distinguishes itself from other *P. putida* strains by the presence of the OCT plasmid, which encodes the alkane hydroxylase system and other proteins involved in alkane oxidation (Chakrabarty, 1973). Over the past three decades, this particular strain (ATCC 29347; named GPo1 in our laboratory) has been investigated in great detail with respect to the enzymology and genetics of alkane oxidation.

The alkane hydroxylase system (Peterson et al., 1966) consists of three components: a 46-kDa hydroxylase, a 19-kDa rubredoxin, and a 48-kDa rubredoxin reductase. The hydroxylase is an integral cytoplasmic membrane protein (Kok et al., 1989b) that contains nonheme iron and requires phospholipids for activity (Ruettinger et al., 1977). It transfers one oxygen atom from molecular oxygen to the substrate (McKenna and Coon, 1970). The other oxygen atom is reduced with electrons supplied by the NADH-dependent rubredoxin reductase (AlkT) (Eggink et al., 1990; Ueda and Coon, 1973a) via the electron carrier rubredoxin (AlkG) (Kok et al., 1989a; Peterson and Coon, 1968).

Work carried out by our group on the genetics of alkane oxidation by *P. oleovorans* has resulted in the model described below and reviewed elsewhere by van Beilen et al. (1994b) (Fig. 1). Two gene regions located on the OCT plasmid, the *alkBFGHJKL* operon and the *alkST* region, encode all the proteins necessary to convert alkanes to fatty acids. The *alkB, alkG*, and *alkT* genes encode the three components of the alkane hydroxylase system: membrane-bound monooxygenase, rubredoxin, and rubredoxin reductase, respectively. The *alkH* gene encodes an NADH-dependent aldehyde dehydrogenase. The alcohol dehydrogenase AlkJ is related to a number of oxidases and soluble cofactor-independent dehydrogenases that are probably linked to the electron transfer chain. AlkK was found to be homologous to several acyl-coenzyme A synthetases, and subsequent studies showed that the *alkK* gene can replace the *fadD* gene of *Escherichia coli*, which encodes an acyl-coenzyme A synthetase. The functions of AlkF and AlkL are not known. All components except alkane hydroxylase, rubredoxin, and the regulator AlkS have equivalents encoded by the chromosomes of *E. coli* and *P. putida*.

The importance of the *P. oleovorans* alkane hydroxylase system and related enzymes in, for example, the degradation of oil is illustrated by the fact that a significant portion (up to 40%) of the naturally occurring hydrocarbon-degrading bacterial populations found

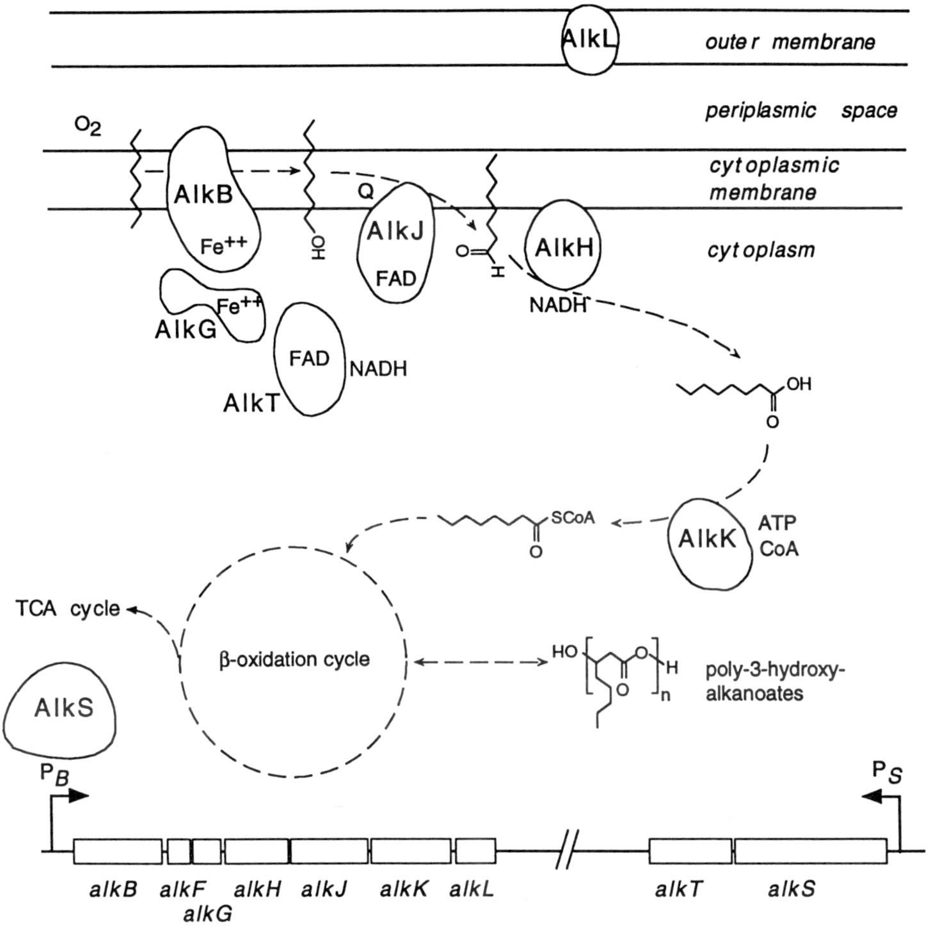

Figure 1. Molecular genetics and pathways of alkane oxidation by *P. oleovorans*. The *alk*-genes are organized in two clusters: the *alkST* locus and the *alkBFGHJKL* operon, both located on the OCT plasmid. Proteins are identified by their gene names. AlkB, alkane hydroxylase; AlkG, rubredoxin; AlkT, rubredoxin reductase; AlkJ, alcohol dehydrogenase; AlkH, aldehyde dehydrogenase; AlkK, acyl-coenzyme A (CoA) synthetase; AlkL, outer membrane protein; AlkS, regulatory protein. TCA, tricarboxylic acid. The *alkF* gene encodes a nonfunctional rubredoxin.

in oil-contaminated areas contains the *alkB* gene (Sotsky et al., 1994). In fact, other bacteria that are able to grow on *n*-alkanes have been isolated and to some extent characterized (van Beilen et al., 1994b), and the available literature indicates that at least some of these strains contain alkane-oxidizing enzyme systems that are similar to the *P. oleovorans* system (Hammer and Liemann, 1976; Kusunose et al., 1967; Van Eyk and Bartels, 1970; Vandecasteele et al., 1983).

With respect to the reaction mechanism of alkane hydroxylase, Fu et al. (1991) used the hypersensitive radical probe *trans*-2-phenyl-1-methylcyclopropane to show that oxidation by alkane hydroxylase proceeds through a nonconcerted radical process: the compound is oxidized to 1-phenyl-3-buten-1-ol, which suggests a relatively stable radi-

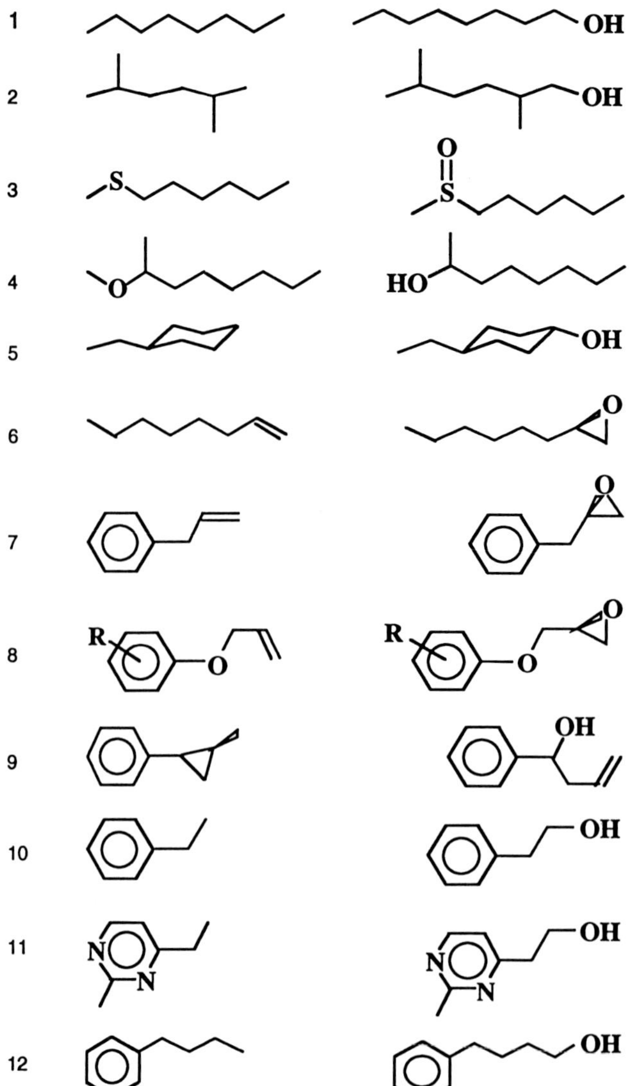

Figure 2. Oxidation reactions catalyzed by the *P. oleovorans* alkane hydroxylase system. References: reaction 1, Baptist et al. (1963); reactions 2, 5, 10, and 12, van Beilen et al. (1994a); reactions 3 and 4, Katopodis et al. (1988); reaction 6, May and Abbott (1972); reaction 7, de Smet et al. (1983); reactions 8 and 9, Fu et al. (1991); reaction 11, Kiener and Zimmermann (1992).

cal intermediate (Fig. 2, reaction 9). The reaction probably involves as oxidizing agent a nonheme iron (V)-oxo species like that proposed for heme-containing monooxygenases (Ortiz de Montellano, 1986). In fact, all reactions mentioned above are also characteristic of heme-containing monooxygenases (see references in Fu et al., 1991).

REGIO- AND STEREOSPECIFIC OXIDATIONS USING THE ALKANE HYDROXYLASE SYSTEM

Besides the hydroxylation of aliphatic and alicyclic compounds (McKenna and Coon, 1970), the alkane hydroxylase system also catalyzes the oxidation of terminal alcohols to their corresponding aldehydes, the demethylation of branched methyl ethers, the sulfoxidation of thioethers, and the epoxidation of terminal olefins (de Smet et al., 1981; Katopodis et al., 1988; Katopodis et al., 1984; May and Abbott, 1972; May and Katopodis, 1986) (Fig. 2).

Several studies have hinted at the utility of the alkane hydroxylase system in the production of fine chemicals such as fatty acids, alcohols, and epoxides (Bosetti et al., 1992; Favre-Bulle et al., 1991; May and Abbott, 1972; Schwartz, 1973; Witholt et al., 1990). The most interesting reaction is the oxidation of compounds with terminal double bonds to the corresponding (*R*)-epoxide with high enantiomeric excess (de Smet et al., 1983; Fu et al., 1991; Johnstone et al., 1986). In most of these studies, intact *P. oleovorans* GPo1 cells, which are well suited for the production of epoxides, were used. However, aliphatic alcohols produced by the alkane hydroxylase are rapidly metabolized because of the presence of active alcohol and aldehyde dehydrogenases in a *P. oleovorans* (Lageveen, 1986). Therefore, Bosetti et al. (1992) introduced plasmid pGEc41, which encodes the alkane hydroxylase system but lacks the alcohol dehydrogenase gene *alkJ* that is part of the *alk* system (Eggink et al., 1987a, 1987b), into *P. putida* PpS81, which lacks the chromosome-encoded medium-chain-length alcohol dehydrogenase activity (AlcA) (Grund et al., 1975), and used this recombinant (PpS8141) to synthesize and accumulate 1-alkanols from linear alkanes.

Using the same recombinant *P. putida* strain, we investigated the in vivo conversion rates of a large number of linear, branched, and cyclic alkanes and alkylbenzenes (van Beilen et al., 1994a). Essentially, substrates are not hydroxylated when a tertiary carbon is present. Substituted cyclic alkanes are oxidized with high stereoselectivity at the 4-*trans* position of the ring relative to the substituents but not at the methyl or ethyl substituents (Fig. 2, reaction 5). Several alkylbenzenes, such as ethylbenzene and its 3- and 4-substituted derivatives, are oxidized at rates close to or superior to the rate for *n*-nonane. A similar reaction, the oxidation of ethyl-substituted five- or six-membered heterocyclic rings, e.g., 5-ethyl-2-methylpyrimidine to 5-hydroxyethyl-2-methylpyrimidine (Fig. 2, reaction 11), was exploited by Kiener and Zimmermann (1992) for the production of synthons for new antibiotics.

Unfortunately, it has not been possible to use *P. oleovorans* for the production of fatty acids, because it utilizes these products as carbon and energy sources, and we have not yet been able to find mutants that are blocked in the β-oxidation pathway. However, we have established that when the *alk* genes are cloned in *E. coli*, the recombinant can carry out the same oxidation reactions. Since the β-oxidation system of *E. coli* is not derepressed by medium-chain-length fatty acids (Overath et al., 1969), *E. coli* recombinants can be used to accumulate these fatty acids. One of the limitations of *E. coli* in two-liquid-phase fermentation systems is that *E. coli* is more sensitive to bulk organic phases. *E. coli* cells are fully viable in the exponential growth phase but lose viability and alkane hydroxylase activity in the stationary phase (Favre-Bulle et al., 1991).

An important factor is the particular host strain used. *E. coli* W3110, which expresses the alkane hydroxylase system to very high levels, was too unstable to be used for continuous production of fatty acids; in contrast, *E. coli* HB101 was perfectly able to maintain plasmid and enzyme activities over periods of more that 1 week (Favre-Bulle et al., 1993).

PHYSIOLOGICAL CHANGES IN *P. OLEOVORANS* AND *E. COLI* IN RESPONSE TO OCTANE

In the studies discussed above, the physiology of the wild-type and recombinant strains in two-liquid phases plays an important role. Electron microscopy studies of *E. coli* and *P. oleovorans* have shown that changes in membrane ultrastructure occur when cells are grown in two-liquid-phase media. Nevertheless, growing cells are relatively immune to the effects of the apolar phase and remain fully viable. Stationary-phase cells show increased damage that is due to exposure to an apolar phase (Preusting et al., 1991), and in *E. coli*, the damage results in a loss of viability and enzyme activity (Favre-Bulle et al., 1991). This problem can be approached by ensuring that cells remain metabolically active, e.g., by maintaining them in continuous cultures. In addition, the expression of the *alk* genes influences the host cell, a fact demonstrated by the genetic instability of many recombinants and the clear signs of stress that induced cells show.

The composition of the membrane lipid fatty acids of *P. oleovorans* grown on octane in continuous cultures shows clear differences from that of the same strain grown in aqueous media (Chen et al., 1995a). These changes include the twofold increase in the unsaturated fatty acid $C_{18:1}$ and the synthesis of *trans*-unsaturated fatty acids (Fig. 3a and 3d), which are not found in most bacteria, including *E. coli*. Changes in the membrane lipid fatty acid composition lead to a decrease in membrane lipid fluidity, as shown by differential scanning calorimetry measurements. The transition temperature of membrane lipids isolated from citrate-grown cells is about 6°C, while the lipid transition temperature of octane-grown cells increases from 24 to 30°C as the growth rate increases (Chen et al., 1995b).

No changes were found in the membrane lipid fatty acid composition when *P. oleovorans* GPo12, a variant of GPo1 cured of the OCT plasmid, was grown in the presence or absence of octane, indicating that octane has no direct effect on membrane composition. However, when recombinant strain GPo12(pGEc47) carrying the *alk* genes

Figure 3. Model for the modification of fatty acid composition during growth of *P. oleovorans* on octane. Changes in fatty acid composition from the standard fatty acid profile observed for citrate-grown cells (a) to the octane-induced profile obtained during growth on octane (d) occur via two different processes: (i) 1-octanol activates the isomerization of *cis*- to *trans*-unsaturated fatty acids by a periplasmic isomerase (I), thus increasing the amount of *trans*-unsaturated fatty acids and resulting in the 1-octanol-induced profile (b); or (ii) induction of the *alk* genes results in insertion of AlkB into the cytoplasmic membrane, which affects fatty acid synthesis and the modification machinery (II), lengthening the mean acyl chain by increasing fatty acid $C_{18:1}$ twofold and resulting in the AlkB-induced profile (c). Growth on octane induces the *alk* genes. This results in the insertion of AlkB and the activation of system II. It also results in a complete alkane hydroxylase (AlkB, AlkG, and AlkT) and production of 1-octanol, which activates isomerase I. The activation of systems I and II leads to the octane-induced fatty acid profile. PP, periplasm; CM, cytoplasmic membrane; CP, cytoplasm; 16:0, hexadecanoic acid; 16:1, 9-hexadecenoic acid;18:1, 11-octadecenoic acid.

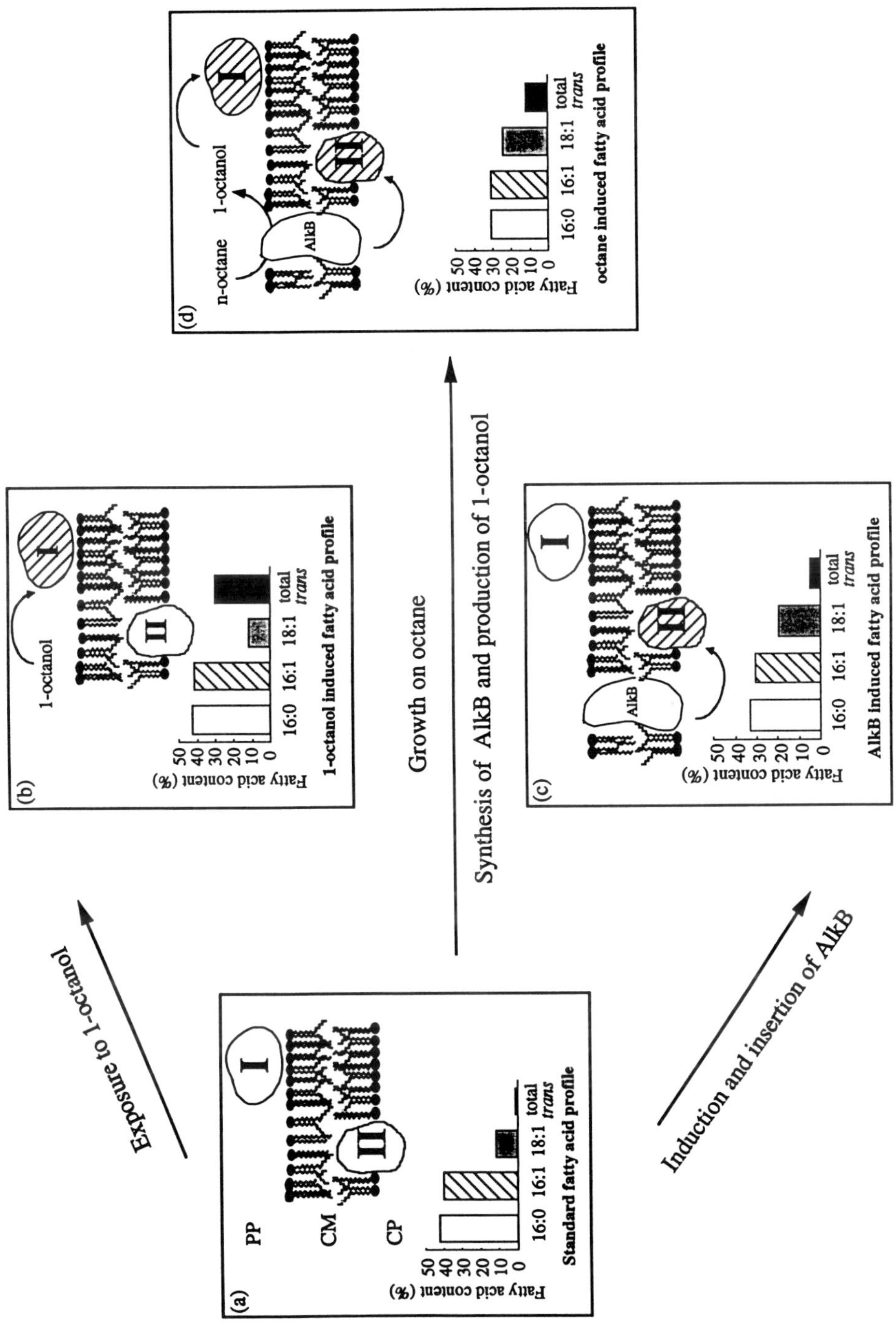
(a)
PP
CM
CP
I
II
Fatty acid content (%)
50
40
30
20
10
0
16:0 16:1 18:1 total trans
Standard fatty acid profile
Exposure to 1-octanol
Induction and insertion of AlkB
(b)
1-octanol
I
II
Fatty acid content (%)
16:0 16:1 18:1 total trans
1-octanol induced fatty acid profile
Growth on octane
Synthesis of AlkB and production of 1-octanol
(c)
I
AlkB
II
Fatty acid content (%)
16:0 16:1 18:1 total trans
AlkB induced fatty acid profile
(d)
n-octane 1-octanol
AlkB
I
II
Fatty acid content (%)
16:0 16:1 18:1 total trans
octane induced fatty acid profile

from the OCT plasmid was grown on octane, it showed the same changes in fatty acid composition as were found for GPo1, indicating that these changes result from induction and expression of the *alk* genes (Fig. 3d).

During growth of GPo1 on octane, the cell produces 35,000 copies of AlkB per cell, an amount that represents 25 to 30% of total cytoplasmic membrane protein. Insertion of large amounts of AlkB into the cytoplasmic membrane might produce the observed fatty acid modifications. This possibility was tested by using an *alkB* gene delection derivative of pGEc47 and the gratuitous inducer dicyclopropylketone, which is not oxidized by the enzyme system. Growth studies showed that induction of AlkB leads to an increase in $C_{18:1}$ but not in the synthesis of *trans*-unsaturated fatty acids (Fig. 3c).

We also examined the effects of octane oxidation products on the fatty acid profile. We found that the *cis*-unsaturated fatty acids were converted to their *trans* isomers after exposure of GPo12 to 1-octanol, which formed during growth of *P. oleovorans* on octane, although the overal fatty acid composition of GPo12, such as the ratio of saturated to unsaturated fatty acids and the mean acyl chain length, remained unchanged (Fig. 3b). Since membrane lipids containing *trans*-unsaturated fatty acids have a higher lipid transition temperature (or lower membrane fluidity) than those containing the *cis* isomers (Cronan and Edward, 1975), a decrease in membrane fluidity due to the synthesis of *trans*-unsaturated fatty acids (Chen et al., 1995b) may compensate for the increase in membrane fluidity caused by 1-octanol. Recently, it was shown that the resistance of several *Pseudomonas* strains to toxic organic solvents such as phenolic compounds (Heipieper et al., 1992), toluene, styrene (Heipieper et al., 1994), and shorter *n*-alkanes ($C \leq 7$) (our unpublished observations) is also accompanied by isomerization of *cis*-unsaturated fatty acids to their *trans* isomers. Thus, formation of the *trans*-unsaturated fatty acids appears to play an important role in the growth of *Pseudomonas* strains in the presence of organic solvents.

In continuous cultures of *P. oleovorans* grown on octane, intracytoplasmic membrane structures have occasionally been observed (Preusting et al., 1991). Since in these cells the membrane protein alkane hydroxylase AlkB is synthesized in large quantities, accounting for 1.5 to 2% of the total cell protein (Eggink et al., 1987a), insertion of AlkB into the cytoplasmic membrane might play a role in the phenomenon. The same phenomenon could be reproduced in *E. coli*: introduction of pGEc47, a broad-host-range

Figure 4. Effects of the expression of alkane hydroxylase on membranes of *E. coli* recombinants. Recombinants were induced in early exponential phase by the addition of dicyclopropylketone (0.05%, vol/vol). Stationary-phase cells were examined. (A) Coomassie blue-stained SDS-polyacrylamide gel showing protein contents of the low-density membrane fraction (lane 1) and the cytoplasmic membrane fraction (lane 2) of induced W3110(pGEc47). The position of AlkB is indicated by an arrow. (B) Freeze-fracture electron micrograph showing vesicles (indicated by arrows) in induced W3110(pGEc47). (C) Sucrose density centrifugation of total membranes of induced W3110(pGEc47) (●) and induced W3110(pGEc47ΔB), the negative control (○). Cells were disrupted by French pressing, and total membranes were isolated. The absorbance at 280 nm (A_{280}) is plotted as a function of the buoyant density. The positions of the low-density membrane fraction (LDF), the cytoplasmic membrane fraction (CM), and the outer membrane fraction (OM) are indicated. (D) Fatty acid profiles of uninduced (□) and induced (■) W3110(pGEc47). The concentrations of individual fatty acids are given as molar percentages of total fatty acid. $C_{12:0}$, dodecanoic acid; $C_{14:0}$, tetradecanoic acid; $C_{16:1}$, 9-hexadecenoic acid; $C_{16:0}$, hexadecanoic acid; $C_{17:0}$ cyc, 9,10-methylenehexadecanoic acid; $C_{18:0}$, octadecanoic acid; $C_{19:0}$ cyc, 11,12-methyleneoctadecanoic acid.

vector which contains the *alk* genes, into *E. coli* DH-1 led to the same level of AlkB as had been found in the original host strain, while *E. coli* W3110 accumulated AlkB to levels corresponding to 10 to 15% of total cell protein. In both strains, this accumulation resulted in the formation of intracytoplasmic vesicles or membrane structures (Fig. 4B) (Nieboer et al., 1993).

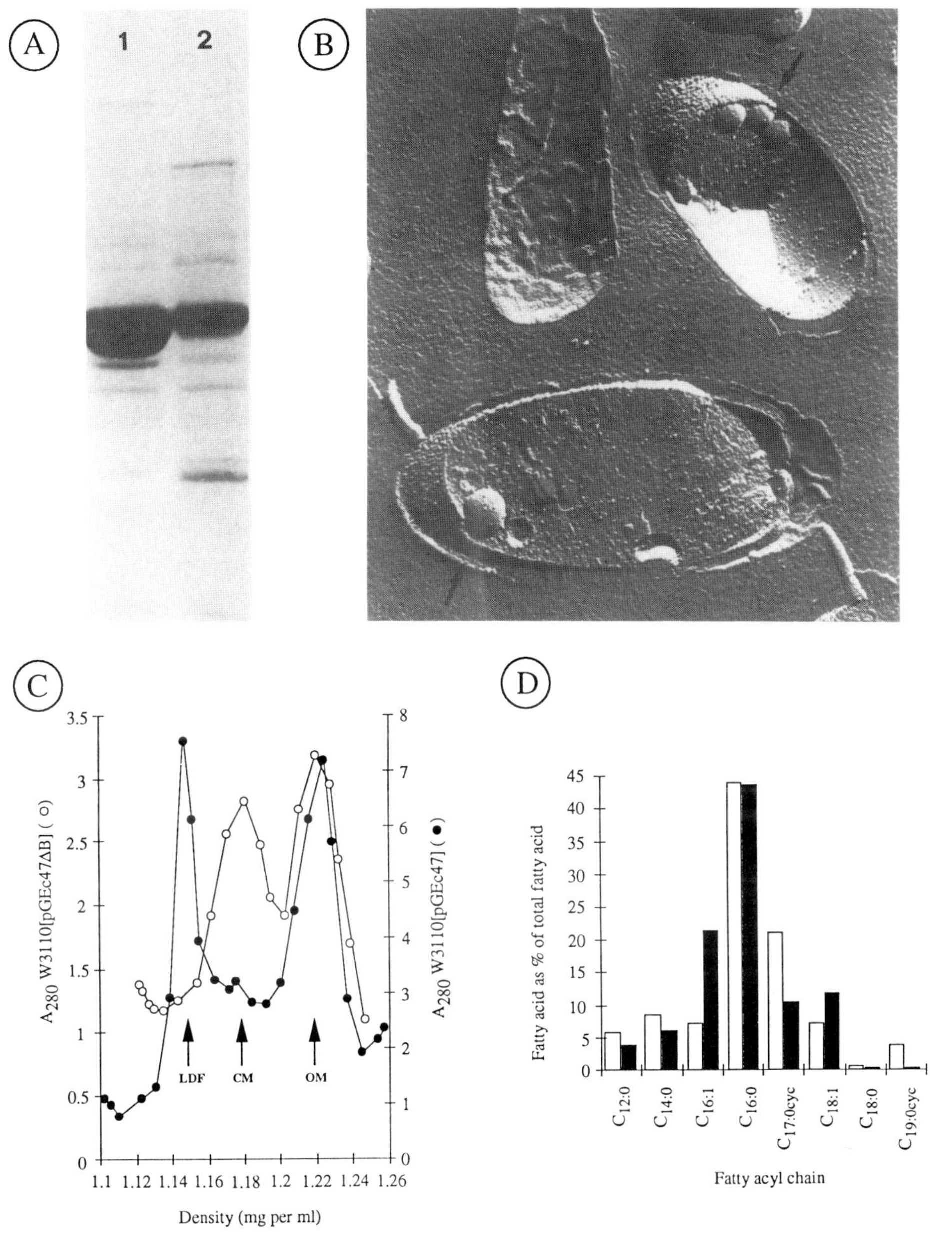

The intracytoplasmic membrane structures could be separated from the cytoplasmic membrane by continuous sucrose density centrifugation. They appeared as a distinct, low-density membrane fraction (Fig. 4C) highly enriched in AlkB (Fig. 4A), as shown by sodium dodecyl sulfate (SDS)-polyacrylamide gel electrophoresis and alkane hydroxylase activity measurements.

Overexpression of AlkB also had clear effects on phospholipid metabolism. Induced *E. coli* W3110(pGEc47) had a two- to threefold-increased phospholipid content and a shift in fatty acid composition toward unsaturated fatty acids (Fig. 4D). The major changes occurred in the unsaturated fatty acids $C_{16:1}$ and $C_{18:1}$, which increased at the expense of $C_{17:0}$ cyc and $C_{19:0}$ cyc.

On the basis of the findings given above, we proposed a model for the effects of octane on *P. oleovorans* and *E. coli* during growth of the cells on octane (Fig. 3) (Chen et al., 1995a). First, AlkB is produced and inserted into the cytoplasmic membrane as a result of induction of the *alk* genes with octane. This insertion activates fatty acid synthesis and its modifying enzymes (system II), which result in an increase in fatty acid $C_{18:1}$ content (Fig. 3a). In *E. coli*, this increase takes place at the expense of the cyclopropane fatty acids (Fig. 4D). At the same time, other *alk* genes are also induced, and octane is oxidized to 1-octanol by the alkane hydroxylase system. Exposure of *P. oleovorans* cells to 1-octanol activates a new isomerase (system I) located in the periplasm (our unpublished results) and catalyzes isomerization of *cis*- to *trans*-unsaturated fatty acids. The combination of these two effects results in the "octane-induced" fatty acid profile (Fig. 3d) seen for *P. oleovorans* grown on octane.

PERSPECTIVES

Wild-type *P. oleovorans* as well as recombinants of *Pseudomonas* spp. and *E. coli* have been applied in continuous and high-cell-density fed batch cultures for the production of both low-molecular-weight compounds (Bosetti et al., 1992; Favre-Bulle et al., 1991; Favre Bulle et al., 1993; Favre-Bulle and Witholt, 1992; Witholt et al., 1990) and poly-(3)-hydroxyalkanoates (Preusting et al., 1993a; Preusting et al., 1993b).

Both in optimized poly-(3)-hydroxyalkanoate production by *P. oleovorans* and in octanoate production by *E. coli* HB101(pGEc47), volumetric productivities equivalent to 4 to 5 tons/year/m^3 of reactor volume were achieved. Reported productivities for industrial continuous bioprocesses range from 1.4 tons/m^3/year for penicillin to 88 tons/m^3/year for gluconic acid, while the average productivity for bulk chemicals like citric acid and lactic acid is around 22 tons/m^3/year (Heijnen et al., 1992). Therefore, the reported productivities for the *alk* system are already in the range of several existing biological production processes. On the other hand, the reported productivity for 1,2-epoxyoctane from 1-octene is equivalent to only 0.75 tons/m^3/year (de Smet et al., 1983) and will have to be improved.

A better knowledge of the effects of *alk* gene expression and growth of bacteria in two-liquid-phase fermentations will help us to identify problems and improve performance. Most recombinants show genetic instability, especially when the *alk* genes are used for cometabolic oxidations. The effects of AlkB expression on cell metabolism indicate that an increase in expression, or biocatalyst activity, must be balanced against the toxic effects of overexpression by choosing the appropriate host or cultivation conditions. An example is *E. coli* HB101(pGEc47), which appears to be quite stable, even in the absence of direct selection for maintenance of the *alk* genes, because it expresses the *alk* genes to levels that are not toxic to the cell.

REFERENCES

Baptist, J. N., R. K. Gholson, and M. J. Coon. 1963. Hydrocarbon oxidation by a bacterial enzyme system. I. Products of octane oxidation. *Biochim. Biophys. Acta* **69:**40–47.

Bosetti, A., J. B. van Beilen, H. Preusting, R. G. Lageveen, and B. Witholt. 1992. Production of primary aliphatic alcohols with a recombinant *Pseudomonas* strain, encoding the alkane hydroxylase enzyme system. *Enzyme Microb. Technol.* **14**:702–708.

Chakrabarty, A. M. 1973. Genetic fusion of incompatible plasmids in *Pseudomonas. Proc. Natl. Acad. Sci. USA* **70:**1641–1644.

Chen, Q., D. B. Janssen, and B. Witholt. 1995a. Growth on octane alters the membrane lipid fatty acids of *Pseudomonas oleovorans* due to the induction of *alkB* and synthesis of octanol. *J. Bacteriol.* **177**:6894–6901.

Chen, Q., A. Nijenhuis, H. Preusting, J. Dolfing, D. B. Janssen, and B. Witholt. 1995b. Effects of octane on the fatty acid composition and transition temperature of *Pseudomonas oleovorans* membrane lipids during growth in liquid phase continuous culture. *Enzyme Microb. Technol.* **17**:647–652.

Cronan, J. E., Jr., and E. P. Gelmann. 1975. Physical properties of membrane lipids; biological relevance and regulation. *Bacteriol. Rev.* **39**:232–256.

de Smet, M.-J., J. Kingma, H. Wynberg, and B. Witholt. 1983. *Pseudomonas oleovorans* as a tool in bioconversions of hydrocarbons: growth, morphology and conversion characteristics in different two-phase systems. *Enzyme Microb. Technol.* **5**:352–360.

de Smet, M.-J., B. Witholt, and H. Wijnberg. 1981. Practical approach to high yield enzymatic stereospecific organic synthesis in multiphase systems. *J. Org. Chem.* **46**:3128–3131.

Eggink, G., H. Engel, G. Vriend, P. Terpstra, and B. Witholt. 1990. Rubredoxin reductase of *Pseudomonas oleovorans*. Structural relationship to other flavoprotein oxidoreductases based on one NAD and two FAD fingerprints. *J. Mol. Biol.* **212:**135–142.

Eggink, G., R. G. Lageveen, B. Altenburg, and B. Witholt. 1987a. Controlled and functional expression of *Pseudomonas oleovorans* alkane utilizing system in *Pseudomonas putida* and *Escherichia coli. J. Biol. Chem.* **262:**17712–17718.

Eggink, G., P. H. van Lelyveld, A. Arnberg, N. Arfman, C. Witteveen, and B. Witholt. 1987b. Structure of the *Pseudomonas putida alkBAC* operon. Identification of transcription and translation products. *J. Biol. Chem.* **262**:6400–6406.

Favre-Bulle, O., T. Schouten, J. Kingma, and B. Witholt. 1991. Bioconversion of n-octane to octanoic acid by a recombinant *Escherichia coli* cultured in a two-liquid phase bioreactor. *Bio/Technology* **9**:367–371.

Favre-Bulle, O., E. Weenink, T. Vos, H. Preusting, and B. Witholt. 1993. Continuous bioconversion of n-octane to octanoic acid by recombinant *Escherichia coli* (alk+) growing in a two-liquid-phase chemostat. *Biotechnol. Bioeng.* **41:**263–272.

Favre-Bulle, O., and B. Witholt. 1992. Biooxidation of n-octane by a recombinant *Escherichia coli* in a two-liquid phase system: effects of medium components on cell growth and alkane oxidation activity. *Enzyme Microb. Technol.* **14**:931–937.

Fu, H., M. Newcomb, and C. H. Wong. 1991. *Pseudomonas oleovorans* monooxygenase catalyzed asymmetric epoxidation of allyl alcohol derivatives and hydroxylation of a hypersensitive radical probe with the radical ring opening state exceeding the oxygen rebound state. *J. Am. Chem. Soc.* **113**:5878–5880.

Grund, A., J. Shapiro, M. Fennewald, P. Bacha, J. Leahy, K. Markbreiter, M. Nieder, and M. Toepfer. 1975. Regulation of alkane oxidation in *Pseudomonas putida. J. Bacteriol.* **123:**546–556.

Hammer, K. D., and F. Liemann. 1976. Primäre Oxydationsmechanismen beim Abbau aliphatischer Kohlenwasserstoffe durch bakterielle Enzymsysteme. *Zentralbl. Bakteriol. Hyg. I Abt. Orig. B* **162**:169–179.

Heijnen, J. J., J. Terwischa van Scheltinga, and A. J. Straathof. 1992. Fundamental bottlenecks in the application of continuous bioprocesses. *J. Biotechnol.* **22**:3–20.

Heipieper, H.-J., R. Diefenbach, and H. Keweloh. 1992. Conversion of *cis* unsaturated fatty acids to *trans*, a possible mechanism for the protection of phenol-degrading *Pseudomonas putida* P8 from substrate toxicity. *Appl. Environ. Microbiol.* **58:**1847–1852.

Heipieper, H.-J., F. J. Weber, J. Sikkema, H. Keweloh, and J. A. M. de Bont. 1994. Mechanism of resistance of whole cells to toxic organic solvents. *Trends Biotechnol.* **12:**409–415.

Johnstone, S. L., G. T. Phillips, B. W. Robertson, P. D. Watts, M. A. Bertola, H. S. Koger, and A. F. Marx. 1986. Stereoselective synthesis of S-(-)-β-blockers via microbially produced epoxide intermediates, p. 387–392. *In* C. Laane, J. Tramper, and M. D. Lilly (ed.), *Biocatalysis in Organic Media.* Elsevier, Amsterdam.

Katopodis, A. G., H. A. Smith, and S. W. May. 1988. New oxyfunctionalization capabilities for ω-hydroxylases: asymmetric aliphatic sulfoxidation and branched ether demethylation. *J. Am. Chem. Soc.* **110**:897–899.

Katopodis, A. G., K. Wimalasena, J. Lee, and S. W. May. 1984. Mechanistic studies on non-heme iron monooxygenase catalysis: epoxidation, aldehyde formation, and demethylation by the ω-hydroxylation system of *Pseudomonas oleovorans. J. Am. Chem. Soc.* **106**:7928–7935.

Kiener, A., and T. Zimmermann. April, 1992. Mikrobiologisches Verfahren zur terminalen Hydroxylierung von Ethylgruppen an aromatischen 5-oder 6 Ring-Heterocyclen. European patent 502 524 A1.

Kok, M., R. Oldenhuis, M. P. G. van der Linden, C. H. C. Meulenberg, J. Kingma, and B. Witholt. 1989a. The *Pseudomonas oleovorans alkBAC* operon encodes two structurally related rubredoxins and an aldehyde dehydrogenase. *J. Biol. Chem.* **264:**5442–5451.

Kok, M., R. Oldenhuis, M. P. G. van der Linden, P. Raatjes, J. Kingma, P. H. van Lelyveld, and B. Witholt. 1989b. The *Pseudomonas oleovorans* alkane hydroxylase gene. Sequence and expression. *J. Biol. Chem.* **264:**5435–5441.

Kusunose, M., J. Matsumoto, K. Ichihara, E. Kusunose, and J. Nozaka. 1967. Requirement for three proteins for hydrocarbon oxidation. *J. Biochem.* **61:**665–667.

Lageveen, R. G. 1986. Ph.D. thesis. University of Groningen, Groningen, The Netherlands.

May, S. W., and B. J. Abbott. 1972. Enzymatic epoxidation. I. Alkane expoxidation by the ω-hydroxylation system of *Pseudomonas oleovorans. Biochem. Biophys. Res. Commun.* **48:**1230–1234.

May, S. W., and A. G. Katopodis. 1986. Oxygenation of alcohol and sulphide substrates by a prototypical nonhaem iron monooxygenase: catalysis and biotechnological potential. *Enzyme Microb. Technol.* **8:**17–21.

McKenna, E. J., and M. J. Coon. 1970. Enzymatic ω-oxidation. IV. Purification and properties of the ω-hydroxylase of *Pseudomonas oleovorans. J. Biol. Chem.* **245:**3882–3889.

Nieboer, M., J. Kingma, and B. Witholt. 1993. The alkane oxidation system of *Pseudomonas oleovorans:* induction of the *alk*-genes in *Escherichia coli* W3110 affects membrane biogenesis and results in overexpression of alkane hydroxylase in a distinct cytoplasmic membrane subfraction. *Mol. Microbiol.* **8:**1039–1051.

Ortiz de Montellano, P. R. 1986. Oxygen activation and transfer, p. 217–271. *In* P. R. Ortiz de Montellano (ed.), *Cytochrome P450. Structure, Mechanism and Biochemistry.* Plenum Press, New York.

Overath, P., G. Pauli, and H. Schairer. 1969. Fatty acid degradation in *Escherichia coli.* An inducible acyl-CoA synthetase, mapping of old-mutations, and the isolation of regulatory mutants. *Eur. J. Biochem.* **7**:559–574.

Peterson, J. A., D. Basu, and M. J. Coon. 1966. Enzymatic ω-oxidation. I. Electron carriers in fatty acid and hydrocarbon hydroxylation. *J. Biol. Chem.* **241:**5162–5164.

Peterson, J. A., and M. J. Coon. 1968. Enzymatic ω-oxidation. III. Purification and properties of rubredoxin, a component of the ω-hydroxylation system of *Pseudomonas oleovorans. J. Biol. Chem.* **243:**329–334.

Preusting, H., W. Hazenberg, and B. Witholt. 1993a. Continuous production of poly(3-hydroxyalkanoates) by *Pseudomonas oleovorans* in a high-cell-density, two-liquid-phase chemostat. *Enzyme Microb. Technol.* **15:**311–316.

Preusting, H., J. Kingma, and B. Witholt. 1991. Physiology and polyester formation of *Pseudomonas oleovorans* in continuous two-liquid phase cultures. *Enzyme Microb. Technol.* **13:**770–780.

Preusting, H., R. van Houten, A. Hoefs, E. Kool van Langenberghe, O. Favre-Bulle, and B. Witholt. 1993b. High cell density cultivation of *Pseudomonas oleovorans*: growth and production of poly(3-hydroxyalkanoates) in two-liquid phase batch and fed-batch systems. *Biotechnol. Bioeng.* **41:**550–556.

Ruettinger, R. T., G. R. Griffith, and M. J. Coon. 1997. Characterization of the ω-hydroxylase of *Pseudomonas oleovorans* as a non-heme iron protein. *Arch. Biochem. Biophys.* **183:**528–537.

Schwartz, R. D. 1973. Octene epoxidation by a cold-stable alkane-oxidizing isolate of *Pseudomonas oleovorans. Appl. Microbiol.* **25:**574–577.

Schwartz, R. D., and C. J. McCoy. 1973. *Pseudomonas oleovorans* hydroxylation-epoxidation system: additional strain improvements. *Appl. Microbiol.* **26:**217–218.

Sotsky, J. B., C. W. Greer, and R. M. Atlas. 1994. Frequency of genes in aromatic and aliphatic biodegradation pathways within bacterial populations from Alaskan sediments. *Can. J. Microbiol.* **40:**981–985.

Stanier, R. Y., N. J. Palleroni, and M. Doudoroff. 1966. The aerobic Pseudomonads: a taxonomic study. *J. Gen. Microbiol.* **43:**159–271.

Ueda, T., and M. J. Coon. 1972. Enzymatic ω-oxidation. VII. Reduced diphosphopyridine nucleotide-rubredoxin reductase: properties and function as an electron carrier in ω-hydroxylation. *J. Biol. Chem.* **247:**5010–5016.

Van Beilen, J. B., J. Kingma, and B. Witholt. 1994a. Substrate specificity of the *Pseudomonas oleovorans* alkane hydroxylase. *Enzyme Microb. Technol.* **16:**161–174.

Van Beilen, J. B., M. G. Wubbolts, and B. Witholt. 1994b. Genetics of alkane oxidation by *Pseudomonas oleovorans. Biodegradation* **5:**161–174.

Vandecasteele, J. P., D. Blanchet, J. P. Tassin, A. M. Bonoamy, and L. Guerrillot. 1983. Enzymology of alkane degradation in *Pseudomonas aeruginosa. Acta Biotechnol.* **3:**339–344.

Van Eyk, J., and T. J. Bartels. 1970. Paraffin oxidation in *Pseudomonas aeruginosa*. II. Gross fractionation of the enzyme systme into soluble and particulate components. *J. Bacteriol.* **104:**1065–1073.

Witholt, B., M. J. de Smet, J. Kingma, J. B. van Beilen, M. Kok, R. G. Lageveen, and G. Eggink. 1990. Bioconversion of aliphatic compounds by *Pseudomonas oleovorans* in multiphase biorectors: background and economic potential. *Trends Biotechnol.* **8:**46–52.

Molecular Biology of Pseudomonads
Edited by T. Nakazawa et al.

Chapter 5

Alternative Pathways for Biodegradation of Alkyl and Alkenylbenzenes

Enrica Galli, Paola Barbieri, Fabrizio Beltrametti, Giovanni Bertoni, Giuseppina Bestetti, Fabrizio Bolognese, Patrizia Di Gennaro, and Elisabetta Zennaro

Benzene, toluene, xylenes, ethylbenzene, and styrene are among the 50 largest-volume industrial chemicals produced in the world. Each of these compounds is produced at a rate of millions of tons per year. They are widely used as fuels and solvents and provide starting materials for the production of resins, polymers, plastics, explosives, agrochemicals, and pharmaceuticals.

Because of their natural ubiquitous presence in the environment and their widespread release through industrial and agricultural activities, the biodegradation of these compounds has been widely studied, because this biodegradation can be considered not only a relevant part of the mineralization processes in nature but also the way through which synthetic pollutants can be removed from the environment (Galli, 1994).

In fact, knowledge of the degradative pathways of aromatic compounds has contributed greatly toward our understanding of xenobiotic biodegradation. It is well known that aromatic hydrocarbons and their substituted derivatives must be modified into *o*-diphenols through different peripheral reactions before ring cleavage can take place. The ability to perform these reactions is an important property of many bacteria, mainly those belonging to genus *Pseudomonas* which utilize aromatic substrates as the sole carbon source, since the main energy-yielding reactions occur only after ring fission. The introduction of one or more substituent groups onto the aromatic nucleus offers the possibility of alternative modes of microbial attack, which implies modification and/or removal of the substituent group before or after ring cleavage, depending on the chemical structure, the position of the substituent, and the selected microorganism (Smith, 1990).

Enrica Galli, Paola Barbieri, Fabrizio Beltrametti, Giuseppina Bestetti, Fabrizio Bolognese, and Patrizia Di Gennaro • Dipartimento di Genetica e di Biologia dei Microrganismi, via Celoria 26, 20133 Milan, Italy. ***Giovanni Bertoni*** • Centro Nacional de Biotecnologia, Campus de Cantoblanco, UAM 28049 Madrid, Spain. ***Elisabetta Zennaro*** • Dipartimento di Biologia Cellulare e dello Sviluppo, p.le A. Moro 5, 00185 Rome, Italy.

BIODEGRADATION OF ALKYLBENZENES

A group of aromatic compounds that usually occur together in gasoline and in diesel and jet fuels are the so-called BTX aromatics, consisting of benzene, its methylated homolog toluene, and the isomeric xylenes.

Several *Pseudomonas* strains have been isolated and described in regard to their abilities to degrade different monalkyl and dialkylbenzenes through alternative biodegradation pathways, namely (i) oxidative attack on the aromatic nucleus, which leads to the formation of alkylcatechols, which are the substrates for ring fission; or (ii) oxidation of the alkyl substituent(s), which leads to the formation of aromatic carboxylic acids, which are further oxidized to dihydroxylated ring fission substrates. Toluene, the simplest of the alkyl-substituted benzenes, is biodegraded by both ring attack and methyl group hydroxylation; five different pathways have been identified among members of the genus *Pseudomonas* (Gibson et al., 1970; Worsey and Williams, 1975; Shields et al., 1989; Whited and Gibson, 1991; Olsen et al., 1994).

The catabolism of dialkylbenzenes (xylenes) appears to be more restricted. The relative positions of the methyl groups on the aromatic ring affect the selection of microorganisms capable of utilizing xylenes through different initial reactions.

Several *Pseudomonas* strains can degrade *meta*- and *para*-xylene through the formation of methylbenzoates, but an alternative pathway that starts with direct hydroxylation of the aromatic ring has been demonstrated with a *Pseudomonas putida* strain and a *Nocardia corallina* strain (Galli et al., 1992). Among the three isomers of xylene, *o*-xylene appears to be the most recalcitrant to biodegradation. Thus far, only a few bacterial strains have been reported to grow on *o*-xylene, and no reports of a strain degrading all three isomers have appeared.

Pseudomonas stutzeri OX1 is able to grow on *o*-xylene and toluene but is unable to grow on *m*- and *p*-xylene (Baggi et al., 1987). *o*-Xylene and toluene are degraded through direct hydroxylation of the aromatic ring to give a mixture of 2,3-dimethylphenol and 3,4-dimethylphenol and a mixture of *o*-cresol, *m*-cresol, and *p*-cresol, respectively.

The enzyme involved in the first step of *o*-xylene and toluene degradation exhibited a broad substrate specificity, being able also to transform benzene, ethylbenzene, *m*-xylene, *p*-xylene, styrene, and naphthalene into their corresponding phenols. Further metabolism of *o*-xylene proceeds via the *meta* pathway. A 28-kb *Eco*RI DNA fragment, designated pFB3401, cloned from the *P. stutzeri* OX1 genomic bank allows *P. putida* PaW340 to convert *o*-xylene and toluene into the corresponding *meta* ring fission products (G. Bertoni, F. Bolognese, P. Barbieri, and E. Galli, unpublished data). In fact, exposure to *o*-xylene or to 2,3- and 3,4-dimethylphenol induced *P. stutzeri* cells to synthesize a catechol 2,3-dioxygenase and produce a semialdehyde-related compound whose spectral properties correspond to those of the 3,4-dimethylcatechol *meta*-cleavage product (Fig. 1). Subcloning and deletion analysis in the *Escherichia coli* vector pGEM-3Z allowed the genes for the conversion of *o*-xylene and toluene into the corresponding catechols to be mapped within a 6-kb region of the pFB3401 insert and made it possible to determine the direction of transcription. A 2-kb *Bam*HI-*Xho*I DNA fragment of the pFB3401 insert that confers the ability to synthesize a catechol 2,3-dioxygenase was also mapped (Fig. 2).

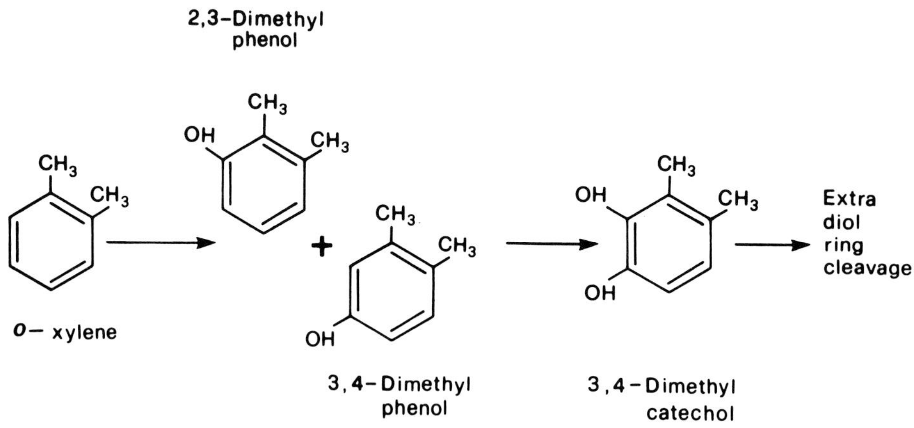

Figure 1. Proposed initial steps for the metabolism of *o*-xylene by *P. stutzeri* OX1 (Baggi et al., 1987).

P. stutzeri OX1 is unable to grow on *p*- and *m*-xylene, but it can use the corresponding methylbenzyl alcohols and toluates in a degradative pathway similar to that encoded by plasmid pWW0 of *P. putida* mt-2, suggesting that the inability to use *m*- and *p*-xylene as growth substrates is due to the fact that strain OX1 is not able to convert these two isomers into the corresponding benzylalcohols. The exposure to *m*- and *p*-xylene leads to a high lethality of the OX1 cells that is apparently caused by the toxic accumulation of 2,4- and 2,5-dimethylphenol. It was possible to isolate from *P. stutzeri* a spontaneous mutant, M1, that has been selected for the ability to grow on *m*- and *p*-xylene but has lost the ability to grow on *o*-xylene. The metabolism of *p*- and *m*-xylene proceeds through the oxidation of the methyl group to the corresponding alcohol (Barbieri et al., 1993).

A revertant strain, R1, was isolated capable of growth on all three isomers. This mutant seemed to have rescued all the metabolic activities of the wild-type OX1 strain while retaining the ability expressed in M1, but undetectable in OX1, to oxidize the methyl group of *m*- and *p*-xylene. R1 cultures degraded *o*-xylene through aromatic-ring hydroxylation to 2,3- and 3,4-dimethylphenol. During growth on *m*- and *p*-xylene, both alcohols and phenols were detected by high-pressure liquid chromatography analysis, but only the benzylalcohols were further metabolized to support growth (Fig. 3).

The growth patterns of R1 cells under different inducing conditions were measured and confirmed the metabolic data. Southern analysis performed on OX1, M1, and R1

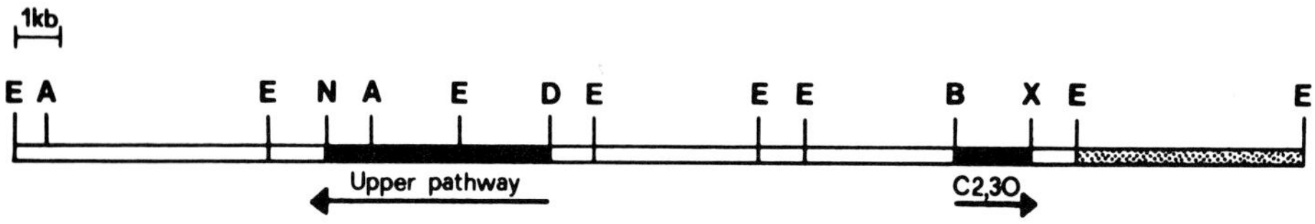

Figure 2. Restriction endonuclease map of a *P. stutzeri* OX1 chromosomal DNA fragment able to confer on *P. putida* PaW340 cells the ability to convert *o*-xylene and toluene into the corresponding *meta*-cleavage products. E, *Eco*RI; A, *Apa*I; N, *Not*I; D, *Dra*I; B, *Bam*HI; X, *Xho*I (Bertoni et al., unpublished data).

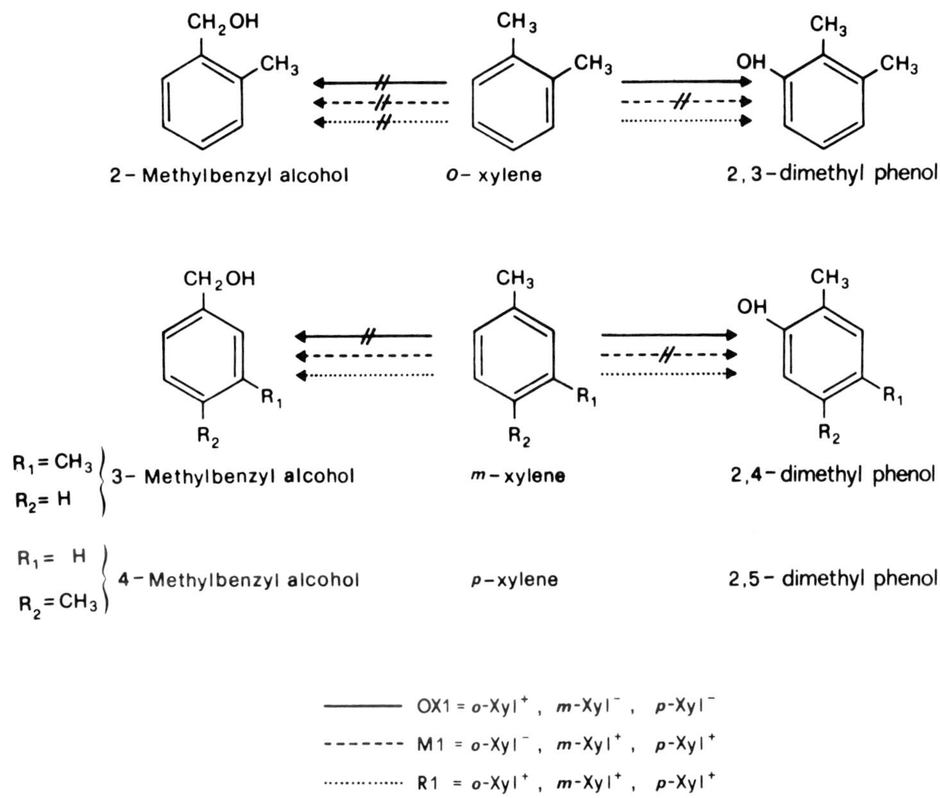

Figure 3. Alternative pathways for *o*-xylene or *m*- and *p*-xylene degradation in *P. stutzeri* OX1 and its mutants M1 and R1. The symbol // indicates an inability to carry out the biotransformation (Barbieri et al., 1993).

with two probes derived from the OX1 DNA fragment containing genes for the early degradative steps of *o*-xylene and from the pWW0 upper-pathway operon, respectively, allowed us to map on the chromosome of M1 the insertion of a 3-kb sequence of unknown origin in the region containing the sequences involved in *o*-xylene initial attack, thus explaining the loss of ability to grow on *o*-xylene. This insertion sequence is missing in the wild-type OX1 strain and in R1. On the other hand, strain OX1 showed an insertion of 3 kb in a region containing homologous sequences of the upper-pathway genes of *m*- and *p*-xylene degradation. This 3-kb sequence is apparently deleted in M1 and R1, both of which are able to grow on *m*- and *p*-xylene.

In conclusion, chromosomal rearrangements probably due to insertion-deletion of a 3-kb sequence lead to the activation of catabolic pathways that are preexisting but not functional, or to the extinction of other pathways that may be potentially suicidal under some conditions. Insofar as the introduction of one or more substituent groups onto a benzene ring leads to alternative modes of microbial attack, we may conclude that in strain R1, the two metabolic pathways do not seem to be incompatible, probably because of a balance between the amount of substrate that was metabolized in a productive way and the amount that was transformed into toxic intermediates.

BIODEGRADATION OF ALKENYLBENZENES

The simplest member of the alkenylbenzene class of aromatic compounds is styrene. The petrochemical industry produces enormous quantities of styrene as a starting material for the production of plastics, synthetic rubber, and resins, but styrene is also produced naturally, mainly by the decarboxylation of cinnamic acid (Warhurst and Fewson, 1994).

The metabolism of styrene in humans has been widely investigated because of the toxic effects of metabolic activation (Bond, 1989). There are many reports of bacteria able to grow on styrene (Shirai and Hisatsuka, 1979; Baggi et al., 1983; Hartmans et al., 1990). However, data concerning the bacterial catabolic pathways of styrene are poor, and only recently have the enzymatic activities of some styrene-degrading strains been identified and partially characterized.

Two main styrene catabolic routes have been proposed (Fig. 4): the first involves the oxidation of the side chain to phenylacetate, and the second involves an initial attack on the aromatic nucleus. As far as alkenyl-group oxidation is concerned, an initial monooxygenation to epoxystyrene, which is subsequently isomerized to phenylacetaldehyde, has been proposed.

Side Chain Modification

Hartmans et al. (1990) isolated a *P. putida* mutant that accumulates epoxystyrene, thus demonstrating that this compound is a real intermediate of styrene oxidation in that strain. 2-Phenylethanol has been associated with microbial degradation of styrene, as this compound is often present in culture broths of styrene-grown cells, and a 2-phenylethanol dehydrogenase activity can be detected in their cell extracts (Hartmans et al., 1989).

Pseudomonas fluorescens ST, which is able to grow on styrene, was previously partially characterized. The proposed catabolic pathway consists of an initial oxidation of the alkenyl lateral chain to phenylacetaldehyde and phenylacetate (Baggi et al., 1983). Recently, *P. fluorescens* ST genes involved in the first steps of styrene degradation were isolated and the intermediates produced by recombinant clones were identified (Marconi et al., 1996). Some recombinant cosmids generated from a genomic library of strain ST allowed *P. putida* PaW340 to grow on styrene (Fig. 5).

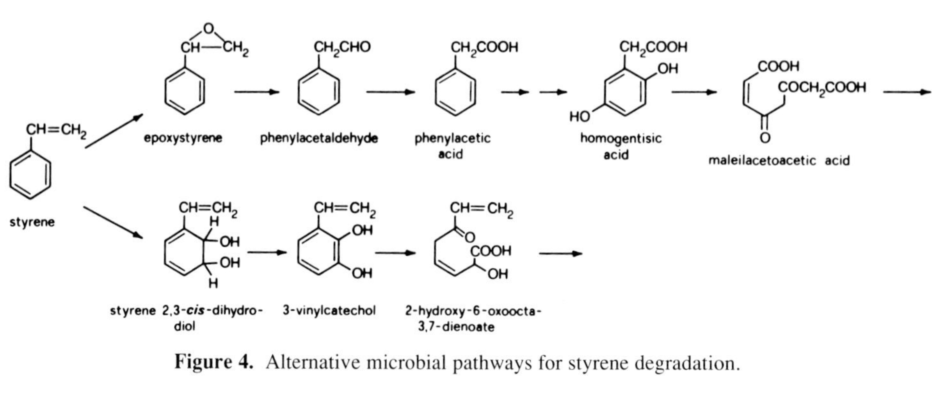

Figure 4. Alternative microbial pathways for styrene degradation.

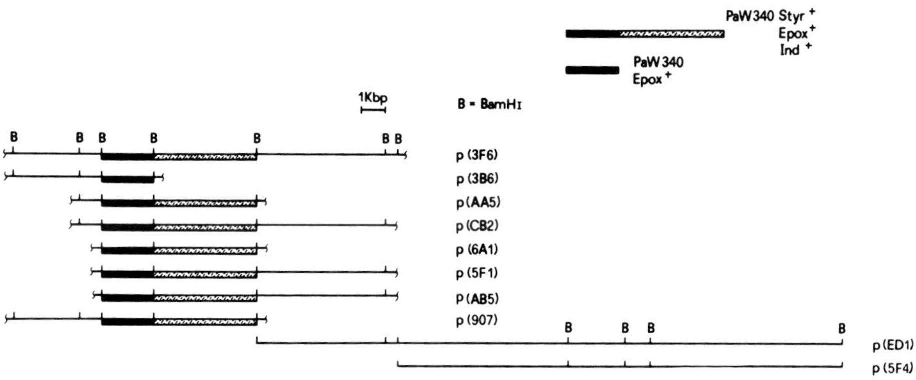

Figure 5. Restriction endonuclease map of *P. fluorescens* ST chromosomal DNA fragments cloned in pLAFR3 able to confer on *P. putida* PaW340 the ability to convert styrene into epoxystyrene and epoxystyrene into phenylacetaldehyde or 2-phenylethanol (Marconi et al., 1996).

The genes encoding the styrene monooxygenase, which is involved in the conversion of styrene to epoxystyrene, and the isomerase responsible for the conversion of epoxystyrene to phenylacetaldehyde have been cloned and localized within a 2.3- to 3-kb DNA fragment (Fig. 5). Enzymatic assays of the cloned catabolic gene products confirmed that *P. fluorescens* ST degrades styrene through oxidation of the alkenyl chain. The first step involves conversion of the vinyl group by a monooxygenase to epoxystyrene, which has been directly identified. This reaction is dependent on the presence of the 3-kb *P. fluorescens* ST genomic fragment (Fig. 5). The 2.3-kb fragment is sufficient to confer on *E. coli* tranformants the capability of converting epoxystyrene to phenylacetaldehyde or 2-phenylethanol (Fig. 6).

Direct transformation of epoxystyrene into 2-phenylethanol was suggested by Shirai and Hisatsuka (1979), whereas Hartmans et al. (1989) proposed that this transformation proceeds in two steps that involve phenylacetaldehyde as an intermediate. We have demonstrated that 2-phenylethanol can be produced directly from the reduction of epoxystyrene by an epoxystyrene reductase encoded by the 2.3-kb fragment. However, in strain ST, 2-phenylethanol is not an obligatory intermediate of styrene degradation, since we selected ST mutants that had lost the ability to grow on 2-phenylethanol but fully retained the ability to grow on styrene. Unlike the production of 2-phenylethanol, the formation of phenylacetaldehyde is independent of inoculation conditions and occurs at a very high rate.

As far as the further metabolism of phenylacetate is concerned, it has already been demonstrated that strain ST metabolizes this compound to *o*-hydroxyphenylacetic acid, which is further channeled into the homogentisate pathway (Baggi et al., 1983) (Fig. 6).

Ring Modification

The initial attack on the aromatic ring of styrene was described for a strain of *Rhodococcus rhodochrous* by Warhurst et al. (1994). 3-Vinylcatechol was produced. This compound undergoes a complete *meta*-cleavage pathway accompanied by the loss of acrylic acid (Fig. 4).

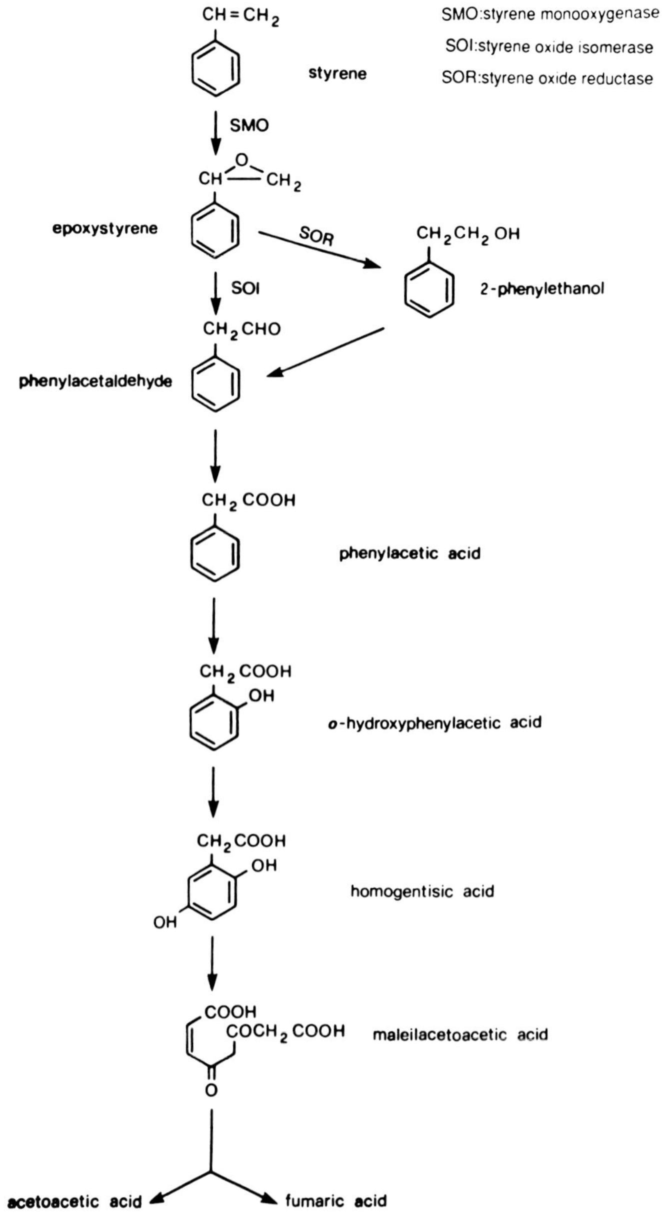

Figure 6. Metabolic pathway of styrene in *P. fluorescens* ST (Baggi et al., 1983).

Ring modifications of other members of this class of aromatic hydrocarbons have not been investigated extensively. However, strains of *Pseudomonas* able to metabolize α- and β-methylstyrene have been described. *Pseudomonas convexa* S107B1 is able to biotransform α-methylstyrene (isopropenylbenzene) into an unusual dihydrodiol, the *cis*-1,2-dihydroxy-3-isopropenyl-3-cyclohexene. The same strain biotransforms β-methylstyrene (α-propenylbenzene) into phenylpropionaldehyde and benzoate. The different modes of attack by the same strain may be due to the different chemical structures of the substituent groups (Omori et al., 1974).

The initial steps of α-methylstyrene biodegradation by *Pseudomonas aeruginosa* DS13 imply a direct hydroxylation of the aromatic ring to give both *cis*-1,2-dihydroxy-3-isopropenyl-3-cyclohexene and isopropylcatechol, which is further cleaved by a 2,3-dioxygenase (Golovleva et al., 1992). There is also evidence of microbial attack on the isopropenyl substituent by the accumulation of α-phenylacrylic acid and α,α′-phenylmethylglycol, which are not further degraded.

In general, despite the chemical analogy between styrene and α-methylstyrene, the bacterial strains capable of degrading styrene are not able to use α-methylstyrene, and vice versa. However, a *P. putida* strain isolated in the presence of α-methylstyrene as the sole carbon and energy source has been reported to biotransform styrene (Bestetti et al., 1989). Metabolic analyses of the wild-type strain and some mutants allowed the elucidation of the initial steps of α-methylstyrene metabolism into 2-phenyl-2-propen-1-ol through direct hydroxylation of the alkenyl group or into a *cis*-dihydrodiol through aromatic ring hydroxylation (Fig. 7). 2-Phenyl-2-propen-1-ol is not metabolized further and accumulates in the cultures, while the diol is oxidized to a catechol and then undergoes a *meta* cleavage; the *cis*-diol is also partially reduced to a *cis*-1,2-dihydroxy-3-isopropenyl-3-cyclohexene, which is not further metabolized. The same strain was found to be able to grow on styrene and other aromatic hydrocarbons (e.g., toluene, benzene, ethylbenzene) through the formation of the corresponding *cis*-diols, which are completely metabolized. In the case of styrene, the formation of a tetrahydrodiol and a side chain oxidation product was also demonstrated, confirming the ability of this strain to use different initial reactions to attack aromatic hydrocarbons. It may be assumed that the

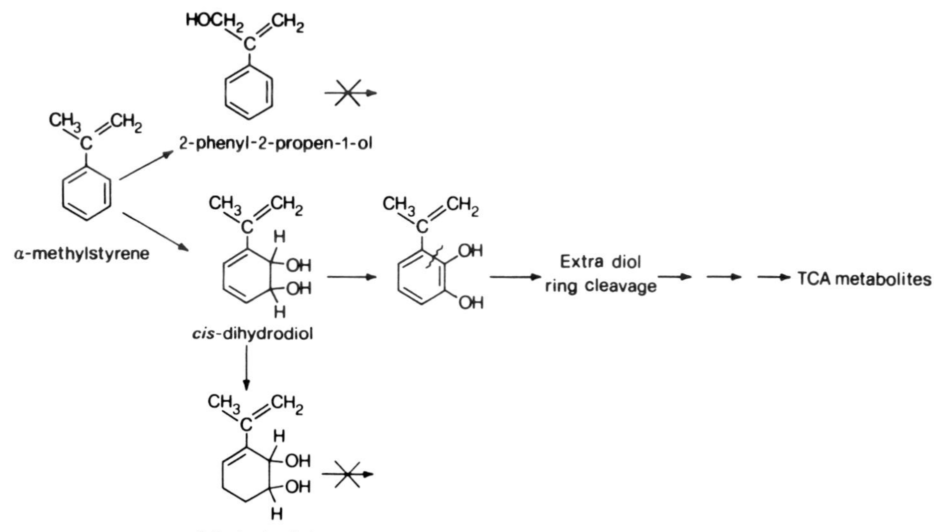

Figure 7. Early metabolic steps of α-methylstyrene by *P. putida* MST (Bestetti et al., 1989). TCA, tricarboxylic acid cycle.

enzyme responsible for aromatic-ring hydroxylation is a dioxygenase with broad substrate specificity, which allows the strain to biotransform a large number of monosubstituted hydrocarbons, including chlorobenzene and chlorophenols (Bestetti et al., 1992). Modification of the side chain could be due to a distinct monooxygenase or to the same dioxygenase that is responsible for aromatic-ring hydroxylation.

CONCLUDING REMARKS

Presently available information on the biodegradation of alkyl and alkenyl benzenes confirms the metabolic versatility of *Pseudomonas* strains, which is based on the development of different peripheral reactions through substrate range extension of the initial conversion enzymes. These bacteria demonstrate great potential in evolving new and desired pathways by recruiting and combining different catabolic activities through genetic mechanisms that contribute to metabolic adaptation.

Acknowledgments. This work was supported by the Target Project on Biotechnology and Bioinstrumentation, Consiglio Nazionale delle Ricerche.

REFERENCES

Baggi, G., P. Barbieri, E. Galli, and S. Tollari. 1987. Isolation of a *Pseudomonas stutzeri* strain that degrades *o*-xylene. *Appl. Environ. Microbiol.* **53**:2129–2131.

Baggi, G., M. M. Boga, D. Catelani, E. Galli, and V. Treccani. 1983. Styrene catabolism by a strain of *Pseudomonas fluorescens*. *Syst. Appl. Microbiol.* **4**:141–147.

Barbieri, P., L. Palladino, P. Di Gennaro, and E. Galli. 1993. Alternative pathways for *o*-xylene or *m*-xylene and *p*-xylene degradation in a *Pseudomonas stutzeri* strain. *Biodegradation* **4**:71–80.

Bestetti, G., E. Galli, C. Benigni, F. Orsini, and F. Pelizzoni. 1989. Biotransformation of styrenes by a *Pseudomonas putida*. *Appl. Microbiol. Biotechnol.* **30**:252–256.

Bestetti, G., E. Galli, B. Leoni, F. Pelizzoni, and G. Sello. 1992. Regioselective hydroxylation of chlorobenzene and chlorophenols by a *Pseudomonas putida*. *Appl. Microbiol. Biotechnol.* **37**:260–263.

Bond, J. A. 1989. Review of the toxicology of styrene. *Crit. Rev. Toxicol.* **19**:227–249.

Galli, E. 1994. The role of microorganisms in the environment decontamination, p. 235–246. *In* A. Renzoni, N. Mattei, L. Lari, and M. C. Fossi (ed.), *Contaminants in the Environment*. CRC Press, Inc., Boca Raton, Fla.

Galli, E., P. Barbieri, and G. Bestetti. 1992. Potential of pseudomonads in the degradation of methylbenzenes, p. 268–276. *In* E. Galli, S. Silver, and B. Witholt (ed.), *Pseudomonas: Molecular Biology and Biotechnology*. American Society for Microbiology, Washington, D.C.

Gibson, D. T., M. Hensley, H. Yoshioka, and T. J. Mabry. 1970. Formation of (+)-*cis*-2,3-dihydroxy-1-methylcyclohexa-4,6-diene from toluene by *Pseudomonas putida*. *Biochemistry* **9**:1626–1630.

Golovleva, L. A., O. V. Maltseva, and I. P. Solyanikova. 1992. Metabolism of foreign compounds in *Pseudomonas* spp., p. 231–238. *In* E. Galli, S. Silver, and B. Witholt (ed.), *Pseudomonas: Molecular Biology and Biotechnology*. American Society for Microbiology, Washington, D.C.

Hartmans, S., J. P. Smits, M. J. van der Werf, F. Volkering, and J. A. M. de Bont. 1989. Metabolism of styrene oxide and 2-phenylethanol in the styrene-degrading *Xanthobacter* strain 124X. *Appl. Environ. Microbiol.* **55**:2850–2855.

Hartmans, S., J. P. Smits, M. J. van der Werf, and J. A. M. de Bont. 1990. Bacterial degradation of styrene involving a novel flavin adenine dinucleotide-dependent styrene monooxygenase. *Appl. Environ. Microbiol.* **56:**1347–1351.

Marconi, A. M., F. Beltrametti, G. Bestetti, F. Solinas, M. Ruzzi, E. Galli, and E. Zennaro. 1996. Cloning and characterization of styrene-catabolic genes from *Pseudomonas fluorescens* strain ST. *Appl. Environ. Microbiol.* **62**:121–127.

Olsen, R. H., J. J. Kukor, and B. Kaphammer. 1994. A novel toluene-3-monooxygenase pathway cloned from *Pseudomonas pickettii* PKO1. *J. Bacteriol.* **176**:3749–3756.

Omori, T., Y. Igami, and Y. Minoda. 1974. Microbial oxidation of α-methylstyrene and β-methylstyrene. *Agric. Biol. Chem.* **38**:409–415.

Shields, M. S., O. Montgomery, P. J. Chapman, S. M. Cuskey, and P. H. Pritchard. 1989. Novel pathway of toluene catabolism in the trichloroethylene degrading bacterium G4. *Appl. Environ. Microbiol.* **55**:1624–1629.

Shirai, K., and K. Hisatsuka. 1979. Isolation and identification of styrene assimilating bacteria. *Agric. Biol. Chem.* **43**:1595–1596.

Smith, M. R. 1990. The biodegradation of aromatic hydrocarbons by bacteria. *Biodegradation* **1**:191–206.

Warhurst, A. M., F. K. Clarke, R. A. Hill, R. A. Holt, and C. A. Fewson. 1994. Metabolism of styrene by *Rhodococcus rhodochrous* NCIMB 13259. *Appl. Environ. Microbiol.* **60**:1137–1145.

Warhurst, A. M., and C. A. Fewson. 1994. Microbial metabolism and biotransformation of styrene. *J. Appl. Bacteriol.* **77**:597–606.

Whited, G. M., and D. T. Gibson. 1991. Toluene-4-monooxygenase, a three-component enzyme system that catalyzes the oxidation of toluene to *p*-cresol in *Pseudomonas mendocina* KR1. *J. Bacteriol.* **173**:3010–3016.

Worsey, M. J., and P. A. Williams. 1975. Metabolism of toluene and xylenes by *Pseudomonas putida (arvilla)* mt-2: evidence for a new function of the TOL plasmid. *J. Bacteriol.* **124**:7–13.

Molecular Biology of Pseudomonads
Edited by T. Nakazawa et al.

Chapter 6

Genes and Enzymes for γ-Hexachlorocyclohexane Degradation in *Sphingomonas paucimobilis* UT26

Yuji Nagata, Masao Fukuda, Keisuke Miyauchi, and Masamichi Takagi

γ-Hexachlorocyclohexane (HCH, BHC, lindane) is a halogenated organic insecticide that was once used worldwide for agriculture and public health. Because of the compound's toxicity and persistence in soil, the use of γ-HCH has been prohibited in many countries. However, for economic reasons, some countries still use γ-HCH, and new sites are being contaminated by γ-HCH and its stereoisomers (a technical mixture of HCH consists of α, β, γ, and δ isomers) (Iwata et al., 1993).

γ-HCH is degraded rapidly under anaerobic conditions, but it is considered extremely persistent in upland soil. *Sphingomonas* (formerly *Pseudomonas*) *paucimobilis* SS86 was isolated from an upland experimental field to which γ-HCH has been applied once a year for 12 years (Senoo and Wada, 1989). We isolated a mutant of SS86, named UT26, that has nalidixic acid resistance as a genetic marker (Imai et al., 1989). SS86 and UT26 utilize γ-HCH as a sole source of carbon and energy under aerobic conditions.

The degradation pathways of γ-HCH are of interest because of the compound's structural features: a cyclohexane skeleton and a highly chlorinated state. In this chapter, we describe the enzymes and genes involved in the early degradation steps of γ-HCH in *S. paucimobilis* UT26.

DEGRADATION PATHWAY OF γ-HCH IN UT26

γ-HCH is converted by two steps of dehydrochlorination via γ-pentachlorocyclohexene (PCCH) to 1,3,4,6-tetrachloro-1,4-cyclohexadiene (1,4-TCDN), which is then metabolized to 2,5-dichloro-2,5-cyclohexadiene-1,4-diol (2,5-DDOL) by two steps of hydrolytic dehalogenation via 2,4,5-trichloro-2,5-cyclohexadiene-1-ol (2,4,5-DNOL) (Nagasawa et al., 1993b; Fig. 1). Through this series of reactions, two dead-end products, 1,2,4-trichlorobenzene (1,2,4-TCB) and 2,5-dichlorophenol (2,5-DCP), are also produced from the unstable intermediates (1,4-TCDN and 2,4,5-DNOL, respectively).

Yuji Nagata, Keisuke Miyauchi, and Masamichi Takagi • Department of Biotechnology, The University of Tokyo, Bunkyo-ku, Tokyo 113, Japan. ***Masao Fukuda*** • Department of Bioengineering, Nagaoka University of Technology, Kamitomioka, Nagaoka, Niigata 940-21, Japan.

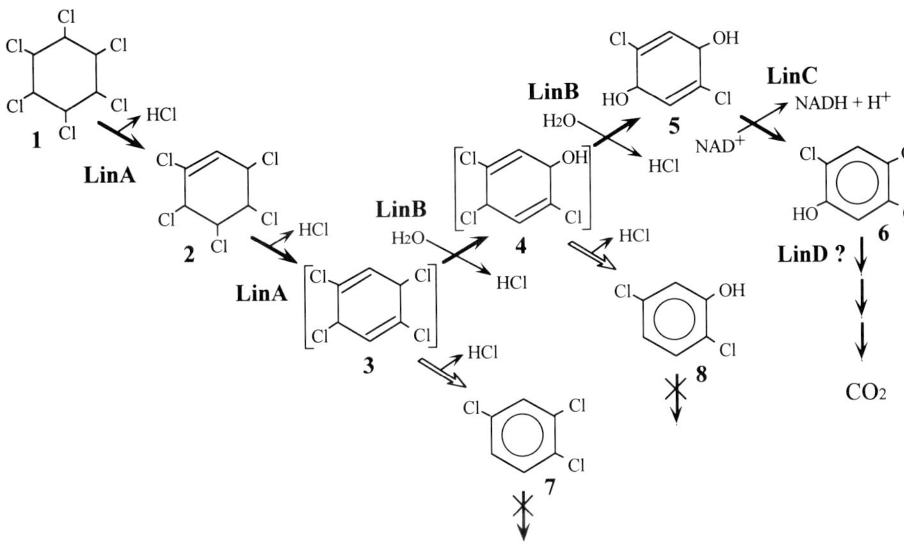

Figure 1. Proposed assimilation pathway of γ-HCH in *S. paucimobilis* UT26. Compounds: 1, γ-HCH (γ -BHC, lindane); 2, γ-PCCH; 3, 1,4-TCDN; 4, 2,4,5-DNOL; 5, 2,5-DDOL; 6, 2,5-DCHQ; 7, 1,2,4-TCB; 8, 2,5-DCP. Because two intermediates (in brackets; compounds 3 and 4) are chemically unstable, they were not identified. Compounds 3 and 4 are proposed to be transformed to stable compounds (7 and 8, respectively) by nonenzymatic reactions (open arrows). Compounds 7 and 8 are not further degraded by UT26.

2,5-DDOL is further degraded to 2,5-dichlorohydroquinone (2,5-DCHQ), and finally, 2,5-DCHQ is mineralized (Nagasawa et al., 1993b).

GENES INVOLVED IN γ-HCH DEGRADATION

The broad-host-range cosmid vector pKS13 (Kimbara et al., 1989) was used for the construction of a gene library of UT26 in *Escherichia coli* HB101. Each clone of the library in *E. coli* was mobilized into *Pseudomonas putida* PpY101 (Kimbara et al., 1989) by triparental mating. The resultant library in *P. putida* was screened for γ-HCH and its degradation metabolites by gas chromatography with an electron capture detector.

We cloned four genes involved in the degradation of γ-HCH in UT26 (Table 1). The *linA* gene encodes γ-HCH dehydrochlorinase (LinA), which is responsible for the conversion of γ-HCH to 1,4-TCDN via γ-PCCH (Imai et al., 1991, 1992). The *linB* gene encodes 1,4-TCDN halidohydrolase (LinB), which is responsible for the conversion of 1,4-TCDN to 2,5-DDOL (Nagata et al., 1993b). The *linC* gene encodes 2,5-DDOL dehydrogenase (LinC), which is responsible for the conversion of 2,5-DDOL to 2,5-DCHQ (Nagata et al., 1994). Recently, we cloned and sequenced a new gene (*linD*) which is directly involved in 2,5-DCHQ degradation (K. Miyauchi, Y. Nagata, and M. Takagi, unpublished data), but the reaction(s) carried out by the gene product is still unknown. The *linA*, *linB*, and *linC* genes are constitutively expressed, while the *linD* gene is inducible in UT26 (Miyauchi et al., unpublished data).

Table 1. Four genes or products involved in γ-HCH degradation in *S. paucimobilis* UT26

Name	Gene	Gene product				Gene expression in UT26	Reference
	Size (bp)	G+C content (%)	No. of amino acid residues	Deduced mol wt (10^3)	Function		
linA	465	53.0	155	17.3	Dehydrochlorinase	Constitutive	Imai et al., 1991
linB	885	62.5	295	33.1	Halidohydrolase	Constitutive	Nagata et al., 1993
linC	750	64.3	250	25.6	Dehydrogenase	Constitutive	Nagata et al., 1994
linD	1,038	61.0	346	38.4	Unknown	Inducible	Miyauchi et al., unpublished data

The G+C content of the *linA* gene is considerably lower than that in each of the other three genes (*linB, linC,* and *linD*) and the genomic DNA of the *S. paucimobilis* strains (65%) (Palleroni, 1984), suggesting that the *linA* gene may have originated from another organism with a lower G+C content. No cosmid clone that contains more than one of these four genes was isolated, suggesting that these four genes (*linA, linB, linC,* and *linD*) are present separately from each other in the UT26 genome. These four genes are at the least not organized as an operon. Genes involved in catabolic pathways usually form operons in prokaryotic cells (van der Meer et al., 1992), but the genes involved in the early degradation steps of γ-HCH seem to be a rare exception. Similar cases were reported with respect to 2,4-dinitrotoluene degradation by *Pseudomonas* sp. strain DNT (Suen and Spain, 1993) and pentachlorophenol degradation by *Flavobacterium* sp. strain ATCC 39823 (Orser et al., 1993a; Orser et al., 1993b). In these cases (including that of UT26), genes that take part in some other function(s) may be involved.

In the following sections, properties of the genes we have cloned and the corresponding enzymes are discussed in detail.

γ-HCH DEHYDROCHLORINASE (LinA)

A database search for the *linA* gene failed to find any significantly homologous sequences. Southern blot analyses using the *linA* gene as a probe against total DNAs of several related strains revealed no homologous sequence (Imai et al., 1991). The origin of the *linA* gene is of great interest but is still unknown.

The *linA* gene was highly expressed in *E. coli,* and the gene product (LinA) was purified to homogeneity (Nagata et al., 1993a). In addition to γ-HCH and γ-PCCH, α- and δ-isomers of HCH and α-PCCH were dehydrochlorinated by LinA; however, β-HCH was not (Nagata et al., 1993a). These results are consistent with those obtained using resting UT26 cells (Nagasawa et al., 1993a). It is suggested that dehydrochlorination by LinA occurs stereoselectively at a *trans* and diaxial pair of hydrogen and chlorine. The other chlorinated compounds tested were not dehydrochlorinated by purified enzyme (Nagata et al., 1993a), indicating that the substrate specificity of LinA is narrow.

Dehydrochlorinase is an enzyme that eliminates HCl from the substrate molecule, leading to the formation of a double bond (Fetzner and Lingens, 1994; Janssen et al., 1994). The properties of three dehydrochlorinases (including LinA) were reported (Table 2). A eukaryotic dehydrochlorinase isolated from *Musca domestica* catalyzes the monodehydrochlorination of 1,1,1-trichloro-2,2-bis (*p*-chlorophenyl) ethane (DDT) (Lipke and Kearns, 1959; Clark and Shanaan, 1984). 3-Chloro-D-alanine dehydrochlorinase was isolated from *P. putida* (Nagasawa et al., 1982). LinA, however, is very different from these two other dehydrochlorinases. DDT dehydrochlorinase and 3-chloro-D-alanine dehydrochlorinase require glutathione and pyridoxal 5′-phosphate, respectively, for their activities, while LinA does not require any cofactors. Purified LinA did not show glutathione *S*-transferase or DDT dehydrochlorinase activity in the presence of glutathione. Thus, it seems most likely that LinA is not a glutathione *S*-transferase-type enzyme. LinA is supposed to be a unique dehydrochlorinase, and its mechanism of dehydrochlorination is of great interest.

Table 2. Properties of three dehydrochlorinases

Source of dehydrochlorinase	Mol wt	Subunit		Cofactor[a]	Optimum pH	Expression	Substrate(s)	Reference(s)
		No.	Mol wt					
S. paucimobilis (LinA)	64,000	4 identical	16,500	None	7.5	Constitutive	γ-HCH, γ-PCCH	Nagata et al., 1993a, b
P. putida	76,000	2 identical	38,000	PLP	9.0	Inducible	3-Chloro-D-alanine	Nagasawa et al., 1982
M. domestica (housefly)	120,000	4 identical	30,000	GSH	7.4	Not known	DDT, γ-HCH	Lipke and Kearns, 1959; Clark and Shanaan, 1984

[a] PLP, pyridoxal 5′-phosphate; GSH, glutathione.

1,4-TCDN HALIDOHYDROLASE (LinB)

The deduced amino acid sequence of LinB showed significant similarity to the sequences of three types of α/β-hydrolase fold enzymes (Ollis et al., 1992), haloalkane dehalogenase (DhlA) from *Xanthobacter autotrophicus* GJ10 (Janssen et al., 1989), haloacetate dehalogenase (DehH1) from *Moraxella* sp. strain B (Kawasaki et al.,1992), and serine hydrolases represented by 2-hydroxymuconic semialdehyde hydrolase (DmpD) from *Pseudomonas* sp. strain CF600 (Nordlund and Shingler, 1990). The identities between these enzymes and LinB were 29.3, 22.6, and 20.5%, respectively. Although Renilla-luciferin 2-monooxygenase (LUCI) from *Renilla reniformis* (Lorenz et al., 1991) showed the highest identity to LinB (41.2%), it seems not to be a monooxygenase. Instead, because of the deduced amino acid sequence, LUCI is considered a member of the α/β-hydrolase family. LinB also showed significant similarity to part of the epoxide hydrolases from eukaryotic cells (Knehr et al., 1993; Grant et al., 1993; Beetham et al., 1993). Recently, a novel human serine hydrolase that showed similarity to bacterial serine hydrolases (BphD, DmpD, TodF, XylF, etc.) was reported (Puente and López-Otín, 1995). The evolutionary and functional relationships of these bacterial and eukaryotic hydrolases need further study.

Because DhlA showed the highest level of similarity to LinB among these three types of hydrolases (except for LUCI), the two sequences were aligned (Fig. 2). The results of this alignment suggested that LinB has the activity of haloalkane halidohydrolase. We purified the LinB overproduced in *E. coli* to homogeneity (Y. Nagata, K. Miyauchi, and M. Takagi, unpublished data). The molecular mass of LinB was calculated as 30 kDa by gel filtration chromatography and 32 kDa by electrophoresis on a sodium dodecyl sulfate-polyacrylamide gel, indicating that LinB is a monomeric enzyme (Table 3). Not only monochloroalkanes (C = 3 to 12) but also dichloroalkanes, bromoalkanes, iodoalkanes, and chlorinated aliphatic alcohols were good substrates for LinB, suggest-

```
LinB  M------------SLGAKPFGEKKFIEIKG---RRMAYIDEGTGDP---ILFQHGNPTSSYLWRNIMPHCAGLG-RLIAC   61
DhlA  MINAIRTPDQRFSNLDQYPFSPNYLDDLPGYPGLRAHYLDEGNSDAEDVFLCLHGEPTWSYLYRKMIPVFAESGARVIAP   80

                                                       +
LinB  DLIGMGDSDKLDPSGPERYAYAEHRDYLDALWEALDLGDRVVLVVHDWGSALGFDWARRHRERVQGIAYMEAIAM--PIE   139
DhlA  DFFGFGKSDK--PVDEEDYTFEFHRNFLLALIERLDLRN-ITIVVQDWGGFLGLTLPMADPSRFKRLIIMNACLMTDPVT   157
                                                     Nucleophilic Asp region

LinB  ---WADFPEQDRDLFQAFRSQAGEELVLQDNVFVEQVLPGLILRPLSEAEMAAYREPFLAAEARRPTLSWPRQIPIAGTP   216
DhlA  QPAFSAFVTQPADGFTAWKY----DLVTPSDLRLDQFMKRWA-PTLTEAEASAYAAPFPDTSYQAGVRKFPKMVAQRDQA   232
                             Cap domain region

                                 +                                   +
LinB  -ADVVAIARDY--AGWLSESPIPKLFINAEPGALTTGRMRDFCRTWPNQTEITVAGAHFIQEDSPDEIGAAIAAFVRRLRPA 295
DhlA  CIDISTEAISFWQNDWNGQTFMAIGMKDKLLGPDVMYPMKALINGCPEPLEIADAG-HFVQEFGEQVAREALKHFAE---TE 310
                                                                    His region
```

Figure 2. Comparison of deduced amino acid sequences of LinB and DhlA. The alignment was made by using Clustal V (Higgins et al., 1992). Amino acid residues are indicated by the one-letter code, and gaps have been introduced to obtain optimum alignment between the proteins. The DhlA sequence is derived from the data of Janssen et al. (1989). Amino acid residues that are conserved in the sequences compared are shown as white letters against a black background. Residues marked with plus signs form the putative active center of DhlA (Asp-124, Asp-260, and His-289) (Franken et al., 1991). The boxed residue is proposed to be important for the substrate specificity of these enzymes (Damborsky, 1995; see text for details).

Table 3. Comparison between two haloalkane halidohydrolases, LinB and DhlA

Enzyme	Source	Molecular mass (kDa) by: SDS-PAGE[a]	Molecular mass (kDa) by: Gel filtration	Length of deduced amino acid sequence	Optimum pH	Expression	Subunit	Substrates	Reference
LinB	*S. paucimobilis* UT26	32	30	33	8.2	Constitutive	Monomer	1-Chloro-*n*-alkanes (C_3 to C_{10}); α,ω-dichloro-*n*-alkanes (C_3 to C_9); 1-bromo-*n*-alkanes; 1-iodo-*n*-alkanes; α-chloro-ω-alkanols	Nagata et al., unpublished data
DhlA	*X. autotrophicus* GJ10	36	31	35	8.2	Constitutive	Monomer	1-Chloro-*n*-alkanes (C_1 to C_4); α,ω-dichloro-*n*-alkanes (C_2 to C_3); 1-bromo-*n*-alkanes; 1-iodo-*n*-alkanes	Keuning et al., 1985

[a]SDS-PAGE, sodium dodecyl sulfate-polyacrylamide gel electrophoresis.

ing that LinB is one of the haloalkane dehalogenases with a broad specificity for substrates. These results indicate that LinB has properties similar to those of DhlA ((Keuning et al., 1985) except for substrate specificity (Table 3). In brief, LinB prefers long-chain haloalkanes as substrates, while DhlA prefers short-chain haloalkanes. The three-dimensional structure of LinB is predictable (Damborsky et al., 1995) because LinB shows significant sequence similarity to DhlA, whose three-dimensional structure has been determined (Franken et al., 1991; Verschueren et al., 1993a; Verschueren et al., 1993b). The deduced active-site residue of DhlA (Asp-124, which is a nucleophilic residue essential for catalysis) is also conserved in LinB (Asp-108). Other residues around the active site are predicted. One of these (Trp-175 in DhlA numbering) is probably changed to Phe (or Gln) in LinB. The importance of this Trp residue for catalysis of 1,2-dichloroethane in DhlA was examined by quantum chemistry calculations (Damborsky et al., personal communication). The change of Trp to Phe increased the reaction barrier from 21 to 28 kcal/mol (1 kcal = 4,184 J) and at the same time increased the energy of the products (2-chloroethanol and chlorine ion) from −12 to −4 kcal/mol. This result suggested that the presence of Phe instead of Trp is one of the most important differences between these two enzymes and may contribute to the difference in substrate specificity.

2,5-DDOL DEHYDROGENASE (LinC)

The deduced amino acid sequence of LinC showed significant similarity to that of the short-chain alcohol dehydrogenase superfamily (Jörnvall et al., 1981; Neidle et al., 1992; Persson et al., 1991; Fig. 3). These enzymes are thought to contain two highly conserved regions (Neidle et al., 1992; Persson et al., 1991). The first conserved region is located at the N terminus of each enzyme. The predicted structures of several dehydrogenases show that this region consists of alternating regions of β-sheet and α-helix (β–α–β); this region

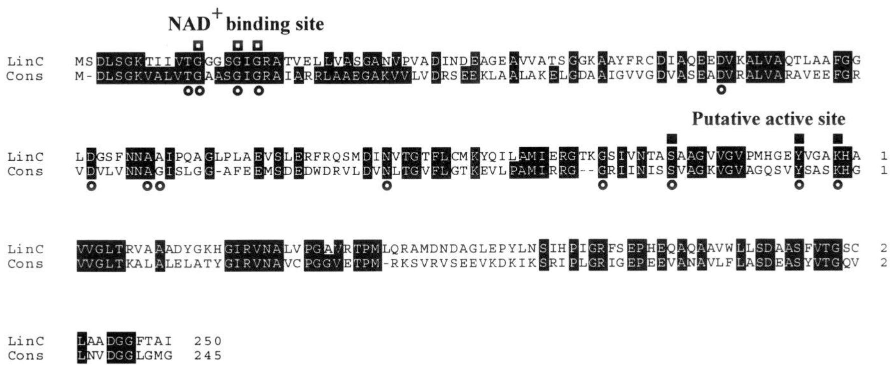

Figure 3. Comparison of the deduced amino acid sequence of LinC and the consensus amino acid sequence of the short-chain alcohol dehydrogenase family, which is derived from Neidle et al. (1992). Amino acid residues that are conserved in the LinC sequence are shown as white letters against a black background. Residues that are highly conserved in different types of short-chain dehydrogenases (Persson et al., 1991) are marked with circles. Putative active-site residues and putative NAD⁺ binding site residues are marked with solid or open squares, respectively (Rossmann et al., 1975).

has been proposed to be part of the NAD^+ binding site. The second homologous region can be seen around positions 150 and 154 of the consensus sequence. Two amino acids, tyrosine at position 150 and lysine at position 154, are highly conserved among the short-chain alcohol dehydrogenase family. The tyrosine residue is conserved among all of them, while the lysine residue is not. Ensor and Tai (1991) demonstrated that the substitution of tyrosine for alanine abolished the 15-hydroxyprostaglandin dehydrogenase activity. In the deduced amino acid sequence of LinC, the amino acid residues mentioned above are highly conserved (Fig. 3), suggesting that LinC has the activity of NAD^+-dependent dehydrogenation.

Members of the short-chain alcohol dehydrogenase family are distributed in organisms from bacteria to humans. A question thus arises concerning the substrate specificities of these enzymes. In preliminary data, we tested whether another short-chain dehydrogenase enzyme has LinC activity (=2,5-DDOL dehydrogenase activity). *E. coli* expressing BphB (biphenyl-*cis*-diol dehydrogenase; Fukuda et al., 1994) or BnzB (*cis*-benzene glycol dehydrogenase; Irie et al., 1987), also known as TodD (*cis*-toluene dihydrodiol dehydrogenase; Zylstra and Gibson, 1989), did not show the activity.

2,5-DCHQ DEGRADATION PATHWAY

UT26 converts γ-HCH to 1,2,4-TCB, 2,5-DCP, and 2,5-DCHQ (Fig. 1). However, UT26 seems to degrade and assimilate only 2,5-DCHQ (Nagasawa et al., 1993b). (Chloro)hydroquinone is reported as an intermetabolite in the degradation pathway of some aromatic compounds such as pentachlorophenol (Uotila et al., 1992; Orser, 1993b), 2,4,6-trichlorophenol (Latus et al., 1995), 2,4,5-trichlorophenol (Joshi and Gold, 1993), and other mono-, di-, and trichlorophenols (Zaborina et al., 1995). In the degradation of 2,4,5-trichlorophenoxyacetic acid by *Burkholderia cepacia* AC1100, 2,5-DCHQ is reported to be an intermetabolite (Daubaras and Chakrabarty, 1992; Daubaras et al., 1995). (Chloro)trihydroxybenzene is identified as a ring fission substrate in these examples (Uotila, 1993; Daubaras and Chakrabarty, 1992; Daubaras et al., 1995; Latus et al., 1995; Zaborina et al., 1995). However, other reports indicate that hydroquinone is a direct ring fission substrate (Larway and Evans, 1965; Darby et al., 1987; Spain and Gibson, 1991; Jones et al., 1995). Although the metabolic pathway of 2,5-DCHQ in UT26 has not been determined, the (chloro)hydroquinone degradation pathway seems to be widespread in organisms from prokaryotes to eukaryotes. The "hydroquinone pathway" is considered to be one of the significant pathways for metabolism of aromatic compounds. In UT26, 2,5-DCHQ degradation activity is expressed inducibly (Nagata et al., 1996).

Recently, we cloned a gene (named *linD*) that is directly involved in 2,5-DCHQ degradation (Miyauchi et al., unpublished data). However, no homologous sequence was identified in the database, suggesting that research on the hydroquinone pathway is still incomplete at the molecular genetic level.

CONCLUSIONS AND PROSPECTS

We have demonstrated a unique degradation pathway of γ-HCH in UT26 and have cloned genes involved in this pathway. It seems that the pathway from γ-HCH to 2,5-DCHQ is especially specific for γ-HCH degradation in UT26. The 2,5-DCHQ degra-

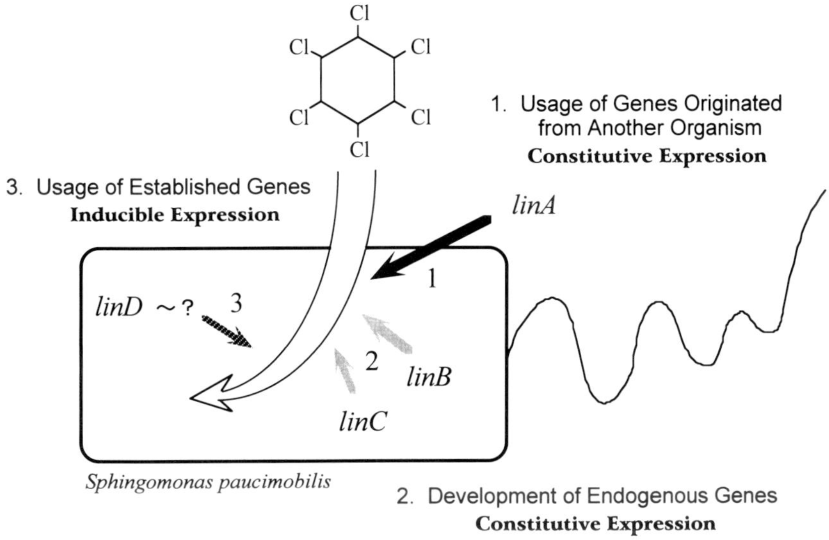

Figure 4. Proposed mechanism of adaptive acquisition of assimilation ability for γ-HCH in *S. paucimobilis* UT26. See the text for details.

dation pathway seems to be widely distributed in nature, as described above. We propose a model for adaptive acquisition of γ-HCH assimilation ability in *S. paucimobilis* UT26 (Fig. 4). For the first attack on γ-HCH, UT26 seems to use a gene that originated from another organism (*linA*). Then UT26 degrades the intermetabolites, which seem to be relatively common substrates, by developing variants of endogenous genes (*linB* and *linC*). Finally, for the common substrate (2,5-DCHQ), UT26 uses established genes that are expressed inducibly. We believe there might be other aerobic γ-HCH degradation pathways that have not yet been identified. Comparison of the γ-HCH degradation pathway in UT26 with such pathways in other organisms will be of interest.

Our current understanding can be applied for the bioremediation of a contaminated environment. UT26 grows slowly when γ-HCH is supplied as the sole source of carbon and energy. Because the genes for γ-HCH degradation that we cloned could be overproduced in other organisms, it is possible to create strains that degrade γ-HCH more effectively. The γ-HCH degradation pathway in UT26, however, is inefficient, because two dead-end products (1,2,4-TCB and 2,5-DCP) are produced (Fig. 1). Enhancement of LinB activity in UT26 and introduction of the *linA* gene into a strain that can assimilate 1,2,4-TCB, such as *Pseudomonas* sp. strain P51 (van der Meer et al., 1991), are strategies for creating strains that degrade γ-HCH more effectively than UT26 does.

Acknowledgments. We thank Jiri Damborsky for unpublished data and helpful discussions. This work was supported in part by a Grant-in-Aid for Scientific Research from the Ministry of Education, Science, and Culture of Japan. This work was performed using the facilities of the Biotechnology Research Center, The University of Tokyo.

REFERENCES

Beetham, J. K., T. Tian, and B. D. Hammock. 1993. cDNA cloning and expression of a soluble epoxide hydrolase from human liver. *Arch. Biochem. Biophys.* **305:**197–201.

Clark, A. G., and N. A. Shanaan. 1984. Evidence that DDT-dehydrochlorinase from the house fly is a glutathione S-transferase. *Pesticide Biochem. Physiol.* **22:**249–261.

Damborský, J., A. T. Bull, and D. J. Hardman. 1995. Homology modelling of haloalkane dehalogenase of *Sfingomonas paucimobilis* UT26. *Biologia* (Bratislava) **50:**523–528.

Darby, J. M., D. G. Taylor, and D. J. Hopper. 1987. Hydroquinone as the ring-fission substrate in the catabolism of 4-ethylphenol and 4-hydroxyacetophenone *by Pseudomonas putida* JD1. *J. Gen. Microbiol.* **133:**2137–2146.

Daubaras, D., and A. M. Chakrabarty. 1992. The environment, microbes and bioremediation: microbial activities modulated by the environment. *Biodegradation* **3:**125–135.

Daubaras, D. L., C. D. Hershberger, K. Kitano, and A. M. Chakrabarty. 1995. Sequence analysis of a gene cluster involved in metabolism of 2,4,5-trichlorophenoxyacetic acid by *Burkholderia cepacia* AC1100. *Appl. Environ. Microbiol.* **61:**1279–1289.

Ensor, C. M., and H.-H. Tai. 1991. Site-directed mutagenesis of the conserved tyrosine 151 of human placental NAD^+-dependent 15-hydroxyprostaglandin dehydrogenase yields a catalytically inactivate enzyme. *Biochem. Biophys. Res. Commun.* **176:**840–845.

Fetzner, S., and F. Lingens. 1994. Bacterial dehalogenases: biochemistry, genetics, and biotechnological applications. *Microbiol. Rev.* **58:**641–685.

Franken, S. M., H. J. Rozeboom, K. H. Kalk, and B. W. Dijkstra. 1991. Crystal structure of haloalkane dehalogenase: an enzyme to detoxify halogenated alkanes. *EMBO J.* **10:**1297–1302.

Fukuda, M., Y. Yasukochi, Y. Kikuchi, Y. Nagata, K. Kimbara, H. Horiuchi, M. Takagi, and K. Yano. 1994. Identification of the *bphA* and *bphB* genes of *Pseudomonas* sp. strain KKS102 involved in degradation of biphenyl and polychlorinated biphenyls. *Biochem. Biophys. Res. Commun.* **202:**850–856.

Grant, D. F., D. H. Storms, and B. D. Hammock. 1993. Molecular cloning and expression of murine liver soluble epoxide hydrolase. *J. Biol. Chem.* **268:**17628–17633.

Higgins, D. G., A. J. Bleasby, and R. Fuchs. 1992. Clustal V: improved software for multiple sequence alignment. *Comput. Appl. Biosci.* **8:**189–191.

Imai, R., Y. Nagata, M. Fukuda, M. Takagi, and K. Yano. 1991. Molecular cloning of a *Pseudomonas paucimobilis* gene encoding a 17-kilodalton polypeptide that eliminates HCl molecules from γ-hexachlorocyclohexane. *J. Bacteriol.* **173:**6811–6819.

Imai, R., Y. Nagata, M. Fukuda, K. Yano, and M. Takagi. 1992. Isolation and characterization of a dehydrochlorinase gene for the degradation of γ-hexachlorocyclohexane in *Pseudomonas paucimobilis,* p. 292–300. *In* E. Galli, S. Silver, and B. Witholt (ed.), *Pseudomonas: Molecular Biology and Biotechnology*. American Society for Microbiology, Washington, D.C.

Imai, R., Y. Nagata, K. Senoo, H. Wada, M. Fukuda, M. Takagi, and K. Yano. 1989. Dehydrochlorination of γ-hexachlorocyclohexane (γ-BHC) by γ-BHC-assimilating *Pseudomonas paucimobilis. Agric. Biol. Chem.* **53:**2015–2017.

Irie, S., S. Doi, T. Yorifuji, M. Takagi, and K. Yano. 1987. Nucleotide sequencing and characterization of the genes encoding benzene oxidation enzymes of *Pseudomonas putida. J. Bacteriol.* **169:**5174–5179.

Iwata, H., S. Tanabe, N. Sakai, and R. Tatsukawa. 1993. Distribution of persistent organochlorines in the oceanic air and surface seawater and the role of ocean on their global transport and fate. *Environ. Sci. Technol.* **27:**1080–1098.

Janssen, D. B., F. Pries, and J. R. van der Ploeg. 1994. Genetics and biochemistry of dehalogenating enzymes. *Annu. Rev. Microbiol.* **48:**163–191.

Janssen, D. B., F. Pries, J. van der Ploeg, B. Kazemier, P. Terpstra, and B. Witholt. 1989. Cloning of 1,2-dichloroethane degradation genes of *Xanthobacter autotrophicus* GJ10 and expression and sequencing of the *dhlA* gene. *J. Bacteriol.* **171:**6791–6700.

Jones, K. H., P. W. Trudgill, and D. J. Hopper. 1995. Evidence of two pathways for the metabolism of phenol by *Aspergillus fumigatus. Arch. Microbiol.* **163:**176–181.

Jörnvall, H., M. Persson, and J. Jeffery. 1981. Alcohol and polyol dehydrogenase are both divided into two protein types, and structural properties cross-relate the different enzyme activities within each type. *Proc. Natl. Acad. Sci. USA* **78:**4226–4230.

Joshi, D. K., and M. H. Gold. 1993. Degradation of 2,4,5-trichlorophenol by the lignin-degrading basidiomycete *Phanerochaete chrysosporium*. *Appl. Environ. Microbiol.* **59:**1779–1785.

Kawaski, H., K. Tsuda, I. Matsushita, and K. Tonomura. 1992. Lack of homology between two haloacetate dehalogenase genes encoded on a plasmid from *Moraxella* sp. strain B. *J. Gen. Microbiol.* **138:**1317–1323.

Keuning, S., D. B. Janssen, and B. Witholt. 1985. Purification and characterization of hydrolytic haloalkane dehalogenase from *Xanthobacter autotrophicus* GJ10. *J. Bacteriol.* **163:**635–639.

Kimbara, K., T. Hashimoto, M. Fukuda, T. Koana, M. Takagi, M. Oishi, and K. Yano. 1989. Cloning of two tandem genes involved in degradation of 2,3-dihydroxybiphenyl to benzoic acid in the polychlorinated biphenyl-degrading soil bacterium *Pseudomonas* sp. strain KKS102. *J. Bacteriol.* **171:**2740–2747.

Knehr, M., H. Thomas, M. Arand, T. Gebel, H.-D. Zeller, and F. Oesch. 1993. Isolation and characterization of a cDNA encoding rat liver cytosolic epoxide hydrolase and its functional expression in *Escherichia coli*. *J. Biol. Chem.* **268:**17623–17627.

Larway, P., and W. C. Evans. 1965. Metabolism of quinol and resorcinol by soil Pseudomonads. *Biochem. J.* **95:**52P.

Latus, M., H.-J. Eberspächer, and F. Lingens. 1995. Purification and characterization of hydroxyquinol 1,2-dioxygenase from *Azotobacter* sp. strain GP1. *Appl. Environ. Microbiol.* **61:**2453–2460.

Lipke, H., and C. W. Kearns. 1959. DDT dehydrochlorinase. *J. Biol. Chem.* **234:**2123–2132.

Lorenz, W. W., R. O. McCann, M. Longiaru, and M. J. Cormier. 1991. Isolation and expression of a cDNA encoding *Renilla reniformis* luciferase. *Proc. Natl. Acad. Sci. USA* **88:**4438–4442.

Nagasawa, S., R. Kikuchi, Y. Nagata, M. Takagi, and M. Matsuo. 1993a. Aerobic mineralization of γ-HCH by *Pseudomonas paucimobilis* UT26. *Chemosphere* **26:**1719–1728.

Nagasawa, S., R. Kikuchi, Y. Nagata, M. Takagi, and M. Matsuo. 1993b. Stereochemical analysis of γ-HCH degradation by *Pseudomonas paucimobilis* UT26. *Chemosphere* **26:**1187–1201.

Nagasawa, T., H. Ohkishi, B. Kawasaki, H. Yamano, H. Hosono, Y. Tani, and H. Yamada. 1982. 3-Chloro-D-alanine chloride-lyase (deaminating) of *Pseudomonas putida* CR 1-1. *J. Biol. Chem.* **257:**13749–13756.

Nagata, Y., T. Hatta, R. Imai, K. Kimbara, M. Fukuda, K. Yano, and M. Takagi. 1993a. Purification and characterization of γ-hexachlorocyclohexane (γ-HCH) dehydrochlorinase (LinA) from *Pseudomonas paucimobilis*. *Biosci. Biotechnol. Biochem.* **57:**1582–1583.

Nagata, T., K. Miyauchi, S.-K. Suh, A. Futamura, and M. Takagi. 1996. Isolation and characterization of Tn*5*-induced mutants of *Sphingomonas paucimobilis* defective in 2,5-dichlorohydroquinone degradation. *Biosci. Biotechnol. Biochem.* **60:**689–691.

Nagata, Y., T. Nariya, R. Ohtomo, M. Fukuda, K. Yano, and M. Takagi. 1993b. Cloning and sequencing of a dehalogenase gene encoding an enzyme with hydrolase activity involved in the degradation of γ-hexachlorocyclohexane (γ-HCH) in *Pseudomonas paucimobilis*. *J. Bacteriol.* **175:**6403–6410.

Nagata, Y., R. Ohtomo, K. Miyauchi, M. Fukuda, K. Yano, and M. Takagi. 1994. Cloning and sequencing of a 2,5-dichloro-2,5-cyclohexadiene-1,4-diol dehydrogenase gene involved in the degradation of γ-hexachlorocyclohexane in *Pseudomonas paucimobilis*. *J. Bacteriol.* **176:**3117–3125.

Neidle, E., C. Hartnett, L. N. Ornston, A. Bairoch, M. Rekik, and S. Harayama. 1992. *cis*-Diol dehydrogenase encoded by the TOL pWW0 plasmid *xylL* gene and the *Acinetobacter calcoaceticus* chromosomal *benD* gene are members of the short-chain alcohol dehydrogenase superfamily. *Eur. J. Biochem.* **204:**113–120.

Nordlund, I., and V. Shingler. 1990. Nucleotide sequences of the *meta*-cleavage pathway enzymes 2-hydroxymuconic semialdehyde dehydrogenase and 2-hydroxymuconic semialdehyde hydrolase from *Pseudomonas* CF600. *Biochim. Biophys. Acta.* **1049:**227–230.

Ollis, D. L., E. Cheah, M. Cygler, B. Dijkstra, F. Frolow, S. M. Franken, M. Harel, S. J. Remington, I. Silman, J. Schrag, J. L. Sussman, K. H. G. Verschueren, and A. Goldman. 1992. The α/β hydrolase fold. *Protein Eng.* **5:**197–211.

Orser, C. S., J. Dutton, C. Lange, P. Jablonski, L. Xun, and M. Hargis. 1993a. Characterization of a *Flavobacterium* glutathione S-transferase gene involved in reductive dechlorination. *J. Bacteriol.* **175:**2640–2644.

Orser, C. S., C. C. Lange, L. Xun, T. C. Zahrt, and B. J. Schneider. 1993b. Cloning, sequencing analysis, and expression of the *Flavobacterium* pentachlorophenol-4-monooxygenase gene in *Escherichia coli*. *J. Bacteriol.* **175:**411–416.

Palleroni, N. J. 1984. Genus I. *Pseudomonas*, p. 141–199. *In* N. R. Krieg and J. G. Holt (ed.), *Bergey's Manual of Systematic Bacteriology*, vol. 1. The Williams & Wilkins Co., Baltimore.

Persson, B., M. Krook, and H. Jörnvall. 1991. Characteristics of short-chain alcohol dehydrogenases and related enzymes. *Eur. J. Biochem.* **200:**537–543.

Puente, X. S., and C. López-Otín. 1995. Cloning and expression analysis of a novel human serine hydrolase with sequence similarity to prokaryotic enzymes involved in the degradation of aromatic compounds. *J. Biol. Chem.* **270:**12926–12932.

Rossmann, M. G., A. Liljas, C.-I. Brändén, and L. J. Banaszak. 1975. Evolutionary and structural relationship among dehydrogenases, p. 61–102. *In* P. D. Boyer (ed.), *The Enzymes*, 3rd ed., vol. 11. Academic Press Inc., New York.

Senoo, K., and H. Wada. 1989. Isolation and identification of an aerobic γ-HCH-decomposing bacterium from soil. *Soil Sci. Plant Nutr.* **35:**79–87.

Spain, J. C., and D. T. Gibson. 1991. Pathway for biodegradation of *p*-nitrophenol in a *Moraxella* sp. *Appl. Environ. Microbiol.* **57:**812–819.

Suen, W.-C., and J. C. Spain. 1993. Cloning and characterization of *Pseudomonas* sp. strain DNT genes for 2,4-dinitrotoluene degradation. *J. Bacteriol.* **175:**1831–1837.

Uotila, J. 1993. Dehalogenases for polyhalogenated aromatic compounds in *Rhodococcus chlorophenolicus* PCP-1 and *Mycobacterium fortuitum* CG-2. Ph.D. thesis. University of Helsinki, Helsinki, Finland.

Uotila, J. S., V. H. Kitunen, T. Saastamoinen, T. Cotte, M. M. Häggblom, and M. S. Salkinoja-Salonen. 1992. Characterization of aromatic dehalogenases of *Mycobacterium fortuitum* CG-2. *J. Bacteriol.* **174:**5669–5675.

van der Meer, J. R., W. M. de Vos, S. Harayama, and A. J. B. Zehnder. 1992. Molecular mechanisms of genetic adaptation to xenobiotic compounds. *Microbiol. Rev.* **56:**677–694.

van der Meer, J. R., A. R. W. vanNeerven, E. J. deVries, W. M. deVos, and A. J. B. Zehnder. 1991. Cloning and characterization of plasmid-encoded genes for the degradation of 1,2-dichloro-, 1,4-dichloro-, and 1,2,4-trichlorobenzene of *Pseudomonas* sp. strain P51. *J. Bacteriol.* **173:**6–15.

Vershueren, K. H. G., S. M. Franken, H. J. Rozeboom, K. H. Kalk, and B. W. Dijkstra. 1993a. Refined X-ray structures of haloalkane dehalogenase at pH 6.2 and pH 8.2 and implications for the reaction mechanism. *J. Mol. Biol.* **232:**856–872.

Verschueren, K. H. G., F. Siljée, H. J. Rozeboom, K. H. Kalk, and B. W. Dijkstra. 1993b. Crystallographic analysis of the catalytic mechanism of haloalkane dehalogenase. *Nature* (London) **363:**693–698.

Zaborina, O., M. Latus, J. Eberspächer, L. A. Golovleva, and F. Lingens. 1995. Purification and characterization of 6-chlorohydroxyquinol 1,2-dioxygenase from *Streptomyces rochei* 303: comparison with an analogous enzyme from *Azotobacter* sp. strain GP1. *J. Bacteriol.* **177:**229–234.

Zylstra, G. J., and D. T. Gibson. 1989. Toluene degradation by *Pseudomonas putida* F1. *J. Biol. Chem.* **264:**14940–14946.

Molecular Biology of Pseudomonads
Edited by T. Nakazawa et al.

Chapter 7

Biodegradation of Chlorobenzoates

Dennis D. Focht

Chlorobenzoates are introduced into the environment as herbicides (2,3,6-trichlorobenzoate, dicamba, tricamba, and chloramiben) or as degradation products of polychlorinated biphenyls (PCBs). They are not priority pollutants, and many bacteria have been reported to utilize them as growth substrates. Consequently, their biodegradation in the environment has generally been accepted as a fait accompli. However, enrichment cultures of chlorobenzoate degraders, particularly dichlorobenzoate degraders, are not readily obtained, and the *clc* genes, which code for the traditional pathway of chlorobenzoate catabolism, are uncommon. Moreover, novel catabolic pathways not encoded by the *clc* genes were recently discovered. These developments raise the questions of how chlorobenzoates are actually decomposed in the environment.

PATHWAYS OF CHLOROBENZOATE METABOLISM

Conversion to Chlorocatechols and the *ortho*-Fission Pathway

The *ortho*-fission pathway involves rupture of chlorocatechols between the two hydroxyl groups brought about by catechol 1,2-dioxygenase with the formation of chlorinated *cis-cis* muconate. Dehalogenation occurs after lactonization. This pathway is the oldest known and the most studied, and it is covered in detail elsewhere (Parsek et al., this volume).

Hydrolytic Dehalogenation to Hydroxybenzoates

Hydrolytic dehalogenation was first described for *Pseudomonas* sp. strain CBS3 (Keil et al., 1981) and *Arthrobacter* sp. (Marks et al., 1984) and involves the nucleophilic displacement of chlorine by a hydroxyl. Molecular oxygen is not involved. The reaction is generally limited to 4-chlorobenzoate, although conversion of 3,4-dichlorobenzoate by successive hydrolytic dehalogenations to carboxybenzoquinone (Adriaens and Focht, 1991) has been reported.

Dennis D. Focht • Department of Soil and Environmental Sciences, University of California, Riverside, California 92521.

Reductive Dehalogenation

Reductive dehalogenation involves the displacement of an aryl chlorine by a hydrogen, possibly by a hydride intermediate. The best-characterized system involves a three-member consortium of obligate anaerobes and has been reviewed extensively by Mohn and Tiedje (1992). Although reductive dehalogenations are generally carried out under extreme reducing conditions, they have been observed during conversion of 2,3-dichlorobenzoate to 4-chlorocatechol by *Pseudomonas aeruginosa* JB2 (Hickey and Focht, 1990) and of 2,4-dichlorobenzoate to 4-chlorobenzoate by *Alcaligenes denitrificans* NTB-1 (van den Tweel et al., 1987).

Dioxygenolytic Dehalogenation

Dioxygenation of the aromatic ring at a chlorine-bearing carbon results in an unstable chlorohydrodiol that spontaneously eliminates HCl and forms the corresponding catechol directly. This reaction, common mostly to *o*-chlorobenzoates, differs from the oxidation of benzoate or of 3- or 4-chlorobenzoate by not requiring a dioldehydrogenase (Hernandez et al., 1991). A similar reaction involves the conversion of 3-chlorobenzoate to protocatechuate; the genes encoding this pathway have no similarity to the *clc* genes (Nakatsu and Wyndham, 1993).

o-CHLOROBENZOATE METABOLISM

o-Chlorobenzoate degraders differ from 3- and 4-chlorobenzoate degraders in having a dioxygenase that is distinctly different from the benzoate dioxygenase. In *Pseudomonas putida* P111, the *o*-chlorobenzoate dioxygenase is plasmid encoded, but the *clc* genes are chromosomally encoded (Brenner et al., 1993). Adaptation from *o*- to *m*-chlorobenzoates resulted in deletions of the plasmid and eventual loss of ability to grow on *o*-chlorobenzoates. The inability of *o*-chlorobenzoate-grown cells to grow on 3,5-dichlorobenzoate was attributed to their inability to induce a functional dioldehydrogenase (Hernandez et al., 1991). Recent characterization of the three-component *o*-chlorobenzoate dioxygenase in *P. aeruginosa* 142 indicates a striking similarity to the sequence homology of the biphenyl dioxygenase (Romanov and Hausinger, 1994).

THE PARADIGM OF CHLOROCATECHOL CATABOLISM

The basic pathways for the three isomeric monochlorobenzoates are shown in Fig. 1 through 3, and those for di- and trichlorobenzoates are shown in Table 1. 3-Chlorocatechol is a suicidal inactivator for catechol-2,3-dioxygenase (i.e., the *meta*-fission pathway) because of the formation of an acyl halide, which acetylates the enzyme (Bartles et al., 1984). Hence, the *ortho*-fission pathway is the preferred route. Although 4-chlorocatechol is processed through the *ortho*-fission pathway by bacteria having *clc* genes, recent studies (Arensdorf and Focht, 1994, 1995; Higson and Focht, 1992; McCullar et al., 1994) show that it can also be processed through the *meta*-fission pathway because an acyl halide is not formed (Fig. 4). Nevertheless, bacteria that utilize this pathway must be able to dehalogenate chloroacetate (or, more likely, the acetyl-coenzyme A ester), which is the final product formed from

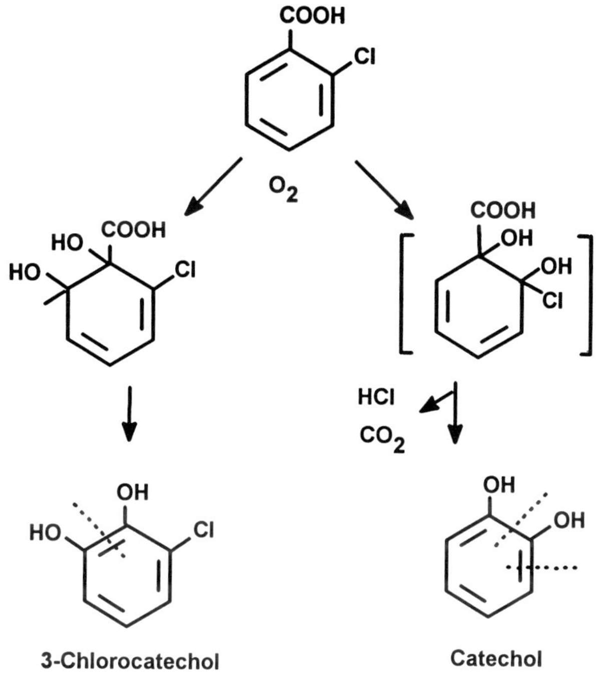

Figure 1. Degradation of 2-chlorobenzoate through the benzoate dioxygenase (left) and *o*-chlorobenzoate dioxygenase (right) pathways. Note the spontaneous loss of chloride and the formation of catechol by the latter mechanism.

the oxidation of chloroacetaldehyde or the decarboxylation of chloropyruvate. Failure to do this would cause disruption of the tricarboxylic acid cycle by incorporation of chlorinated intermediates or by direct inhibition of chloroacetate on *cis*-aconitase activity. Chloroacetate dehalogenases have been well characterized (Hardman and Slater, 1981; Kawasaki et al., 1981a, b): the conversion to glycolate is similar to the hydrolytic dehalogenation of 4-chlorobenzoate to 4-hydroxybenzoate in the require-

Table 1. Biodegradation of polychlorinated benzoates[a]

Substrate	Products prior to ring fission[b]	Dehalogenation[c]
2,3-DCBa	2,3-Dichloro-1-carboxy-1,6-diol→4-chlorocatechol	Reductive (2)
2,4-DCBa	4-CBa→	Reductive (2)
2,5-DCBa	4-Chlorocatechol→	Dioxygenolytic (2)
3,4-DCBa	3-Chloro-4-hydroxybenzoate→carboxy-3,4-benzoquinone→	Hydrolytic (4)
	via protocatechuate pathway	Hydrolytic (3)
3,5-DCBa	3,5-Dichloro-1-carboxy-1,2-diol→3,5-dichlorocatechol	Aliphatic (3, 5) (after ring fission)
2,3,5-TCBa	3,5-Dichlorocatechol	Dioxygenolytic (2)
2,3,6-TCBa	2,5-DCBa	Reductive (2)

[a] CBa, chlorobenzoate; DCBa, dichlorobenzoate; TCBa, trichlorobenzoate.
[b] Products are listed in sequential order of metabolism.
[c] Numbers in parentheses refer to the original position(s) of the chlorine substituent(s) on the aromatic ring (Focht, 1993).

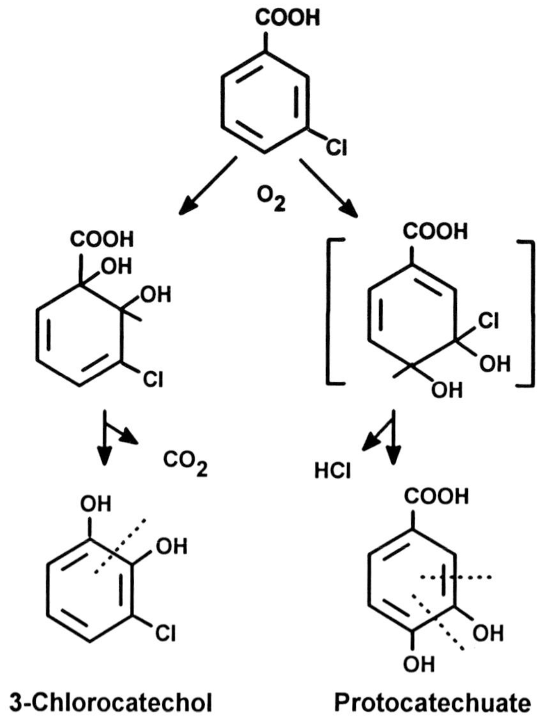

Figure 2. Degradation of 3-chlorobenzoate by the standard benzoate dioxygenase and chlorocatechol pathway (left) and by a novel dioxygenase (Nakatsu and Wyndham, 1993) that causes spontaneous loss of chloride and formation of protocatechuate (right).

ment for acetyl-coenzyme A and ATP (Copley and Crooks, 1992). Nevertheless, 39 of 40 biphenyl-utilizing bacteria that use the *meta*-fission pathway are unable to utilize chloroacetates as growth substrates (Hernandez et al., 1995).

The ability of bacteria to process all catechols, with the exception of 3-chlorocatechol, raises the possibility of chlorobenzoates being degraded through a productive *meta*-fission pathway. Moreover, chlorobenzoate degraders, namely, those having the *clc* genes, are not commonly found in soil or pristine aquatic environments. The two observations may be unrelated, yet a reductionist approach to the argument is germane in addressing how chlorobenzoates may be metabolized in the environment.

ARE *clc* GENES REALLY NECESSARY FOR DEGRADATION OF CHLOROBENZOATES IN THE ENVIRONMENT?

Let us begin from a historical perspective with 2,4-dichlorophenoxyacetic acid (2,4-D). This xenobiotic compound was the first to be studied in soil for its effects on soil microbiota (Martin, 1946) and microbiotic acclimation during degradation (Whiteside and Alexander, 1960). It was the first xenobiotic compound demonstrated to be clearly biodegradable to innocuous products of the tricarboxylic acid cycle (Duxbury et al., 1970; Tiedje and Alexander, 1969; Tiedje et al., 1969) and one of the first to provide the

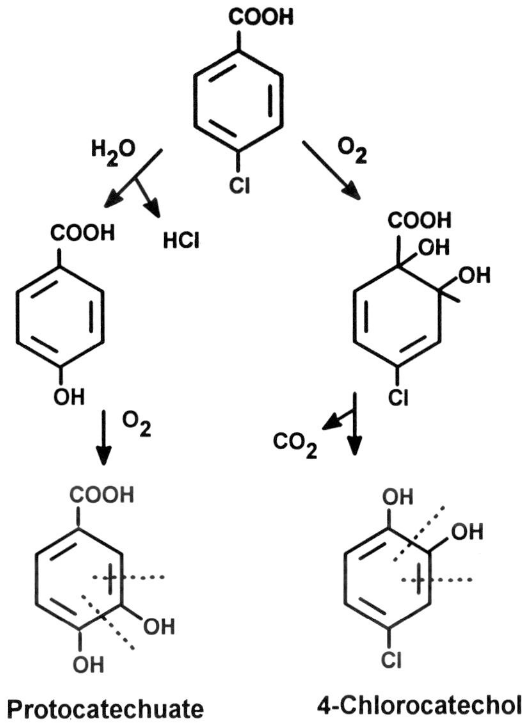

Figure 3. Degradation of 4-chlorobenzoate by a hydrolytic route (left) and by the benzoate dioxygenase pathway (right). Note that productive *ortho*- and *meta*-fission routes are possible in both cases.

molecular basis for the organization of catabolic genes (Pemberton et al., 1979). 2,4-D does not persist in the environment, yet enrichment cultures are extremely difficult to obtain by comparison to toluene or biphenyl degraders, which use the *meta*-fission pathway. For example, the first 2,4-D degrader described in the literature (Loos et al., 1967) required more than 1 year in enrichment culture before it could be isolated (J.-M. Bollag, personal communication). The *tfdA* and *tfdB* genes, which code for the removal of the ether linkage and the subsequent oxidation of 2,4-dichlorophenol to 3,5-dichlorocatechol, respectively, appear to be common in the environment and may actually code for lignin degradation. However, the *tfdCDEF* genes (the equivalent of *clc* genes) were not found among the same samples from soil, wastewater, and river water (Amy et al., 1985; Holben et al., 1992) but were common to wastewater (Amy et al., 1985). This finding suggests that the *clc* genes may have been recruited by genetic exchange and selection pressure, which would be greater in contaminated environments than in agricultural soils because of the higher concentration and influx of xenobiotic compounds in the former.

Thus, the possibility that 2,4-D is degraded through a productive *meta*-fission pathway cannot be precluded according to the scheme shown in Fig. 5. Note that distal *meta* fission of 3,5-dichlorocatechol, in contrast to proximal cleavage, does not generate an acyl halide. Somewhere overlooked in the dogma of chlorocatechol metabolism is a

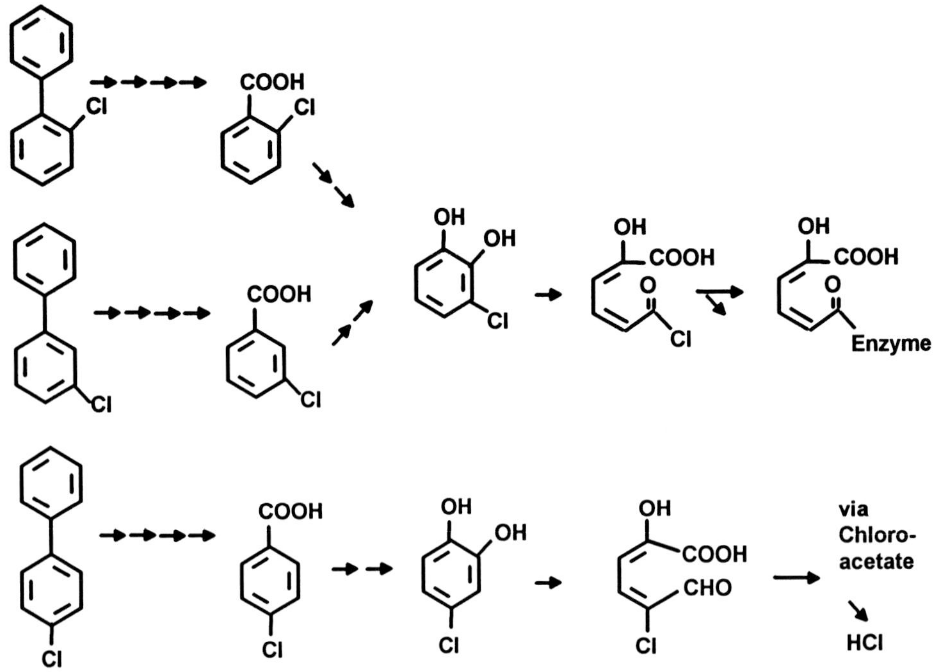

Figure 4. Exclusive *meta*-fission pathway used for growth of *P. putida* P166 on 2-, 3-, and 4-chlorobiphenyl. Redrawn from Arensdorf and Focht (1994).

study done 25 years ago by Horvath (1970), in which the distal *meta* cleavage of 3,5-dichlorocatechol was clearly demonstrated.

Alcaligenes eutrophus JMP 134, originally isolated by enrichment with 2,4-D (Don and Pemberton, 1981), metabolizes chlorocatechols through the *ortho*-fission pathway. However, the organism is induced for the *meta*-fission pathway by growth on methyl phenols (cresols) (Pieper et al., 1995). Although 2,4-D clearly induces the *ortho*-fission pathway, cells grown on *o*-cresol metabolize 3,5-dichlorocatechol through the *meta*-fission pathway (S.-C. Koh and M. V. McCullar, unpublished data).

A COMPLETE *meta*-FISSION PATHWAY FOR MINERALIZATION OF CHLOROBIPHENYLS

The same five-carbon fragment produced from hydrolysis of the ring fission product in the biphenyl pathway (Fig. 6) is also generated from the *meta*-fission pathway of catechol. The genes are identical to the *xyl* and *dmp* genes, which code for the metabolism of xylenes and dimethylphenols, respectively. The nomenclature adopted by Carrington et al. (1994) uses *bphH*, *bphI*, and *bphJ* for the genes coding for the steps shown in Fig. 6. Thus, the enzymes of this pathway might fortuitously process the chlorinated analogs of 4-chlorobenzoate catabolism.

Pseudomonas sp. strain 166 (Arensdorf and Focht, 1994) was recently shown to metabolize all three monochlorobiphenyls, including chlorobenzoates, exclusively through

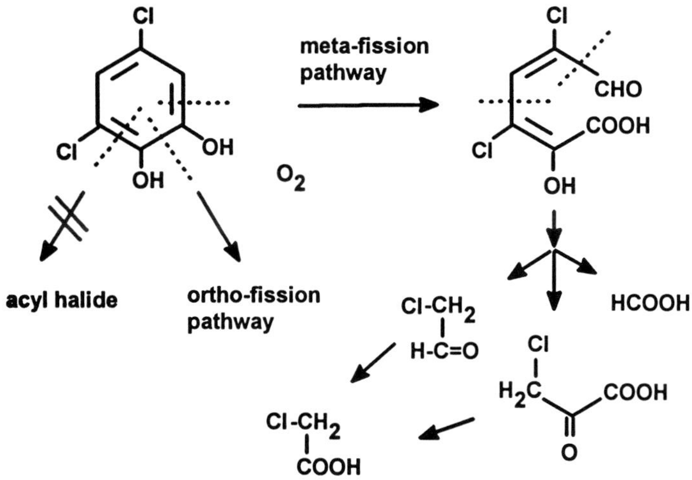

Figure 5. Possible ring fission pathways for 3,5-dichlorocatechol, a metabolite of 2,4-D and 3,5-dichlorobenzoate degradation. Note the central importance of chloroacetate when the *meta*-fission pathway is used.

a *meta*-fission pathway (Fig. 4). In the case of 4-chlorobenzoate, suicidal products were not formed, and viable cell counts for growth on biphenyl and on 4-chlorobiphenyl were comparable. Although the turbidities of all cultures during growth were comparable, viable cell counts were about 100-fold less in cultures grown on 2- or 3-chlorobiphenyl than in those grown on biphenyl because of the suicidal *meta* fission of 3-chlorocatechol. Nevertheless, a low steady-state density of viable cells (<10^8 cells ml^{-1}) was adequate to effect stoichiometric release of chloride from the growth substrate.

Pseudomonas acidovorans M3GY is a recombinant organism uniquely able to utilize 3,4′-dichlorobiphenyl as a sole carbon source, having acquired the complementary *bph* and *clc* genes and those encoding for chloroacetate degradation from three parental strains (McCullar et al., 1994). Although the organism metabolizes the growth substrate through

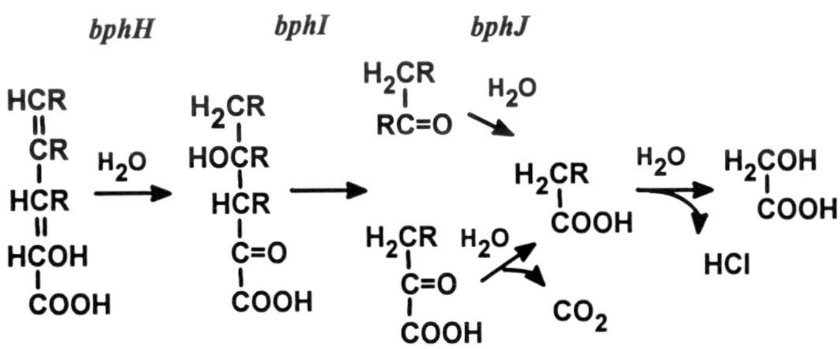

Figure 6. The *meta*-fission pathway for degradation of the five-carbon aliphatic acid produced through the benzoate and biphenyl pathways. The same pathway is used for *meta* fission of 4-chlorocatechol.

4-chlorobenzoate by using a *meta*-fission pathway exclusively, it nevertheless retains the *clc* genes and the ability to utilize 3-chlorobenzoate. A mutant strain lacking the *clc* genes and unable to utilize 3-chlorobenzoate produces 3-chlorocatechol from 3,4′-dichlorobiphenyl, which indicates that oxidation of both rings occurs (McCullar, 1995). The inability to detect 3-chlorobenzoate or 3-chlorocatechol in the wild-type recombinant strain was probably due to the rapid rates of conversion of these compounds. Hence, the *clc* genes may be quite relevant in removal of 3-chlorocatechol, which is a potent inhibitor of phenylcatechol dioxygenase (Adams et al., 1992).

GENETIC EXCHANGE IN SOIL AND THE RELEVANCE OF CHLOROBENZOATE DEGRADATION

Genetic exchange readily occurs in situ among introduced bacteria (Berg and Trevors, 1990; Chamier et al., 1993; Selvaratnam and Gealt, 1992) and among indigenous strains (Fulthorpe and Wyndham, 1989; Kinkle et al., 1993; Pertsova et al., 1984). Fulthorpe and Wyndham (1989, 1991) showed that the *cba* region of pBR60, which codes for 3-chlorobenzoate metabolism, was transferred to the aquatic community from the inoculant, which did not survive after disappearance of the substrate. Genetic exchange could be advantageous to biodegradation of recalcitrant compounds in the environment, because it allows for more rapid evolution of microorganisms than could occur by mutation alone. Thus, inoculation of soil with the "missing genes" (e.g., *clc* genes) may give rise to recombinants that contain the two complementary catabolic pathways.

The enhanced mineralization of PCBs in soil brought about by the addition of biphenyl was demonstrated 10 years ago in Altamont soil (Brunner et al., 1985; Focht and Brunner, 1985). The apparent lag in $^{14}CO_2$ production in comparison to CO_2 production from biphenyl was attributed to the succession of populations of chlorobenzoate degraders. However, it has since been observed that, in contrast to biphenyl degraders (Bedard et al., 1986; Furukawa et al., 1978; Hernandez et al., 1995), chlorobenzoate degraders are not indigenous soil bacteria (Focht and Shelton, 1987; Fulthorpe and Wyndham, 1989; Hickey et al., 1993; Pertsova et al., 1984) and that chlorobenzoates accumulate during in situ bioremediation of PCBs (Flanagan and May, 1993). Moreover, inoculation of Altamont soil with *P. putida* P111 and *P. aeruginosa* JB2, both of which harbor the *clc* genes, effected significantly higher levels of $^{14}CO_2$ than those in uninoculated soils (Hickey et al., 1993). This increase in mineralization of PCBs was attributed to the formation of recombinant strains having both the *bph* and the *clc* genes. Recent work has established that the recombinants are the result of genetic exchange from indigenous biphenyl utilizers to the chlorobenzoate inoculants and that the Altamont soil does not contain indigenous chlorobenzoate utilizers or DNA that hybridizes to the *clc* gene probe (Focht et al., submitted). Although a complete *meta*-fission pathway for PCB degradation may occur in the soil, this pathway may not be as efficacious as one coupled with the *ortho*-fission pathway.

REFERENCES

Adams, R. H., C. M. Huang, F. K. Higson, V. Brenner, and D. D. Focht. 1992. Construction of a 3-chlorobiphenyl-utilizing recombinant from an intergeneric mating. *Appl. Environ. Microbiol.* **58:**647–654.

Adriaens, P., and D. D. Focht. 1991. Cometabolism of 3,4-dichlorobenzoate by *Acinetobacter* sp. strain 4-CB1. *Appl. Environ. Microbiol.* **57:**173–179.

Amy, P. S., J. W. Schulke, L. M. Frazier, and R. J. Seidler. 1985. Characterization of aquatic bacteria and cloning of genes specifying partial degradation of 2,4-dichlorophenoxyacetic acid. *Appl. Environ. Microbiol.* **49:**1237–1245.

Arensdorf, J. J., and D. D. Focht. 1994. Formation of chlorocatechol *meta*-cleavage products by a pseudomonad during metabolism of monochlorobiphenyls. *Appl. Environ. Microbiol.* **60:**2884–2889.

Arensdorf, J. J., and D. D. Focht. 1995. A *meta*-cleavage pathway for 4-chlorobenzoate, an intermediate in the metabolism of 4-chlorobiphenyl by *Pseudomonas cepacia* P166. *Appl. Environ. Microbiol.* **61:**443–447.

Bartles, I., H.-J. Knackmuss, and W. Reineke. 1984. Suicide inactivation of catechol-2,3-dioxygenase from *Pseudomonas putida* MT-2 by 3-halocatechols. *Appl. Environ. Microbiol.* **47:**500–505.

Bedard, D. L., R. Unterman, L. H. Bopp, M. J. Brennan, M. L. Haberl, and C. Johnson. 1986. Rapid assay for screening and characterizing microorganisms for the ability to degrade polychlorinated biphenyls. *Appl. Environ. Microbiol.* **51:**761–768.

Berg, G., and J. T. Trevors. 1990. Bacterial conjugation between *Escherichia coli* and *Pseudomonas* spp. donor and recipient cells in soil. *J. Ind. Microbiol.* **5:**79–84.

Brenner, V., B. S. Hernandez, and D. D. Focht. 1993. Variation in chlorobenzoate catabolism by *Pseudomonas putida* P111 as a consequence of genetic alterations. *Appl. Environ. Microbiol.* **59:**2790–2794.

Brunner, W., F. H. Sutherland, and D. D. Focht. 1985. Enhanced biodegradation of polychlorinated biphenyls in soil by analog enrichment and bacterial inoculation. *J. Environ. Qual.* **14:**324–328.

Carrington, B., A. Lowe, L. E. Shaw, and P. A. Williams. 1994. The lower pathway operon for benzoate catabolism in biphenyl-utilizing *Pseudomonas* sp. strain IC and the nucleotide sequence of the *bphE* gene for catechol 2,3-dioxygenase. *Microbiology* **140:**499–508.

Chamier, B., M. G. Lorenz, and W. Wackernagel. 1993. Natural transformation of *Acinetobacter calcoaceticus* by plasmid DNA adsorbed on sand and groundwater aquifer material. *Appl. Environ. Microbiol.* **59:**1662–1667.

Copley, S. D., and G. P. Crooks. 1992. Enzymic dehalogenation of 4-chlorobenzoyl coenzyme-A in *Acinetobacter* sp. strain 4-CB1. *Appl. Environ. Microbiol.* **58:**1385–1387.

Don, R. H., and J. M. Pemberton. 1981. Properties of six pesticide degradation plasmids isolated from *Alcaligenes paradoxus* and *Alcaligenes eutrophus*. *J. Bacteriol.* **145:**681–686.

Duxbury, J. M., J. M. Tiedje, M. Alexander, and J. E. Dawson. 1970. 2,4-D metabolism: enzymatic conversion of chloromaleylacetic acid to succinic acid. *J. Agric. Food Chem.* **18:**199–201.

Flanagan, W. P., and R. J. May. 1993. Metabolite detection as evidence for naturally occurring aerobic PCB biodegradation in Hudson River sediments. *Environ. Sci. Technol.* **27:**2207–2212.

Focht, D. D. 1993. Microbial degradation of chlorinated biphenyls, p. 341–407. *In* J.-M. Bollag and G. Stozky (ed.), *Soil Biochemistry*, vol. 8. Marcel Dekker, New York.

Focht, D. D., and W. Brunner. 1985. Kinetics of biphenyl and polychlorinated biphenyl metabolism in soil. *Appl. Environ. Microbiol.* **50:**1058–1063.

Focht, D. D., D. B. Searles, and S.-C. Koh. Genetic exchange in soil between introduced chlorobenzoate degraders and indigenous biphenyl degraders. Submitted for publication.

Focht, D. D., and D. Shelton. 1987. Growth kinetics of *Pseudomonas alcaligenes* C-O relative to inoculation and 3-chlorobenzoate metabolism in soil. *Appl. Environ. Microbiol.* **53:**1846–1849.

Fulthorpe, R. R., and R. C. Wyndham. 1989. Survival and activity of a 3-chlorobenzoate-catabolic genotype in a natural system. *Appl. Environ. Microbiol.* **55:**1584–1590.

Fulthorpe, R. R., and R. C. Wyndham. 1991. Transfer and expression of the catabolic plasmid pBRC60 in wild bacterial recipients in a freshwater ecosystem. *Appl. Environ. Microbiol.* **57:**1546–1553.

Furukawa, K., F. Matsumura, and K. Tonomura. 1978. *Alcaligenes* and *Acinetobacter* strains capable of degrading polychlorinated biphenyls. *Agric. Biol. Chem.* **42:**543–548.

Hardman, D. J., and J. H. Slater. 1981. Dehalogenases in soil bacteria. *J. Gen. Microbiol.* **123:**117–128.

Hernandez, B. S., J. J. Arensdorf, and D. D. Focht. 1995. Catabolic characteristics of biphenyl-utilizing isolates which cometabolize PCBs. *Biodegradation* **6:**75–82.

Hernandez, B. S., F. K. Higson, R. Kondrat, and D. D. Focht. 1991. Metabolism of and inhibition by chlorobenzoates in *Pseudomonas putida* P111. *Appl. Environ. Microbiol.* **57:**3361–3366.

Hickey, W. J., and D. D. Focht. 1990. Degradation of mono-, di-, and trihalogenated benzoic acids by *Pseudomonas aeruginosa* JB2. *Appl. Environ. Microbiol.* **56:**3842–3850.

Hickey, W. J., D. B. Searles, and D. D. Focht. 1993. Enhanced mineralization of polychlorinated biphenyls in soil inoculated with chlorobenzoate-degrading bacteria. *Appl. Environ. Microbiol.* **59:**1194–1200.

Higson, F. K., and D. D. Focht. 1992. Utilization of 3-chloro 2-methylbenzoic acid by *Pseudomonas cepacia* MB2 through the *meta*-fission pathway. *Appl. Environ. Microbiol.* **58:**2501–2504.

Holben, W. E., B. M. Schroeter, V. G. M. Calabrese, R. H. Olsen, J. K. Kukor, A. E. Biederbeck, A. E. Smith, and J. M. Tiedje. 1992. Gene probe analysis of soil microbial populations selected by amendment with 2,4-dichlorophenoxyacetic acid. *Appl. Environ. Microbiol.* **58:**3941–3969.

Horvath, R. S. 1970. Co-metabolism of methyl- and chloro-substituted catechols by an *Achromobacter* sp. possessing a new *meta*-cleaving oxygenase. *Biochem. J.* **119:**871–876.

Kawasaki, H., N. Tone, and K. Tonomura. 1981a. Plasmid-determined dehalogenation of haloacetates in *Moraxella* species. *Agric. Biol. Chem.* **45:**29–34.

Kawasaki, H., N. Tone, and K. Tonomura. 1981b. Purification and properties of haloacetate halidohydrolase specified by plasmid from *Moraxella* sp. strain B. *Agric. Biol. Chem.* **45:**35–42.

Keil, H., U. Klages, and F. Lingens. 1981. Degradation of 4-chlorobenzoate by *Pseudomonas* sp. CBS3: induction of catabolic enzymes. *FEMS Microbiol. Lett.* **10:**213–215.

Kinkle, B. K., M. J. Sadowsky, E. L. Schmidt, and W. C. Koskinen. 1993. Plasmids pJP4 and r68.45 can be transferred between populations of *Bradyrhizobia* in nonsterile soil. *Appl. Environ. Microbiol.* **59:**1762–1766.

Loos, M. A., J.-M. Bollag, and M. Alexander. 1967. Phenoxyacetate herbicide detoxication by bacterial enzymes. *J. Agric. Food Chem.* **15:**858–863.

Marks, T. S., A. R. W. Smith, and A. V. Quirk. 1984. Degradation of 4-chlorobenzoic acid by *Arthrobacter* sp. *Appl. Environ. Microbiol.* **48:**1020–1025.

Martin, J. P. 1946. The hormone weed killer 2,4-D. *Calif. Citrogr.* **31:**248, 264–265.

McCullar, M. V. 1995. Biodegradation of 3,4′-dichlorobiphenyl by recombinant bacterium *Pseudomonas acidovorans* M3GY. Ph.D. thesis. University of California, Riverside.

McCullar, M. V., V. Brenner, R. H. Adams, and D. D. Focht. 1994. Construction of a novel polychlorinated biphenyl-degrading bacterium: utilization of 3,4′-dichlorobiphenyl by *Pseudomonas acidovorans* M3GY. *Appl. Environ. Microbiol.* **60:**3833–3839.

Mohn, W. W., and J. M. Tiedje. 1992. Microbial reductive dehalogenation. *Microbiol. Rev.* **56:**482–507.

Nakatsu, C. H., and R. C. Wyndham. 1993. Cloning and expression of the transposable chlorobenzoate-3,4-dioxygenase genes of *Alcaligenes* sp. strain BR60. *Appl. Environ. Microbiol.* **59:**3625–3633.

Pemberton, J. M., B. Corney, and R. H. Don. 1979. Evolution and spread of pesticide degrading ability among soil micro-organisms, p. 287–300. *In* K. N. Timmis and A. Pühler (ed.), *Plasmids of Medical, Environmental, and Commercial Importance.* Elsevier/North-Holland Biomedical Press, Amsterdam.

Pertsova, R. N., F. Kunc, and L. A. Golovleva. 1984. Degradation of 3-chlorobenzoate in soil by pseudomonads carrying biodegradative plasmids. *Folia Microbiol.* **29:**242–247.

Pieper, D. H., K. Stadler-Fritzsche, H.-J. Knackmuss, and K. N. Timmis. 1995. Formation of dimethylmuconolactones from dimethylphenols by *Alcaligenes eutrophus* JMP 134. *Appl. Environ. Microbiol.* **61:**2159–2165.

Romanov, V., and R. P. Hausinger. 1994. *Pseudomonas aeruginosa* 142 uses a three-component ortho-halobenzoate 1,2-dioxygenase for metabolism of 2,4-dichloro- and 2-chlorobenzoate. *J. Bacteriol.* **176:**3368–3374.

Selvaratnam, S., and M. A. Gealt. 1992. Recombinant plasmid gene transfer in amended soil. *Water Res.* **26:**39–43.

Tiedje, J. M., and M. Alexander. 1969. Enzymatic cleavage of the ether bond of 2,4-dichlorophenoxyacetate. *J. Agric. Food Chem.* **17:**1080–1084.

Tiedje, J. M., J. M. Duxbury, M. Alexander, and J. E. Dawson. 1969. 2,4-D metabolism: pathway of degradation of chlorocatechols by *Arthrobacter* sp. *J. Agric. Food Chem.* **17:**1021–1026.

van den Tweel, W. J. J., J. B. Kok, and J. A M. de Bont. 1987. Reductive dechlorination of 2,4-dichlorobenzoate to 4-chlorobenzoate and hydrolytic dehalogenation of 4-chloro-, 4-bromo-, and 4-iodobenzoate by *Alcaligenes denitrificans* NTB-1. *Appl. Environ. Microbiol.* **53:**810–815.

Whiteside, J. S., and M. Alexander. 1960. Measurement of microbiological effects of herbicides. *Weeds* **8:**204–213.

Molecular Biology of Pseudomonads
Edited by T. Nakazawa et al.

Chapter 8

Construction of Hybrid Operons Conferring Expanded Capability for Degrading Aromatic Hydrocarbons and Chlorinated Compounds

Kensuke Furukawa, Nobutada Kimura, Ryo Iwakiri, Akito Nishi, and Akiko Suyama

Soil bacteria have adaptively evolved by modifying key enzymes to utilize a variety of aromatic compounds that are present in the environment (van der Meer et al., 1992; Wyndham et al., 1994). Recent studies revealed that dioxygenases involved in the initial oxygenation of aromatic hydrocarbons are multicomponent enzymes; their corresponding subunits show high degrees of homology and seem to have a common ancestry (Harayama et al., 1992). It is also known that large subunits of terminal dioxygenase (an iron-sulfur protein) are critically involved in the substrate specificity of aromatic ring dioxygenases (Furukawa et al., 1993). In this context, we have tried to construct hybrid dioxygenases by replacing subunit components of structurally similar but functionally different enzymes. Here we describe recombinant strains expressing composite dioxygenases that show wide ranges and higher degrees of degradation capability for various aromatic hydrocarbons and chlorinated compounds such as trichloroethylene (TCE).

COMPONENTS RESPONSIBLE FOR SUBSTRATE SPECIFICITY IN THE CATABOLISM OF BIPHENYL AND TOLUENE

Biphenyl-utilizing bacteria are widely distributed in the environment; they degrade polychlorinated biphenyls (PCBs) by cometabolism (Furukawa, 1982, 1994; Bedard et al., 1986). Several biphenyl catabolic genes (*bph*) have been cloned, and the sequences of *bph* genes coding for initial oxidation have been determined for several *Pseudomonas* strains (Taira et al., 1992; Erickson and Mondello, 1992; Kikuchi et al., 1994) and more recently for a gram-positive *Rhodococcus* strain (Masai et al., 1995). One such strain, *Pseudomonas pseudoalcaligenes* KF707, possesses a chromosomal *bph* operon consisting of *bphA1 bphA2 bphA3 bphA4 bphB bphC bphX0 bphX1 bphX2 bphX3 bphD* (Fig. 1),

Kensuke Furukawa, Nobutada Kimura, Ryo Iwakiri, Akito Nishi, and Akiko Suyama • Department of Agricultural Chemistry, Kyushu University, Hakozaki, Fukuoka 812-81, Japan.

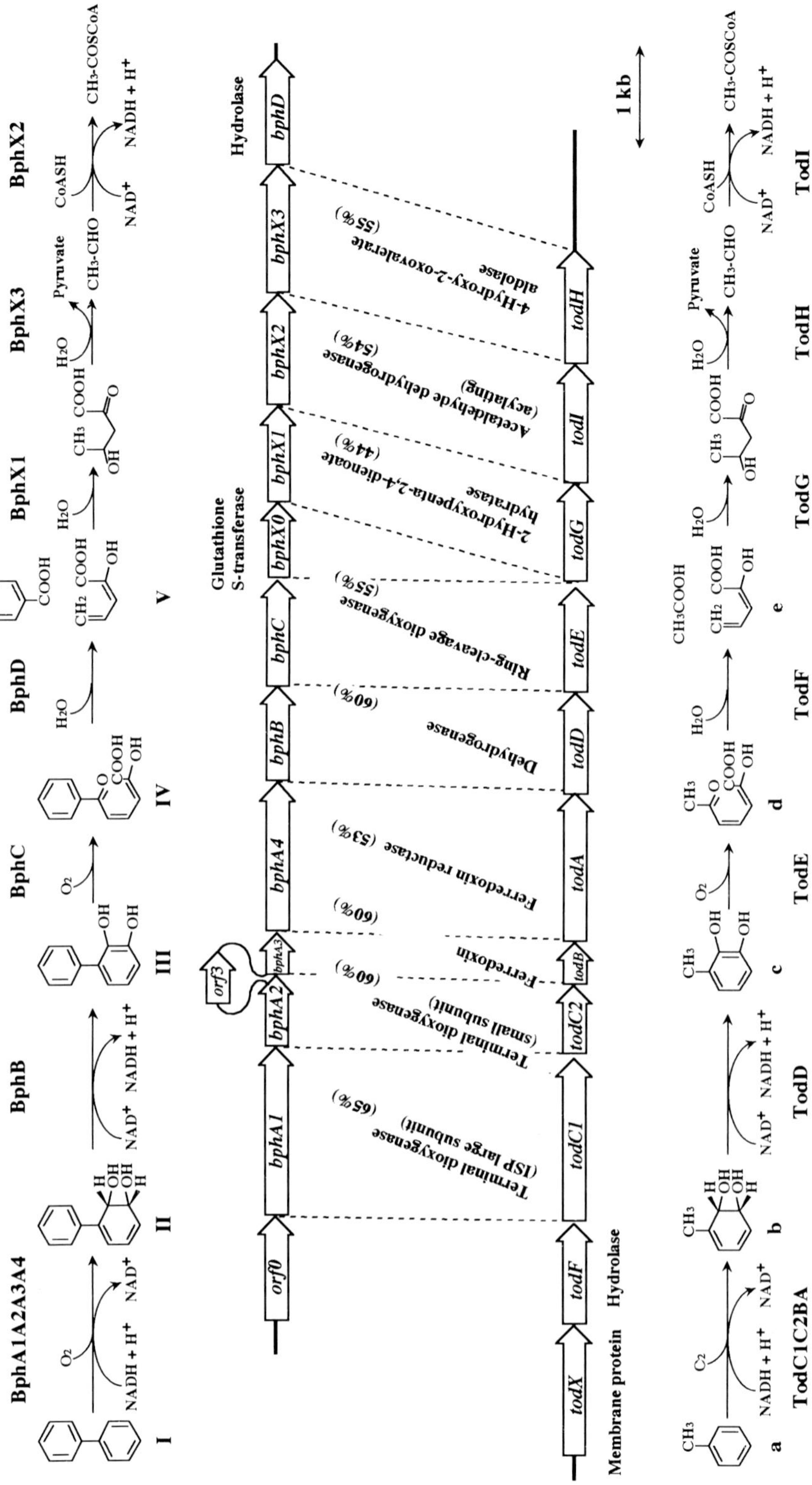

BphA1A2A3A4
BphB
BphC
BphD
BphX1
BphX3
BphX2
I
II
III
IV
V
Hydrolase
Glutathione S-transferase
orf0
bphA1
bphA2
orf3
bphA3
bphA4
bphB
bphC
bphX0
bphX1
bphX2
bphX3
bphD
Terminal dioxygenase (ISP large subunit) (65%)
Terminal dioxygenase (small subunit)
Ferredoxin (60%)
Ferredoxin reductase (53%)
Dehydrogenase (60%)
Ring-cleavage dioxygenase (55%)
2-Hydroxypenta-2,4-dienoate hydratase (44%)
Acetaldehyde dehydrogenase (acylating) (54%)
4-Hydroxy-2-oxovalerate aldolase (55%)
1 kb
todX
todF
todC1
todC2
todB
todA
todD
todE
todG
todI
todH
Membrane protein
Hydrolase
a
b
c
d
e
TodC1C2BA
TodD
TodE
TodF
TodG
TodH
TodI

where *bphA1 bphA2 bphA3 bphA4* encodes a multicomponent biphenyl dioxygenase: *bphA1* codes for a large subunit of terminal dioxygenase, *bphA2* codes for a small subunit of terminal dioxygenase, *bphA3* codes for ferredoxin, and *bphA4* codes for ferredoxin reductase (Taira et al., 1992). Biphenyl dihydrodiol (2,3-dihydroxy-4-phenylhexa-4,6-diene [compound II in Fig. 1]) dehydrogenase is encoded by *bphB; bphC* encodes 2,3-dihydroxybiphenyl (compound III in Fig. 1) dioxygenase, and *bphD* encodes a 2-hydroxy-6-oxo-6-phenylhexa-2,4-dienoate (compound IV in Fig. 1) hydrolase. The *bphX1 bphX2 bphX3* cluster is involved in the conversion of 2-hydroxy-penta-2,4-dienoate (compound V in Fig. 1) to acetyl-coenzyme A, as in *Pseudomonas* sp. strain LB400 (Hofer et al., 1994). Also *bphX0* is nearly identical to *bphK* of LB400, which encodes gluthathione *S*-transferase.

Toluene-utilizing *Pseudomonas putida* F1 possesses a toluene catabolic operon (*tod*) that is similar to the KF707 *bph* operon in terms of gene organization and the nucleotide sequence of the corresponding genes (Zylstra and Gibson, 1989; Wang et al., 1995) (Fig. 1). Part of the *tod* operon contains *todF todC1 todC2 todB todA todD todE*, where the cluster *todC1 todC2 todB todA* encodes a multicomponent toluene dioxygenase: *todC1* codes for a large subunit of terminal dioxygenase, *todC2* codes for a small subunit of terminal dioxygenase, *todB* codes for ferredoxin, and *todA* codes for ferredoxin reductase. *todD* encodes toluene dihydrodiol dehydrogenase, and *todF* encodes the toluene *meta*-cleavage compound hydrolase. The amino acid sequences of the corresponding enzymes encoded by the *bph* and *tod* operons are approximately 60% identical. In contrast, *bphD* and *todF*, which encode the respective hydrolases, have only 35.1% identity (Hirose et al., 1994).

The biphenyl-utilizing strain KF707 does not grow on toluene as a sole source of carbon and energy (Furukawa et al., 1993). In order to investigate the inability of KF707 to utilize toluene, *Escherichia coli* JM109 cells carrying *bphA1 bphA2 bphA3 bphA4 bphB bphC* were incubated with toluene: no toluene was converted. The same strain, however, converted toluene-*cis*-dihydrodiol (1-methyl-2,3-dihydroxy-4,6-cyclodiene [compound b in Fig. 1] into the ring *meta*-cleavage compound. These results indicate that BphA (biphenyl dioxygenase) cannot initiate the conversion of toluene but that BphB (biphenyl dihydrodiol dehydrogenase) can convert toluene-*cis*-dihydrodiol to 3-methylcatechol (compound c in Fig. 1), which is subsequently cleaved by BphC (2,3-dihydroxybiphenyl dioxygenase) to form 2-hydroxy-6-oxo-hepta-2,4-dienoic acid (compound d in Fig. 1). However, BphD (2-hydroxy-6-oxo-6-phenylhexa-2,4-dienoic acid hydrolase) failed to hydrolyze 2-hydroxy-6-oxo-hepta-2,4-dienoic acid (compound IV in Fig. 1). On the other hand, toluene-utilizing *P. putida* F1 did not grow on biphenyl but was able to convert biphenyl into the *meta*-cleavage 2-hydroxy-6-oxo-6-phenylhexa-2,4-dienoic acid, indicating that toluene dioxygenase (TodC1 TodC2 TodB TodA), toluene dihydrodiol dehydrogenase (TodD), and 3-methylcatechol dioxygenase (TodE) are all active for the conversion of biphenyl to 2-hydroxy-6-oxo-6-phenylhexa-2,4-dienoic acid but that 2-hydroxy-6-oxo-hepta-2,4-dienoic acid hydrolase (TodF) did not attack 2-

Figure 1. Comparison of the *bph* operon of *P. pseudoalcaligenes* KF707 and the *tod* operon of *P. putida* F1. Data are from Zylstra and Gibson (1989), Taira et al. (1992), and Wang et al. (1995). The roles of *orf-0* and *orf-3* in the KF707 *bph* operon are unknown. CoASH, coenzyme A; ISP, iron sulfur protein.

hydroxy-6-oxo-6-phenylhexa-2,4-dienoic acid. On the basis of functional analyses of *bph* and *tod* genes, we introduced a *tod* gene component(s) into KF707 or *bph* genes into F1 in *trans*. The introduction of *todC1 todC2* or even *todC1* alone via a broad-host-range plasmid vector pML122 (Labes et al., 1990) allowed KF707 to grown on toluene (Fig. 2) (Furukawa et al., 1993). On the other hand, the introduction of *bphD* (the KF707 2-hydroxy-6-oxo-6-phenylhexa-2,4-dienoic acid hydrolase gene) into the toluene utilizer *P. putida* F1 permitted growth on biphenyl. These results indicate that the large subunits of terminal dioxygenases (encoded by *bphA1* and *todC1*) and the ring *meta*-cleavage compound hydrolases (encoded by *bphD* and *todF*) are critically involved in their discrete metabolic specificities.

CONSTRUCTION AND FUNCTIONAL ANALYSIS OF Bph-Tod HYBRID DIOXYGENASES

Since biphenyl dioxygenase and toluene dioxygenase show a high degree of sequence homology (approximately 60%) in spite of their discrete substrate specificity, we constructed hybrid *bph-tod* gene clusters by replacing the genes for large and small subunits of terminal dioxygenases (Hirose et al., 1994). *E. coli* cells expressing the hybrid dioxygenases TodC1–BphA2-BphA3-BphA4, TodC1-TodC2–BphA3-BphA4, and BphA1–TodC2–BphA3-BphA4 were able to convert various aromatic hydrocarbons, in-

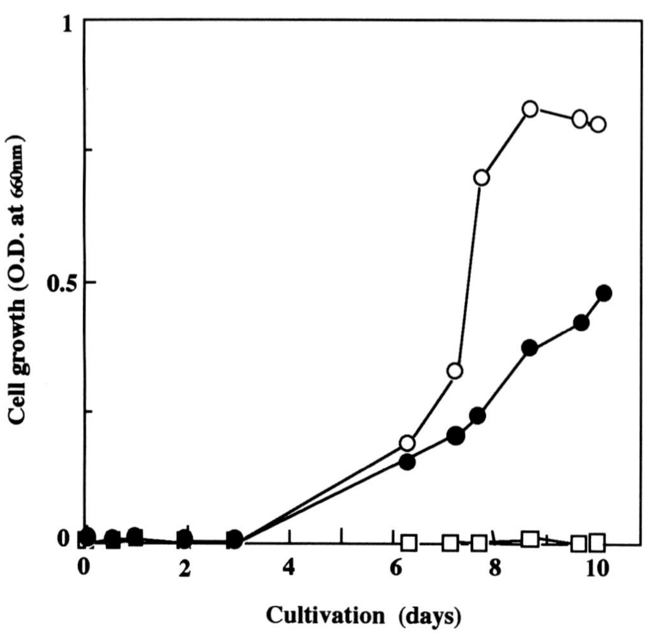

Figure 2. Growth of biphenyl-degrading *P. pseudoalcaligenes* KF707 recombinant strains on toluene. Results shown are for KF707 without plasmid (□), KF707(pMLCl carrying *todC1*) (●), and KF707(pMLC1C2 carrying *todC1 todC2*) (○). O.D., optical density.

cluding benzene, toluene, naphthalene, and biphenyl (Fig. 2). These results indicate that the terminal dioxygenase composed of TodC1-BphA2 and BphA1-TodC2 forms functionally active dioxygenases associated with BphA3 (ferredoxin) and BphA4 (ferredoxin reductase). The hybrid dioxygenase composed of either TodC1–BphA2-BphA3-BphA4 or TodC1-TodC2–BphA3-BphA4 showed a wide range of substrate specificities similar to those of the original toluene dioxygenase. On the other hand, the hybrid BphA1–TodC2–BphA3-BphA4 showed oxidative activities for the same compounds, but the extent of oxidation was low and varied, depending on the substrates (Fig. 3).

TCE has been recognized as one of the most significant environmental pollutants in soil and groundwater. A recent study showed that TCE could be degraded by aerobic bacteria (Nelson et al., 1987). Wackett and Gibson (1988) showed that toluene dioxygenase of *P. putida* F1 plays a role in the degradation of TCE. This was confirmed with *E. coli* carrying the structural genes (*todC1 todC2 todB todA*) for toluene dioxygenase (Zylstra

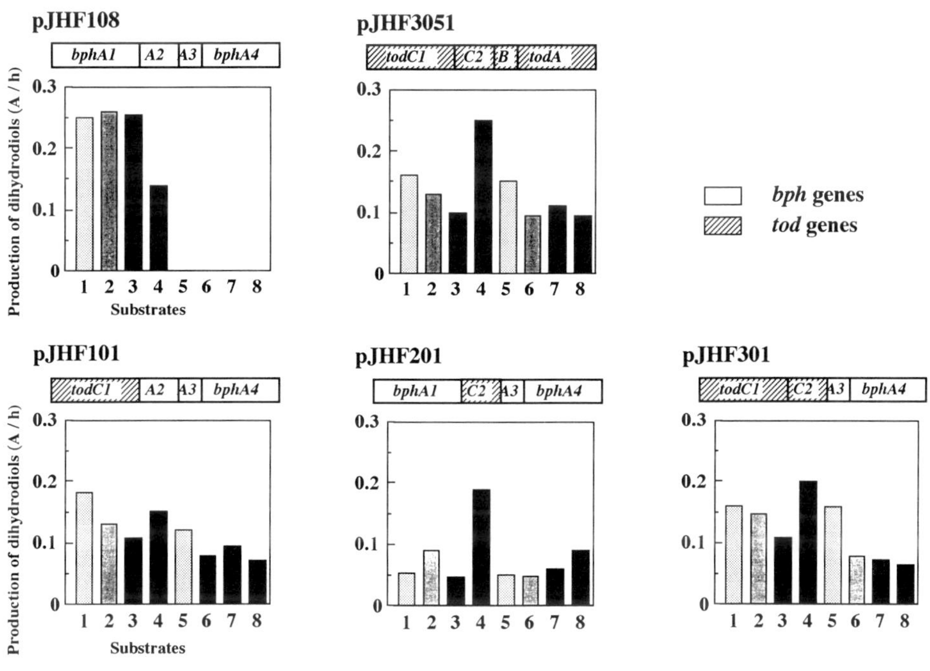

Figure 3. Production of dihydrodiol compounds from biphenyl, benzene, and their derivatives by *E. coli* recombinants. Cells (absorbance at 660 nm = 1.0) carrying pJHF108 (containing *bphA1 bphA2 bphA3 bphA4*), pJHF3051 (containing *todC1 todC2 todB todA*), pJHF101 (containing *todC1 bphA2 bphA3 bphA4*), pJHF201 (containing *bphA1 todC2 bphA3 bphA4*), and pJHF301 (containing *todC1 todC2 bphA3 bphA4*) were incubated with various aromatic hydrocarbons at final concentrations of 0.5 mM. The increase in absorbance (A) derived from the production of the respective dihydrodiol compounds was measured. Absorbances: bar 1, 303 nm for biphenyl; bar 2, 306 nm for 4-chlorobiphenyl; bar 3, 307 nm for 4-methylbiphenyl; bar 4, 259 nm for diphenylmethane; bar 5, 262 nm for naphthalene; bar 6, 275 nm for toluene; bar 7, 275 nm for *p*-chlorotoluene; bar 8, 260 nm for benzene.

et al., 1989). Since we have constructed *E. coli* strains carrying hybrid *bph-tod* genes, we examined the degradation of TCE (Furukawa et al., 1994). Most interestingly, *E. coli* cells expressing a hybrid TodC1–BphA2-BphA3-BphA4 dioxygenase degraded TCE much faster than did *E. coli* cells expressing the original toluene dioxygenase (TodC1-TodC2-TodB-TodA) or the original biphenyl dioxygenase (BphA1-BphA2-BphA3-BphA4). *E. coli* cells expressing TodC1-TodC2–BphA3-BphA4 showed intermediate activity for TCE degradation. However, BphA1–TodC2–BphA3-BphA4–expressing cells failed to degrade TCE.

The reason for the wide catabolic capabilities of various hybrid dioxygenases remains to be elucidated. Protein analysis in native polyacrylamide gels showed that TodC1-BphA2 is formed as a heterodimer, while TodC1-TodC2 and BphA1-TodC2 are associated as heterotetramers (Fig. 4). It will be interesting to learn whether heterodimeric structures enhance the affinity between enzyme and substrates or an efficient electron flow from NADH.

ENGINEERING *PSEUDOMONAS* BY INTEGRATING *todC1* INTO CHROMOSOMAL *bph* OPERONS

Since *E. coli* expressing the hybrid dioxygenase genes *todC1, bphA2, bphA3*, and *bphA4* showed a wide substrate range for degradation of various aromatic hydrocarbons and TCE, we attempted to introduce *todC1* into biphenyl-utilizing *Pseudomonas* strains. For this purpose, the *orf-0, todC1, bphA2, bphA3*, and *bphA4* genes were subcloned into a suicide vector, pSUP102 (Simon et al., 1989), and the resultant plasmid, pSUP102-*bph/tod*, was introduced into *E. coli* S17-1 (Simon et al., 1983) (Fig. 5). Strain S17-1 carrying pSUP102-*bph/tod* and the parent strain, biphenyl-utilizing *P. pseudoalcaligenes*

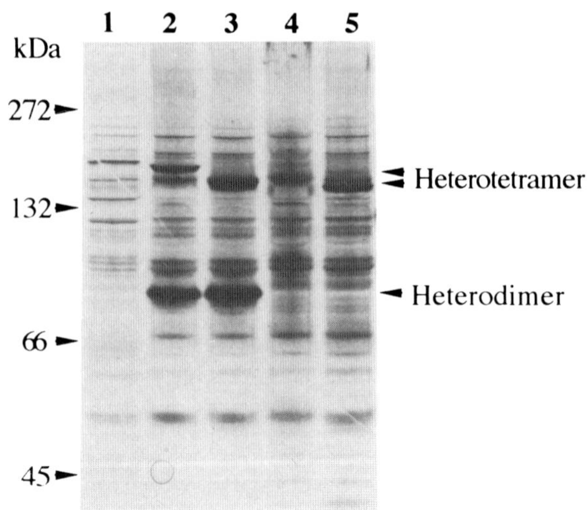

Figure 4. Native polyacrylamide gel electrophoresis of cell extracts overexpressed by the hybrid *bph-tod* gene cluster. Lanes: 1, pUC118 vector; 2, pJHF108 (*bphaI bphA2 bphA3 bphA4*): 3, pJHF101 (*todC1 bphA2 bphA3 bphA4*); 4, pJHF201 (*bphA1 todC2 bphA3 bphA4*); 5, pJHF301 (*todC1 todC2 bphA3 bphA4*).

KF707, were filter mated, and colonies that could grow on toluene were obtained. These were single- and double-crossover recombinants in which the *orf-0* region (upstream) and/or the *bphA2 bphA3 bphA4* region (downstream of the *todC1* insertion) were recombined (Fig. 5). The same hybrid genes were also introduced into another biphenyl-utilizing *P. putida* strain, KF715, which possesses a *bph* operon very similar to that of KF707 except that the *bphX0 bphX1 bphX2 bphX3* region is absent (Hayase et al., 1990). Strains KF707 and KF715 utilized only biphenyl and biphenyl derivatives such as 4-methylbiphenyl and diphenylmethane, and *P. putida* F1 grew on only toluene and benzene. Both single- and double-crossover recombinants having *todC1* within the *bph* operon grew well on biphenyl and benzene-toluene. Moreover, such recombinant strains were capable of degrading TCE very efficiently. The parent biphenyl degraders, KF707 and KF715, could not degrade TCE at all. Strain F1 degraded TCE rather slowly by the action of toluene dioxygenase. However, both single- and double-crossover recombinants of KF707 and KF715 degraded TCE (10 μg/ml, 77 μM) completely in 4 h when they were grown on biphenyl and even when they were grown on sodium succinate and toluene (Fig. 6). It is worth noting that the double-crossover strain KF7139 (derived from KF715) possesses a *bph-tod* hybrid operon with genes from three different strains: *todC1* from strain F1, some region of *bphA1 bphA2 bphA3 bphA4* from KF707, and other downstream *bph* genes from KF715 (Fig. 5). Since recombinant strains having *todC1* within the *bph* operon attack both aromatic rings and ethylene, we examined the degradation of chlorostyrene, which possesses both an aromatic moiety and an ethylene group (Fig. 7). The major metabolites from 2-chlorostyrene were 2-hydroxy-2-(2-chlorophenyl)-ethylalcohol (compound II in Fig. 7) and l-ethyl-2,3-dihydroxy-6-chloro-cyclo-4,6-diene (compound III in Fig. 7), indicating that the TodC1–BphA2-BphA3-BphA4 hybrid dioxygenase attacked the aromatic moiety and the ethylene group simultaneously.

SELF-MOBILIZATION OF THE *bph-tod* HYBRID OPERON

The biphenyl catabolic pathway of *P. putida* KF715 is chromosomally encoded (Hayase et al., 1990). The entire set of pathway genes, including an upper operon coding for the conversion of biphenyl to benzoic acid and a lower operon coding for the benzoate *meta*-cleavage pathway, was obtained from a cosmid genomic library. The upper and lower operons were separated by ca. 7 kb of DNA (K. Furukawa et al., unpublished data). When the KF715 cells were grown in rich medium, the pathway was highly prone to deletion. The deletion apparently took place at the region of the upper operon or at the region including both upper and lower operons. More interestingly, it was found that more than 70 kb of DNA, including the upper and lower pathways, could be transferred by conjugation from strain KF715 to *P. putida* AC30. The *bph* genes were integrated into the chromosome of the recipient. Such transconjugants gained the ability to grow on biphenyl as a sole source of carbon and energy. Furthermore, the chromosomally integrated *bph* genes in strain AC30 were also highly prone to deletion when these genes were mobilized back to the chromosome of a *bph* deletion mutant of KF715 or to *P. putida* KT2440.

Since we have constructed a double-crossover strain (KF7139) in which *bphA1* is replaced by *todC1* within the KF715 *bph* operon (Fig. 5), we checked whether the hybrid operon is self-transmissible to other strains. For some unknown reason, the transfer

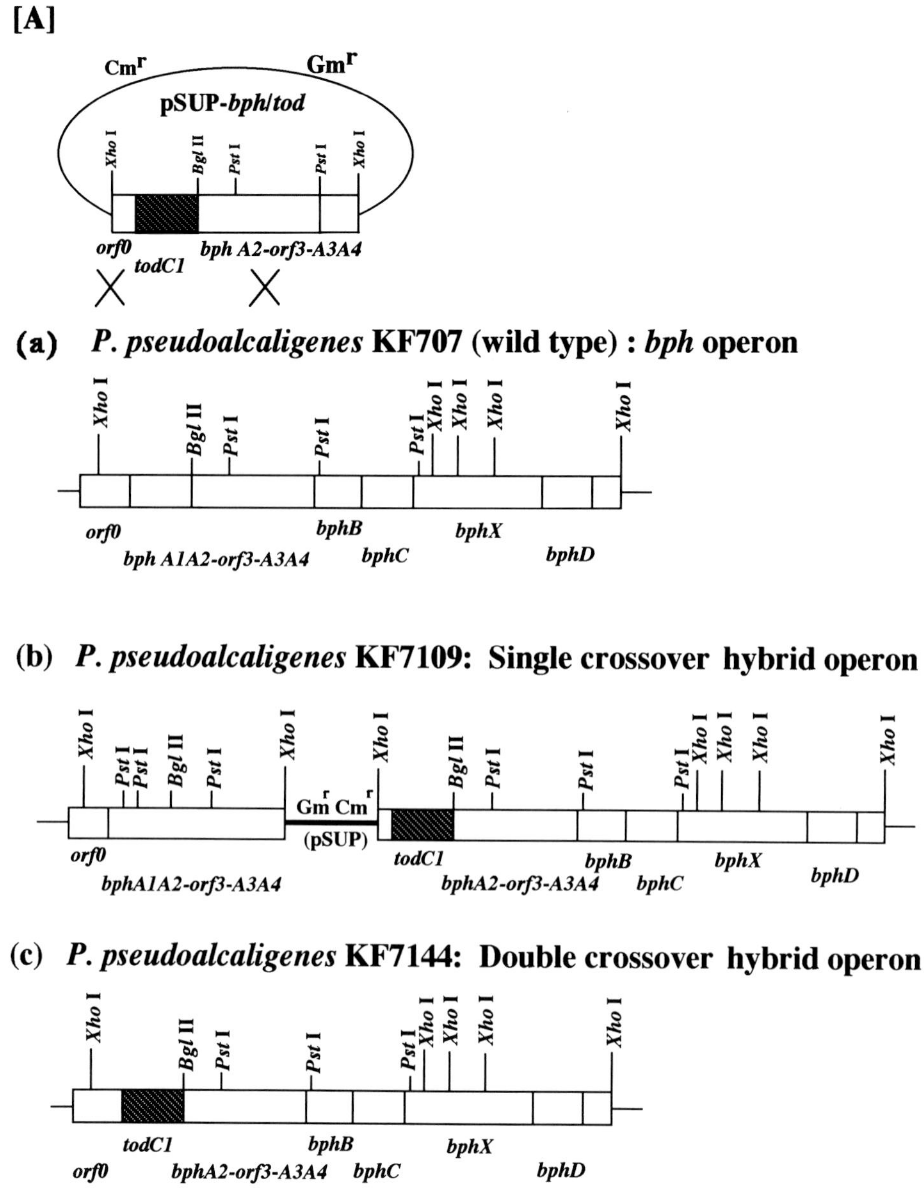

Figure 5. Schematic representation of single- and double-crossover hybrid operons in which *todC1* of *P. putida* F1 (solid bars) is integrated into the chromosomal *bph* operons of *P. pseudoalcaligenes* KF707 (open bars) (A) and *P. putida* KF715 (hatched bars) (B). (a) *bph* operon of KF707; (b) single-crossover hybrid operon in which the *bphA2 orf-3 bphA3 bphA4* region of pSUP-*bph/tod* was recombined with the KF707 chromosomal *bph* gene; (c) double-crossover hybrid operon in which both the *orf-0 and bphA2 orf-3 bphA3 bphA4* regions of pSUP-*bph/tod* were recombined with the KF707 chromosomal *bph* genes; (d) *bph* operon of KF715; (e) single-crossover hybrid operon in which the *orf-0* region of pSUP-*bph/tod* was recombined with the KF715 locus; (f) double-crossover hybrid *bph* operon in which both the *orf-0* and the *bphA2 bphA3 bphA4* regions of pSUP-*bph/tod* were recombined with KF715 chromosomal *bph* genes.

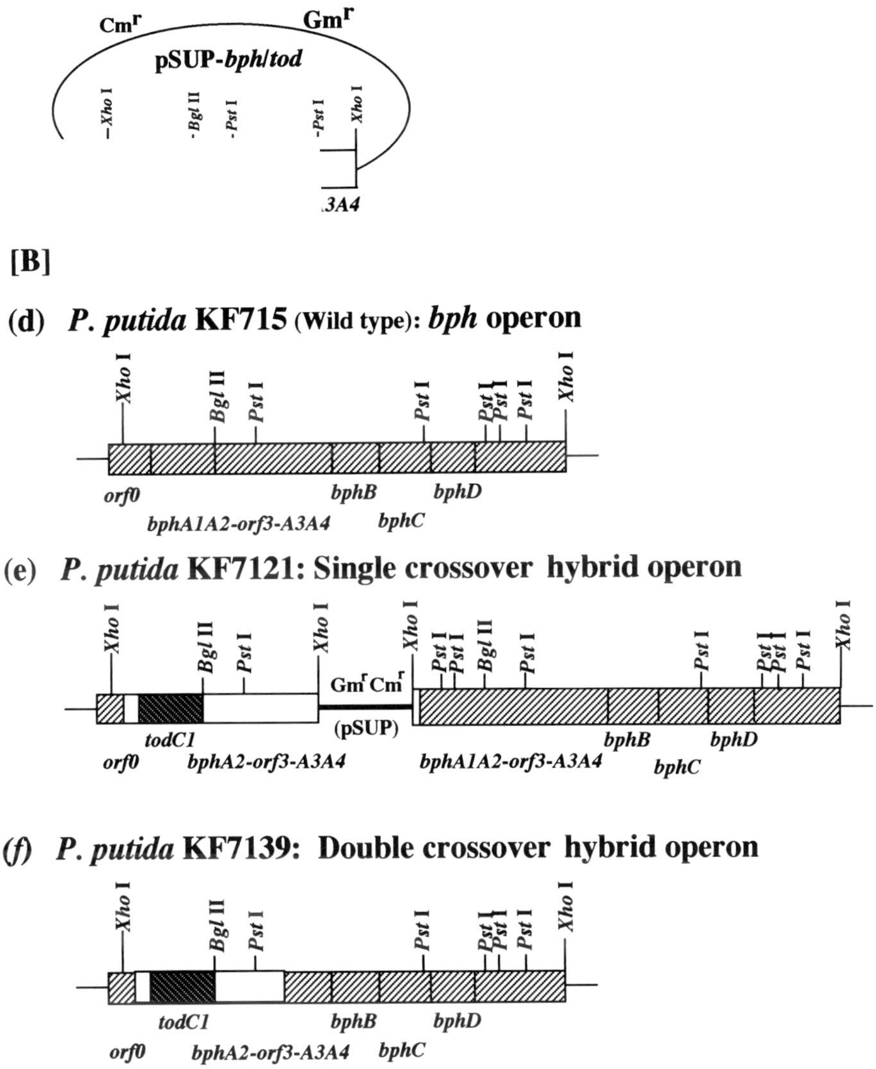

Figure 5. *Continued*

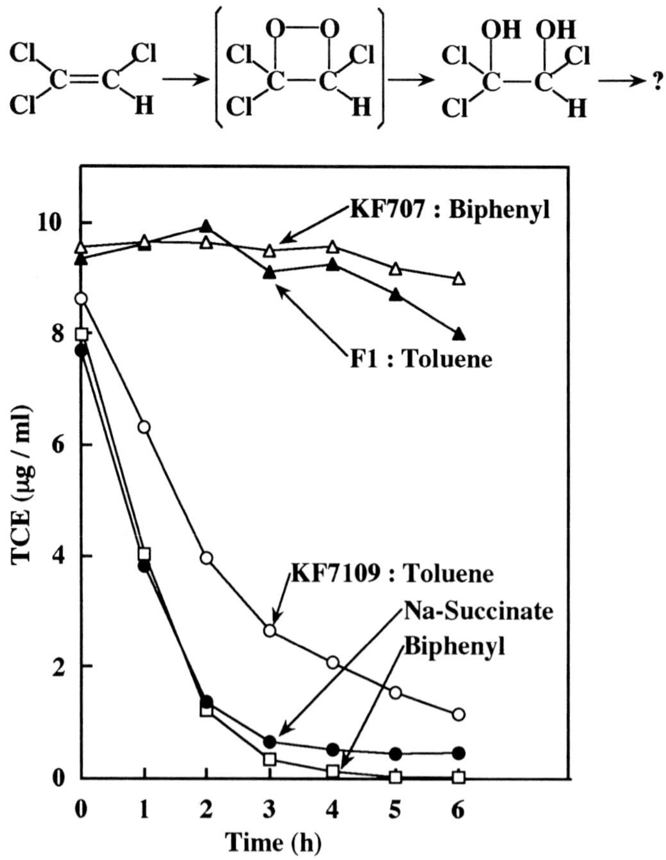

Figure 6. Degradation of TCE by *P. pseudoalcaligenes* KF707, *P. putida* F1, and *P. pseudoalcaligenes* KF7109 (KF707 derivative) in which *todC1* is integrated into the KF707 *bph* operon by single crossover (see Fig. 5). Strains were grown with the indicated substrates. The possible degradation pathway of TCE is shown.

frequency of the *bph-tod* hybrid operon was greatly reduced, but *P. putida* AC30 was able to be a recipient and gained the ability to utilize biphenyl and benzene.

CONSTRUCTION OF CHIMERIC BIPHENYL DIOXYGENASES AND FUNCTIONAL ANALYSIS

The biphenyl dioxygenase of *P. pseudoalcaligenes* KF707 introduces two atoms of molecular oxygen at positions 2 and 3 on the non-chlorinated or lesser chlorinated ring of PCB (2,3-dioxygenation). On the other hand, the *Pseudomonas* sp. strain LB400 biphenyl dioxygenase introduces O_2 at positions 3 and 4 (3,4-dioxygenation) or positions 2 and 3, depending on the chlorine substitution of PCB congeners (Bedard et al., 1986; Bedard et al., 1987). Thereby LB400 shows wide substrate ranges for PCB degradation (Erickson and Mondello, 1993; Gibson et al., 1993). KF707 degraded 2,5,4′-

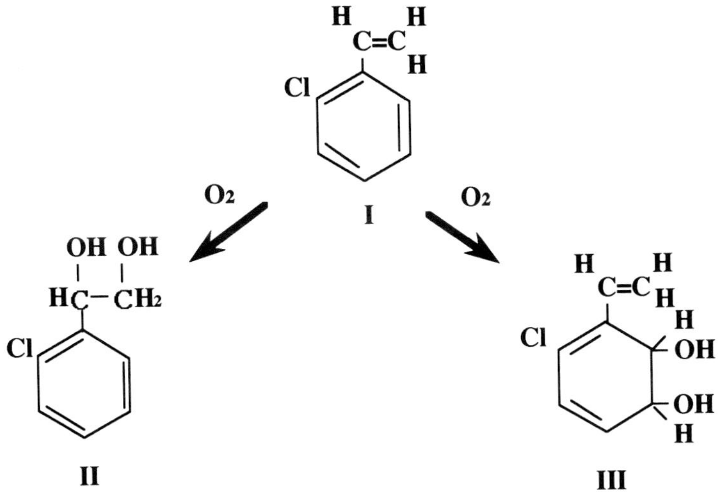

Figure 7. Degradation of 2-chlorostyrene by *E. coli* cells expressing *todC1 bphA2 bphA3 bphA4*. Compounds: I, 2-chlorostyrene; II, 2-hydroxy-2-(2-chlorophenyl)-ethylalcohol; III, 1-ethyl-2,3-dihydroxy-6-chloro-cyclo-4,6-diene.

trichlorobiphenyl through 2,3-dioxygenation and accumulated the ring *meta*-cleavage yellow compound, but the same strain did not attack 2,5,2′,5′-tetrachlorobiphenyl. On the other hand, LB400 oxidized both 2,5,4′-tri- and 2,5,2′,5′-tetrachlorobiphenyl to dihydrodiols and partly dihydroxy compounds with dechlorination through 3,4-dioxygenation (Haddock et al., 1995). In spite of the functional difference, the gene organization and nucleotide sequences of the biphenyl dioxygenase genes of the two strains are surprisingly identical or nearly identical. The identities of amino acid sequences in the corresponding proteins are as follows: BphA1, 95.6%; BphA2, 99.5%; BphA3, 100%; BphA4, 100%. The sequences of other enzymes, such as BphB (100%), BphC (99.9%), and BphD (96.9%), are also nearly identical. KF707-BphA1 (458 amino acids) and LB400-BphA1 (459 amino acids) show 20 amino acid differences. We constructed chimeric biphenyl dioxygenases by replacing KF707-*bphA1* with LB400-*bphA1* within the KF707 *bph* gene cluster. An *E. coli* strain expressing a hybrid biphenyl dioxygenase consisting of BphA1 (LB400)–BphA2-BphA3-BphA4 (KF707) oxidized 2,5,4′-tri- and 2,5,2′,5′-tetrachlorobiphenyl through 3,4-dioxygenation. A chimeric BphA1 composed of the N-terminal half from KF707-BphA1 and the C-terminal half of LB400-BphA1, in which eight amino acid substitutions were introduced into a KF707-BphA1 background, was also functional for 3,4-dioxygenation of 2,5,4′-tri- and 2,5,2′,5′-tetrachlorobiphenyl. Erickson and Mondello (1993) changed four amino acids of the LB400 BphA1 to those of the KF707 enzyme. The resultant enzyme retained the broad substrate specificity of the LB400 enzyme and showed the superior ability of the KF707 enzyme to degrade double-*para*-substituted congeners. These results indicate that relatively few amino acid residues are involved in the 2,3- or 3,4-dioxygenation activity or thereby in great differences in the primary degradation of PCB.

CONCLUSIONS

The genes coding for multicomponent aromatic ring dioxygenases have a common ancestry. Our studies showed that large subunits of terminal dioxygenases were critically involved in substrate specificity. The replacement of *bphA1* by *todC1* in chromosomal *bph* operons by single- and/or double-crossover recombinations expanded the substrate ranges of the recombinant strains for the degradation of many aromatic hydrocarbons, such as biphenyl, diphenylmethane, toluene, benzene, and styrene. Most interestingly, the same recombinant strains degraded TCE very efficiently. The construction of various chimeric dioxygenases from two functionally different biphenyl dioxygenases and subsequent site-directed mutagenesis allowed us to analyze the amino acid residues responsible for 2,3-dioxygenation and/or 3,4-dioxygenation activities for PCB degradation. Thus, modifications of large subunits of terminal dioxygenases or shuffling of subunits among various aromatic ring dioxygenases may allow us to enhance and expand the dioxygenase activities for naturally occurring and xenobiotic compounds.

REFERENCES

Bedard, D. L., M. L. Haberl, R. J. May, and M. J. Brennan. 1987. Evidence for novel mechanism of polychlorinated biphenyl metabolism in *Alcaligenes eutrophus* H850. *Appl. Environ. Microbiol.* **53:**1103–1112.

Bedard, D. L., R. Unterman, L. H. Bopp, M. H. Brennan, M. L. Haberl, and C. Johnson. 1986. Rapid assay for screening and characterizing microorganisms for the ability to degrade polychlorinated biphenyls. *Appl. Environ. Microbiol.* **51:**761–768.

Erickson, B. D., and F. J. Mondello. 1992. Nucleotide sequencing and transcriptional mapping of the genes encoding biphenyl dioxygenase, a multicomponent polychlorinated biphenyl-degrading enzyme in *Pseudomonas* strain LB400. *J. Bacteriol.* **174:**2903–2912.

Erickson, B. D., and F. J. Mondello. 1993. Enhanced biodegradation of polychlorinated biphenyls after site-directed mutagenesis of a biphenyl dioxygenase gene. *Appl. Environ. Microbiol.* **59:**3858–3862.

Furukawa, K. 1982. Microbial degradation of polychlorinated biphenyls, p. 33–57. *In* A. M. Chakrabarty (ed.), *Biodegradation and Detoxification of Environmental Pollutants.* CRC Press, Inc., Boca Raton, Fla.

Furukawa, K. 1994. Molecular genetics and evolutionary relationship of PCB-degrading bacteria. *Biodegradation* **5:**289–300.

Furukawa, K., J. Hirose, S. Hayashida, and K. Nakamura. 1994. Efficient degradation of trichloroethylene by a hybrid aromatic ring dioxygenase. *J. Bacteriol.* **176:**2121–2123.

Furukawa, K., J. Hirose, A. Suyama, T. Zaiki, and S. Hayashida. 1993. Gene components responsible for discrete substrate specificity in the metabolism of biphenyl (*bph* operon) and toluene (*tod* operon). *J. Bacteriol.* **175:**5224–5232.

Gibson, D. T., D. L. Cruden, J. D. Haddock, G. J. Zylstra, and J. M. Brand. 1993. Oxidation of polychlorinated biphenyls by *Pseudomonas* sp. LB400 and *Pseudomonas pseudoalcaligenes* KF707. *J. Bacteriol.* **175:**4561–4564.

Haddock, J. D., J. R. Horton, and D. T. Gibson. 1995. Dihydroxylation and dechlorination of chlorinated biphenyls by purified biphenyl dioxygenase from *Pseudeomonas* sp. strain LB400. *J. Bacteriol.* **177:**20–26.

Harayama, S., M. Kok, and E. L. Neidle. 1992. Functional and evolutionary relationships among diverse oxygenases. *Annu. Rev. Microbiol.* **46:**565–601.

Hayase, N., K. Taira, and K. Furukawa. 1990. *Pseudomonas putida* KF715 *bphABCD* operon encoding biphenyl and polychlorinated biphenyl degradation: cloning, analysis, and expression in soil bacteria. *J. Bacteriol.* **172:**1160–1164.

Hirose, J., A. Suyama, S. Hayashida, and K. Furukawa. 1994. Construction of hybrid biphenyl (*bph*) and toluene (*tod*) genes for functional analysis of aromatic ring dioxygenase. *Gene* **138:**27–33.

Hofer, B., S. Backhaus, and K. N. Timmis. 1994. The biphenyl/polychlorinated biphenyl-degradation locus (*bph*) of *Pseudomonas* sp. LB400 encodes four additional metabolic enzymes. *Gene* **144:**9–16.

Kikuchi, Y., Y. Yasukochi, Y. Nagata, M. Fukuda, and M. Takagi. 1994. Nucleotide sequence and functional analysis of the *meta*-cleavage pathway involved in biphenyl and polychlorinated biphenyl degradation in *Pseudomonas* sp. strain KKS102. *J. Bacteriol.* **176:**4269–4276.

Labes, M., A. Pühler, and R. Simon. 1990. A new family of RSF1010-derived expression and *lac*-fusion broad-host-range vectors for Gram-negative bacteria. *Gene* **89:**37–46.

Masai, E., A. Yamada, J. H. Healy, T. Hatta, K. Kimbara, M. Fukuda, and K. Yano. 1995. Characterization of biphenyl catabolic genes of gram-positive polychlorinated biphenyl degrader *Rhodococcus* sp. strain RHA1. *Appl. Environ. Microbiol.* **61:**2079–2085.

Nelson, M. J., S. O. Montgomery, W. R. Mahaffey, and P. H. Prichard. 1987. Biodegradation of trichloroethylene and involvement of an aromatic biodegradative pathway. *Appl. Environ. Microbiol.* **53:**949–954.

Simon, R., U. Priefer, and A. Pühler. 1983. A broad host range mobilization system for in vivo genetic engineering: transposon mutagenesis in gram negative bacteria. *Bio/Technology* **1:**784–791.

Simon, R., J. Quandt, and W. Klipp. 1989. New derivatives of transposons Tn*5* suitable for mobilization of replicons, generation of operon fusion and induction of genes in Gram-negative bacteria. *Gene* **80:**161–169.

Taira, K., J. Horose, S. Hayashida, and K. Furukawa. 1992. Analysis of *bph* operon from polychlorinated biphenyl-degrading strain of *Pseudomonas pseudoalcaligenes* KF707. *J. Biol. Chem.* **267:**4844–4853.

van der Meer, J. R., W. M. de Vos, S. Harayama, and A. J. B Zehnder. 1992. Molecular mechanism of genetic adaptation to xenobiotic compounds. *Microbiol. Rev.* **56:**677–694.

Wackett, L., and D. T. Gibson. 1988. Degradation of trichloroethylene by toluene dioxygenase in whole-cell studies with *Pseudomonas putida* F1. *Appl. Environ. Microbiol.* **54:**1703–1708.

Wang, Y., M. Rawlings, D. T. Gibson, D. Labbe, H. Bergeron, R. Brousseau, and P. C. K. Lau. 1995. Identification of a membrane protein and truncated LysR-type regulator associated with the toluene degradation pathway in *Pseudomonas putida* F1. *Mol. Gen. Genet.* **246:**570–579.

Wyndham, R. C., A. E. Cashore, C. H. Nakatsu, and M. C. Peel. 1994. Catabolic transposons. *Biodegradation* **5:**323–342.

Zylstra, G. J., and D. T. Gibson. 1989. Toluene degradation by *Pseudomonas putida* F1: nucleotide sequence of the *todC1C2BADE* genes and their expression in *Escherichia coli*. *J. Biol. Chem.* **264:**14940–14946.

Zylstra, G. J., L. P. Wackett, and D. T. Gibson. 1989. Trichloroethylene degradation by *Escherichia coli* containing the cloned *Pseudomonas putida* F1 toluene dioxygenase genes. *Appl. Environ. Microbiol.* **55:**3162–3166.

Molecular Biology of Pseudomonads
Edited by T. Nakazawa et al.

Chapter 9

Development of Hybrid Strains for the Mineralization of Chloroaromatics

Jürgen Havel, Thomas Kasberg, Stefan R. Kaschabek, Heiner Mokroß, Detlef Müller, and Walter Reineke

The ability of microorganisms to degrade organic substances has been used for more than 100 years in the biological treatment of wastewater streams. The entire population of existing microbes has the capacity to degrade nearly all naturally occurring substances. Without these degradative capabilities, no circulation of compounds would be possible in nature, and biological waste treatment would not exist.

Bacteria are well adapted to the utilization of natural substances. However, some synthetic chemicals have turned out to be extremely persistent. Whether a synthetic compound is metabolized by microorganisms depends partly on environmental conditions such as humidity, oxygen supply, temperature, and pH, but also on specific properties of the compound such as structure, water solubility, and vapor pressure. Xenobiotics, which resemble naturally occurring compounds, usually do not lead to problems concerning degradation. On the other hand, structures that strongly deviate from natural patterns are often recalcitrant.

In addition to other classes of compounds, chlorinated aromatics belong to this group of problematic compounds. Well-known examples are the polychlorinated biphenyls, the chlorinated dibenzo-*p*-dioxins, and dibenzofurans. In regard to overall amounts, chlorobenzenes and chlorophenols are more important, since at present, 700,000 and 150,000 tons, respectively, are produced worldwide per year. For the biological cleanup of waste or of soils contaminated with such compounds, microorganisms with the ability to use chloroaromatics as sources of carbon and energy would be helpful. The following methods may be used in order to obtain active cultures: (i) enrichment from soil or water samples; (ii) in vivo construction by conjugative gene transfer; and (iii) in vitro construction by genetic engineering.

In the following discussion, only in vivo construction is considered. The advantages of this technique over the others are pointed out. The genetic basis and biochemical aspects of the development of hybrid organisms by cell-cell contact are discussed.

Jürgen Havel, Thomas Kasberg, Stefan R. Kaschabek, Heiner Mokroß, Detlef Müller, and Walter Reineke • Bergische Universität, Gesamthochschule Wuppertal, Chemische Mikrobiologie, Gaußstraße 20, D-42097 Wuppertal, Germany.

HOW DO WE GET ORGANISMS THAT USE CHLOROAROMATICS AS GROWTH SUBSTRATES?

The incubation of aromatic-compound-degrading bacteria with analogous chlorinated substrates often leads to black-colored products, which turn out to be autooxidation products of dead-end metabolites. In most cases, the reason for these products can be found in the absence of enzyme sequences able to transform chlorocatechols, which occur during degradation of the chlorinated aromatic. The establishment of a complete sequence for the degradation of chloroaromatics in one strain should lead to a new strain able to use these compounds as growth substrates. This idea is summarized in Fig. 1. A hybrid path-

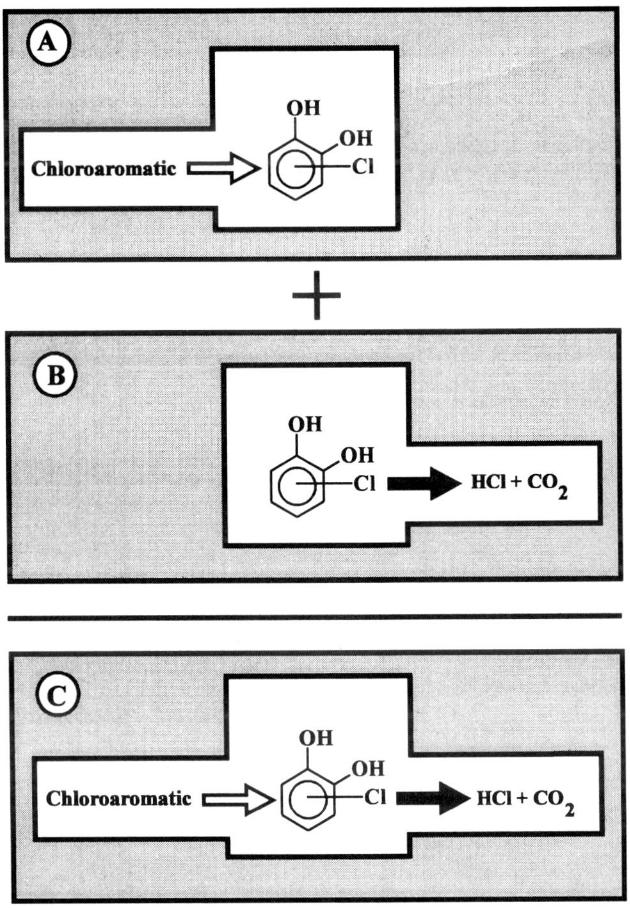

Figure 1. Principle of the development of hybrid pathways (C) for the degradation of chloroaromatics by the combination of two segments (A and B), with chlorocatechol as the central intermediate (according to Reineke and Knackmuss, 1979). (A) Peripheral enzyme sequence of aromatic-compound-degrading strains able to convert chloroaromatics to chlorocatechols; (B) central enzyme sequence for chlorocatechols, the modified *ortho* pathway such as that in *Pseudomonas* sp. strain B13.

way for chloroaromatics that leads to chloride, CO_2, and biomass results from the combination of two pathways: (i) a peripheral sequence taken from an aromatic-compound-degrading strain that is able to transform chlorinated aromatics up to the stage of chlorocatechols, and (ii) a chlorocatechol-degrading central sequence, the so-called modified *ortho* pathway.

HOW CAN GENE TRANSFER BE PUT INTO PRACTICE?

For the necessary enzymes to be produced, the appropriate genetic information must be transferred from one strain into another. Table 1 shows that a multitude of degradative sequences are encoded on plasmids. Most of these plasmids are transferable via conjugation. The plasmids contain genes for peripheral pathways as well as central ones. The detection of plasmids may be difficult in some cases; however, even then, transfer by conjugation can be demonstrated. In some bacterial strains, the genes for certain degradative sequences are located on the chromosome or on nonconjugative plasmids. With a few exceptions, these strains can be used only as acceptors for additional DNA. In a typical assay for conjugative gene transfer, the participating organisms are brought into close contact, usually on a solid complex medium, and this contact enables them to exchange genetic material. Afterward, the population is transferred onto selective medium in order to develop the desired properties.

WHAT IS THE STRUCTURE OF THE GENES?

This discussion must be limited to selected pathways. The genes of biphenyl and xylene degradation are chosen as two examples of peripheral pathways because of their importance in the degradation of xenobiotics and the multitude of data available on these pathways. Information on the genetics of the central pathway for chlorocatechol degradation is also presented.

The organization of the genes of biphenyl degradation, usually denoted *bph*, has been clarified in various laboratories. Figure 2 shows 12 structural genes of the peripheral pathway of biphenyl degradation lying alongside the central *meta* pathway. (The importance of the central *meta* pathway is explained later.) As far as we know, one transcript is formed from the *bph* gene cluster. There are many similarities but also some differences in the organization of the operons. Differences exist, for example, in the compositions of the clusters of well-investigated strains like KSS102 on the one hand and strains like LB400 and KF707 on the other hand. The order of structural genes is identical in strains LB400 and KF707. Difficulties arise from different nomenclatures for the genes.

The method of regulation of biphenyl-degrading pathways is not yet known.

Among the genes for peripheral pathways, the *xyl* genes, which are on the TOL plasmid pWW0, are the best characterized. These genes, which are essential for the total degradation of toluene and xylenes, form two functional units, the upper operon and the *meta*, or lower, operon. A simplified model is given in Fig. 3. The upper operon, *xylCMABN*, encodes three enzymes that oxidize toluene and xylenes to benzoate and toluates, respectively. The function of the protein encoded by *xylN* is unknown. The promoter of the upper pathway genes, Pu, is regulated positively by the regulatory gene *xylR*. This gene contains the information for a protein that enhances transcription after

Table 1. Degradative plasmids relevant to the construction of chloroaromatic-compound-degrading hybrid strains

Plasmid	Size (kb)	Conjugative	Incompatibility group[a]	Substrates	Reference(s)
Peripheral pathways					
TOL	117	+	P-9	Xylenes, toluene, toluate	Bayley et al., 1979; Lehrbach et al., 1982, 1983a, 1983b; Williams and Murray, 1974
NAH7	83	+	P-9	Naphthalene via salicylate	Bayley et al., 1979; Dunn and Gunsalus, 1973; Lehrbach et al., 1983b; Schell, 1983; Yen and Gunsalus, 1983, Yen et al., 1983
pWW60-1	87	+	P-9	Naphthalene via salicylate	Cane and Williams, 1982
pDTG1	83	+	P-9	Naphthalene via salicylate	Serdar and Gibson, 1989
SAL1	85	+	P-9	Salicylate	Bayley et al., 1979; Chakrabarty, 1972; Lehrbach et al., 1983b; Yen and Gunsalus, 1983; Yen et al., 1983
pKF1	82	–	ND	Biphenyl via benzoate	Furukawa and Chakrabarty, 1982
pWW100	~200	–	ND	Biphenyl via benzoate Methylbiphenyls via toluates	Lloyd-Jones et al., 1994
pWW110	>200	ND	ND	Biphenyl via benzoate Methylbiphenyls via toluates	Carrington et al., 1994
pCITI	100	ND	ND	Aniline	Anson and Mackinnon, 1984
pEB	253	ND	ND	Ethylbenzene	Bestetti and Galli, 1984
pRE4	105	ND	ND	Isopropylbenzene	Eaton and Timmis, 1986a, 1986b
pWW174	200	+	ND	Benzene	Winstanley et al., 1987
pHMT112	112	ND	ND	Benzene	Tan and Mason, 1990
pEST1005	44	ND	ND	Phenol	Kivisaar et al., 1990
pVI150	Mega	+	P-2	Phenol, cresols, 3,4-dimethylphenol	Bartilson et al., 1990; Shingler et al., 1989
Central pathways					
pAC25	117	+	P-9	3-Chlorobenzoate	Chatterjee et al., 1981b
pJP4	77	+	P-1	3-Chlorobenzoate, 2,4-D	Don and Pemberton, 1981
pBR60	85	+	ND	3-Chlorobenzoate	Wyndham et al., 1988
pRC10	45	ND	ND	2,4-D	Chaudhry and Huang, 1988
pP51	100	–	ND	1,2,4-Trichlorobenzene	van der Meer et al., 1991c
pMAB1	90	ND	ND	2,4-D	Bhat et al., 1994

[a]ND, not determined.

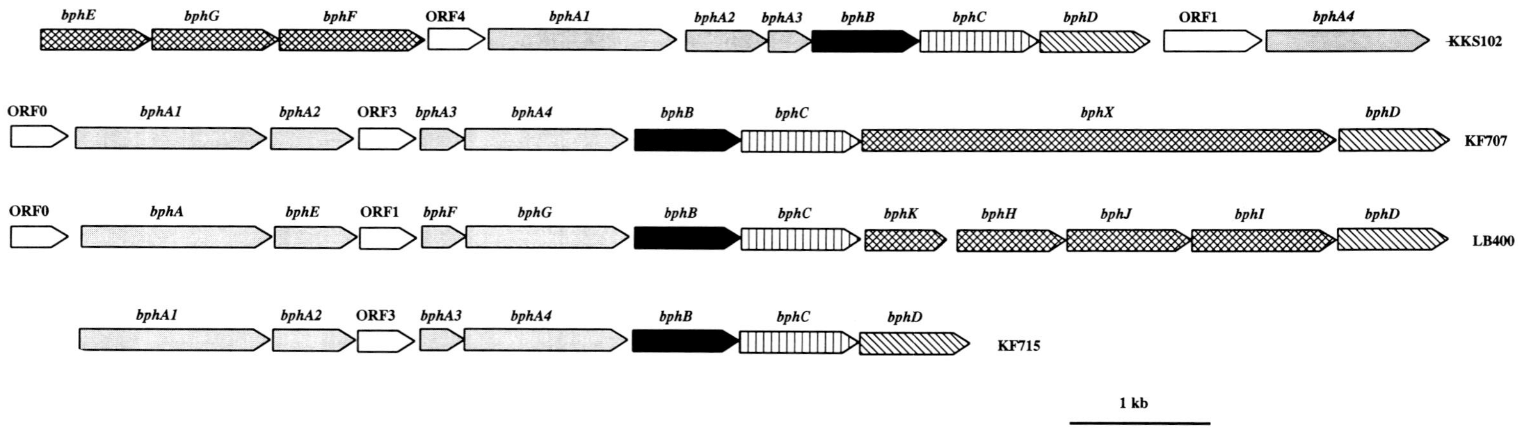

Figure 2. Operon structures of the genes of the biphenyl degradation pathways in strains KKS102, KF707, LB400, and KF715 (*bph* for biphenyl). Each arrow corresponds to a gene or an open reading frame (ORF). Homologous genes are shaded the same way. The genes of biphenyl 2,3-dioxygenase (*bphA1-4*, *bphAEFG*) are gray, those of biphenyldihydrodiol dehydrogenase (*bphB*) are black, those of the phenylcatechol 1,2-dioxygenase (*bphC*) are striped, and those coding for hydrolases (*bphD*) are marked with diagonals. The genes of strains KKS102, KF707, and LB400 that code for enzymes of the *meta* pathway (*bphE*, *bphF*, *bphG*, *bphX*, *bphK*, *bphH*, *bphJ*, and *bphI*) are marked by cross-hatching. Information was compiled from Erickson and Mondello (1992), Fukuda et al. (1994), Furukawa et al. (1987), Hayase et al. (1990), Hofer et al. (1993, 1994), Kikuchi et al. (1994a, 1994b), Kimbara et al. (1989), and Taira et al. (1988, 1992).

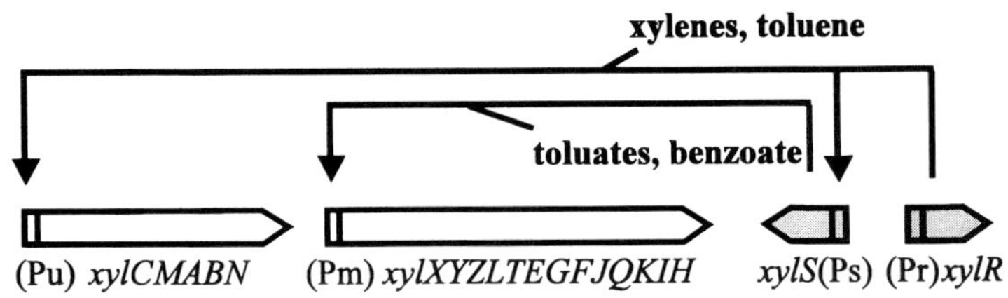

Figure 3. Simplified model of the regulation of *xyl* (xylene) gene operons. The upper operon (*xylCMABN*) encodes xylene monooxygenase, benzylalcohol dehydrogenase, and benzaldehyde dehydrogenase, while 13 enzymes are encoded by the *meta* operon (*xylXYZLTEGFJQKIH*). These enzymes include toluate 1,2-dioxygenase, toluate-dihydrodiol dehydrogenase, and catechol 2,3-dioxygenase. Regulator genes *xylS* and *xylR* are shown in gray. Promoter regions are marked by small boxes. Arrows indicate induction by XylR and XylS regulatory proteins in concert with the respective aromatic effectors. Data are from Harayama et al. (1986), Holtel et al. (1990), Inouye et al. (1984a, 1984b), Mermod et al. (1984), and Ramos et al. (1986, 1987).

the binding of an inducing molecule (toluene, *m*-xylene, or one of the respective benzyl alcohols). Subsequently, benzoate and toluate are transformed into the respective catechols, which are mineralized by the enzymes of the *meta* pathway. These enzymes are encoded by the genes of the *meta* operon. Misunderstandings are caused by nonuniform use of the term *meta* to define both the operon and the biochemical pathway. The *meta* operon contains the genes *xylXYZ* and *xylL*, which encode the enzymes toluate 1,2-dioxygenase and toluatedihydrodiol dehydrogenase, which belong to the peripheral pathway in the biochemical sense. Biochemically, the central, *meta* pathway starts with the degradation of catechol. No fewer than nine enzymes are coordinately expressed from the promoter Pm in this polycistronic operon. For efficient expression of the *meta* operon by the promoter Pm, the product of the *xylS* gene is needed. Inducing compounds like benzoate and toluate bind to XylS, bringing about an activated form.

We emphasize that both operons and both regulatory genes are indispensable for the transformation of toluenes to catechols. All the necessary genes are jointly transferred during plasmid exchange. Problems might arise, since not only the genes of peripheral sequences but also information for pathways disturbing the degradation of chloroaromatics, for example, the central *meta* pathway, are transferred. This point is discussed below.

The plasmids that contain the genes for degradation of chlorocatechols have been well investigated. The structures of the corresponding operons are nearly identical in spite of the different origins of the bacteria (Fig. 4). The *clc* and *tcb* genes, for example, are identically organized, and the *tfdCDEF* operon differs from these genes only in the absence of an open reading frame between *tfdD* and *tfdE*. The presumably regulatory genes *tfdR*, *clcR*, and *tcbR* are oriented in the opposite direction. Not only the structures of the operons of the *clc*, *tcb*, and *tfd* genes are similar: a comparison of the sequences shows a strong identity between the corresponding enzymes of the different bacteria. The gene products of the regulatory genes act as positive regulators. However, which substances are the effectors that activate the regulatory proteins remains unclear. Because of several analogies to the regulation of the "normal" 3-oxoadipate pathway with *cis,cis*-muconate as the effector, chlorinated muconates are thought to play this role in the modified *ortho* pathway.

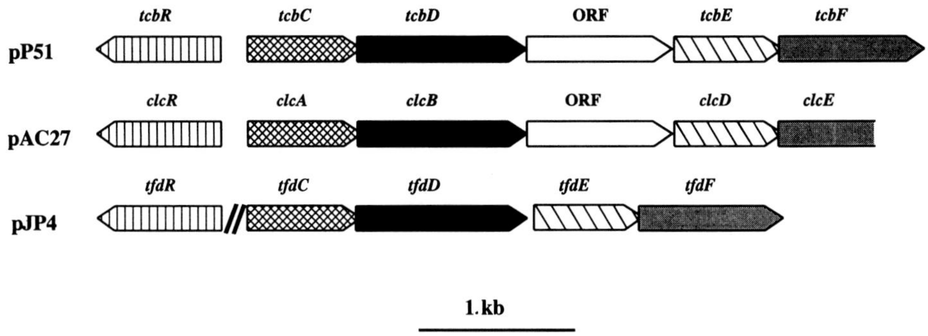

Figure 4. Operon structures of genes of the modified *ortho* pathway with adjacent regulatory genes (*tcb* [trichlorobenzene], *clc* [chlorocatechol], and *tfd* [two-four-D]). Each arrow corresponds to a gene or an open reading frame (ORF). Homologous genes are marked the same way. Genes for chlorocatechol 1,2-dioxygenase (*tcbC, clcA, tfdC*) are cross-hatched, those for chloromuconate cycloisomerase (*tcbD, clcB, tfdD*) are black, those for dienelactone hydrolase (*tcdE, clcD, tfdE*) are marked with diagonals, and those for maleylacetate reductase (*tcdF, clcE, tfdF*) are gray. The regulator genes *tcbR, clcR* and *tfdR* are marked with vertical stripes. *tfdR* is located several kilobases upstream of *tfdCDEF*. Arrows without tips denote overlap of the reading frames. Information was compiled from Coco et al. (1993), Frantz and Chakrabarty (1987), Kasberg et al. (1995), Leveau et al. (1994), Matrubutham and Harker (1994), Perkins et al. (1990), van der Meer et al. (1991a), and van der Meer et al. (1991b).

HOW DOES A DEGRADATIVE PATHWAY LOOK IN DETAIL?

The degradation of aromatic compounds involves many reaction steps that can be grouped into a few different types of reactions. Degradative sequences analogous to those demonstrated for the degradation of mononuclear aromatics like aniline, benzene, benzoate, salicylate, and toluene and for binuclear compounds like biphenyl, dibenzofuran, dibenzo-*p*-dioxin, and naphthalene are present (Fig. 5). These peripheral pathways converge at the stage of substituted diphenols like catechol.

The following is an important principle: an aromatic compound without a hydroxyl group is activated through a dioxygenase using molecular oxygen. Subsequently, the resulting *cis*-dihydrodiol is converted by a dehydrogenase to give a 1,2-diphenol, regain-

Figure 5. Peripheral degradation sequences for aromatics relevant to the development of hybrid strains that use chloroaromatics. 1, Naphthalene; 2, dibenzofuran; 3, dibenzo-*p*-dioxin; 4, benzene; 5, phenol; 6, aniline; 7, biphenyl; 8, toluene; 9, salicylate; 10, benzoate. Path 4 is also used for toluene and ethylbenzene, and xylenes are degraded via path 8, so methyl- or ethyl-substituted metabolites result, respectively. Catechol or the methyl- and ethyl-substituted analogs, the central metabolites, are degraded via the *meta* pathway. The cleavage of C-C bonds is marked by a line of stars. The information is compiled from Bachofer and Lingens (1975), Bayly and Wigmore (1973), Catelani et al. (1971, 1973), Catelani and Colombi (1974), Engesser et al. (1989), Fortnagel et al. (1989, 1990), Gibson et al. (1968, 1970a, 1970b, 1973), Harms et al. (1990), Lunt and Evans (1970), Pothuluri and Cerniglia (1994), Reiner (1971), Reiner and Hegeman (1971), Strubel et al. (1991), Wittich et al. (1992), and Worsey and Williams (1975).

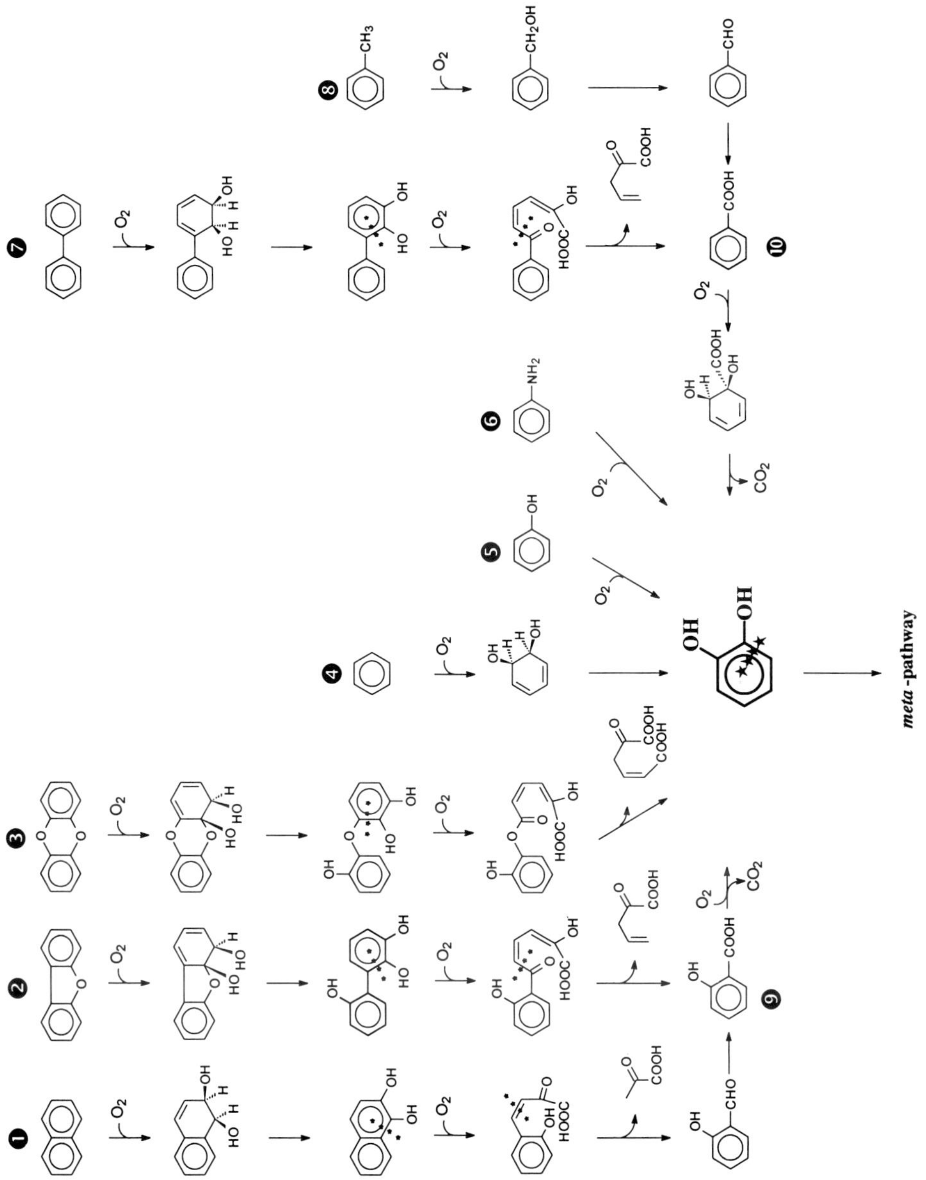

ing the aromatic state. The resulting diphenol acts as substrate for ring cleavage, often *meta* cleavage, which requires another mole of molecular oxygen. In mononuclear aromatics, the ring-cleaving dioxygenation is considered part of the central pathway. During the degradation of binuclear aromatics, the formation and cleavage of 1,2-diphenol takes place twice. The *cis*-dihydrodiols, which appear during the degradation of dibenzo-*p*-dioxin and dibenzofuran, are unstable because they are hemiacetals. Therefore, the ether bond is cleaved spontaneously, and a dehydrogenase is not necessary. During aniline degradation, the stage of diphenol is reached by the action of an aniline dioxygenase that eliminates NH_3 at the same time. In this case as well, no dehydrogenase is needed.

The peripheral degradation of a multitude of aromatics converges at the stage of catechol or chlorocatechols if the chlorinated compounds are degraded via the sequences mentioned.

The reaction steps of the central degradation pathway of chlorocatechols are shown in Fig. 6. Ring cleavage by chlorocatechol 1,2-dioxygenase with consumption of molecular oxygen results in formation of the corresponding *cis,cis*-muconate. Further degradation by a chloromuconate cycloisomerase leads to a lactone, which eliminates chlorine as HCl from position 4 or 5, bringing about the formation of an exocyclic double bond. In this way, dienelactone is formed, and this dienelactone is transformed into the corresponding chloromaleylacetate via hydrolytic cleavage. Maleylacetate reductase, whose original function is the reduction of the double bond, is able to eliminate a possible chlorine substituent from position 2. The degradative pathways of catechol and chlorocatechols converge at the stage of oxoadipates.

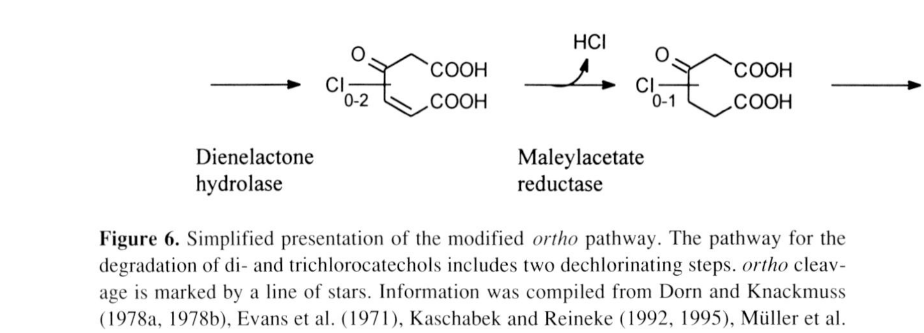

Figure 6. Simplified presentation of the modified *ortho* pathway. The pathway for the degradation of di- and trichlorocatechols includes two dechlorinating steps. *ortho* cleavage is marked by a line of stars. Information was compiled from Dorn and Knackmuss (1978a, 1978b), Evans et al. (1971), Kaschabek and Reineke (1992, 1995), Müller et al. (1996), Sander et al. (1991), Schmidt and Knackmuss (1980), Schwien et al. (1988), Tiedje et al. (1969), Vollmer et al. (1993, 1994), and Vollmer and Schlömann (1995).

IS THE ENZYME SPECIFICITY OF DEGRADATIVE SEQUENCES BROAD ENOUGH FOR DEGRADATION OF A MULTITUDE OF CHLOROAROMATIC COMPOUNDS?

It is not a matter of course that all enzymes of a strain that has been enriched with a nonchlorinated aromatic compound also show activity with chlorinated compounds. In this section, information on the specificity of the enzymes of the toluene and biphenyl degradation pathways is discussed.

The oxygenation of different chlorotoluenes has been investigated in *Pseudomonas putida* PaWl, a strain that uses xylenes as growth substrates. Only 3-chloro- and 4-chlorotoluene are transformed at high rates, while no or only low activity is found with other chlorotoluenes.

Benzylalcohol and benzaldehyde dehydrogenase show broader specificities (Table 2), but again, a chlorine substituent in the *ortho* position leads to a drastic decrease in substrate conversion rate.

Three types of enzymes that dioxygenate chlorinated benzoates are known (Table 3). *Alcaligenes eutrophus* and *Pseudomonas* sp. strain B13 possess similar benzoate 1,2-dioxygenases with narrow specificities. In addition to benzoate, only 3-chlorobenzoate is converted. In contrast, the toluate 1,2-dioxygenase of *P. putida* PaWl transforms all tested chlorobenzoates except 2-chlorobenzoate. The corresponding isoenzyme from *Pseudomonas* sp. strain WR401, an *o*-toluate degrader, is finally no bottleneck even for 2-chlorobenzoate. The data indicate that steric hindrance, instead of electronic effects of chlorosubstituents, is responsible for the various activities found with different chlorobenzoates.

The dihydrodihydroxybenzoate dehydrogenases occurring in *A. eutrophus*, *Pseudomonas* sp. strain B13, and *P. putida* PaWl are characterized by a broad substrate specificity and the ability to transform all dihydrodiols tested to the corresponding catechols (Table 4).

Table 2. Dehydrogenation of benzylalcohols and benzaldehydes[a]

Substrate	Dehydrogenation, V_{max} rel (%)[b] *of P. putida* PaW1 on *m*-xylene
Benzylalcohol	100
2-Chlorobenzylalcohol	10
3-Chlorobenzylalcohol	65
4-Chlorobenzylalcohol	100
2,4-Dichlorobenzylalcohol	7
2,6-Dichlorobenzylalcohol	<1
3,4-Dichlorobenzylalcohol	50
3,5-Dichlorobenzylalcohol	40
Benzaldehyde	100
2-Chlorobenzaldehyde	5
3-Chlorobenzaldehyde	200
4-Chlorobenzaldehyde	210
2,6-Dichlorobenzaldehyde	<1
3,4-Dichlorobenzaldehyde	195

[a] Data from Brinkmann and Reineke (1992).

[b] Relative maximum rate of metabolism (V_{max} rel) was determined by comparing the rate for the nonsubstituted substrate (100%) with that for the substituted substrate in a cell-free assay. Growth substrate is *m*-xylene.

Table 3. Dioxygenation of benzoates by *A. eutrophus* B9, *Pseudomonas* sp. strain B13, *P. putida* PaW 1, and *Pseudomonas* sp. strain WR401[a]

Substrate	Dioxygenation of benzoate, V_{max} rel (%)[b]			
	B9, benzoate	B13, 3-chlorobenzoate	PaW1, *m*-toluate	WR401, *o*-toluate
Benzoate	100	100	100	100
2-Chlorobenzoate	0	<1	<1	85
3-Chlorobenzoate	15	31	48	114
4-Chlorobenzoate	<1	<1	32	50
3,4-Dichlorobenzoate	<1	ND	9	ND
3,5-Dichlorobenzoate	<1	<1	10	ND

[a] Data are from Reineke and Knackmuss (1978a) and Engelberts et al. (1989).

[b] Relative maximum rate of metabolism (V_{max} rel) was determined by comparing the rate for the nonsubstituted substrate (100%) with that for the substituted substrate in a whole-cell assay. Growth substrates are given below strain names. ND, not determined.

Concerning the dioxygenation of chlorobiphenyls, congeners chlorinated in only one ring were transformed at a high rate by biphenyl-degrading strains. On the other hand, substrates carrying chlorine substituents in both rings, like 2,2′-dichloro- or 4,4′-dichlorobiphenyl, are converted at low rates only.

At present, only a small number of chlorinated phenylcatechols are available. Therefore, data on the specificity of the following enzymes of the biphenyl-degrading pathway are to be considered fragmentary. 2′-Chloro-, 3′-chloro-, and 4′-chlorophenylcatechol are metabolized at high rates, while a substituent located in the diphenolic ring, as shown for 4-chloro- and 5-chlorophenylcatechol, leads to a drastic decrease in the transformation rate. Substrate specificity turns out to be more or less similar in the biphenyl-degrading strains *P. putida* BN10, *Pseudomonas* sp. strain JHR, strain Dan, and *A. eutrophus* AE992.

The hydrolase reaction is slowed down by a chlorine substituent next to the position of cleavage, as shown for 3-chloro-2-hydroxy-6-oxo-6-phenylhexa-2,4-dienoate. It was unexpected to find that 3′,5′-dichloro-2-hydroxy-6-oxo-6-phenylhexa-2,4-dienoate, which

Table 4. Dehydrogenation of dihydrodihydroxybenzoates[a]

Substrate	Dehydrogenation, V_{max} rel (%)[b]		
	P. putida PaW1, *m*-toluate	*A. eutrophus*, benzoate	*Pseudomonas* sp. strain B13, 3-chlorobenzoate
Dihydrodihydroxybenzoate	100	100	100
3-Chlorodihydrodihydroxybenzoate	23	16	43
4-Chlorodihydrodihydroxybenzoate	35	32	30
5-Chlorodihydrodihydroxybenzoate	57	95	75
3,5-Dichlorodihydrodihydroxybenzoate	23	ND	16

[a] Data from Reineke and Knackmuss (1978b) and A. Stolz and W. Reineke (unpublished results).

[b] Relative maximum rate of metabolism (V_{max} rel) was determined by comparing the rate for the nonsubstituted substrate (100%) with that for the substituted substrate in a cell-free assay or with purified enzyme. Growth substrates are given below strain names. ND, not determined.

carries substituents only in the ring not participating in the reaction, is hydrolyzed at a low rate, while the same substituents in positions 3′ and 4′ have only a minor influence.

Until now, data on the conversion of chlorobiphenyls through the biphenyl pathway have provided a conclusive explanation for the observation of a bottleneck concerning effective degradation of polychlorinated biphenyl congeners chlorinated in both rings. For the moment, the extent to which other properties of these congeners, like solubility or vapor pressure, are responsible for the reduction of the transformation rate remains unclear.

Some data on the specificity of enzymes of the modified *ortho* pathway are given in Tables 5, 6, and 7. The chlorocatechol 1,2-dioxygenases as well as the chloromuconate cycloisomerases catalyze reactions analogous to those catalyzed by catechol 1,2-dioxygenase and muconate cycloisomerase, which are enzymes that participate in the degradation of nonchlorinated aromatics. The main difference between catechol and chlorocatechol 1,2-dioxygenases can be found in the high affinities and activities of the latter toward 3-chloro-, 4-chloro-, and 3,5-dichlorocatechol. Some kind of adaptation is observed, especially to the chlorocatechol that occurs during degradation of the enrichment substrate.

In a similar way, chloromuconate cycloisomerase accepts 2-chloro- and 3-chloro-*cis,cis*-muconate in addition to *cis,cis*-muconate, whereas muconate cycloisomerase shows very low affinities and activities toward the chlorinated substrates. The chloromuconate cycloisomerase of 2,4-dichlorophenoxyacetic acid (2,4-D)-degrading strains develops some activity toward *cis,cis*-muconate but only a very low affinity. This enzyme is highly specific to the 2,4-dichloro-*cis,cis*-muconate that appears during 2,4-D degradation.

Dienelactone hydrolase is not able to transform the corresponding metabolite of the 3-oxoadipate pathway, 3-oxoadipate enollactone. In the same way, 3-oxoadipate enollactone hydrolase fails to convert *cis*- and *trans*-dienelactone. Therefore, dienelactone hydrolase cannot be considered simply a 3-oxoadipate enollactone hydrolase with a low substrate specificity. Some enzymes of the degradation pathway of chlorinated aromatics are highly specialized so that they are no longer able to convert the nonchlorinated metabolites.

Maleylacetate reductase has no equivalent in the 3-oxoadipate pathway. This enzyme transforms many chlorinated substrates.

ARE PERIPHERAL DEGRADATION SEQUENCES INDUCED BY CHLORINATED COMPOUNDS?

In addition to enzyme specificity, the induction of enzymes can be a bottleneck during the degradation of chlorinated aromatics. Overall, only a few data exist on the effector specificity of degradative pathways. Tables 8 and 9 summarize our information about the induction of the upper and *meta* operons, which are encoded on the TOL plasmid, by different chlorinated substrate analogs. Furthermore, the induction of the first enzyme of the 3-chlorobenzoate degradation pathway has been investigated.

Two different methods, the reporter gene technique and induction with whole cells, lead to similar results concerning the effector specificity of the proteins XylR and XylS. In the whole-cell assay, 3-chloro- and 3,4-dichlorotoluene and their corresponding benzoates gave rise to problems because black autooxidation products inhibited the enzymes, mimicking a low induction state. All toluenes tested were effectors for XylR,

Table 5. Ring cleavage of catechols[a]

Substrate	1,2-Dioxygenation of catechols, V_{max} rel (%)[b]									
	B13, benzoate (C12O)	JMP134 (C12O)	B13, chloro-benzoate (CC12O)	AC866, 3-chlorobenzoate	CA28, 3-chloroaniline	BRI 6011, 2,5-dichlorobenzoate	JMP134, 2,4-D (CC12O)	CSV90, 2,4-D	HV3, 4-chloro-2-methylphenoxyacetate	PS12, 1,2,4-trichlorobenzene
Catechol	100	100	100	100	100	100	100	100	100	100
3-Chlorocatechol	<1	2	164	131	186	125	124	159	130	210
4-Chlorocatechol	11	14	120	80	140	92	122	136	116	190
3,5-Dichlorocatechol	<1	1	148	89	172	55	181	224	287	155

[a] Sources of data: for *Pseudomonas* sp. strain B13, Dorn and Knackmuss (1978a, 1978b) and Reineke and Knackmuss (1980); for *A. eutrophus* JMP134, Pieper et al. (1988); for *P. putida* AC866, Broderick and O'Halloran (1991); for *Pseudomonas acidovorans* CA28, Hinteregger et al. (1992); for *Alcaligenes denitrificans* BRI 6011, Miguez et al. (1993); for *Pseudomonas cepacia* CSV90, Bhat et al. (1993); for *Pseudomonas* sp. strain HV3, Kilpi et al. (1983); and for *Pseudomonas* sp. strain PS12, Sander et al. (1991).

[b] Relative maximum rate of metabolism (V_{max} rel) was determined by comparing the rate for the nonsubstituted subtrate (100%) with that for the substituted substrate. Growth substrates are given below strain names. C12O, catechol 1,2-dioxygenase, used in the degradation of aromatics, CC12O, chlorocatechol 1,2-dioxygenase, induced for the degradation of chloroaromatics.

Table 6. Lactonization of muconates[a]

Substrate	Lactonization of muconates, V_{max} rel (%)[b]		
	B13, benzoate	B13, 3-chlorobenzoate	JMP134, 2,4-D
Muconate	100	100	100[c]
2-Chloromuconate	<1	180	30
3-Chloromuconate	7	201	230
2,4-Dichloromuconate	ND	ND	125

[a] Sources of data: for *Pseudomonas* sp. strain B13, Schmidt and Knackmuss (1980); for *A. eutrophus* JMP134, Kuhm et al. (1990).

[b] Relative maximum rate of metabolism (V_{max} rel) was determined by comparing the rate for the nonsubstituted substrate (100%) with that for the substituted substrate. Growth substrates are given below strain names. ND, not determined.

[c] Low affinity.

thus indicating a broad effector specificity of XylR. It is remarkable that 2-chlorotoluene, although a bad substrate for xylene oxygenase, is the best effector.

In XylS protein, a different degree of substitution in positions 2, 3, and/or 4 is possible without loss of effector activity. The binding site of XylS seems to exclude a disubstitution with one substituent in the *ortho* position. Simultaneous substitution at positions 3 and 5 negatively influences the effector activity, too.

Only 3-chlorobenzoate is a good inducer for the peripheral pathway of strain B13, whereas 4-chloro- and 3,5-dichlorobenzoate do not function as inducing compounds.

Data on induction of the central modified *ortho* pathway are not yet available.

IS THE TRANSFER OF DNA ALONE SUFFICIENT TO PRODUCE A FUNCTIONING HYBRID PATHWAY?

Some examples of the construction of chlorobenzoate-, chlorotoluene-, and chlorobiphenyl-degrading strains will answer the question of whether DNA transfer alone can produce a functioning hybrid pathway.

Table 7. Reduction of maleylacetates[a]

Substrate	Reduction of maleylacetates, V_{max} rel (%)[b]			
	B13, benzoate	B13 3-chlorobenzoate	RHO1, 1,4-dichlorobenzene	JMP134, 2,4-D
Maleylacetate	NA	100	100	100
2-Chloromaleylacetate	NA	84	81	75
3-Chloromaleylacetate	NA	72	71	69
5-Chloromaleylacetate	NA	2	2	9
2,3-Dichloromaleylacetate	NA	63	34	ND
2,5-Dichloromaleylacetate	NA	3	3	ND

[a] Sources of data: for *Pseudomonas* sp. strain B13, Reineke (1984) and Kaschabek and Reineke (1995); for *Pseudomonas aeruginosa* RHO1, Müller et al. (1996); and for *A. eutrophus* JMP134, Müller et al. (1996).

[b] Relative maximum rate of metabolism (V_{max} rel) was determined by comparing the rate for the nonsubstituted substrate (100%) with that for the substituted substrate. Growth substrates are given below strain names. NA, no activity; ND, not determined.

Table 8. Induction of benzylalcohol dehydrogenase as a representative enzyme of the upper pathway of *P. putida* PaWl[a] and analysis of *xylR* gene product specificity by use of Pu::*lacZ* fusion technique[b]

Substrate	Induction ratio of activity[c]	
	BAD	β-GAL
Toluene	44	10
2-Chlorotoluene	85	18
3-Chlorotoluene	7[d]	17
4-Chlorotoluene	17	16
2,4-Dichlorotoluene	60	ND
2,5-Dichlorotoluene	ND	9
2,6-Dichlorotoluene	49	4
3,4-Dichlorotoluene	11[d]	ND
3,5-Dichlorotoluene	20	ND

[a] Data from Brinkmann and Reineke (1992).
[b] Data from Abril et al. (1989).
[c] Cells were grown on 20 mM acetate and incubated for 12 h with 20 mM acetate or acetate plus toluenes introduced via the vapor phase. Cell extracts were assayed for benzylalcohol dehydrogenase (BAD) activity and β-galactosidase (β-GAL) levels. Ratios are of levels in cells treated with inducer to levels in cells not treated with inducer. ND, not determined.
[d] Brown coloration: nonspecific inhibition or destruction of activity.

A multitude of information resulted from the experiments with *Pseudomonas* sp. strain B13 and *P. putida* PaWl that led to hybrid strains able to grow with 4-chloro- and 3,5-dichlorobenzoate (Fig. 7). Strain B13 was enriched with 3-chlorobenzoate (Dorn et al., 1974), and it converts this substrate to 3-chloro- and 4-chlorocatechol, which are mineralized via the modified *ortho* pathway. Strain B13 is not able to use 4-chloro- and 3,5-dichlorobenzoate as growth substrates, since its benzoate 1,2-dioxygenase has a narrow specificity and does not convert these compounds. However, the expected metabolites, 4-chloro- and 3,5-dichlorocatechol, can be mineralized by strain B13. The toluate 1,2-dioxygenase of *P. putida* PaWl, which is encoded on the TOL plasmid, has a broader substrate specificity than the corresponding B13 enzyme and accepts 4-chloro- and 3,5-dichlorobenzoate as substrates. Transconjugants of the mating between *Pseudomonas* sp. strain B13 as the acceptor (a streptomycin-resistant derivative was used) and *P. putida* PaWl as the donor showed the phenotype of strain B13 with the additional ability to grow with *m*- and *p*-toluate (strain WR211). However, this hybrid strain was not able to utilize 4-chlorobenzoate. The biochemical explanation of this behavior is given below. Mutants like strain WR216 that are able to grow with 4-chlorobenzoate could easily be obtained from strain WR211 by using solid medium with 4-chlorobenzoate as sole source of carbon. It was surprising to find that this strain is unable to grow with the toluates. These results clearly show that plasmid transfer is necessary but not sufficient for the development of a new degradative pathway.

Transconjugants like WR241 were obtained by mating strains B13 and PaWl and then selecting directly for growth with 4-chlorobenzoate. The transconjugants occurred at a frequency similar to the result of the single steps during selection for strains WR211 and WR216. Investigation of the substrates used by strains like WR241 showed that strain B13 had functioned as the acceptor in the mating.

On the other hand, strain B13 can also serve as the donor for the genes of the modified *ortho* pathway. This was shown in a mating between strain B13 and a streptomycin-

Table 9. Induction of benzoate 1,2-dioxygenase and toluate 1,2-dioxygenase as representative enzymes of the benzoate pathway of *Pseudomonas* sp. strain B13 and the toluate pathway of *P. putida* PaWl[a] and analysis of the *xylS* gene product specificity by use of the Pm::*lacZ* fusion technique[b]

Substrate	Induction ratio of activity[c]		
	Strain B13, oxygen uptake	Strain PaW1, oxygen uptake	Strain PaW1, β-GAL
Benzoate	ND	ND	12
2-Chlorobenzoate	2	ND	14
3-Chlorobenzoate	14	5[d]	11
4-Chlorobenzoate	1	6	5
2,4-Dichlorobenzoate	ND	ND	1
2,5-Dichlorobenzoate	ND	ND	1
2,6-Dichlorobenzoate	ND	ND	1
3,4-Dichlorobenzoate	1	1[d]	4
3,5-Dichlorobenzoate	1	1.5	1

[a] Data from A. Stolz and W. Reineke (unpublished results).
[b] Data from Ramos et al. (1986).
[c] Cells were grown on 20 mM acetate and incubated for 12 h with 20 mM acetate or acetate plus benzoates (5 mM). Cells were assayed for oxygen uptake with benzoate (strain B13) or 4-chlorobenzoate (strain PaW1). Ratios are of levels in cells treated with inducer to levels in cells not treated with inducer. β-GAL, β-galactosidase; ND not determined.
[d] Brown coloration: nonspecific inhibition or destruction of activity.

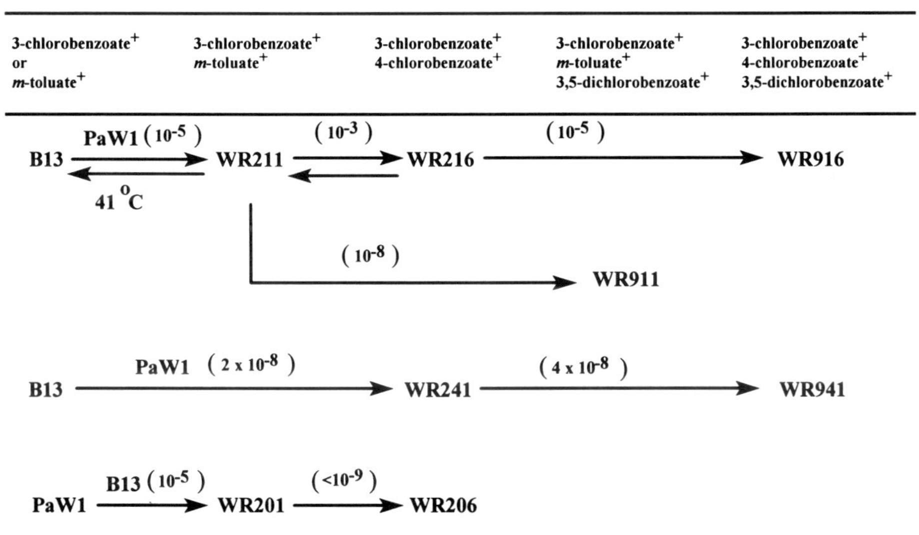

Figure 7. Genealogy of hybrid strains that degrade various chlorobenzoates and that result from matings between PaW1 and streptomycin-resistant B13 and between B13 and streptomycin-resistant PaW1. Phenotypes given at the top are valid for all strains in the respective columns below. Frequencies given in parentheses are defined as the numbers of transconjugants per donor cell or as spontaneous mutations on selective substrate. Data are from Reineke and Knackmuss (1979) and A. Stolz and W. Reineke (unpublished data).

resistant derivative of strain PaWl. Transconjugants like strain WR201 occurred at a frequency similar to that observed in the matings leading to strains like WR211 if the medium contained 3-chlorobenzoate for selection of the genes encoding chlorocatechol degradation and streptomycin for counterselection against donor strain B13. These strains showed the phenotype of strain PaWl as well as the ability to grow with 3-chlorobenzoate. However, no growth with 4-chlorobenzoate could be observed.

Strains like WR206, which acquired the potential to use 4-chlorobenzoate as the growth substrate, occurred at a very low frequency. This result explains why exclusively transconjugants have been obtained with strain B13 as the acceptor of the TOL plasmid when strains B13 and PaWl were mated and selected for growth with 4-chlorobenzoate, without use of drug resistance to select against the donor strain.

In addition to bottlenecks concerning the turnover of substrates, the induction of a pathway by a novel compound sometimes does not take place. One example of such a failure occurs with 3,5-dichlorobenzoate, which fails to induce toluate 1,2-dioxygenase in strains WR211, WR216, and WR241. In contrast, the compound is an effector in strains WR911, WR916, and WR941, which have occurred on solid medium containing 3,5-dichlorobenzoate from strains WR211, WR216, and WR241, respectively. Strains such as WR911 retained an *m*-toluate$^+$ phenotype.

At this point it can be ascertained that the degradations of 3-chloro- and 3,5-dichlorobenzoate and *m*-toluate are compatible, while those of 4-chlorobenzoate and *m*-toluate seem to exclude each other in the system investigated.

The conclusions given above may be interpreted as follows. Since the desired peripheral sequences as well as the *meta* pathway are encoded on plasmids, misrouting of chlorocatechols into the *meta* pathway must be avoided in the hybrid strains. This necessity will be discussed for the ring cleavage substrates 3-chloro-, 4-chloro-, and 3,5-dichlorocatechol (Fig. 8). The critical element for degradation through the *ortho* pathway in hybrid strains is the presence or absence of both ring-cleaving dioxygenases and the activity against and affinity for chlorocatechols. The *meta*-cleaving catechol 2,3-dioxygenase is present at a high basic level and is induced by substrates such as toluate in *P. putida* PaWl. In contrast, product induction by *cis,cis*-muconate has been demonstrated for *ortho*-cleaving catechol 1,2-dioxygenase. The inducer of the chlorocatechol 1,2-dioxygenase has not been determined but is presumed to be 2-chloro- or 2,4-dichloro-*cis,cis*-muconate.

Misrouting of 3-chlorocatechol into the *meta* pathway can be avoided as follows. Both ring-cleaving dioxygenases exhibit activity with 3-chlorocatechol. Catechol 2,3-dioxygenase forms from 3-chlorocatechol an acylchloride that reacts in the catalytic site of the enzyme and results in a nonreversible, so-called suicide inactivation of the enzyme. Further conversion of 3-chlorocatechol into the *meta* pathway is thereby prevented, and thus, induction of 1,2-dioxygenase can occur.

A quite different mechanism is necessary to avoid misrouting of 4-chlorocatechol. In this case, no acylchloride is formed, and therefore, the induction of catechol 2,3-dioxygenase causes a constant misrouting of 4-chlorocatechol into the *meta* pathway. Consequently, no inducer of *ortho*-cleaving chlorocatechol 1,2-dioxygenase is formed. The *meta* pathway can be prevented on the gene level, however, since the gene for catechol 2,3-dioxygenase, *xylE*, can be inactivated by an insertion or a point mutation (Jeenes et al., 1982; P. A. Williams, personal communication).

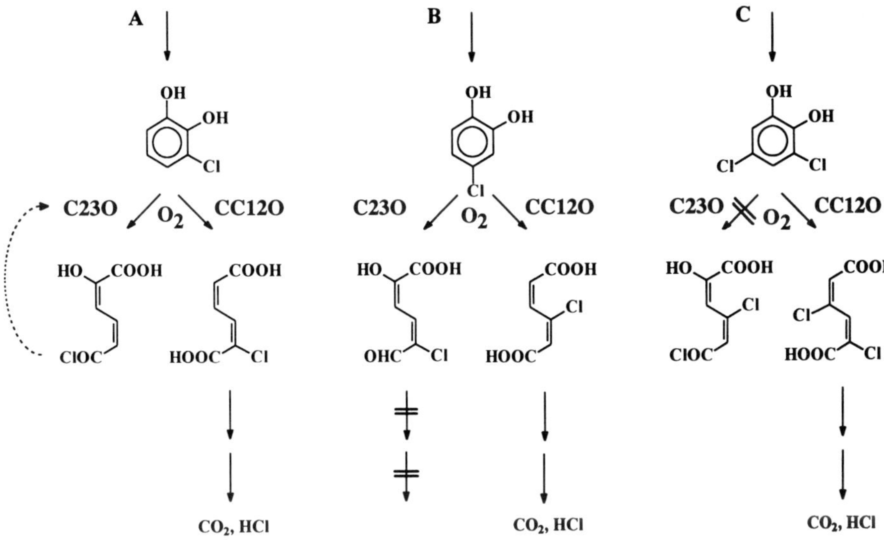

Substrate	C23O		CC12O	
	V_{max} rel. (%)	K_m or K_i (μM)	V_{max} rel. (%)	K_m (μM)
Catechol	100		100	
3-Chlorocatechol	5	23	164	
4-Chlorocatechol	80		120	
3,5-Dichlorocatechol	<1	14,000	148	0.3

Figure 8. Divergent pathways for chlorocatechols in hybrid strains and some kinetic data on the respective ring-cleaving enzyme: (A) 3-chlorocatechol; (B) 4-chlorocatechol; (C) 3,5-dichlorocatechol. The dashed arrow illustrates the reaction of acylchloride with catechol 2,3-dioxygenase. (Left) *meta* cleavage by catechol 2,3-dioxygenase (C23O); (right) *ortho* cleavage by chlorocatechol 1,2-dioxygenase (CC12O) and total degradation, with elimination of chloride. Data are from Bartels et al. (1984), Dorn and Knackmuss (1978b), Reineke and Knackmuss (1980), and W. Reineke (unpublished data). V_{max} rel., relative maximum rate of conversion.

By analogy to the suicide inactivation mechanism observed for 3-chlorocatechol, an acylchloride was also expected to be formed from 3,5-dichlorocatechol via catechol 2,3-dioxygenase. However, misrouting of 3,5-dichlorocatechol into the *meta* pathway did not occur, since catechol 2,3-dioxygenase exhibited low activity and low affinity with the compound. In contrast, chlorocatechol 1,2-dioxygenase showed high activity and high affinity toward 3,5-dichlorocatechol.

We emphasized that natural mechanisms eliminate the unsuitable *meta* pathway. The utilization of whole plasmids, which leads to the transfer of all genes encoding a peripheral pathway, including the essential regulatory proteins, does not create a problem, although genes encoding the *meta* pathway are cotransferred.

3-Chlorotoluene:

PaWl (TOL) x B13 ($3CBA^+$) ⟶ WR1412 ($3CT^+$)

4-Chlorotoluene:

PaWl (TOL) x B13 ($3CBA^+$) ⟶ WR1441 ($4CT^+$)

3,5-Dichlorotoluene:

PaWl (TOL) x B13 ($3CBA^+$) ⟶ WR1426 ($35DCT^+$)

(2-Chlorotoluene:)

PaWl (TOL) x JH230 ($2CBA^+$) ⟶ WR233 ($3CT^+$, $4CT^+$, $2CBL^+$, $2CT^-$)

Figure 9. Genealogy of chlorotoluene-degrading strains (Brinkmann and Reineke, 1992). Abbreviations: 2CBA and 3CBA, 2-chloro- and 3-chlorobenzoate, respectively; 2CT, 3CT, 4CT, and 35DCT, 2-chloro-, 3-chloro-, 4-chloro-, and 3,5-dichlorotoluene, respectively; 2CBL, 2-chlorobenzylalcohol.

When strains PaWl and B13 were mated and selected for growth with 3-chloro- and 4-chlorotoluene, strains such as WR1412 or WR1441 occurred at a high frequency (Fig. 9). Strains such as WR1426, with the ability to grow with 3,5-dichlorotoluene, were obtained from the same mating. The investigation of the enzymes clearly indicates that TOL plasmid-encoded enzymes, including toluate 1,2-dioxygenase and those of the modified *ortho* pathway, are used by hybrid strains for growth with the chlorotoluenes.

Since strain JH230 is able to grow with 2-chlorobenzoate, this strain was thought to be the right partner to mate with strain PaWl in order to obtain 2-chlorotoluene-degrading hybrid strains. 3-Chlorotoluene-positive strains such as WR233 resulted at a low frequency from the mating between strains PaWl and JH230. However, strain WR233 fails to use 2-chlorotoluene as the growth substrate. Since it is able to grow with 2-chlorobenzylalcohol, and since 2-chlorotoluene is an effective inducer of the upper pathway, xylene oxygenase seems to be the sole bottleneck to be overcome, but until now we have failed to overcome it.

In contrast to the examples mentioned above, for some chloroanalogous substrates, the respective peripheral pathways do not bring about conversion to chlorocatechols. In this case, more than the mating of two strains is necessary. Moreover, a "novel" pathway has to be constructed in one organism by using segments from at least three organisms. Such a mating is summarized schematically for various chlorobiphenyls in Fig. 10 and 11. However, the nature of some events that have to take place during the development is presently unknown.

WHAT CONCLUSIONS CAN BE DRAWN FROM THE DATA PRESENTED?

The development of hybrid pathways by DNA transfer with whole degradative plasmids has been demonstrated for various mono- and dichlorosubstituted aromatics (Fig. 12). The procedure is superior in its technical simplicity and effective positive selection. In comparison to the enrichment of chloroaromatic-compound-

3-Chlorobiphenyl:

BN10 (BiP^+) x B13 ($3CBA^+$, Sm^r) ——*——→ B131 ($3CBiP^+$) ***($3x10^{-7}$ per donor)***

B13 ($3CBA^+$) x BN10 (BiP^+, Nal^r) ——2*——→ BN210 ($3CBiP^+$) ***($3x10^{-5}$ per donor)***

4-Chlorobiphenyl:

PaW1 ($4MBA^+$) x BN210 ($3CBiP^+$, Nal^r) ——3*——→ KE210 ($4CBiP^+$)

2-Chlorobiphenyl:

1) B13 ($3CBA^+$) x WR401 ($3MSA^+$, $2MBA^+$) ——2*——→ WR612 ($5CSA^+$) ——4*——→ JH230 ($2CBA^+$)

2) JHR (BiP^+) x JH230 ($2CBA^+$, Sm^r, Nal^r) ——*——→ JHR2 ($3CBiP^+$, $4CBiP^+$, $2CBA^+$, $35CBA^+$) ***($1x10^{-7}$ per donor)***

3) JHR2 ——5*——→ JHR22 ($2CBiP^+$, $3CBiP^+$, $4CBiP^+$, $24CBiP^+$, $35CBiP^+$)

Figure 10. Genealogy of chlorobiphenyl-degrading strains (K. Engelberts, unpublished data; Hartmann et al., 1989; Havel and Reineke, 1991; Mokross et al., 1990; D. Springael, unpublished data). The frequency of transfer (given in parentheses) is defined as the number of transconjugants per donor cell. Abbreviations: BiP, biphenyl; 2CBiP, 3CBiP, 4CBiP, 24CBiP, and 35CBiP, 2-chloro-, 3-chloro-, 4-chloro-, 2,4-dichloro-, 3,5-dichlorobiphenyl, respectively; 2CBA, 3CBA, and 4MBA, 2-chloro-, 3-chloro-, and 4-methylbenzoate, respectively; 3MSA and 5CSA, 3-methyl- and 5-chlorosalicylate, respectively; Sm, streptomycin; Nal, nalidixic acid. Symbols: *, transfer of genes encoding biphenyl degradation; 2*, transfer of genes encoding the modified *ortho* pathway for chlorocatechols; 3*, transfer of TOL plasmid; 4*, selection for growth with 2-chlorobenzoate; 5*, selection for growth with 2-chlorobiphenyl.

degrading strains from contaminated sources, which often takes a couple of months, hybrid strains can be developed by well-aimed mating within 1 to 4 weeks, since the organisms with suitable pathway segments are inoculated together on solid medium, making gene transfer easy. However, the selection steps must be done in the right order. It is important to establish the chlorocatechol degradative sequence in the beginning of the development of the hybrid strains, since otherwise, the accumulated chlorocatechols will harm the cells.

In principle, similar strains can also be constructed by using genetic engineering techniques. The major disadvantage of that technique is the huge mass of research necessary before the in vitro construction experiment leading to hybrid strains can be done. Cloning of structural as well as regulatory genes has to be followed by establishment in a suitable host. An additional disadvantage is the higher instability of the resulting strains in comparison to hybrid strains obtained by the in vivo process.

It is highly probable that strains that have been obtained from enrichment cultures and are able to use a chloroaromatic as the growth substrate result from gene transfer. This has been shown for a strain degrading 1,2,4-trichlorobenzene that was enriched from

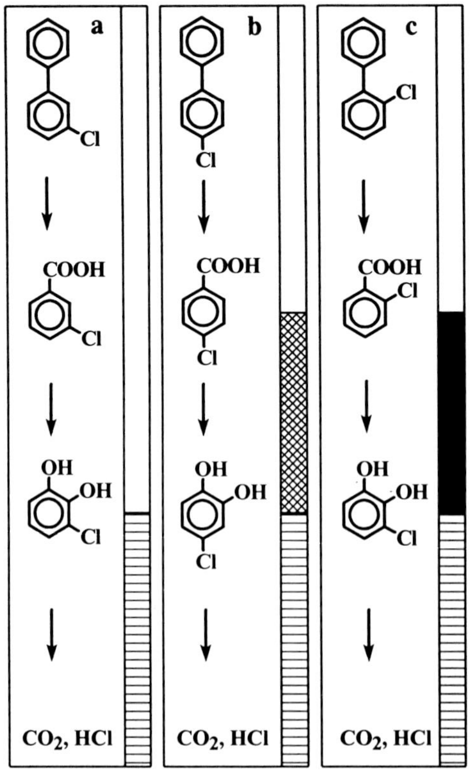

Figure 11. Hybrid pathways for the mineralization of chlorobiphenyls in hybrid strains BN210 and 3CBip$^+$ (a); KE210, 3CBip$^+$, and 4CBip$^+$ (b); and JHR22, 2CBip$^+$, 3CBip$^+$, 4CBip$^+$, 24CBip$^+$, and 35CBip$^+$ (c). The color or hatching on the right side of the pathway characterizes the origin of that pathway segment in the hybrid strains: open bars, biphenyl-degrading strains JHR (c) or BN10 (a,b); cross-hatched bars, *p*-toluate-degrading strain PaW1; solid bars, *o*-toluate-degrading strain WR401; hatched bars, modified *ortho* pathway of strain B13.

sediment of the Rhine River. Van der Meer et al. (1991d) found that a transposon carrying genes that code for the two initial enzymes in the degradation of 1,2,4-trichlorobenzene is part of plasmid pP51, so when the transposon sequence was combined with the chlorocatechol sequence, a hybrid pathway was formed. This clearly indicates that in vivo construction also happens in nature.

Thus far, the dibenzofuran and dibenzo-*p*-dioxin degradation sequences mentioned in Fig. 5 have not been used successfully to develop hybrid strains. One future task should be the degradation of higher-chlorinated biphenyls. New strains that can be used for in vivo construction should harbor a peripheral pathway with the ability to effectively convert biphenyls chlorinated in both rings. However, these strains must also be the right partners in matings with strains such as B13.

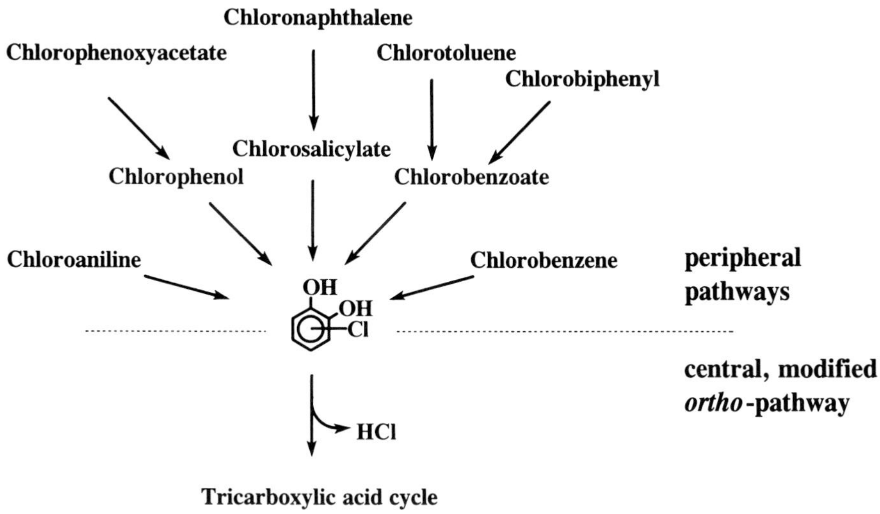

Figure 12. Hybrid pathways for the mineralization of chloroaromatics developed by in vivo construction (Abril et al., 1989; Brinkmann and Reineke, 1992; Chapman, 1988; Chatterjee and Chakrabarty, 1982; Chatterjee et al., 1981a, 1981c; Hartmann et al., 1989; Havel and Reineke, 1991; Latorre et al., 1984; Liu and Chapman, 1983; Mokross et al., 1990; Oltmanns et al., 1988; Reineke and Knackmuss, 1979; Reineke et al., 1982a, 1982b; Schwien and Schmidt, 1982; Timmis et al., 1985).

Acknowledgments. This review was supported by the European Union under the ENVIRONMENT Programme, contract EV5V-CT92-0192, and by the Deusche Forschungsgemeinschaft under contract Re659/3.

REFERENCES

Abril, M.-A., C. Michan, K. N. Timmis, and J. L. Ramos. 1989. Regulator and enzyme specificities of the TOL plasmid-encoded upper pathway for degradation of aromatic hydrocarbons and expansion of the substrate range of the pathway. *J. Bacteriol.* **171:**6782–6790.

Anson, J. G., and G. Mackinnon. 1984. Novel *Pseudomonas* plasmid involved in aniline degradation. *Appl. Environ. Microbiol.* **48:**868–869.

Bachofer, R., and F. Lingens. 1975. Conversion of aniline into pyrocatechol by a *Nocardia* sp.: incorporation of oxygen-18. *FEBS Lett.* **50:**288–290.

Bartels, I., H.-J. Knackmuss, and W. Reineke. 1984. Suicide inactivation of catechol 2,3-dioxygenase from *Pseudomonas putida* mt-2 by 3-halocatechols. *Appl. Environ. Microbiol.* **47:**500–505.

Bartilson, M., I. Nordlund, and V. Shingler. 1990. Location and organization of the dimethylphenol catabolic genes of *Pseudomonas* CF600. *Mol. Gen. Genet.* **220:**294–300.

Bayley, S. A., D. W. Morris, and P. Broda. 1979. The relationship of degradative and resistance plasmids of *Pseudomonas* belonging to the same incompatibility group. *Nature* (London) **280:**338–339.

Bayly, R. C., and G. J. Wigmore. 1973. Metabolism of phenol and cresols by mutants of *Pseudomonas putida*. *J. Bacteriol.* **113:**1112–1120.

Bestetti, G., and E. Galli. 1984. Plasmid-coded degradation of ethylbenzene and 1-phenylethanol in *Pseudomonas fluorescens*. *FEMS Microbiol. Lett.* **21:**165–168.

Bhat, M. A., T. Ishida, K. Horiike, C. S. Vaidyanathan, and M. Nozaki. 1993. Purification of 3,5-dichlorocatechol 1,2-dioxygenase, a nonheme iron dioxygenase and a key enzyme in the biodegradation of a herbicide, 2,4-dichlorophenoxyacetic acid (2,4-D), from *Pseudomonas cepacia* CSV90. *Arch. Biochem. Biophys.* **300:**738–746.

Bhat, M. A., M. Tsuda, K. Horiike, M. Nozaki, C. S. Vaidyanathan, and T. Nakazawa. 1994. Identification and characterization of a new plasmid carrying genes for degradation of 2,4-dichlorophenoxyacetate from *Pseudomonas cepacia* CSV90. *Appl. Environ. Microbiol.* **60:**307–312.

Brinkmann, U., and W. Reineke. 1992. Degradation of chlorotoluenes by in vivo constructed hybrid strains: problems of enzyme specificity, induction and prevention of *meta*-pathway. *FEMS Microbiol. Lett.* **96:**81–88.

Broderick, J. B., and T. V. O'Halloran. 1991. Overproduction, purification, and characterization of chlorocatechol dioxygenase, a non-heme iron dioxygenase with broad substrate tolerance. *Biochemistry* **30:**7349–7358.

Cane, P. A., and P. W. Williams. 1982. The plasmid-coded metabolism of naphthalene and 2-methylnaphthalene in *Pseudomonas* strains: phenotypic changes correlated with structural modification of the plasmid pWW60-1. *J. Gen. Microbiol.* **128:**2281–2290.

Carrington, B., A. Lowe, L. E. Shaw, and P. A. Williams. 1994. The lower pathway operon for benzoate catabolism in biphenyl-utilizing *Pseudomonas* sp. strain IC and the nucleotide sequence of the *bphE* gene for catechol 2,3-dioxygenase. *Microbiology* **140:**499–508.

Catelani, D., and A. Colombi. 1974. Metabolism of biphenyl structure and physicochemical properties of 2-hydroxy-6-oxo-6-phenylhexa-2,4-dienoic acid the *meta*-cleavage product from 2,3-dihydroxybiphenyl by *Pseudomonas putida. Biochem. J.* **143:**431–434.

Catelani, D., A. Colombi, C. Sorlini, and V. Treccani. 1973. Metabolism of biphenyl. 2-Hydroxy-6-oxo-6-phenylhexa-2,4-dienoate: the *meta*-cleavage product from 2,3-dihydroxybiphenyl by *Pseudomonas putida. Biochem. J.* **134:**1063–1066.

Catelani, D., C. Sorlini, and V. Treccani. 1971. The metabolism of biphenyl by *Pseudomonas putida. Experientia* **27:**1173–1174.

Chakrabarty, A. M. 1972. Genetic basis of the biodegradation of salicylate in *Pseudomonas. J. Bacteriol.* **112:**815–823.

Chapman, P. J. 1988. Constructing microbial strains for degradation of halogenated aromatic hydrocarbons. *Basic Life Sci.* **45:**81–95.

Chatterjee, D. K., and A. M. Chakrabarty. 1982. Genetic rearrangements in plasmids specifying total degradation of chlorinated benzoic acids. *Mol. Gen. Genet.* **188:**279–285.

Chatterjee, D. K., S. T. Kellogg, K. Furukawa, J. J. Kilbane, and A. M. Chakrabarty. 1981a. Genetic approaches to the problems of toxic chemical pollution, p. 199–212. *In* A. G. Walton (ed.), *Recombinant DNA*. Elsevier, Amsterdam.

Chatterjee, D. K., S. T. Kellogg, S. Hamada, and A. M. Chakrabarty. 1981b. Plasmid specifying total degradation of 3-chlorobenzoate by a modified *ortho* pathway. *J. Bacteriol.* **146:**639–646.

Chatterjee, D. K., S. T. Kellogg, D. R. Watkins, and A. M. Chakrabarty. 1981c. Plasmids in the biodegradation of chlorinated aromatic compounds, p. 519–528. *In* S. B. Levy, R. C. Clowes, and E. L. Koenig (ed.), *Molecular Biology, Pathogenicity, and Ecology of Bacterial Plasmids*. Plenum Press, New York.

Chaudhry, G. R., and G. H. Huang. 1988. Isolation and characterization of a new plasmid from a *Flavobacterium* sp. which carries the genes for degradation of 2,4-dichlorophenoxyacetate. *J. Bacteriol.* **170:**3897–3902.

Coco, W. M., R. K. Rothmel, S. Henikoff, and A. M. Chakrabarty. 1993. Nucleotide sequence and initial functional characterization of the *clcR* gene encoding a LysR family activator of the *clcABD* chlorocatechol operon in *Pseudomonas putida. J. Bacteriol.* **175:**417–427.

Don, R. H., and J. M. Pemberton. 1981. Properties of six pesticide degradation plasmids isolated from *Alcaligenes eutrophus. J. Bacteriol.* **145:**681–686.

Dorn, E., and H.-J. Knackmuss. 1978a. Chemical structure and biodegradability of halogenated aromatic compounds. Two catechol 1,2-dioxygenases from a 3-chlorobenzoate-grown pseudomonad. *Biochem. J.* **174:**73–84.

Dorn, E., and H.-J. Knackmuss. 1987b. Chemical structure and biodegradability of halogenated aromatic compounds. Substituent effects on 1,2-dioxygenation of catechol. *Biochem. J.* **174:**85–94.

Dorn, E., M. Hellwig, W. Reineke, and H.-J. Knackmuss. 1974. Isolation and characterization of a 3-chlorobenzoate degrading pseudomonad. *Arch. Microbiol.* **99:**61–70.

Dunn, N. W., and I. C. Gunsalus. 1973. Transmissible plasmid coding early enzymes of naphthalene oxidation in *Pseudomonas putida. J. Bacteriol.* **114:**974–979.

Eaton, R. W., and K. N. Timmis. 1986a. Characterization of a plasmid-specified pathway for catabolism of isopropylbenzene in *Pseudomonas putida* RE204. *J. Bacteriol.* **168:**123–131.

Eaton, R. W., and K. N. Timmis. 1986b. Spontaneous deletion of a 20-kilobase DNA segment carrying genes specifying isopropylbenzene metabolism in *Pseudomonas putida* RE204. *J. Bacteriol.* **168:**428–430.

Engelberts, K., E. Schmidt, and W. Reineke. 1989. Degradation of *o*-toluate by *Pseudomonas* sp. strain WR401. *FEMS Microbiol. Lett.* **59:**35–38.

Engesser, K. H., V. Strubel, K. Christoglou, P. Fischer, and H. G. Rast. 1989. Dioxygenolytic cleavage of aryl ether bonds: 1,10-dihydro-1,10-dihydroxyfluoren-9-one, a novel arene dihydrodiol as evidence for angular dioxygenation of dibenzofuran. *FEMS Microbiol. Lett.* **65:**205–210.

Erickson, B. D., and F. J. Mondello. 1992. Nucleotide sequencing and transcriptional mapping of the genes encoding biphenyl dioxygenase, a multicomponent polychlorinated-biphenyl-degrading enzyme in *Pseudomonas* strain LB400. *J. Bacteriol.* **174:**2903–2912.

Evans, W. C., B. S. W. Smith, H. N. Fernley, and J. I. Davies. 1971. Bacterial metabolism of 2,4-dichlorophenoxyacetate. *Biochem. J.* **122:**543–551.

Fortnagel, P., H. Harms, R.-M. Wittich, S. Krohn, H. Meyer, V. Sinnwell, H. Wilkes, and W. Francke. 1990. Metabolism of dibenzofuran by *Pseudomonas* sp. strain HH69 and the mixed culture HH27. *Appl. Environ. Microbiol.* **56:**1148–1156.

Fortnagel, P., R.-M. Wittich, H. Harms, S. Schmidt, S. Franke, V. Sinnwell, H. Wilkes, and W. Francke. 1989. New bacterial degradation of the biaryl ether structure. Regioselective dioxygenation prompts cleavage of ether bonds. *Naturwissenschaften* **76:**523–524.

Frantz, B., and A. M. Chakrabarty. 1987. Organization and nucleotide sequence determination of a gene cluster involved in 3-chlorocatechol degradation. *Proc. Natl. Acad. Sci. USA* **84:**4460–4464.

Fukuda, M., Y. Yasukouchi, Y. Kikuchi, Y. Nagata, K. Kimbara, H. Horiuchi, M. Takagi, and K. Yano. 1994. Identification of the *bphA* and *bphB* genes of *Pseudomonas* sp. strain KKS102 involved in degradation of biphenyl and polychlorinated biphenyls. *Biochem. Biophys. Res. Commun.* **202:**850–856.

Furukawa, K., N. Arimura, and T. Miyazaki. 1987. Nucleotide sequence of the 2,3-dihydroxybiphenyl dioxygenase gene of *Pseudomonas pseudoalcaligenes*. *J. Bacteriol.* **169:**427–429.

Furukawa, K., and A. M. Chakrabarty. 1982. Involvement of plasmids in total degradation of chlorinated biphenyls. *Appl. Environ. Microbiol.* **44:**619–626.

Gibson, D. T., G. E. Cardini, F. C. Maseles, and R. E. Kallio. 1970a. Incorporation of oxygen-18 into benzene by *Pseudomonas putida*. *Biochemistry* **9:**1631–1635.

Gibson, D. T., M. Hensley, H. Yoshioka, and R. J. Mabry. 1970b. Formation of (+)-*cis*-2,3-dihydroxy-1-methylcyclohexa-4,6-diene from toluene by *Pseudomonas putida*. *Biochemistry* **9:**1626–1630.

Gibson, D. T., J. R. Koch, and R. E. Kallio. 1968. Oxidative degradation of aromatic hydrocarbons by microorganisms. I. Enzymatic formation of catechol from benzene. *Biochemistry* **1:**2653–2662.

Gibson, D. T., R. L. Roberts, M. C. Wells, and V. M. Kobal. 1973. Oxidation of biphenyl by a *Beijerinckia* species. *Biochem. Biophys. Res. Commun.* **50:**211–219.

Harayama, S., R. A. Leppick, M. Rekik, N. Mermod, P. R. Lehrbach, and K. N. Timmis. 1986. Gene order of the TOL catabolic plasmid upper pathway operon and oxygenation of both toluene and benzyl alcohol by the *xylA* product. *J. Bacteriol.* **167:**455–461.

Harms, H., R.-M. Wittich, V. Sinnwell, H. Meyer, P. Fortnagel, and W. Francke. 1990. Transformation of dibenzo-*p*-dioxin by *Pseudomonas* sp. strain HH69. *Appl. Environ. Microbiol.* **56:**1157–1159.

Hartmann, J., K. Engelberts, B. Nordhaus, E. Schmidt, and W. Reineke. 1989. Degradation of 2-chlorobenzoate by in vivo constructed hybrid pseudomonads. *FEMS Microbiol. Lett.* **61:**17–22.

Havel, J., and W. Reineke. 1991. Total degradation of various chlorobiphenyls by cocultures and in vivo constructed hybrid pseudomonads. *FEMS Microbiol. Lett.* **78:**163–170.

Hayase, N., K. Taira, and K. Furukawa. 1990. *Pseudomonas putida* KF715 *bphABCD* operon encoding biphenyl and polychlorinated biphenyl degradation: cloning, analysis, and expression of soil bacteria. *J. Bacteriol.* **172:**1160–1164.

Hinteregger, C., M. Loidl, and F. Streichsbier. 1992. Characterization of isofunctional ring-cleaving enzymes in aniline and 3-chloroaniline degradation of *Pseudomonas acidovorans* CA28. *FEMS Microbiol. Lett.* **97:**261–266.

Hofer, B., S. Backhaus, and K. N. Timmis. 1994. The biphenyl/polychlorinated biphenyl-degradation locus (*bph*) of *Pseudomonas* sp. LB400 encodes four additional metabolic enzymes. *Gene* **144:**9–16.

Hofer, B., L. D. Eltis, D. N. Dowlings, and K. N. Timmis. 1993. Genetic analysis of a *Pseudomonas* locus encoding a pathway for biphenyl/polychlorinated biphenyl degradation. *Gene* **130:**47–55.

Holtel, A., M.-A. Abril, S. Marques, K. N. Timmis, and J. L. Ramos. 1990. Promoter-upstream activator sequences are required for expression of the *xylS* gene and upper-pathway operon on the *Pseudomonas* TOL plasmid. *Mol. Microbiol.* **4:**1551–1556.

Inouye, S., Y. Ebina, A. Nakazawa, and T. Nakazawa. 1984a. Nucleotide sequence surrounding transcription initiation site of *xylABC* operon on TOL plasmid of *Pseudomonas putida*. *Proc. Natl. Acad. Sci. USA* **81:**1688–1691.

Inouye, S., A. Nakazawa, and T. Nakazawa. 1984b. Nucleotide sequence promoter region of the *xylDEFG* operon on TOL plasmid of *Pseudomonas putida*. *Gene* **29:**323–330.

Jeenes, D. J., W. Reineke, H.-J. Knackmuss, and P. A. Williams. 1982. TOL plasmid pWW0 in constructed halobenzoate-degrading *Pseudomonas* strains: enzyme regulation and DNA structure. *J. Bacteriol.* **150:**180–187.

Kasberg, T., D. L. Daubaras, A. M. Chakrabarty, D. Kinzelt, and W. Reineke. 1995. Evidence that operons *tcb, tfd,* and *clc* encode maleylacetate reductase, the fourth enzyme of the modified *ortho* pathway. *J. Bacteriol.* **177:**3885–3889.

Kaschabek, S. R., and W. Reineke. 1992. Maleylacetate reductase of *Pseudomonas* sp. strain B13: dechlorination of chloromaleylacetates, metabolites in the degradation of chloroaromatic compounds. *Arch. Microbiol.* **159:**412–417.

Kaschabek, S. R., and W. Reineke. 1995. Maleylacetate reductase of *Pseudomonas* sp. strain B13: specificity of substrate conversion and halide elimination. *J. Bacteriol.* **177:**320–325.

Kikuchi, Y., Y. Nagata, M. Hinata, K. Kimbara, M. Fukuda, K. Yano, and M. Takagi. 1994a. Identification of the *bphA4* gene encoding ferredoxin reductase involved in biphenyl and polychlorinated biphenyl degradation in *Pseudomonas* sp. strain KKS102. *J. Bacteriol.* **176:**1689–1694.

Kikuchi, Y., Y. Yasukochi, Y. Nagata, M. Fukuda, and M. Takagi. 1994b. Nucleotide sequence and functional analysis of the *meta*-cleavage pathway involved in biphenyl and polychlorinated biphenyl degradation in *Pseudomonas* sp. strain KKS102. *J. Bacteriol.* **176:**4269–4276.

Kilpi, S., V. Backström, and M. Korhola. 1983. Degradation of catechol, methylcatechols and chlorocatechols by *Pseudomonas* sp. HV3. *FEMS Microbiol. Lett.* **18:**1–5.

Kimbara, K., T. Hashimoto, M. Fukuda, T. Koana, M. Takagi, M. Oishi, and K. Yano. 1989. Cloning and sequencing of two tandem genes involved in degradation of 2,3-dihydroxybiphenyl to benzoic acid in the polychlorinated biphenyl-degrading soil bacterium *Pseudomonas* sp. strain KKS102. *J. Bacteriol.* **171:**2740–2747.

Kivisaar, M., R. Horak, L. Kasak, A. Heinaru, and J. Habicht. 1990. Selection of independent plasmids determining phenol degradation in *Pseudomonas putida* and the cloning and expression of genes encoding phenol monooxygenase and catechol 1,2-dioxygenase. *Plasmid* **24:**25–36.

Kuhm, A. E., M. Schlömann, H.-J. Knackmuss, and D. H. Pieper. 1990. Purification and characterization of dichloromuconate cycloisomerase from *Alcaligenes eutrophus* JMP134. *Biochem. J.* **266:**877–883.

Latorre, J., W. Reineke, and H.-J. Knackmuss. 1984. Microbial metabolism of chloroanilines: enhanced evolution by naturally genetic exchange. *Arch. Microbiol.* **140:**159–165.

Lehrbach, P. R., D. J. Jeenes, and P. Broda. 1983a. Characterization by molecular cloning or insertion mutants in TOL catabolic functions. *Plasmid* **9:**112–125.

Lehrbach, P. R., I. McGregor, J. M. Ward, and P. Broda. 1983b. Molecular relationships between *Pseudomonas* Inc P-9 degradative plasmids TOL, NAH, and SAL. *Plasmid* **10:**164–174.

Lehrbach, P. R., J. M. Ward, P. Meutien, and P. Broda. 1982. Physical mapping of TOL plasmids pWW0 and pND2 and various R plasmid-TOL derivatives from *Pseudomonas* spp. *J. Bacteriol.* **152:**1280–1283.

Leveau, J. H. J., W. M. de Vos, and J. R. van der Meer. 1994. Analysis of the binding site of the LysR-type transcriptional activator TcbR on the *tcbR* and *tcbC* divergent promoter sequences. *J. Bacteriol.* **176:**1850–1856.

Liu, T., and P. J. Chapman. 1983. Degradation of halogenated aromatic acids and hydrocarbons by *Pseudomonas putida*. *Abstr. Annu. Meet. Am. Soc. Microbiol.*, K211, p. 212.

Lloyd-Jones, G., C. de Jong, R. C. Ogden, W. A. Duetz, and P. A. Williams. 1994. Recombination of *bph* (biphenyl) catabolic genes from plasmid pWW100 and their deletion during growth on benzoate. *Appl. Environ. Microbiol.* **60:**691–696.

Lunt, D., and W. C. Evans. 1970. The microbial metabolism of biphenyl. *Biochem. J.* **118:**54p.

Matrubutham, U., and A. R. Harker. 1994. Analysis of duplicated gene sequence associated with *tfdR* and *tfdS* in *Alcaligenes eutrophus* JMP134. *J. Bacteriol.* **176:**2348–2353.

Mermod, N., P. R. Lehrbach, W. Reineke, and K. N. Timmis. 1984. Transcription of the TOL plasmid toluate catabolic pathway operon of *Pseudomonas putida* is determined by a pair of co-ordinately and positively overlapping promoters. *EMBO J.* **3:**2461–2466.

Miguez, C. B., C. W. Greer, and J. M. Ingram. 1993. Purification and properties of chlorocatechol 1,2-dioxygenase from *Alcaligenes denitrificans* BRI 6011. *Can. J. Microbiol.* **39:**1–5.

Mokross, H., E. Schmidt, and W. Reineke. 1990. Degradation of 3-chlorobiphenyl by in vivo constructed hybrid pseudomonads. *FEMS Microbiol. Lett.* **71:**179–186.

Müller, D., M. Schlömann, and W. Reineke. 1996. Maleylacetate reductases in chloroaromatic-degrading bacteria using the modified *ortho* pathway: comparison of catalytic properties. *J. Bacteriol.* **178:**298–300.

Oltmanns, R. H., H. G. Rast, and W. Reineke. 1988. Degradation of 1,4-dichlorobenzene by constructed and enriched strains. *Appl. Microbiol. Biotechnol.* **28:**609–616.

Perkins, E. J., M. P. Gordon, O. Caceres, and P. F. Lurquin. 1990. Organization and sequence analysis of the 2,4-dichlorophenol hydroxylase and dichlorocatechol oxidative operons of plasmid pJP4. *J. Bacteriol.* **172:**2351–2359.

Pieper, D. H., W. Reineke, K.-H. Engesser, and H.-J. Knackmuss. 1988. Metabolism of 2,4-dichlorophenoxyacetic acid, 4-chloro-2-methylphenoxyacetic acid and 2-methylphenoxyacetic acid by *Alcaligenes eutrophus* JMP134. *Arch. Microbiol.* **150:**95–102.

Pothuluri, J. V., and C. E. Cerniglia. 1994. Microbial metabolism of polycyclic aromatic hydrocarbons, p. 92–124. *In* G. R. Chaudhry (ed.), *Biological Degradation and Bioremediation of Toxic Chemicals*. Dioscorides Press, Portland, Ore.

Ramos, J. L., N. Mermod, and K. N. Timmis. 1987. Regulatory circuits controlling transcription of TOL plasmid operon encoding *meta*-cleavage pathway for degradation of alkylbenzoates by *Pseudomonas*. *Mol. Microbiol.* **1:**293–300.

Ramos, J. L., A. Stolz, W. Reineke, and K. N. Timmis. 1986. New effector specificities in regulators of gene expression: TOL plasmid *xylS* mutants and their use to engineer expansion of the range of aromatics degraded by bacteria. *Proc. Natl. Acad. Sci. USA* **83:**8467–8471.

Reineke, W. 1984. Microbial degradation of halogenated aromatic compounds, p. 319–360. *In* D. T. Gibson (ed.), *Microbial Degradation of Organic Compounds*. Marcel Dekker, New York.

Reineke, W., D. J. Jeenes, P. A. Williams, and H.-J. Knackmuss. 1982a. TOL plasmid pWW0 in constructed halobenzoate-degrading *Pseudomonas* strains: prevention of *meta* pathway. *J. Bacteriol.* **150:**195–201.

Reineke, W., and H.-J. Knackmuss. 1978a. Chemical structure and biodegradability of halogenated aromatic compounds. Substituent effects on 1,2-dioxygenation of benzoic acid. *Biochim. Biophys. Acta* **542:**412–423.

Reineke, W., and H.-J. Knackmuss. 1978b. Chemical structure and biodegradability of halogenated aromatic compounds. Substituent effects on dehydrogenation of 3,5-cyclohexadiene-1,2-diol-1-carboxylic acid. *Biochim. Biophys. Acta* **542:**424–429.

Reineke, W., and H.-J. Knackmuss. 1979. Construction of haloaromatics utilising bacteria. *Nature* (London) **277:**385–386.

Reineke, W., and H.-J. Knackmuss. 1980. Hybrid pathway for chlorobenzoate metabolism in *Pseudomonas* sp. B13 derivatives. *J. Bacteriol.* **142:**467–473.

Reineke, W., S. W. Wessels, M. A. Rubio, J. Latorre, U. Schwien, E. Schmidt, M. Schlömann, and H.-J. Knackmuss. 1982b. Degradation of monochlorinated aromatics following transfer of genes encoding chlorocatechol catabolism. *FEMS Microbiol. Lett.* **14:**291–294.

Reiner, A., M. 1971. Metabolism of benzoic acid by bacteria: 3,5-cyclohexadiene-1,2-diol-1-carboxylic acid is an intermediate in the formation of catechol. *J. Bacteriol.* **108:**89–94.

Reiner, A. M., and G. D. Hegeman. 1971. Metabolism of benzoic acid by bacteria. Accumulation of (-)-3,5-cyclohexadiene-1,2-diol-1-carboxylic acid by a mutant strain of *Alcaligenes eutrophus*. *Biochemistry* **10:**2530–2536.

Sander, P., R.-M. Wittich, P. Fortnagel, H. Wilkes, and W. Francke. 1991. Degradation of 1,2,4-trichloro- and 1,2,4,5-tetrachlorobenzene by *Pseudomonas* strains. *Appl. Environ. Microbiol.* **57:**1430–1440.

Schell, M. A. 1983. Cloning and expression in *Escherichia coli* of the naphthalene degradation genes from plasmid NAH7. *J. Bacteriol.* **153:**822–829.

Schmidt, E., and H.-J. Knackmuss. 1980. Chemical structure and biodegradability of halogenated aromatic compounds. Conversion of chlorinated muconic acids into maleoylacetic acid. *Biochem. J.* **192:**339–347.

Schwein, U. E. Schmidt. 1982. Improved degradation of monochlorophenols by a constructed strain. *Appl. Environ. Microbiol.* **44:**33–39.

Schwien, U., E. Schmidt, H.-J. Knackmuss, and W. Reineke. 1988. Degradation of chlorosubstituted aromatic compounds by *Pseudomonas* sp. strain B13: fate of 3,5-dichlorocatechol. *Arch. Microbiol.* **150:**78–84.

Serdar, C. M., and D. T. Gibson. 1989. Isolation and characterization of altered plasmids in mutant strains of *Pseudomonas putida* NCIB 9816. *Biochem. Biophys. Res. Commun.* **164:**764–771.

Shingler, V., F. C. H. Franklin, M. Tsuda, D. Holroyd, and M. Bagdasarian. 1989. Molecular analysis of a plasmid-encoded phenol hydroxylase from *Pseudomonas* CF600. *J. Gen. Microbiol.* **135:**1083–1092.

Strubel, V., K. H. Engesser, P. Fischer, and H.-J. Knackmuss. 1991. 3-(2-Hydroxyphenyl)catechol as substrate for proximal *meta* ring cleavage in dibenzofuran degradation by *Brevibacterium* sp. strain DPO 1361. *J. Bacteriol.* **173:**1932–1937.

Taira, K., N. Hayase, N. Arimura, S. Yamashita, T. Miyazaki, and K. Furukawa. 1988. Cloning and nucleotide sequence of the 2,3-dihydroxybiphenyl dioxygenase gene from the PCB-degrading strain of *Pseudomonas paucimobilis* Q1. *Biochemistry* **27:**3990–3996.

Taira, K., J. Hirose, S. Hayashida, and K. Furukawa. 1992. Analysis of *bph* operon from the polychlorinated biphenyl-degrading strain of *Pseudomonas pseudoalcaligenes* KF707. *J. Biol. Chem.* **267:**4844–4853.

Tan, H.-M., and J. R. Mason. 1990. Cloning and expression of the plasmid-encoded benzene dioxygenase genes from *Pseudomonas putida* ML2. *FEMS Microbiol. Lett.* **72:**259–264.

Tiedje, J. M., J. M. Duxbury, M. Alexander, and J. E. Dawson. 1969. 2,4-D metabolism: pathway of degradation of chlorocatechols by *Arthrobacter* sp. *J. Agric. Food Chem.* **17:**1021–1026.

Timmis, K. N., P. R. Lehrbach, S. Harayama, R. H. Don, N. Mermod, S. Bas, R. Leppik, A. J Weightman, W. Reineke, and H.-J. Knackmuss. 1985. Analysis and manipulation of plasmid encoded pathways for the catabolism of aromatic compounds by soil bacteria, p. 719–739. *In* D. R. Helinski, S. N. Cohen, D. B. Clewell, D. A. Jackson, and A. Hollaender (ed.), *Plasmids in Bacteria.* Plenum Press, New York.

van der Meer, J. R., R. I. L. Eggen, A. J. B. Zehnder, and W. M. de Vos. 1991a. Sequence analysis of the *Pseudomonas* sp. strain P51 *tcb* gene cluster, which encodes metabolism of chlorinated catechols: evidence for specialization of catechol 1,2-dioxygenases for chlorinated substrates. *J. Bacteriol.* **173:**2425–2434.

van der Meer, J. R., A. C. J. Frijters, J. H. J. Leveau, R. I. L. Eggen, A. J. B. Zehnder, and W. M. de Vos. 1991b. Characterization of the *Pseudomonas* sp. strain P51 gene *tcbR*, a LysR-type transcriptional activator of the *tcbCDEF* chlorocatechol oxidation operon, and analysis of the regulatory region. *J. Bacteriol.* **173:**3700–3708.

van der Meer, J. R., A. R. W. van Neerven, E. J. de Vries, W. M. de Vos, and A. J. B. Zehnder. 1991c. Cloning and characterization of plasmid-encoded genes for the degradation of 1,2-dichloro-, 1,4-dichloro-, and 1,2,4-trichlorobenzene of *Pseudomonas* sp. strain P51. *J. Bacteriol.* **173:**6–15.

van der Meer, J. R., A. J. B Zehnder, and W. M. de Vos. 1991d. Identification of a novel composite transposable element, Tn*5280*, carrying chlorobenzene dioxygenase genes of *Pseudomonas* sp. strain P51. *J. Bacteriol.* **173:**7077–7083.

Vollmer, M. D., P. Fischer, H.-J. Knackmuss, and M. Schlömann. 1994. Inability of muconate cycloisomerases to cause dehalogenation during conversion of 2-chloro-*cis,cis*-muconate. *J. Bacteriol.* **176:**4366–4375.

Vollmer, M. D., and M. Schlömann. 1995. Conversion of 2-chloro-*cis,cis*-muconate and its metabolites 2-chloro- and 5-chloromuconolactone by chloromuconate cycloisomerase of pJP4 and pAC27. *J. Bacteriol.* **177:**2938–2941.

Vollmer, M. D., K. Stadler-Fritzsche, and M. Schlömann. 1993. Conversion of 2-chloromaleylacetate in *Alcaligenes eutrophus* JMP134. *Arch. Microbiol.* **159:**182–188.

Williams, P. A., and K. Murray. 1974. Metabolism of benzoate and methylbenzoates by *Pseudomonas putida (arvilla)* mt-2: evidence for the existence of a TOL plasmid. *J. Bacteriol.* **120:**416–423.

Winstanley, C., S. C. Taylor, and P. A. Williams. 1987. pWW174: a large plasmid from *Acinetobacter calcoaceticus* encoding benzene catabolism by the β-ketoadipate pathway. *Mol. Microbiol.* **1:**219–227.

Wittich, R.-M., H. Wilkes, V. Sinnwell, W. Francke, and P. Fortnagel. 1992. Metabolism of dibenzo-*p*-dioxin by *Sphingomonas* sp. strain RW1. *Appl. Environ. Microbiol.* **58:**1005–1010.

Worsey, M. J., and P. A. Williams. 1975. Metabolism of toluene and xylenes by *Pseudomonas putida (arvilla)* mt-2: evidence for a new function of the TOL plasmid. *J. Bacteriol.* **124:**7–13.

Wyndham, R. C., R. K. Singh, and N. A. Straus. 1988. Catabolic instability, plasmid gene deletion and recombination in *Alcaligenes* sp. BR60. *Arch. Microbiol.* **150:**237–243.

Yen, K.-M., and I. C. Gunsalus. 1983. Plasmid gene organization: naphthalene/salicylate oxidation. *Proc. Natl. Acad. Sci. USA* **79:**874–878.

Yen, K.-M., M. Sullivan, and I. C. Gunsalus. 1983. Electron microscope heteroduplex mapping of naphthalene oxidation genes on the NAH7 and SAL1 plasmids. *Plasmid* **9:**105–111.

Molecular Biology of Pseudomonads
Edited by T. Nakazawa et al.

Chapter 10

Pseudomonads Designed for Bioremediation and Circumvention of Undesirable Routes

Bernd Hofer, Rafael Blasco, Mallavarapu Megharaj, Michael Seeger, David McKay, Rolf-Michael Wittich, Dietmar H. Pieper, and Kenneth N. Timmis

Halogenated aromatic compounds such as polychlorinated biphenyls (PCBs) and dioxins constitute a major class of anthropogenic environmental pollutants that are highly persistent. Microorganisms exhibit an exceptional range of evolutionary potential that enables them to grow at the expense of a wide spectrum of noxious compounds. The evolution of new catabolic pathways for xenobiotics is generally considered to occur by adaptation of preexisting pathways (Clarke, 1984). Many catabolic enzymes for natural substrates exhibit a relaxed specificity (Ramos et al., 1987) that facilitates this evolution. Organisms capable of degrading haloaromatics, for example, often produce two sets of isoenzymes, one constituting a pathway for the halogen-free natural substrate and the other constituting a pathway for the xenobiotic.

The aerobic degradation of a wide range of aromatic compounds involves their being channeled toward one of a few key dihydroxylated intermediates such as catechol, gentisate, or protocatechuate, which are the substrates for cleavage of the aromatic ring. For haloaromatics, the major degradative route involves conversion to the corresponding halocatechols, intradiol (*ortho*) cleavage of the aromatic ring, and halide elimination during a subsequent reaction. This so-called modified *ortho*-cleavage pathway is thought to essentially parallel the classical 3-oxoadipate pathway, and enzymes of both pathways have been assumed to carry out analogous reactions (Dorn and Knackmuss, 1978a, 1978b; Schmidt and Knackmuss, 1980). However, investigations in our laboratory show that this is not generally the case. An unexpected decarboxylation in the degradative route of the key metabolite 4-chlorocatechol (4-CC) that was catalyzed by an enzyme of the ubiquitous 3-oxoadipate pathway led to the formation of an antibiotic that is ordi-

Bernd Hofer, Michael Seeger, David McKay, Rolf-Michael Wittich, Dietmar H. Pieper, and Kenneth N. Timmis • Division of Microbiology, National Research Centre for Biotechnology, Mascheroder Weg 1, 38124 Braunschweig, Germany. ***Rafael Blasco*** • Departamento de Bioquimica y Biologia Molecular, Universidad de Cordoba, Avenida S. Alberto Magno S/N, 14071 Cordoba, Spain. ***Mallavarapu Megharaj*** • Department of Microbiology, University of Otago, POB 56, Dunedin, New Zealand.

narily plant derived and is toxic to microorganisms. This finding provides one explanation for the ecotoxicity of some chloroaromatics. In an attempt to circumvent the problem of poor survival of the potent PCB degrader *Pseudomonas* sp. strain LB400 in nonsterile contaminated soil and to achieve mineralization of the chlorinated benzoates (CBAs) formed by the breakdown of PCBs, recombinant strains were constructed by transfer of genes encoding the well-characterized PCB degradative pathway of LB400 into a pseudomonad capable of utilizing several CBAs.

ANTIBIOTIC FORMATION FROM XENOBIOTICS

Incubation of 4-CC with catechol 1,2-dioxygenase (C12O I) and muconate cycloisomerase, two enzymes of the 3-oxoadipate pathway that are purified from the 3-chlorobenzoate(3-CBA)-degrading bacterium *Pseudomonas* sp. strain B13, gave rise to an unexpected novel metabolite. Although C12O I formed 3-chloro-*cis,cis*-muconate from 4-CC, muconate cycloisomerase, the next enzyme of the classical pathway, did not convert this ring cleavage product to *cis*-dienelactone, as does chloromuconate cycloisomerase, but to a product which by gas chromatography-mass spectrometry (GC-MS), ^{1}H-nuclear magnetic resonance, and spectrophotometric characterization was identified as 4-methylenebut-2-en-4-olide, or protoanemonin (Fig. 1), a natural antibiotic. Formation of protoanemonin was also observed when cell extracts from cultures of other bacteria expressing the 3-oxoadipate pathway (e.g., benzoate-grown *Pseudomonas putida* KT2442 or *Sphingomonas* sp. strain RW1, salicylate-grown *P. putida* RW10) were incubated with 4-CC, indicating a general metabolic conversion catalyzed by muconate cycloisomerizing enzymes. Disappearance of protoanemonin was negligible, suggesting that the antibiotic is a dead-end product of the classical *ortho*-cleavage pathway.

In contrast to cells induced for biosynthesis of the 3-oxaoadipate pathway (or type I) enzymes, 3-CBA-grown cells of strain B13 that are induced for the biosynthesis of the 3-oxoadipate and modified *ortho* pathway (or type II) enzymes did not produce protoanemonin. In this case, maleylacetate resulting from subsequent catabolic steps

Figure 1. Aerobic degradation of haloaromatic compounds. (A) Initial steps in the degradation of certain chloroaromatics. The end products of these upper pathways are generally further metabolized to catechols, which are regarded as central intermediates (Reineke and Knackmuss, 1988). (B) Metabolism of catechols by the classical and modified 3-oxoadipate pathways. While enzymes of the classical pathway metabolize catechol, enzymes of the modified pathway are responsible for the metabolism of CCs. The scheme shows the previously proposed intermediates (Dorn and Knackmuss, 1978a, 1978b; Reineke, 1984; Reineke and Knackmuss, 1988; Schmidt and Knackmuss, 1980) and protoanemonin. Reactions are indicated as follows. Small solid arrows in panel A represent enzymes for the metabolism of bicyclic aromatics. Open arrows between panels A and B indicate enzymes for the metabolism of mononuclear aromatics to catechol. Large solid arrows in panel B indicate reactions catalyzed by enzymes of the 3-oxoadipate pathway (type I enzymes). Finally, open arrows in panel B designate reactions catalyzed by enzymes of the modified *ortho* pathway (type II enzymes). The enzymes involved are catechol 1,2-dioxygenase type I (C12O I), catechol 1,2-dioxygenase type II (C12O II), muconate cycloisomerase (MCI), chloromuconate cycloisomerase (CMCI), muconolactone isomerase (MI), enollactone hydrolase (ELH), dienelactone hydrolase (DLH), and maleylacetate reductase (MAR).

A

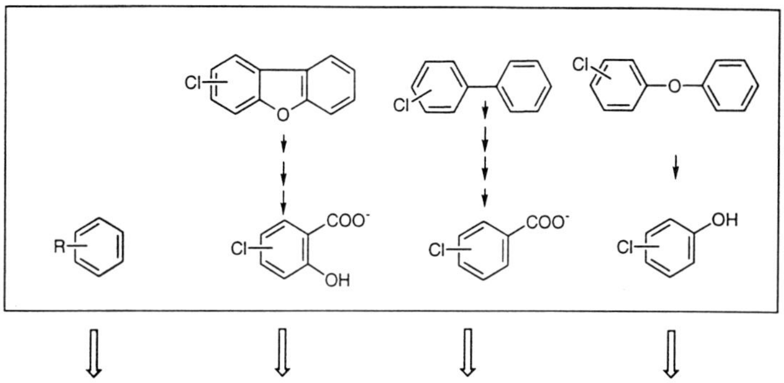

Cl
O
COO⁻
OH
R

B

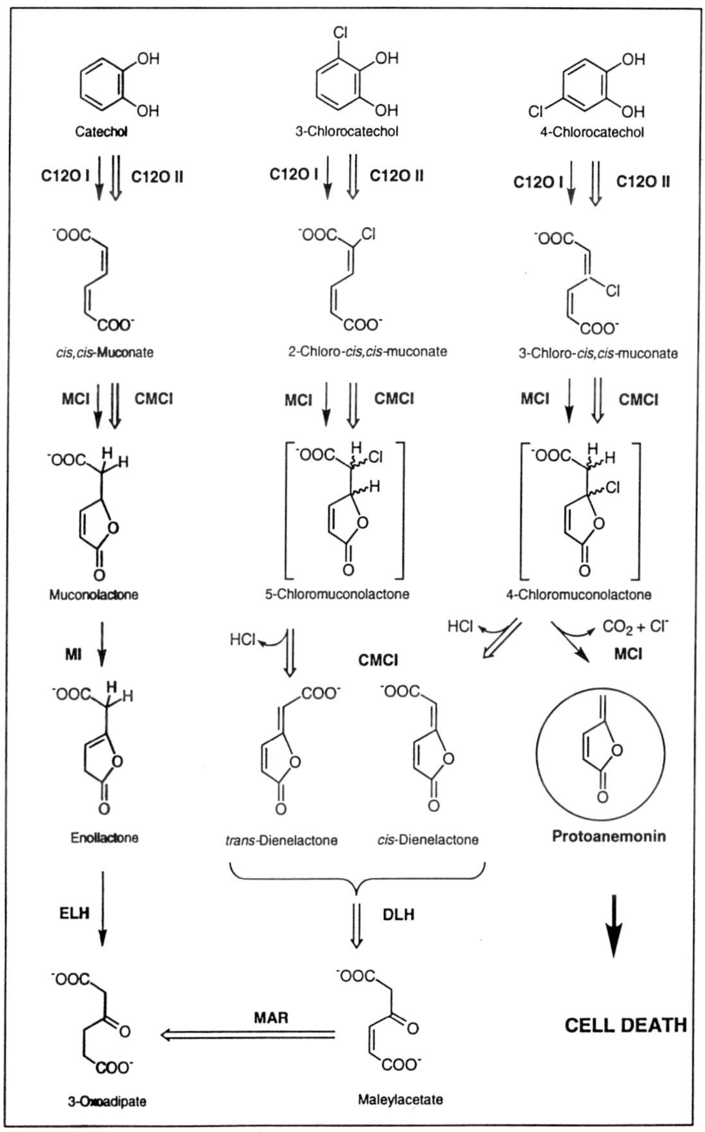

Catechol
3-Chlorocatechol
4-Chlorocatechol
C12O I
C12O II
cis,cis-Muconate
2-Chloro-cis,cis-muconate
3-Chloro-cis,cis-muconate
MCI
CMCI
Muconolactone
5-Chloromuconolactone
4-Chloromuconolactone
HCl
CO2 + Cl⁻
MI
Enollactone
trans-Dienelactone
cis-Dienelactone
Protoanemonin
ELH
DLH
MAR
CELL DEATH
3-Oxoadipate
Maleylacetate

catalyzed by chloromuconate cycloisomerase and dienelactone hydrolase (Fig. 1) was the only product observed.

ECOTOXICITY OF PROTOANEMONIN FORMATION

Protoanemonin has been known since 1945 as a constituent of plants of the *Ranunculaceae* family that is antibiotically active against a wide spectrum of microorganisms (Seegal and Holden, 1945). Formation of this antibiotic might thus be an important factor in the observed toxicity of chloroaromatic pollutants. The compound was enzymatically synthesized and found to exhibit antibiotic activity against bacterial strains of interest for bioremediation as well as against indigenous soil microorganisms. When applied to soil, 75 or 150 ppm of protoanemonin reduced the active microflora (quantitated by dehydrogenase activity) by 40 or 60%, respectively, within 2 days. Eukaryotic microorganisms were more sensitive than prokaryotes, as shown by a more rapid decline in viable counts of fungi and algae than of bacteria. Protoanemonin disappeared completely from nonsterile soil but was fully recoverable from sterile soil, suggesting microbial degradation of the compound.

Although many bacteria are able to attack xenobiotics, incomplete degradation of more highly substituted compounds is frequently observed. PCBs, for example, are typically converted into the corresponding CBAs as dead-end products that are then excreted. These products may subsequently be further metabolized by other members of the microbial community to the respective CCs and then to protoanemonin, with the attendant ecotoxicological consequences for the microbial population. The poor survival observed for some PCB degraders and other strains selected for soil bioremediation (Havel and Reineke, 1992; Harkness et al., 1993) and the positive effect on such survival achieved by coinoculation with CBA degraders (Sondossi et al., 1992; Hickey et al., 1993) are consistent with this hypothesis.

We observed a significant drop in bacterial viability when potential precursors of protoanemonin, such as 4-chlorobiphenyl (4-CB), 4-CBA, or 4-CC, were applied either to pure cultures that had been grown on benzoate (3-oxoadipate pathway induced) or to soil microcosms into which PCB degraders had been introduced (Fig. 2B). With liquid cultures, protoanemonin accumulated in the supernatant as viability dropped. In soil experiments, only minute amounts of the antibiotic were detected. This low recovery is assumed to be due to the ability of a fraction of the natural microflora to metabolize this compound, because protoanemonin could be quantitatively recovered from sterilized soil. The decline of viable counts in soil paralleled the decrease in concentration of the applied chloroaromatics. No toxicity was observed when the soil was treated with a nonchlorinated analog (Fig. 2B), sterilized prior to treatment (Fig. 2A), or coinoculated with a CBA degrader (Fig. 2C). The 4-CBA cometabolizer *P. putida* KT2442, harboring the TOL plasmid which encodes a *meta*-cleavage pathway, also protected against 4-CBA toxicity (Fig. 2C). This rules out possible toxicity due to misrouting of catabolites into that pathway.

These results strongly suggest that protoanemonin formation is a major cause of the ecotoxicity exerted by some chlorinated xenobiotics. If a general problem in haloaromatic-contaminated environments is the formation of protoanemonin, a potential solution seems to be to combine the pathways that are able to degrade pollutants as far as halobenzoates

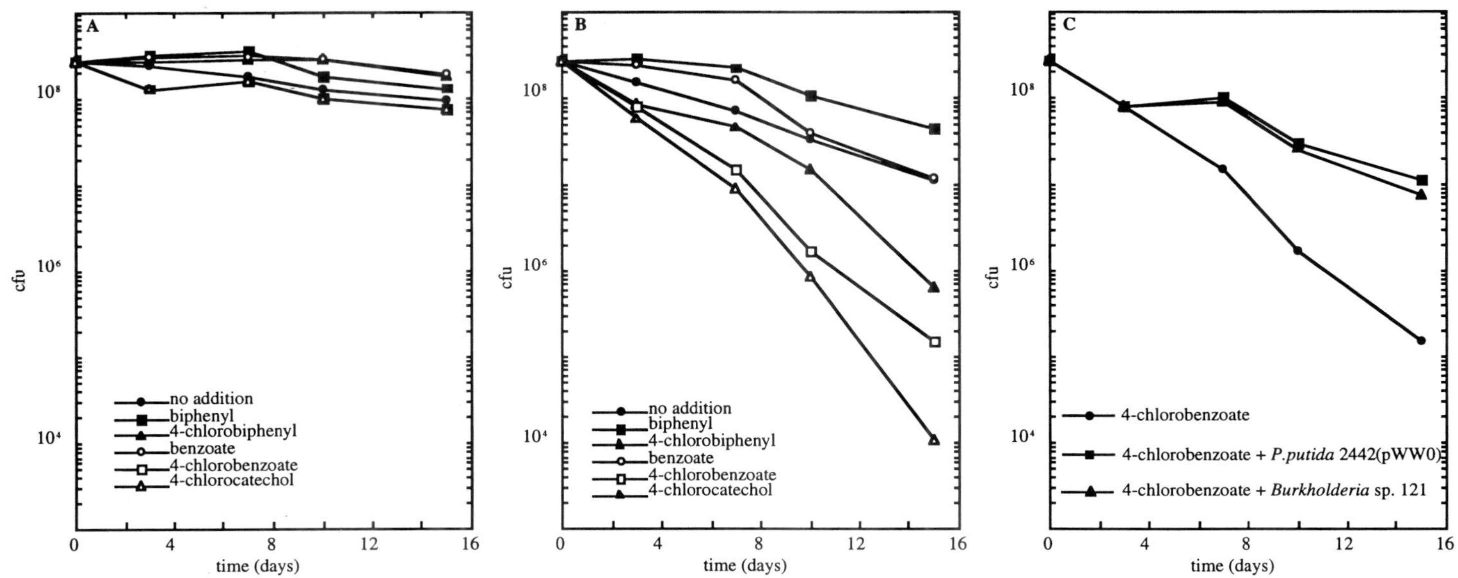

Figure 2. Survival of a PCB degrader in contaminated soil. *Pseudomonas* sp. strain LB400 bacteria containing a mini-Tn*5 lacZ*-Km transposon were added to sterilized (A) and nonsterilized (B) soil amended with 1 mg of probable precursors of protoanemonin (4-CB, 4-CBA, and 4-CC) and their unchlorinated analogs per g of soil. The viability of *Pseudomonas* sp. strain LB400 was determined at the indicated intervals by using Luria broth–5-bromo-4-chloro-3-indolyl-β-D-galactopyranoside plates with or without kanamycin. The effect of 4-CBA on the viability of *Pseudomonas* sp. strain LB400 in nonsterilized soil was studied in the presence of the CBA degrader *Burkholderia* sp. strain 121 (DSM 8961) and the 4-CBA cometabolizer *P. putida* KT2442(pWW0). Data points represent means of three independent experiments.

with "lower" pathways that prevent formation and/or accumulation of protoanemonin. This combination should not only increase survival of the degraders in such environments but also contribute to a more complete degradation of the halogenated xenobiotic. Genes encoding a pathway for PCB degradation have been isolated in this laboratory (Dowling et al., 1993). In the following sections, we describe this pathway and its introduction into a CBA-degrading pseudomonad.

GENETIC AND CATABOLIC CHARACTERIZATION OF AN AEROBIC PCB-DEGRADATIVE PATHWAY

Pseudomonas sp. strain LB400 is known for its ability to deplete a particularly wide range of chlorinated biphenyls (CBs) (Bopp, 1986). A 12.5-kb DNA segment from this strain that is involved in the breakdown of biphenyls (Mondello, 1989; Dowling et al., 1993) was genetically characterized by restriction mapping, subcloning, verification of protein biosynthesis, monitoring of enzymatic activities, and DNA sequencing (Hofer et al., 1993, 1994). The results are summarized in Fig. 3A. To date, functions can be assigned to 11 genes. The *bphA1A2A3A4* genes (also named *bphAEFG* [Erickson and Mondello, 1992]; in the following, collectively referred to as *bphA*) encode the ring-hydroxylating dioxygenase system that belongs to class IIB of such enzymes and is composed of the dioxygenase itself, consisting of two different subunits, and a short electron transport chain comprising a ferredoxin and a ferredoxin reductase. The *bphBCD* genes encode three enzymatic activities that are required for the residual steps of the "upper" pathway of biphenyl degradation that lead to benzoate and an aliphatic C_5 compound, 2-hydroxypenta-2,4-dienoate (Fig. 3B). The *bphHIJ* genes encode three enzymes that catabolize the latter metabolite to pyruvate and acetyl-coenzyme A (Fig. 3B). The product of *bphK* possesses glutathione *S*-transferase activity, as confirmed by conjugation of 1-chloro-2,4-dinitrobenzene with glutathione (Hofer et al., 1994). Its role in biphenyl metabolism is less clear. However, a number of biphenyl-degrading microorganisms have been shown to contain an analogous gene (F. Bartels, K. N. Timmis, and B. Hofer, unpublished data). In addition to the genes described, the 12.5-kb segment contains two open reading frames (ORFs) of unknown function. The ORF located between *bphA2* and *bphA3* is not required for catabolism of biphenyl to 2-hydroxy-6-oxo-6-phenylhexa-2,4-dienoate (Fig. 3B) by a closely related pathway from *Pseudomonas pseudoalcaligenes* KF707 (Furukawa et al., 1992). Expression of *bph* genes is induced by growth of the parental organism on biphenyl (Mondello, 1989). Results by Erickson and Mondello (1992) suggest that a transcriptional start site that is subject to positive regulation by biphenyl is located about 0.9 kb upstream of *bphA1*.

In order to investigate the degradative abilities of *bph*-encoded enzymes with respect to the breakdown of CBs, efficient heterologous expression systems were established. After cloning of *bph* genes downstream of a strong bacteriophage T7 late promoter, most polypeptides constituting the enzymes of the upper pathway could be obtained as the most abundant soluble proteins in *Escherichia coli*. *bph* gene expression in this host, which was expected to be devoid of enzymatic activities able to metabolize CBs, was used to study the catabolic potential of the isolated pathway (Seeger et al., 1995).

GC-MS analysis of products formed by a strain encoding only the ring-hydroxylating dioxygenase (BphA) showed that some congeners attacked in a substituted ring were

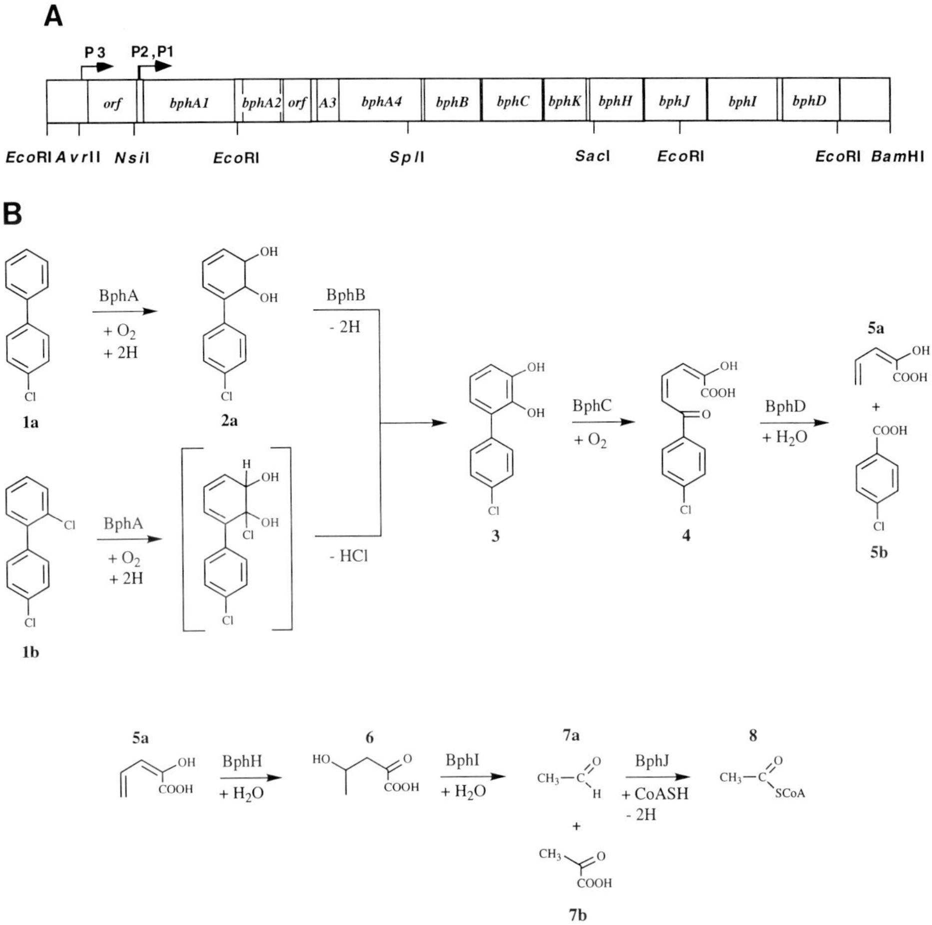

Figure 3. Genetics and biochemistry of (chloro)biphenyl degradation mediated by the *bph* locus of *Pseudomonas* sp. strain LB400. (A) Map of the locus. Cistrons encode metabolic enzymes as follows: *bphA1A2A3A4*, biphenyl-2,3 dioxygenase system; *bphB*, biphenyl-2,3-dihydro-2,3-diol-2,3 dehydrogenase; *bphC*, 2,3-dihydroxybiphenyl-1,2 dioxygenase; *bphK*, glutathione *S*-transferase; *bphH*, 2-hydroxypenta-2,4-dienoate hydratase; *bphJ*, acetaldehyde dehydrogenase (acylating); *bphI*, 4-hydroxy-2-oxovalerate aldolase; *bphD*, 2-hydroxy-6-oxo-6-phenylhexa-2,4-dienoate hydrolase. The fragment shown is 12.5 kb long. P1, P2, and P3 indicate the probable locations of promoters active in *Pseudomonas* spp. or *E. coli* (Erickson and Mondello, 1992). (B) Reactions catalyzed by the encoded enzymes. Metabolites: **1a,** 4-CB; **1b**, 2,4′-dichlorobiphenyl; **2a**, 4-chlorobiphenyl-2′,3′-dihydro-2′,3′-diol;′ **3**, 4-chloro-2′,3′-dihydroxybiphenyl; **4,** 2-hydroxy-6-oxo-6-(4′-chlorophenyl)-hexa-2,4-dienoic acid; **5a,** 2-hydroxypenta-2,4-dienoic acid; **5b**, 4-CBA; **6**, 4-hydroxy-2-oxovaleric acid; **7a**, acetaldehyde; **7b**, pyruvic acid; **8**, acetyl-coenzyme A. CoASH, coenzyme A.

Table 1. Degradation of CBs by *bphABCD*-encoded upper pathway of *Pseudomonas* sp. strain LB400[a]

CB	CBA formed	Dechlorination of oxidized CB ring
2-	2-	NA
3-	3-	NA
4-	4-	NA
2,3-	2,3-	NA
2,4-	2,4	NA
2,5-	2,5-	NA
2,6-	ND	NA
2,2′-	2-	++
2,3′-	3-	+
2,4′-	4-	++
3,3′-	3-	–
3,4′-	4-	–
4,4′-	ND	–
2,3,5-	2,3,5-	NA
2,3,2′-	2,3-	++
2,5,2′-	2,5-	+
3,4,2′-	3,4-	++

[a] ND, not detected; NA, not applicable; ++, complete dechlorination; +, partial dechlorination; –, no dechlorination.

dechlorinated during this initial oxidation (Table 1). Dehalogenation took place by elimination of hydrochloric acid, which directly, i.e., without participation of the normally required dehydrogenase BphB, gave rise to chlorinated dihydroxybiphenyls. So far, dechlorination has been observed only at chlorinated *ortho*-carbons. Dechlorination of CBs has also been reported to occur in vitro when isolated BphA is used (Haddock et al., 1995). Dehalogenation of aromatic compounds has been described for other ring-hydroxylating oxygenases, including halobenzoate dioxygenases (Ahmad et al., 1991; Fetzner et al., 1992; Romanov and Hausinger, 1994).

Formation of CBAs from CBs was monitored by high-pressure liquid chromatography with UV using a recombinant *E. coli* strain harboring *bphABCD* (Table 1). Expression of the cloned pathway genes directed complete or partial breakdown to CBAs of all mono- and dichlorinated biphenyls except 2,6- and 4,4′-dichlorobiphenyl. Of the trichlorinated CBs assayed, only those that possessed either a non- or a mono-*ortho*-chlorinated ring were degraded to benzoates. Normally, the CBA formed originated from initial oxidation of the less-chlorinated ring. When both rings were monochlorinated, the preference of ring attack leading to CBA formation was as follows: 2-chlorinated > 3-chlorinated > 4-chlorinated. As can be seen in Table 1, the *bph*-encoded pathway from strain LB400 is able to break down a number of CBs to CBAs that *P. putida* P111 has been reported to use as sole carbon and energy sources (Hernandez et al., 1991). Therefore, we tried to use this strain as recipient for the *bph* gene cluster.

TRANSFER OF THE PCB-DEGRADATIVE PATHWAY TO A CBA-MINERALIZING MICROORGANISM

Three different gene cassettes were constructed and used for transfer into *P. putida* P111. Cassette *bph*-1 contains the entire 12.5-kb fragment (Fig. 3A), cassette *bph*-2 is a deletion derivative of *bph*-1 that does not contain the first ORF and the biphenyl-regulated promoter, and cassette *bph*-3 is a restructured segment that contains only the genes encoding the upper pathway plus the ORF between *bphA2* and *bphA3*. These cassettes were inserted into a mobilizable delivery vector containing a Tn*5*-based artificial minitransposon (de Lorenzo et al., 1990). Because the delivery vector is able to replicate only in specialized strains that synthesize the π protein (Miller and Mekalanos, 1988), establishment of the *bph* genes within the recipient cell requires their integration into the P111 genome. Mating mixtures were selected for growth on 2-CB. Growth was observed only in transfer experiments involving cassettes *bph*-1 and *bph*-2. The presence of *bph* genes was independently verified by PCR.

With clones containing cassette *bph*-1 or *bph*-2, the genetic stability of the *bph*-encoded pathway during growth for about 100 generations under nonselective conditions was monitored by determining the percentage of cells expressing *bphC*. All *bph*-2 clones had virtually completely lost BphC activity after about 20 generations. Four clones containing cassette *bph*-1 were BphC$^-$ after approximately 70 generations, but five clones of this type were completely stable during the course of the experiment. They were chosen for further investigations. The molecular basis for the instability of *bph*-2 and some *bph*-1 clones is currently unknown.

The presence of the entire *bph*-1 cassette in the five stable clones was confirmed by PCR and by assays for *bphABCD*-encoded enzymatic activities (Table 2). Integration into the recipient's genome may be due either to transposition involving the Tn*5* ends or to another double- or single-crossover recombinatorial event. PCR using primers hybridizing to the transposase gene of the delivery vector, which is located outside of the artificial transposon, indicated the presence of vector sequences other than those originating from the mini-Tn*5* element in all five clones (Table 2). Thus, integration of the *bph* genes probably was not mediated by the Tn*5* system.

The level of *bph* gene expression and its response to growth on biphenyl or succinate as sole carbon source was assessed via determination of BphC activity in cell extracts. Although somevariation was found among the different recombinants, BphC specific activities after growth on either succinate or biphenyl were comparable for the P111 derivatives (Table 2) and strain LB400 (not shown) and were about 20-fold higher after growth on biphenyl. Although cassette *bph*-1 probably contains a biphenyl-inducible promoter, it is presently unclear whether the presumably required regulator protein(s) is

Table 2. Characteristics of stable P111::*bph* recombinants[a]

Strain	Enzyme activity		PCR result			BphC activity ratio (biphenyl/ succinate)	Growth on:			
	BphABC	BphD	*bphA*	*bphD*	*tnp*		2-CB	4-CB	2,2′-CB	2,4′-CB
P111	–	–	–	–	–		–	–	ND	ND
C11	+	+	+	+	+	17	+	+	+	+
C12	+	+	+	+	+	25	+	+	+	+
C13	+	+	+	+	+	19	+	+	+	+

[a]ND, not determined.

supplied by the recipient or whether the ORF preceding *bphA1* plays a role. This ORF encodes an amino acid sequence that shows some similarity to the sequences of transcriptional regulators. As Table 2 shows, the recombinants were also able to use congeners other than 2-CB as sole carbon sources. The potential of these substrates to act as inducers has yet to be assessed.

It was shown that the *bph*-encoded pathway can be stably, inducibly, and functionally integrated into strain P111. Future studies will include detailed investigations of CB catabolism as well as CBA catabolism by the recombinants, because it has recently been shown that intermediates from either pathway may interfere with substrate flux through the combined degradative route (Guilbeault et al., 1994; Lloyd-Jones et al., 1994).

Acknowledgments. We thank Manfred Nimtz and Victor Wray for performing GC-MS and nuclear magnetic resonance analyses, Michael Schlömann for fruitful discussions, and Silke Backhaus for excellent technical assistance. This work was supported by the Federal Ministry of Research and Technology (award 0319-433A). R.B. was supported by the Spanish Ministerio de Educación y Ciencia and the European Environmental Research Organization. M.S. was supported by doctoral fellowships from the Deutscher Akademischer Austauschdienst (Bonn, Germany) and the Consejo Nacional de Ciencia y Tecnología (Santiago, Chile). K.N.T. gratefully acknowledges generous support by the Fonds der Chemischen Industrie.

REFERENCES

Ahmad, D., M. Sylvestre, and M. Sondossi. 1991. Subcloning of *bph* genes from *Pseudomonas testosteroni* and *Escherichia coli*: evidence for dehalogenation during initial attack on chlorobiphenyls. *Appl. Environ. Microbiol.* **57**:2880–2887.

Bopp, L. H. 1986. Degradation of highly chlorinated PCBs by *Pseudomonas* strain LB400. *J. Ind. Microbiol.* **1**:23–29.

Clarke, P. H. 1984. The evolution of degradative pathways, p.11–27. *In* D. T. Gibson (ed.), *Microbial Degradation of Organic Compounds*. Marcel Dekker, New York.

de Lorenzo, V., M. Herrero, U. Jakubzik, and K. N. Timmis. 1990. Mini-Tn*5* transposon derivatives for insertion mutagenesis, promoter probing, and chromosomal insertion of cloned DNA in gram-negative eubacteria. *J. Bacteriol.* **11**:6568–6572.

Dorn, E., and H.-J. Knackmuss. 1978a. Chemical structure and biodegradability of halogenated aromatic compounds. Two catechol 1,2-dioxygenases from a 3-chlorobenzoate grown pseudomonad. *Biochem. J.* **174**:73–84.

Dorn, E., and H.-J. Knackmuss. 1978b. Chemical structure and biodegradability of halogenated aromatic compounds. Substituent effects on 1,2-dioxygenation of catechol. *Biochem J.* **174**:85–94.

Dowling, D. N., R. Pipke, and D. F. Dwyer. 1993. A DNA module encoding *bph* genes for the degradation of polychlorinated biphenyls (PCBs). *FEMS Microbiol. Lett.* **113**:149–154.

Erickson, B. D., and F. J. Mondello. 1992. Nucleotide sequencing and transcriptional mapping of the genes encoding biphenyl dioxygenase, a multicomponent polychlorinated-biphenyl-degrading enzyme in *Pseudomonas* strain LB400. *J. Bacteriol.* **174**:2903–2912.

Fetzner, S., R. Müller, and F. Lingens. 1992. Purification and some properties of 2-halobenzoate 1,2-dioxygenase, a two component enzyme system from *Pseudomonas cepacia* 2CBS. *J. Bacteriol.* **174**:279–290.

Furukawa, K., S. Hayashida, and K. Taira. 1992. Biochemical and genetic basis for the degradation of polychlorinated biphenyls in soil bacteria, p. 259–267. *In* E. Galli, S. Silver, and B. Witholt (ed.), *Pseudomonas: Molecular Biology and Biotechnology*. American Society for Microbiology, Washington, D.C.

Guilbeault, B., M. Sondossi, D. Ahmad, and M. Sylvestre. 1994. Factors affecting the enhancement of PCB degradative ability of soil microbial populations. *Int. Biodeterior. Biodegrad.* **33**:73–91.

Haddock, J. D., J. R. Horton, and D. T. Gibson. 1995. Dihydroxylation and dechlorination of chlorinated biphenyls by purified biphenyl 2,3-dioxygenase from *Pseudomonas* sp. strain LB400. *J. Bacteriol.* **177**:20–26.

Harkness, M. R., J. B. McDermott, D. A. Abramowicz, J. J. Salvo, W. P. Flanagan, M. L. Stephens, F. J. Mondello, R. J. May, J. H. Lobos, K. M. Carroll, M J. Brennan, A. A. Bracco, K. M. Fish, G. L. Warner, P. R. Wilson, D. K. Dietrich, D. T. Lin, C. B. Morgan, and W. L. Gately. 1993. In situ stimulation of aerobic PCB biodegradation in Hudson river sediments. *Science* **259**:503–507.

Havel, J., and W. Reineke. 1992. Degradation of Aroclor 1221 and survival of strains in soil microcosms. *Appl. Microbiol. Biotechnol.* **38**:129–134.

Hernandez, B. S., F. K. Higson, R. Kondrat, and D. D. Focht. 1991. Metabolism of and inhibition by chlorobenzoates in *Pseudomonas putida* P111. *Appl. Environ. Microbiol.* **57**:3361–3366.

Hickey, W. J., D. B. Searles, and D. D. Focht. 1993. Enhanced mineralization of polychlorinated biphenyls in soil inoculated with chlorobenzoate-degrading bacteria. *Appl. Environ. Microbiol.* **59**:1194–1200.

Hofer, B., S. Backhaus, and K. N. Timmis. 1994. The biphenyl/polychlorinated biphenyl-degradation locus (*bph*) of *Pseudomonas* sp. LB400 encodes four additional metabolic enzymes. *Gene* **144**:9–16.

Hofer, B., L. D. Eltis, D. N. Dowling, and K. N. Timmis. 1993. Genetic analysis of a *Pseudomonas* locus encoding a pathway for biphenyl/polychlorinated biphenyl degradation. *Gene* **130**:47–55.

Lloyd-Jones, G., C. de Jong, R. C. Ogden, W. A. Duetz, and P. A. Williams. 1994. Recombination of the *bph* (biphenyl) catabolic genes from plasmid pWW100 and their deletion during growth on benzoate. *Appl. Environ. Microbiol.* **60**:691–696.

Miller, V. L., and J. J. Mekalanos. 1988. A novel suicide vector and its use in construction of insertion mutations: osmoregulation of outer membrane proteins and virulence determinants in *Vibrio cholerae* requires *toxR*. *J. Bacteriol.* **170**:2575–2583.

Mondello, F. J. 1989. Cloning and expression in *Escherichia coli* of *Pseudomonas* strain LB400 genes encoding polychlorinated biphenyl degradation. *J. Bacteriol.* **171**:1725–1732.

Ramos, J. L., A. Wasserfallen, K. Rose, and K. N. Timmis. 1987. Redesigning metabolic routes: manipulation of TOL plasmid pathway for catabolism of alkylbenzoates. *Science* **235**:593–596.

Reineke, W. 1984. Microbial degradation of halogenated aromatic compounds, p. 319–360. *In* D. T. Gibson (ed.), *Microbial Degradation of Organic Compounds*. Marcel Dekker, New York.

Reineke, W., and H.-J. Knackmuss. 1988. Microbial degradation of haloaromatics. *Annu. Rev. Microbiol.* **42**:263–287.

Romanov, V., and R. Hausinger. 1994. *Pseudomonas aeruginosa* 142 uses a three-component *ortho*-halobenzoate 1,2-dioxygenase for metabolism of 2,4-dichloro- and 2-chlorobenzoate. *J. Bacteriol.* **176**:3368–3374.

Schmidt, E., and H.-J. Knackmuss. 1980. Chemical structure and biodegradability of halogenated aromatic compounds. Conversion of chlorinated muconic acids into maleoylacetic acid. *Biochem. J.* **192**:339–347.

Seegal, B. C., and M. Holden. 1945. The antibiotic activity of extracts of *Ranunculaceae*. *Science* **101**:413–415.

Seeger, M., K. N. Timmis, and B. Hofer. 1995. Conversion of chlorobiphenyls into phenylhexadienoates and benzoates by the enzymes of the upper pathway for polychlorobiphenyl degradation encoded by the *bph* locus of *Pseudomonas* sp. strain LB400. *Appl. Environ. Microbiol.* **61**:2654–2658.

Sondossi, M., M. Sylvestre, and D. Ahmad. 1992. Effects of chlorobenzoate transformation on the *Pseudomonas testosteroni* biphenyl and chlorobiphenyl degradation pathway. *Appl. Environ. Microbiol.* **58**:485–495.

Section III

REGULATORY GENES AND TRANSCRIPTIONAL CIRCUITS

Molecular Biology of Pseudomonads
Edited by T. Nakazawa et al.

Chapter 11

Evolution of Regulatory Systems of Biodegradative Pathways

Matthew R. Parsek, Sally M. McFall, and Ananda M. Chakrabarty

Microorganisms are extraordinary in their ability to adapt to unique environmental niches. This adaptability encompasses the ability to use a wide variety of compounds as energy and carbon sources. In the past 50 years, the agrochemical and chemical industries have manufactured a large number of synthetic compounds which have been introduced into the environment. Many of these compounds are rather short-lived and are broken down quickly in nature. However, some, particularly those with halogenated aromatic rings, are persistent in the environment and pose threats to the ecosystems they contaminate. In areas where contamination persists, bacteria capable of degrading these compounds can be isolated. Typically, *Pseudomonas* species are predominant in this population.

Pseudomonads are capable of degrading many substituted aromatics. The genes that enable them to do this are frequently plasmid borne and have evolved over a relatively short time period. The genes encoding the enzymes capable of metabolizing these substituted aromatic compounds are proposed to have been recruited from preexisting genes of related catabolic pathways. The expression of most of these biodegradative pathways is controlled by one or more regulatory proteins. The evolutionary relationships between different pathway enzymes have been carefully studied. However, little is known about how the cell ensures the expression of a newly evolved catabolic pathway. This article will attempt to address some of the questions regarding the evolution of new regulatory systems.

BIODEGRADATIVE REGULATORY SYSTEMS

Many biodegradative pathways have been analyzed and their respective regulators have been characterized. A variety of regulatory mechanisms are utilized to control the expression of these pathways. Almost every family of regulatory proteins is represented

Matthew R. Parsek • Department of Microbiology, University of Iowa, Iowa City, Iowa 52242. ***Sally M. McFall and Ananda M. Chakrabarty*** • Department of Microbiology and Immunology, University of Illinois at Chicago, Chicago, Illinois 60612.

among the different biodegradative regulators identified thus far (see Table 1). Presumably, pathways that are very similar are more likely to have analogous regulatory systems than those which degrade different compounds by completely unrelated pathways. An evolved biodegradative pathway will probably retain the regulatory mechanism of the ancestral system from which it was derived.

Examples of regulatory genes include the *cat, clc, tfd*, and *tcb* systems involved in the degradation, respectively, of catechol in *Pseudomonas putida* and *Acinetobacter calcoaceticus* (Aldrich et al., 1987; Neidle et al., 1989); of 3-chlorocatechol in *P. putida* (Frantz and Chakrabarty, 1987); of 2,4-dichlorophenoxyacetate in *Alcaligenes eutrophus* (Perkins et al., 1990); and of 1,2,4-trichlorobenzene in *Pseudomonas* sp. strain P51 (van der Meer et al., 1991a). The chromosomal *ortho*-cleavage catechol (*cat*) degradation

Table 1. A selection of biodegradative regulatory proteins, their functions, and the organisms from which they were derived

Regulator	Family	Function	Organism	Reference
xylR	NtrC	Activates expression of TOL plasmid upper pathway	*P. putida*	Abril et al., 1989
dmpR	NtrC	Activates expression of *dmp* operon of phenol-degrading plasmid pVI150	*Pseudomonas* sp. strain CF600	Shingler et al., 1993
phhR	NtrC	Activates expression of phenol- and monomethyl-degrading genes of *P. putida* P35X	*P. putida*	Ng et al., 1995
catR	LysR	Activates expression of chromosomal catechol-degrading *catBC* operon	*P. putida*	Rothmel et al., 1990
catM	LysR	Activates expression of catechol-degrading chromosomal *catBCEFD* operon	*Acinetobacter calcoaceticus*	Romero-Arroyo et al., 1995
clcR	LysR	Activates expression *of clcABD* operon of chlorocatechol-degrading plasmid pAC27	*P. putida*	Coco et al., 1993
tfdR	LysR	Activates expression of 2,4-dichlorophenoxyacetate-degrading operon of plasmid pJP4	*Alcaligenes eutrophus*	Perkins et al., 1990
tcbR	LysR	Activates expression of *tcbCDEF* operon of plasmid pP51 involved in 1,2,4-trichlorobenzene degradation	*Pseudomonas* sp. strain P51	van der Meer et al., 1991a
nahR	LysR	Activates expression of naphthalene-degrading *nah* and *sal* operons of plasmid pNAH7 (among others)	*P. putida*	Schell and Poser, 1989
pcaQ	LysR	Activates expression of genes involved in protocatechuate catabolism	*Agrobacterium tumefaciens*	Parke, 1996
xylS	AraC	Activates expression of TOL plasmid lower pathway	*P. putida*	Ramos et al., 1990
pobR	PobR	Activates expression of chromosomal gene involved in *p*-hydroxybenzoate degradation	*Acinetobacter calcoaceticus*	DiMarco et al., 1993
pcaR	PobR	Activates expression of chromosomal genes involved in protocatechuate catabolism	*P. putida*	Parales and Harwood, 1993
camR	TetR	Represses expression of camphor-degrading genes of the CAM plasmid	*P. putida*	Aramaki et al., 1995
aadR	Crp	Activates expression of chromosomal genes required for anaerobic benzoate and 4-hydroxybenzoate catabolism	*Rhodopseudomonas palustris*	Dispensa et al., 1992

genes may be the ancestral system from which the plasmid-borne pathways are derived. The four systems all share similar catabolic intermediates, genes, genetic organization, and regulatory systems (Daubaras and Chakrabarty, 1992). They are controlled by LysR-type transcriptional regulators that induce expression of pathway genes in the presence of the growth substrates or pathway intermediates. LysR family members generally show high amino acid sequence homology in the N-terminal helix-turn-helix DNA binding motif and bind independently of inducer to a region centered approximately 65 bp upstream of the transcriptional start site of the genes they regulate (Schell, 1993). They are positive regulators that activate expression of the genes they regulate after presumably interacting with an inducer molecule. Another LysR-type biodegradative regulator which is much more distantly related to *catR* is encoded by the *nahR* gene, which regulates naphthalene degradation in *P. putida* (Schell and Wender, 1986).

The *P. putida* regulator, CatR, and the inducer molecule, *cis,cis*-muconate, have been shown to be required for expression of the chromosomal *catBC* operon (Rothmel et al., 1990; Wheelis and Ornston, 1972). DNase I footprinting has shown that in the absence of inducer, CatR binds to a 27-bp region termed the repression binding site. This site is located –79 to –53 relative to the *catBC* transcriptional start site. When the inducer molecule is present, an additional downstream binding site called the activation binding site is protected (–47 to –34) (Parsek et al., 1992) (Fig. 1). Binding of CatR to the activation binding site is cooperative and requires an intact repression binding site. The inducer, *cis,cis*-muconate, also increases the binding affinity of CatR for promoter DNA (Parsek et al., 1992) and is required for *catBC* transcript formation in in vitro transcription assays (Parsek et al., in preparation). Recently, the *catA* gene, which encodes catechol 1,2,-dioxygenase, was cloned and sequenced and found to lie directly downstream of the *catC* gene (Houghton et al., 1995). Insertion of Tn*5* in *catR* blocked the expression of *catA* and *catBC,* but insertion of Tn*5* into *catB* did not effect the expression of *catA* (i.e., there is no polar effect). This indicates that *catR* independently activates the *catBC* operon and the *catA* gene. Gel shift assays that showed CatR can bind to a DNA fragment of *catC* supported this supposition, but this interaction has not been footprinted, nor has promoter activity been demonstrated for this fragment (Houghton et al., 1995).

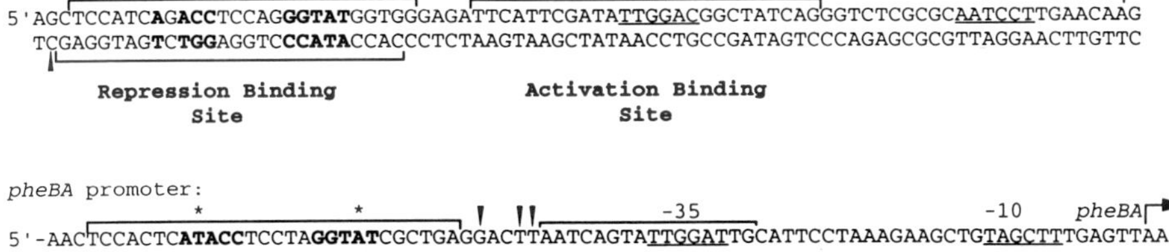

Figure 1. Comparison of the *catBC* and *pheBA* promoter regions. The repression binding site and activation binding site are indicated in the diagram. Sequences protected by CatR from DNase I digestion are depicted by brackets; regions of hypersensitivity are indicated by arrows. The –35 and –10 consensus hexamer sequences are underlined. The CatR inverted recognition repeat is in boldface type. The estimated K_ds of CatR for the *catBC* promoter are –ccm = 7.0×10^{-11} M and +ccm = 3.1×10^{-11} M; the estimated K_ds of CatR for the *pheBA* promoter are –ccm = 5.5×10^{-11} M and +ccm = 2.3×10^{-11} M.

The *catM* gene regulates the chromosomal *catBCIJFD* operon that is involved in catechol degradation in *Acinetobacter calcoaceticus* (Neidle et al., 1989). Originally, CatM was reported to be unique among the LysR family because it was a repressor of the *catBCIJFD* operon on the basis of constitutive phenotypes of two *catM* mutants (Neidle et al., 1989). Recently, it has been demonstrated that this constitutive expression was the result of a mutation in a gene distinct from *catM* and that *catM* is an activator of the *catA* and the *catBCIJFD* operons in response to *cis,cis*-muconate (Romero-Arroyo et al., 1995). CatM has been shown to bind to the operons' promoter regions irrespective of the inducer *cis,cis*-muconate, and methylation protection footprinting showed that CatM bound to a sequence (−72 to −58) that was very similar to the recognition sequence of CatR (Romero-Arroyo, 1992). The similarities in binding sequences and the high DNA homology between *catR* and *catM* (45% identical) despite significant differences in G+C content (*catR*, 65%; *catM*, 44%) strongly indicate that they may have evolved from a common ancestor (Romero-Arroyo et al., 1995).

The 3-chlorocatechol regulator ClcR activates expression of the *clcABD* operon encoded by the plasmid pAC27 (Frantz and Chakrabarty, 1987; Coco et al., 1993). DNase I footprinting showed that ClcR protected a long discontinuous sequence interspersed with hypersensitive bands extending from −74 to −19 relative to the *clcABD* transcriptional start site (Coco et al., 1994). ClcR is thought to interact with an inducer molecule, possibly 2-chloromuconate, which causes a conformational change in the protein. This conformational change may allow ClcR to interact with RNA polymerase and subsequently initiate transcription (Coco et al., 1994).

The regulatory gene *tfdR* controls expression of the *tfdCDEF* operon of the 2,4-dichlorophenoxyacetate-degrading plasmid pJP4 (Perkins et al., 1990). Another gene, *tfdS*, was implicated in the regulation of the *tfdB* gene (Kaphammer and Olsen, 1990). This gene was later reported to be identical to the *tfdR* gene (Matrubutham and Harker, 1994; You and Ghosal, 1995). Gel shift assays demonstrated the interaction of *tfdR* with the *tfdCDEF* promoter region (Matrubutham and Harker, 1994). This interaction has not yet been footprinted.

The *tcbCDEF* operon of the 1,2,4-trichlorobenzene-degrading plasmid pP51 is under control of the regulatory gene *tcbR* (van der Meer et al., 1991a). The TcbR protein has been shown to interact with the *tcbCDEF* promoter by using gel shift assays (van der Meer et al., 1991b) and DNase I footprinting (Leveau et al., 1994). Footprinting demonstrated noncontinuous protection of the *tcbCDEF* promoter DNA from −81 to −17 relative to the transcriptional start site. This footprint contained regions of hypersensitivity throughout the protected area and is very similar to the footprint of ClcR on the *clcABD* promoter region (Coco et al., 1994). This suggests that ClcR and TcbR activate transcription through similar mechanisms. The addition of 1 μM 2-chloromuconic acid or 3-chlorocatechol had no effect on the footprinting pattern, although the more substituted potential inducers, di- and trichloromuconic acids, have not been tested.

The plasmid NAH7 harbors genes specifying naphthalene degradation by way of the *meta*-cleavage pathway (Schell, 1983). These genes are organized into two operons (*sal* and *nah*) that are under control of the *nahR* gene (Yen and Gunsalus, 1985; Schell, 1985). The *nahR* gene product activates expression of these operons in the presence of the inducer salicylate. By use of gel shift assays, NahR was found to bind to the promoter regions of the operon independent of and unaffected by the presence of inducer (Schell and Poser, 1989). DNase I footprinting showed that NahR bound an area −82 to −47 relative to both the *nah* and *sal* transcriptional start sites. The NahR binding sequences at both promoters were approximately 70% identical, and salicylate did not affect the DNase I footprinting pattern (Schell and Poser, 1989). However, in vivo footprinting revealed that guanines downstream of the original DNase I footprinting-defined binding site at the *nah* and *sal* promoters were critical for NahR binding in the presence of inducer (Huang and Schell, 1991). Thus, like CatR, NahR protects sequences downstream from the primary binding site in the presence of inducer. The downstream protection may encompass the −35 consensus promoter sequence. The binding of NahR to downstream sequences may play a role in transcriptional activation by enhancing recognition of the promoter by RNA polymerase, possibly through NahR-RNA polymerase interactions.

The XylR and DmpR gene products belong to the NtrC class of transcriptional regulators and are involved in regulating the upper pathway of the *P. putida* mt-2 TOL plasmid and the phenol-degrading operon of *Pseudomonas* sp. strain CF600, respectively (Abril et al., 1989; Shingler et al., 1993). The NtrC family of transcriptional regulators is characterized by the position of the regulatory binding sites located approximately 120 to 180 bp upstream of the transcriptional start sites of the genes they activate (Morett and Segovia, 1993). Many also activate σ^{54}-dependent promoters after being phosphorylated by an environmental sensor protein. Both DmpR and XylR exhibit modular domain organization characteristic of the NtrC family, but instead of being activated by phosphorylation, they interact directly with their effector molecules to sense a change in the environment (Morett and Segovia, 1993). The amino acid sequences of DmpR and XylR have been shown to be 64% identical, suggesting a common evolutionary origin (Shingler and Moore, 1994). Recently, PhhR, a proposed NtrC family member, has been demonstrated to regulate the chromosomal *meta*-cleavage phenol- and monomethyl phenol-degrading genes in *P. putida* P35X (Ng et al., 1995).

The *xylR* gene product activates the upper pathway promoter of the TOL plasmid (Pu) and the *xylS* promoter (Ps). The *xylS* gene encodes the regulator for the lower pathway of the TOL plasmid (Abril et al., 1989; Marques and Ramos, 1993; Inouye et al., 1987). XylR binds to a region called the upstream activating sequence (UAS) which spans nucleotides −175 to −124 of the Pu promoter and −187 to −136 of the Ps promoter (Inouye et al., 1990; Gomada et al., 1992). The UAS contains an inverted repeat that is thought to be important in sequence-specific recognition, although the exact sequence recognized by XylR is unclear (Fernandez et al., 1994). The activation mechanism is thought to involve the interaction of XylR with an effector molecule (toluene; *m*-, *o*-, and *p*-xylene) which causes a conformational change and repositioning of the N-terminal domain of the protein, exposing residues in the central domain involved in activation (Abril et al., 1989; Fernandez et al., 1995). The general DNA-bending proteins, integration host factor and HU protein, play a role in the activation of the Pu and Ps promoters, respectively (de Lorenzo et al., 1991; Perez-Martin and de Lorenzo, 1995). The activation mechanism of DmpR is not as well characterized, although it is likely very similar to the TOL system. The *dmp* operon has a UAS (−174 to −123) that shows high homology to the TOL plasmid UAS (Shingler et al., 1993). DmpR responds to a very wide range of effector molecules, including phenol, cresols, chlorophenol, and catechol (Shingler and Moore, 1994).

The promoter for the lower pathway (Pm) of the TOL plasmid is regulated by the *xylS* gene product, which shows homology to the AraC family of transcriptional regulators

(Ramos et al., 1990; Mermod et al., 1987). The lower pathway of the TOL plasmid is a *meta*-cleavage pathway responsible for converting benzoate and a number of substituted benzoates to common metabolic intermediates via 2-hydroxymuconic semialdehyde. XylS has been shown to bind to a regulatory element called OM_L/OM_R, which consists of two 15-bp direct repeats separated by 6 bp. This binding element extends from –70 to –35 relative to the transcriptional start of the Pm (Kessler et al., 1993). XylS responds to an effector molecule such as benzoate or 3-methylbenzoate and induces transcription by presumably overcoming a poor –35 consensus RNA polymerase hexamer.

A recently described family of regulators called the PobR family has been identified based on amino acid homology (DiMarco et al., 1993). This family includes the repressor of the acetate operon *iclR* (Sunnarborg et al., 1990) and regulators of *p*-hydroxybenzoate and protocatechuate catabolism (Parales and Harwood, 1993; DiMarco et al., 1993). The *pobR* gene and the substrate *p*-hydroxybenzoate were found to be required for expression of the *pobA* gene, which is responsible for converting *p*-hydroxybenzoate to protocatechuate in *Acinetobacter calcoaceticus* (Doten et al., 1987). The *pobR* gene is divergently transcribed from the *pobA* gene, and the genes are 134 bp apart (DiMarco et al., 1993). *p*-Hydroxybenzoate presumably interacts with PobR since many analogs of *p*-hydroxybenzoate were shown to inhibit induction of *pobA* expression (DiMarco et al., 1993).

The *pcaR* gene activates expression of the protocatechuate pathway *pcaIJ, pcaB, pcaC, pcaD,* and *pcaF* genes in *P. putida* (Hughes et al., 1988). These gene products convert β-carboxy-*cis,cis*-muconate to succinyl-CoA and acetyl-CoA. The *pcaR* gene product requires β-ketoadipate as an inducer molecule for activation of the *pca* genes (Hughes et al., 1988; Parales and Harwood, 1993). Gel shift assays have demonstrated that PcaR binds the *pcaI* promoter region (Romero-Steiner et al., 1994). A 15-bp repeat located in both *pcaI* and *pobA* promoter regions is thought to represent a conserved DNA binding element (Romero-Steiner et al., 1994). The importance of this repeat in the *pca* system was determined using deletions of the promoter region in in vivo expression studies (Parales and Harwood, 1993). This element encompasses the –10 hexamer of both promoter regions, suggesting a novel regulatory mechanism.

The *Agrobacterium tumefaciens pcaQ* gene activates transcription of the *pcaD* gene in the presence of β-carboxy-*cis,cis*-muconate (Parke, 1993). The *pcaD* gene product is responsible for the conversion of β-ketoadipate enol-lactone to β-ketoadipate (Parke and Ornston, 1986). At least three other *pca* genes were not expressed in a *pcaQ* mutant background. The *pcaQ* gene product regulates isofunctional genes of the β-ketoadipate pathway as the *P. putida* regulator, *pcaR*. PcaQ is thought to be unique from *P. putida* PcaR since the inducer molecule is β-carboxy-*cis,cis*-muconate and not β-ketoadipate. This was confirmed when the sequence of *pcaQ* was recently published, and the deduced amino acid sequence indicated that PcaQ is a LysR-type regulator that activates the expression of the *pcaDCHGB* operon (Parke, 1996).

The CAM plasmid of *P. putida* contains genes required for catabolism of the compounds D- and L-camphor (Rheinwald et al., 1973). The negative regulator, CamR, represses expression of the cytochrome P-450cam hydroxylase operon (*camDCAB*) and autorepresses *camR* in the absence of the inducer camphor (Koga et al., 1986). The presence of camphor in the growth medium results in a relief of repression by CamR. The *camR* gene is divergently transcribed from the operon, and the transcriptional start sites are separated by 11 bp (Fujita et al., 1993). CamR has been shown to bind to a 23-bp region encompassing the −10 hexamer of the *camR* gene and partially encompassing the −10 region of the *camDCAB* promoter. CamR protected this region from DNase I attack, and this protection was inhibited by the addition of D-camphor, a substrate of cytochrome P-450cam (Aramaki et al., 1995). The putative helix-turn-helix region of CamR exhibits homology to BM3R1, the transcriptional repressor of *Bacillus megaterium*, which controls the expression of its own gene (*bm3R1*) and the cytochrome P-450_{BM} gene (Aramaki et al., 1995). Because Bm3R1 and CamR repress related genes and have similar footprints on their promoters which are inhibited by the substrates of the cytochrome P-450s of their respective organisms, it has been suggested that they may have derived from a common ancestor that resembled TetR (Aramaki et al., 1995).

Rhodopseudomonas palustris is capable of anaerobically converting many aromatic carboxylic acids to benzoate and 4-hydroxybenzoate, which are further degraded by ring-fusion pathways to acetyl-coenzyme A (Dispensa et al., 1992). The anaerobic pathway for benzoate degradation is significantly different from the aerobic pathway, in that it utilizes a reductive mechanism instead of an oxidative one. The regulatory gene *aadR* was shown to be required for expression of the first enzyme in the pathway, benzoate-coenzyme A ligase, which activates benzoate so that it can be reductively degraded (Dispensa et al., 1992). AadR was required for anaerobic growth on 4-hydroxybenzoate and was shown by sequence analysis to belong to the CRP family of transcriptional activators (Dispensa et al., 1992).

COMMON CHARACTERISTICS OF BIODEGRADATIVE REGULATORY SYSTEMS

Although the previous section emphasized the diversity of biodegradative regulators, there are a number of common features shared by many of these systems. One characteristic shared by most biodegradative regulatory systems is that the genes encoding metabolic pathway enzymes are almost always transcriptionally activated. The environmental sensing mechanism for these systems usually involves a catabolic intermediate of the pathway being regulated, which acts as an inducer molecule. Nearly all the transcriptional activators mentioned are presumed to interact directly with inducer molecules. The inducer has been suggested to cause a conformational change in the regulatory protein that allows it to activate transcriptional initiation (Fernandez et al., 1994; Parsek et al., 1992).

The inducer molecule may provide a degree of regulatory specificity for a biodegradative system. An illustration of this point can be seen with the *cat* and *clc* regulatory schemes. CatR and ClcR are responsible for activating the expression of the *cat* and *clc* operons in the presence of the inducers *cis,cis*-muconate and 2-chloromuconate, respectively. CatR and ClcR have been suggested to be evolutionarily related (Schlaman et al., 1992) and are capable of cross-binding to each other's promoter regions (Parsek et al., 1994a). The specificity of each regulator is determined by its inducer molecule. Although CatR can bind to the promoter region of the *clcABD* operon, full activation requires its own inducer. Specific regulators must evolve with the new pathway in order to utilize a novel catabolic intermediate as an inducer molecule, as in the case of ClcR and 2-chloromuconate. On the other hand, their DNA binding sequence specificities would not necessarily have to change dramatically to ensure expression of the new pathway genes.

Another feature of many biodegradative regulatory systems is the existence of a regulatory cascade. This feature probably results from the need of the cell to be able to coordinately control expression of different genes at different points in the pathway. Examples of this are seen in the catechol and protocatechuate branches of the β-ketoadipate pathway and in the regulation of the TOL plasmid. Conversion of *p*-hydroxybenzoate to trichloroacetic acid (TCA) cycle intermediates requires eight genes that are regulated by at least two different transcriptional activators, PobR and PcaR (Parales and Harwood, 1993). PobR activates expression of *pobA*, which is required for the initial breakdown of *p*-hydroxybenzoate. PcaR regulates the genes which convert β-carboxy-*cis,cis*-muconate to TCA cycle intermediates.

Another example of a regulatory cascade is the catechol branch of the β-ketoadipate pathway which degrades benzoate to TCA cycle intermediates and is regulated by at least three genes. The regulatory *benR* has been implicated in controlling expression of the genes that convert benzoate to catechol (Jeffrey et al., 1992). The *catR* gene product then regulates the genes responsible for degrading catechol to β-ketoadipate enol-lactone. PcaR controls the expression of genes required for the final steps of the pathway where β-ketoadipate enol-lactone is converted to TCA cycle intermediates. A regulatory cascade allows the selective activation of genes at different points in this pathway. Since many catabolic systems feed into the catechol and protocatechuate pathways at different points, this selective activation avoids the uneconomical expression of unnecessary genes.

A regulatory cascade is also seen in the TOL plasmid system. The conversion of toluene and *m*- and *p*-xylenes to the corresponding benzoate and toluates requires the upper pathway gene products. Expression of the upper pathway promoter requires the regulator XylR. XylR also is responsible for the expression of the *xylS* gene which, in turn, controls expression of the TOL plasmid lower pathway operon (Inouye et al., 1987).

EVOLVING A NEW REGULATORY SYSTEM

The adaptation of preexisting catabolic pathways for new compounds requires a corresponding change in the preexisting regulatory system to ensure expression of the new pathway genes. The evolution of a new regulatory system may involve a generation of a new regulator or simply modification of existing regulatory elements (positional or sequence alterations of DNA binding sequences, for example).

Plasmid pEST1226 allows *P. putida* PaW85 to grow on phenol (Kivisaar et al., 1990). The plasmid harbors the *pheBA* operon, which encodes the enzymes for conversion of phenol to *cis,cis*-muconate, as well as two genes of unknown function, ORF1 and ORF2 (Nurk et al., 1991). *cis,cis*-Muconate is then catabolized to TCA cycle intermediates via the chromosomal β-ketoadipate pathway. Expression of the *pheBA* operon was shown to require the chromosomal catechol *catR* regulatory gene (Kasak et al., 1993). Analysis of the *pheBA* promoter and the chromosomal CatR-regulated *catBC* promoter revealed a high degree of sequence identity (Fig. 1). DNase I footprinting and gel shift assays demonstrated that CatR interacts with the *catBC* and *pheBA* promoter regions in a very similar manner in vitro (Parsek et al., 1995). These data suggest that the regulatory mechanisms of the *catBC* and *pheBA* promoters are very similar.

Recently a CatR binding site was found within the *catB* structural gene approximately 164 bp downstream of the transcriptional start site (+164 to +191) of the *catBC* operon (Fig 2A). This site, called the internal binding site, was found to play a possible role in enhancing activation of the *catBC* operon, although its exact role in regulation is under investigation. Interestingly, the *pheBA* promoter region was found to have a CatR binding site downstream of the transcriptional start site as well (+204 to +221) (Fig. 2B), 40 bp before the ATG of ORF1. Apparently, the CatR regulatory mechanism may require binding sites downstream of the promoter region. The ORF1 and *catB* genes share no functional or sequence homology, yet the *pheBA* regulatory system conserved the internal binding site. This indicates that recruitment of the *catBC* promoter region was not the only event that occurred in the evolution of the *pheBA* regulatory system.

The apparent recruitment of the *catR* gene for the regulation of the *pheBA* operon conserved most of the regulatory features of the *catBC* system. Besides DNase I footprinting and gel shift data, this is reflected in CatR DNA bending assays (Parsek et al., 1995). LysR-family members have previously been shown to have inducer-responsive changes in DNA bending at the promoter region which is thought to be important in

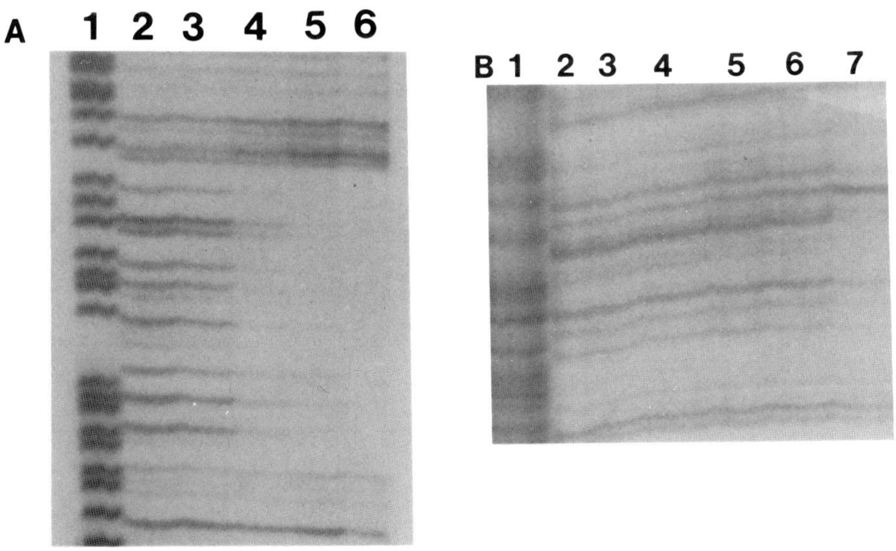

catB internal site:

5'-CCATGAGCAGC**AGACC**CTGGT**GGTAT**TGCGTGTTCG
GGTACTCGTCG**TCTGG**GACCA**CCATA**ACGCACAAGC
+164 +191

pheBA internal site:

5'-TTGGCAAA**ATACC**GCGACCCC**A**CCCACCGAG
AACCGTTT**TATGG**CGCTGGGG**T**GGGTGGCTC
+204 +221

Figure 2. DNase I footprinting of CatR to the *phe* and *cat* system internal binding sites. (A) CatR binding to the *catB* internal binding site. All reactions contain approximately 5 ng of ^{32}P-end-labeled DNA. Lane 1 is a G+A reaction. Lane 2 contains free DNA. Lanes 3 through 6 contain 55 ng, 330 ng, 880 ng, and 3.3 μg of CatR, respectively. The sequences protected by CatR are depicted below in brackets. (B) CatR binding to the *phe* internal site. Lane 1 is a G+A reaction. Lane 2 contains free DNA. Lanes 3 through 7 contain 77 ng, 110 ng, 220 ng, 440 ng, and 880 ng of purified CatR, respectively. The sequences protected from DNase I digestion by CatR are bracketed.

the activation mechanism (Hryniewicz and Kredich, 1994; Wang et al., 1992). This property was examined by using the circular permutation gel shift assay to analyze the interaction of CatR with the *pheBA* and *catBC* promoter regions. CatR was found to bend both the *catBC* and *pheBA* promoter regions (Parsek et al., 1995). In the presence of inducer, CatR introduced almost identical bends in the two promoter regions (37° and 38°, respectively) (Fig. 3B, compare lanes 1 through 5 versus lanes 6 through 10). This may reflect the importance of a fixed, CatR-induced bending angle at the promoter region for activation.

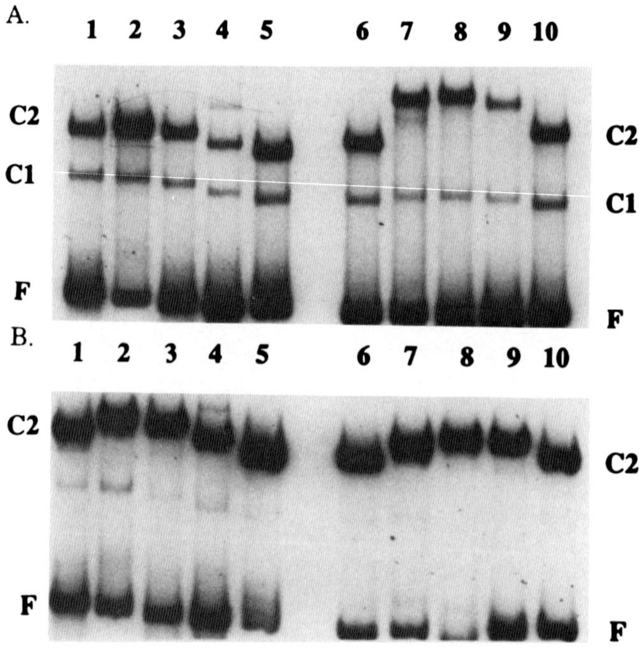

Figure 3. Gel shift assays depicting CatR bending of the *pheBA* and *catBC* promoter regions in the presence and absence of inducer. Five different 228-bp PCR-generated ^{32}P-labeled DNA fragments contained the CatR binding sites positioned at different locations with respect to the end of the DNA fragment. This was done for both the *catBC* and *pheBA* promoter regions. Each reaction contained a fixed amount of protein (5.5 ng) and DNA (10 ng). (A) CatR bending of the *catBC* and *pheBA* promoter regions in the absence of inducer. CatR forms two complexes with both promoter regions (designated C1 and C2). The free DNA is indicated by the letter F. CatR bends the *catBC* promoter DNA (lanes 6 through 10) significantly more than the *pheBA* promoter DNA (lanes 1 through 5). (B) Gel shift assay showing CatR bending of the *catBC* and *pheBA* promoter regions in the presence of inducer. Lanes 1 through 5 and 6 through 10 contain the corresponding DNA fragments as lanes 1 through 5 and 6 through 10 in panel A. CatR forms a single complex (designated C2) with both promoter regions. The degree of CatR-induced bending is very similar for the *catBC* and *pheBA* promoter regions. The inducer significantly relaxes the degree of CatR-induced bending of the *catBC* promoter, but has little effect on the degree of CatR-induced bending of the *pheBA* promoter region.

However, bending of the *catBC* and *pheBA* promoter regions in the absence of inducer is significantly different (59° versus 34°, respectively) (Fig. 3A, compare lanes 1 through 5 versus 6 through 10). Although footprinting and gel shift data indicate very similar CatR-promoter region DNA interactions, the DNA bending data suggest that the nature of these two interactions is different. Whether the divergence of the *pheBA* promoter region simply reflects an inconsequential change in protein-DNA topology or has a functional significance is unclear.

Similarities between the *pheBA* and *catBC* systems are also seen in in vitro transcription assays. Both systems require CatR and inducer for expression of the *catBC* and *pheBA* transcripts (Fig. 4). An intact α-subunit of RNA polymerase has been shown to be required for the expression of many positively regulated systems (Igarishi et al., 1991). This is thought to be mediated by protein-protein contacts between the regulator and RNA polymerase. In vitro transcription reactions conducted with RNA polymerase harboring deletions of the C-terminal region of the α-subunit of RNA polymerase failed to generate transcript in either system (see Fig. 4).

A slight, yet interesting difference between the two systems is the low-level expression of *pheBA* transcript seen in the presence of CatR and in the absence of inducer (Fig. 4B, lane 3). No expression of the *catBC* transcript is seen in the absence of inducer (Fig.

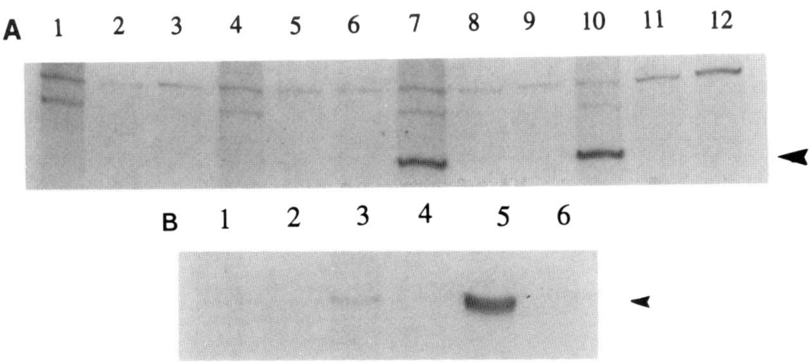

Figure 4. In vitro transcription assay demonstrating requirements for CatR, *cis,cis*-muconate, and the α-subunit of RNA polymerase for expression of the *catBC* and *pheBA* transcripts. (A) In vitro transcription of the *catBC* promoter. Lanes 1, 4, 7, and 10, in vitro transcription assays conducted in the presence of wild-type RNA polymerase. Lanes 2, 5, 8, 11 and 3, 6, 9, 12 contained RNA polymerase-bearing truncations of the α-subunit at amino acid positions 235 and 256, respectively, toward the C-terminal region of the α-subunit. Lanes 1 to 3 lacked both CatR and the inducer *cis,cis*-muconate; lanes 4 to 6 contained 55 ng of purified CatR; lanes 7 to 9 contained 5.5 ng of CatR and 1 mM *cis,cis*-muconate; lanes 10 to 12 contained 55 ng of purified CatR and 1 mM *cis,cis*-muconate. (B) In vitro transcription of the *pheBA* promoter. Lanes 1, 3, and 5 represent reactions conducted in the presence of wild-type RNA polymerase. Lanes 2, 4 and 6 contained RNA polymerase bearing a truncation at position 235 of the C-terminal region of the α-subunit. Lanes 1 and 2 contained RNA polymerase only; lanes 3 and 4 contained 55 ng of purified CatR; lanes 5 and 6 contained 55 ng of purified CatR and 1 mM *cis,cis*-muconate. The *catBC* and *pheBA* transcripts are indicated by arrows. The specific activities of the mutant and wild-type RNA polymerases were normalized using the RNA I transcript of the ColE1 replicon.

4A, lane 4). This may reflect the fact that the CatR-induced bending angle in the *phe* system is very similar in both the presence and absence of inducer, which may allow a low level of *pheBA* expression in the absence of inducer, whereas in the *catBC* system, the significant DNA bend introduced by CatR in the absence of inducer may play a role in repressing expression of the *catBC* transcript.

Another interesting difference between the *catBC* and *pheBA* promoter regions lies in the inverted repeat that serves as a CatR DNA recognition sequence. The *catBC* promoter contains an interrupted, imperfect, inverted repeat within the repression binding site (A$\underline{G}$ACC-N_5-GGT$\underline{A}$T). This imperfect repeat harbors a G-N_{11}-A (underlined) instead of the consensus T-N_{11}-A of the LysR-family DNA binding motifs (Goethals et al., 1992). The *pheBA* promoter has a perfect inverted repeat (A$\underline{T}$ACC-N_5-GGT$\underline{A}$T). A perfect inverted repeat has been shown by site-directed mutagenesis to improve CatR binding in vitro and increase *catBC* expression in vivo (Parsek et al., 1994b). Therefore, it wasn't suprising to find that CatR bound the *pheBA* promoter with greater affinity than the *catBC* promoter region (Parsek et al., 1995). The evolutionary process may have optimized *pheBA* expression by selecting a perfect CatR binding repeat. This may be important to enable the plasmid-borne promoter region to tightly bind CatR.

While the *phe* system appears to have recruited a preexisting regulator, many systems evolve distinct regulatory proteins. This is seen in the previously mentioned plasmid-borne *clc, tfd*, and *tcb* pathways. These systems are presumably derived from the chromosomal catechol degradative pathway. All these pathways have LysR-type regulators (ClcR, TfdR, and TcbR, respectively) that activate transcription of biodegradative operons in the presence of inducers that are pathway intermediates. The *clc, tfd,* and *tcb* pathways are all modified *ortho*-cleavage pathways that consist of chlorinated intermediates which may dictate the necessity of evolving a new regulator. Recruitment of a preexisting regulator is not possible because a unique, substituted pathway intermediate cannot serve as an inducer for CatR (Parsek et al., 1994a).

BIODEGRADATIVE PATHWAY REGULATORY CROSS-TALK

A consequence of closely related regulatory systems coexisting in the same cell is the possibility of regulatory cross-talk. Regulators that recognize similar binding sequences and utilize similar activation mechanisms have been shown to be capable of cross-regulation. This phenomenon has been observed in the NtrC family of transcriptional regulators (Wanner, 1992; Dixon, 1986). The upper pathway of the TOL plasmid was activated by the *Escherichia coli* regulators NtrC and NifA (Dixon, 1986). The *E. coli* and *P. putida* genes are known to be significantly diverged. Therefore, this suggests that the regulatory elements of the NtrC family are functionally conserved.

The DmpR regulator of the phenol-degrading plasmid pVI150 cross-activates the upper pathway promoter of the TOL plasmid (Fernandez et al., 1994). Likewise, the *xylR* gene complements *dmpR* for activation of the *dmp* operon. Analysis of the promoter regions of the TOL upper pathway and *dmp* operon promoters revealed regions of high similarity from approximately −170 to −120 upstream of the transcriptional start sites (Fernandez et al., 1994). These regions contain the regulatory protein binding sites, although in vitro confirmation of cross-binding of the two regulators was not demonstrated. When both regulators were present in the same cell, the TOL plasmid upper pathway showed a broad responsiveness to both regulatory proteins in presence of the appropriate inducers. This implied that the observed cross-regulation was a highly specific event that may be important for broadening the environmental responsiveness of these promoters (Fernandez et al., 1994).

Cross-regulation is also thought to occur in expression of the TOL plasmid lower pathway promoter. This promoter is normally activated by the *xylS* gene product in response to benzoate and benzoate derivatives such as 3-methylbenzoate (Kessler et al., 1993). When *xylS* is not functional, the lower pathway is still responsive to benzoate for induction. This was suggested to be due to cross-activation by the *benR* gene product, the proposed regulator of the chromosomal benzoate catabolic genes (Jeffrey et al., 1992). This theory was later questioned due to the lack of homology between the BenR and XylS proteins and the requirement of the *rpoN* gene for *xylS*-independent activation (Kessler et al., 1994). The TOL plasmid lower pathway promoter is σ^{70} dependent, suggesting that the cross-regulator may be part of a regulatory cascade that involves a σ^{54}-dependent regulator. Therefore, it is possible that the *xylS*-independent expression is not cross-regulation, but a highly specific regulation modulated by different environmental conditions.

The *P. putida* catechol and chlorocatechol regulators, CatR and ClcR, were shown to cross-bind to one another's promoter regions (Parsek et al., 1994a). This was not surprising since both are closely related LysR family regulators and recognize nearly identical inverted repeat recognition sequences (AGACC-N_5-GGTAT for CatR versus ATACC-N_5-CGTAT for ClcR) (Coco et al., 1994). This inverted repeat recognition sequence is similar for the *tcb* and *tfd* systems as well. In fact, TcbR cross-bound to the *tfd* promoter region (van der Meer et al., 1991b). Gel shift assays showed that the cross-binding of CatR and ClcR was nearly as efficient as their binding to their cognate promoters (Parsek et al., 1994a). CatR was shown in vivo to cross-activate the *clcABD* operon in the presence of benzoate. However, ClcR was not able to cross-activate the *catBC* operon. This unusual result may be understood from the DNase I footprinting data of CatR and ClcR cross-binding to each other's promoter regions (Fig. 5). CatR and ClcR show very similar noncontiguous protection patterns on the *clcABD* promoter. On the other hand, CatR and ClcR show completely different protection patterns of the *catBC* promoter region. In the absence of inducer, ClcR protects a large interrupted region which is interspersed with hypersensitivity sites. CatR protects a small defined area in the absence of inducer and demonstrates binding to an additional downstream site in the presence of inducer. Apparently, ClcR does not make functional contacts with the *catBC* promoter region, although it does protect relatively the same area as CatR.

The benefits of biodegradative regulatory cross-talk are obvious. It allows a promoter to respond to a wider variety of inducer molecules, which in turn would allow the cell to elicit a general activation of closely related biodegradative pathways. Cross-talk also provides the cell with a mechanism for coping with the loss of a pathway regulator. Although presumably not as efficient as the native regulator, a cross-regulator would allow the cell to express a particular biodegradative pathway.

On the other hand, the effects of cross-regulation would not always be favorable to the cell. If a regulator is capable of cross-binding to another promoter with high affinity, but is not functional, the cross-regulator could effectively compete with the native regulator and interfere with the expression of the induced genes. This possibility must be considered when new biodegradative pathways and regulators are engineered.

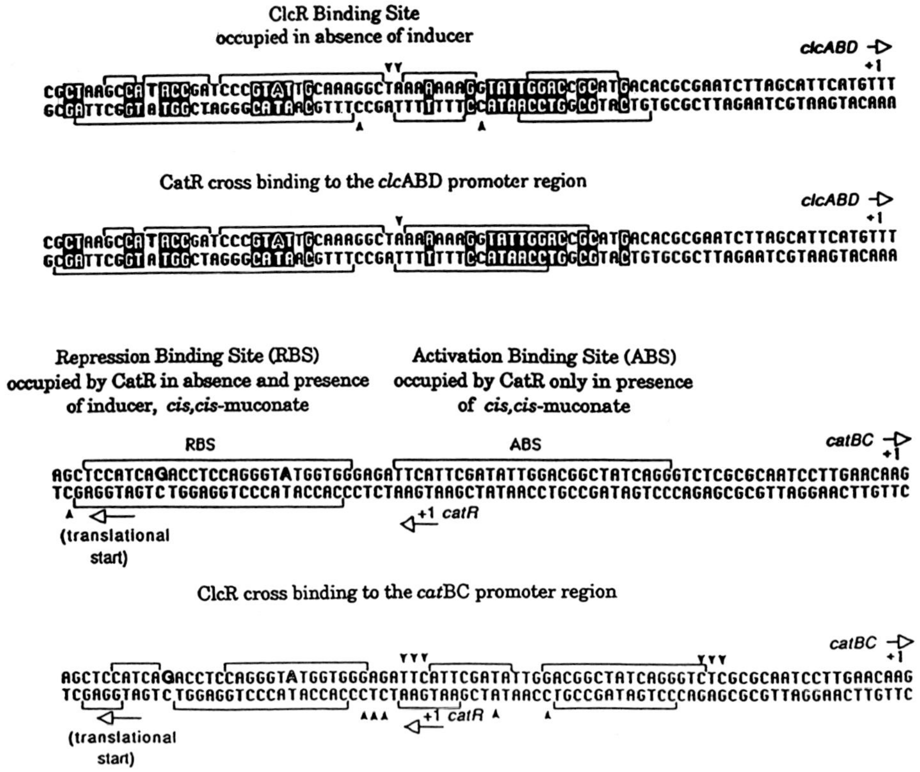

Figure 5. Diagram depicting sequences protected by CatR and ClcR on native and cross-bound promoters. The sequences protected from DNase I digestion are outlined by brackets. Hypersensitivity is depicted by arrows. Highlighted residues in the *clcABD* promoter region represent identical residues in the *catBC* promoter region.

SUMMARY

The regulation of biodegradative systems encompasses a wide variety of regulatory schemes. Many of the familiar transcriptional regulatory families are represented, indicating a great divergence in the evolutionary origins of the different biodegradation systems. Despite the wide divergence, most biodegradative system regulators are transcriptional activators that presumably interact with a pathway intermediate which serves as an inducer molecule. The evolution of new biodegradative pathways with unique pathway intermediates apparently dictates the need to evolve a new regulator which must be able to recognize a new inducer molecule. If newly evolved pathways have catabolic intermediates that are at least partially identical to a preexisting pathway, the regulator of the preexisting pathway can be recruited by the new system. However, the evolution of a new regulator may also involve the slight modification of a closely related regulator. The existence of very similar regulatory systems in the same cell may result in regulatory cross-talk. The significance of regulatory cross-talk is uncertain, but it may be involved in the cell generating a broad induction of similar catabolic genes. Cross-talk could also affect the success of the bioengineering of new biodegradative pathways and their regulators.

Acknowledgments. This work was supported by Public Health Service Grant ES 04050-08 from the National Institute of Environmental Health Sciences and in part by Grant MCB 91-00015 from the National Science Foundation. S.M.M. is supported by The Searle Environmental Health and Safety Fellowship.

REFERENCES

Abril, M. A., C. Michan, K. N. Timmis, and J. L. Ramos. 1989. Regulator and enzyme specificities of the TOL plasmid-encoded upper pathway for degradation of aromatic hydrocarbons and expansion of the substrate range of the pathway. *J. Bacteriol.* **171:**6782–6790.

Aldrich, T. L., B. Frantz, B. Gill, J. F Kilbane, and A. M. Chakrabarty. 1987. Cloning and complete nucleotide sequence determination of the *catB* gene encoding *cis,cis*-muconate lactonizing enzyme. *Gene* **52:**185–195.

Aramaki, H., Y. Sagara, H. Kabata, N. Shimamoto, and T. Horiuchi. 1995. Purification and characterization of a *cam* repressor (CamR) for the cytochrome P-450_{cam} hydroxylase operon of the *Pseudomonas putida* CAM plasmid. *J. Bacteriol.* **177:**3120–3127.

Coco, W. M., M. R. Parsek, and A. M. Chakrabarty. 1994. Purification of the LysR family regulator, ClcR, and its interaction with the *Pseudomonas putida clcABD* chlorocatechol operon promoter. *J. Bacteriol.* **176:**5530–5533.

Coco, W. M., R. Rothmel, S. Henikoff, and A. M. Chakrabarty. 1993. Nucleotide sequence and initial functional characterization of *clcR*, a LysR family activator of the *clcABD* chlorocatechol operon in *Pseudomonas putida*. *J. Bacteriol.* **175:**417–427.

Daubaras, D., and A. M. Chakrabarty. 1992. The environment, microbes and bioremediation: microbial activities modulated by the environment. *Biodegradation* **3:**125–135.

de Lorenzo, V., M. Herrero, M. Metzke, and K. N. Timmis. 1991. An upstream XylR- and IHF-induced nucleoprotein complex regulates the σ^{54}-dependent *Pu* promoter of TOL plasmid. *EMBO J.* **10:**1159–1167.

DiMarco, A. A., B. Averhoff, and L. N. Ornston. 1993. Identification of the transcriptional activator *pobR* and characterization of its role in the expression of *pobA*, the structural gene for *p*-hydroxybenzoate hydroxylase in *Acinetobacter calcoaceticus*. *J. Bacteriol.* **175:**4499–4506.

Dispensa, M., C. T. Thomas, M.-K. Kim, J. A. Perrotta, J. Gibson, and C. S. Harwood. 1992. Anaerobic growth of *Rhodopseudomonas palustris* on 4-hydroxybenzoate is dependent on AadR, a member of the cyclic AMP receptor protein family of transcriptional regulators. *J. Bacteriol.* **174:**5803–5813.

Dixon, R. 1986. The *xylABC* promoter from the *Pseudomonas putida* TOL plasmid is activated by nitrogen regulatory genes in *Escherichia coli*. *Mol. Gen. Genet.* **203:**129–136.

Doten, R. C., K.-L. Ngai, D. J. Mitchell, and L. N. Ornston. 1987. Cloning and genetic organization of the *pca* gene cluster from *Acinetobacter calcoaceticus*. *J. Bacteriol.* **169:**3168–3174.

Fernandez, S., V. de Lorenzo, and J. Perez-Martin. 1995. Activation of the transcriptional regulator XylR of *Pseudomonas putida* by release of repression between functional domains. *Mol. Microbiol.* **16:**205–213.

Fernandez, S., V. Shingler, and V. de Lorenzo. 1994. Cross-regulation by XylR and DmpR activators of *Pseudomonas putida* suggests that transcriptional control of biodegradative operons evolves independently of catabolic genes. *J. Bacteriol.* **176:**5052–5058.

Frantz, B., and A. M. Chakrabarty. 1987. Organization and nucleotide sequence determination of a gene cluster involved in 3-chlorocatechol degradation. *Proc. Natl. Acad. Sci. USA* **84:**4460–4464.

Fujita, M., H. Aramaki, T. Horiuchi, and A. Amemura. 1993. Transcription of the *cam* operon and *camR* genes in *Pseudomonas putida* PpG1. *J. Bacteriol.* **175:**6953–6958.

Goethals, K., M. VanMontagu, and M. Holsters. 1992. Conserved motifs in a divergent *nod* box of *Azorhizobium caulinodans* ORS571 reveal a common structure in promoters regulated by LysR-type proteins. *Proc. Natl. Acad. Sci. USA* **89:**1646–1650.

Gomada, M., S. Inouye, H. Imaishi, A. Nakazawa, and T. Nakazawa. 1992. Analysis of an upstream regulatory sequence required for activation of the regulatory gene *xylS* in xylene metabolism directed by the TOL plasmid of *Pseudomonas putida*. *Mol. Gen. Genet.* **233:**419–426.

Houghton, J. E., T. M. Brown, A. J. Appel, E. J. Hughes, and L. N. Ornston. 1995. Discontinuities in the evolution of *Pseudomonas putida cat* genes. *J. Bacteriol.* **177:**401–412.

Hryniewicz, M., and N. M. Kredich. 1994. Stoichiometry of binding of CysB to the *cysJIH, cysK,* and *cysP* promoter regions of *Salmonella typhimurium. J. Bacteriol.* **176:**3673–3682.

Huang, J., and M. A. Schell. 1991. *In vivo* interactions of the NahR transcriptional activator with its target sequences: inducer mediated changes resulting in transcription activation. *J. Biol. Chem.* **266:**10830–10838.

Hughes, E. J., M. J. Shapiro, J. E. Houghton, and L. N. Ornston. 1988. Cloning and expression of *pca* genes from *Pseudomonas putida* in *Escherichia coli. J. Gen. Microbiol.* **134:**2877–2887.

Igarishi, I., A. Hanamura, K. Makino, H. Aiba, H. Aiba, T. Mizuno, A. Nakata, and A. Ishihama. 1991. Functional map of the α-subunit of *Escherichia coli* RNA polymerase: two modes of transcription activation by positive factors. *Proc. Natl. Acad. Sci. USA* **88:**8958–8962.

Inouye, S., M. Gomada, U. M. X. Sangodkar, A. Nakazawa, and T. Nakazawa. 1990. Upstream regulatory sequences for transcriptional activator XylR in the first operon of xylene metabolism of the TOL plasmid. *J. Mol. Biol.* **216:**251–260.

Inouye, S., A. Nakazawa, and T. Nakazawa. 1987. Expression of the regulatory gene *xylS* on the TOL plasmid is positively controlled by the *xylR* gene product. *Proc. Natl. Acad. Sci. USA* **84:**5182–5186.

Jeffrey, W. H., S. M. Cuskey, P. J. Chapman, S. Resnick, and R. H. Olsen. 1992. Characterization of *Pseudomonas putida* mutants unable to catabolize benzoate: cloning and characterization of *Pseudomonas* genes involved in benzoate catabolism and isolation of a chromosomal DNA fragment able to substitute for *xylS* in activation of the TOL lower-pathway promoter. *J. Bacteriol.* **174:**4986–4996.

Kaphammer, B. K., and R. H. Olsen. 1990. Cloning and characterization of *tfdS*, the repressor-activator gene of *tfdB*, from the 2,4-dichlorophenoxyacetic acid catabolic plasmid pJP4. *J. Bacteriol.* **172:**5856–5862.

Kasak, L., R. Horak, A. Nurk, K. Talvik, and M. Kivisaar. 1993. Regulation of the catechol 1,2-dioxygenase- and phenol monooxygenase-encoding *pheBA* operon in *Pseudomonas putida* PaW85. *J. Bacteriol.* **175:**8038–8042.

Kessler, B., V. de Lorenzo, and K. N. Timmis. 1993. Identification of a *cis*-acting sequence within the *Pm* promoter of the TOL plasmid which confers XylS-mediated responsiveness to substituted benzoates. *J. Mol. Biol.* **230:**699–703.

Kessler, B., S. Marqués, T. Köhler, J. L. Ramos, K. N. Timmis, and V. de Lorenzo. 1994. Cross talk between catabolic pathways in *Pseudomonas putida*: XylS-dependent and -independent activation of the TOL *meta* operon requires the same *cis*-acting sequences within the *Pm* promoter. *J. Bacteriol.* **176:**5578–5582.

Kivisaar, M., R. Horak, L. Kasak, A. Heinaru, and J. Habicht. 1990. Selection of independent plasmids determining phenol degradation in *Pseudomonas putida* and the cloning and expression of the genes encoding phenol monooxygenase and catechol 1,2-dioxygenase. *Plasmid* **24:**25–36.

Koga, H., H. Aramaki, E. Yamaguchi, K. Takeuchi, T. Horiuchi, and I. C. Gunsalus. 1986. *camR*, a negative regulator locus of the cytochrome P-450_{cam} hydroxylase operon. *J. Bacteriol.* **166:**1089–1095.

Leveau, J. H., W. M. de Vos, and J. R. van der Meer. 1994. Analysis of the binding site of the LysR-type transcriptional activator TcbR on the *tcbR* and *tcbC* divergent promoter sequences. *J. Bacteriol.* **176:**1850–1856.

Marques, S., and J. L. Ramos. 1993. Transcriptional control of the *Pseudomonas putida* TOL plasmid catabolic pathways. *Mol. Microbiol.* **9:**923–929.

Matrubutham, U., and A. R. Harker. 1994. Analysis of duplicated gene sequences associated with *tfdR* and *tfdS* in *Alcaligenes eutrophus* JMP134. *J. Bacteriol.* **176:**2348–2353.

Mermod, N., J. L. Ramos, A. Bairoch, and K. N. Timmis. 1987. The *xylS* gene positive regulator of TOL plasmid pWW0: identification, sequence analysis and overproduction leading to constitutive expression of *meta* cleavage operon. *Mol. Gen. Genet.* **207:**349–354.

Morett, E., and L. Segovia. 1993. The σ^{54} bacterial enhancer-binding protein family: mechanism of action and phylogenetic relationship of their functional domains. *J. Bacteriol.* **178:**6067–6074.

Neidle, E. L., C. Hartnett, and L. N. Ornston. 1989. Characterization of *Acinetobacter calcoaceticus catM*, a repressor gene homologous in sequence to transcriptional activator genes. *J. Bacteriol.* **171:**5410–5421.

Ng, L. C., C. L. Poh, and V. Shingler. 1995. Aromatic effector activation of the NtrC-like transcriptional regulator PhhR limits the catabolic potential of the (methyl)phenol degradative pathway it controls. *J. Bacteriol.* **177:**1485–1490.

Nurk, A., L. Kasak, and M. Kivisaar. 1991. Sequence of the gene (*pheA*) encoding phenol monooxygenase from *Pseudomonas* sp. strain EST1001: expression in *Escherichia coli* and *Pseudomonas putida. Gene* **102:**13–18.

Parales, R. E., and C. S. Harwood. 1993. Regulation of the *pcaIJ* genes for aromatic acid degradation in *Pseudomonas putida. J. Bacteriol.* **175:**5829–5838.

Parke, D. 1993. Positive regulation of phenolic catabolism in *Agrobacterium tumefaciens* by the *pcaQ* gene in response to β-carboxy-*cis,cis*-muconate. *J. Bacteriol.* **175:**3529–3535.

Parke, D. 1996. Characterization of PcaQ, a LysR-type transcriptional activator required for catabolism of phenolic compounds from *Agrobacterium tumefaciens. J. Bacteriol.* **178:**266–272.

Parke, D., and L. N. Ornston. 1986. Enzymes of the β-ketoadipate pathway are inducible in *Rhizobium* and *Agrobacterium* spp. and constitutive in *Bradyrhizobium* spp. *J. Bacteriol.* **165:**288–292.

Parsek, M. R., C. D. Hershberger, S. Chugani, A. Ishihama, and A. M. Chakrabarty. Manuscript in preparation.

Parsek, M. R., M. Kivisaar, and A. M. Chakrabarty. 1995. Differential DNA bending introduced by the *Pseudomonas putida* LysR-type regulator, CatR, at the plasmid-borne *pheBA* and chromosomal *catBC* promoters. *Mol. Microbiol.* **15:**819–828.

Parsek, M. R., S. M. McFall, D. L. Shinabarger, and A. M. Chakrabarty. 1994a. Interaction of two LysR-type regulatory proteins CatR and ClcR with heterologous promoters: functional and evolutionary implications. *Proc. Natl. Acad. Sci. USA* **91:**12393–12397.

Parsek, M. R., D. L. Shinabarger, R. K. Rothmel, and A. M. Chakrabarty. 1992. Roles of CatR and *cis,cis*-muconate in activation of the *catBC* operon, which is involved in benzoate degradation in *Pseudomonas putida. J. Bacteriol.* **174:**7798–7806.

Parsek, M. R., R. W. Ye, P. Pun, and A. M. Chakrabarty. 1994b. Critical nucleotides in the interaction of a LysR-type regulator with its target promoter region: *catBC* promoter activation by CatR. *J. Biol. Chem.* **269:**11279–11284.

Perez-Martin, J., and V. de Lorenzo. 1995. The σ^{54}-dependent promoter *Ps* of the TOL plasmid of *Pseudomonas putida* requires HU for transcriptional activation in vivo by XylR. *J. Bacteriol.* **177:**3758–3763.

Perkins, E. J., M. P. Gordon, O. Caceres, and P. F. Lurquin. 1990. Organization and sequence analysis of the 2,4-dichlorophenol hydroxylase and dichlorocatechol oxidative operons of plasmid pJP4. *J. Bacteriol.* **172:**2351–2359.

Ramos, J. L., F. Rojo, and K. N. Timmis. 1990. A family of positive regulators related to the *Pseudomonas putida* TOL plasmid XylS and the *Escherichia coli* AraC activators. *Nucleic Acids Res.* **18:**2149–2152.

Rheinwald, J. G., A. M. Chakrabarty, and I. C. Gunsalus. 1973. A transmissible plasmid controlling camphor oxidation in *Pseudomonas putida. Proc. Natl. Acad. Sci. USA* **70:**885–889.

Romero-Arroyo, C. E. 1992. *In vitro* studies of transcriptional regulation of the *catBCEFD* operon in *Acinetobacter calcoaceticus* by CatM. MS thesis. University of Georgia, Athens.

Romero-Arroyo, C. E., M. A. Schell, G. L. Gaines III, and E. L. Neidle. 1995. *catM* encodes a LysR-type transcriptional activator regulating catechol degradation in *Acinetobacter calcoaceticus. J. Bacteriol.* **177:**5891–5898.

Romero-Steiner, S., R. E. Parales, C. S. Harwood, and J. E. Houghton. 1994. Characterization of the *pcaR* regulatory gene from *Pseudomonas putida*, which is required for the complete degradation of *p*-hydroxybenzoate. *J. Bacteriol.* **176:**5771–5779.

Rothmel, R. K., T. L. Aldrich, J. E. Houghton, W. M. Coco, L. M. Ornston, and A. M. Chakrabarty. 1990. Nucleotide sequencing and characterization of *Pseudomonas putida* CatR: a positive regulator of the *catBC* operon is a member of the LysR family. *J. Bacteriol.* **172:**922–931.

Schell, M. A. 1983. Cloning and expression in *Escherichia coli* of the naphthalene degradation genes from plasmid NAH7. *J. Bacteriol.* **153:**822–828.

Schell, M. A. 1985. Transcriptional control of the *nah* and *sal* hydrocarbon degradation operons by the *nahR* gene product. *Gene* **36:**301–309.

Schell, M. A. 1993. Molecular biology of the LysR family of transcriptional regulators. *Annu. Rev. Microbiol.* **47:**597–626.

Schell, M. A., and E. Poser. 1989. Demonstration, characterization, and mutational analysis of NahR protein binding to the *nah* and *sal* promoters. *J. Bacteriol.* **171:**837–846.

Schell, M. A., and P. E. Wender. 1986. Identification of the *nahR* gene product and nucleotide sequences required for its activation of the *sal* operon. *J. Bacteriol.* **166:**9–14.

Schlaman, H. R. M., R. J. H. Okker, and B. J. J. Lugtenberg. 1992. Regulation of nodulation gene expression by NodD in Rhizobia. *J. Bacteriol.* **174:**5177–5182.

Shingler, V., M. Bartilson, and T. Moore. 1993. Cloning and nucleotide sequence of the gene encoding the positive regulator (DmpR) of the phenol catabolic pathway encoded by pVI150 and identification of DmpR as a member of the NtrC family of transcriptional activators. *J. Bacteriol.* **175:**1596–1604.

Shingler, V., and T. Moore. 1994. Sensing aromatic compounds by the DmpR transcriptional activator of phenol-catabolizing *Pseudomonas* sp. strain CF600. *J. Bacteriol.* **176:**1555–1560.

Sunnarborg, A., D. Klumpp, T. Chung, and D. C. LaPorte. 1990. Regulation of the glyoxylate bypass operon: cloning and characterization of *iclR*. *J. Bacteriol.* **172:**2642–2649.

van der Meer, J. R., R. I. L. Eggen, A. J. B. Zehnder, and W. M. de Vos. 1991a. Sequence analysis of the *Pseudomonas* sp. strain P51 *tcb* gene cluster, which encodes metabolism of chlorinated catechols: evidence for specialization of catechol 1,2-dioxygenases for chlorinated substrates. *J. Bacteriol.* **173:**2425–2434.

van der Meer, J. R., A. C. J. Frijters, J. H. J. Leveau, R. I. L. Eggen, A. J. B Zehnder, and W. M. de Vos. 1991b. Characterization of the *Pseudomonas* sp. strain P51 gene *tcbR*, a LysR-type transcriptional activator of the *tcbCDEF* chlorocatechol oxidative operon, and analysis of the regulatory region. *J. Bacteriol.* **173:**3700–3708.

Wang, L., J. D. Helmann, and S. C. Winans. 1992. The *Agrobacterium tumefaciens* transcriptional activator OccR causes a bend at a target promoter, which is partially relaxed by a plant tumor metabolite. Cell **69:**659–667.

Wanner, B. L. 1992. Is cross regulation by phosphorylation of two-component response regulator proteins important in bacteria? *J. Bacteriol.* **174:**2053–2058.

Wheelis, M. L., and L. N. Ornston. 1972. Genetic control of enzyme induction in the β-ketoadipate pathway of *Pseudomonas putida*: deletion mapping of *cat* mutations. *J. Bacteriol.* **108:**790–795.

Yen, K.-M., and I. C. Gunsalus. 1985. Regulation of naphthalene catabolic plasmid NAH7. *J. Bacteriol.* **162:**1008–1013.

You, I.-S., and D. Ghosal. 1995. Genetic and molecular analysis of a regulatory region of the herbicide 2,4-dichlorophenoxyacetate catabolic plasmid pJP4. *Mol. Microbiol.* **16:**321–331.

Molecular Biology of Pseudomonads
Edited by T. Nakazawa et al.

Chapter 12

Metabolic and Regulatory Check Points in Phenol Degradation by *Pseudomonas* sp. Strain CF600

Victoria Shingler

Aromatic compounds constitute a large group of environmental pollutants that are persistent because of the stability of the aromatic ring. In general, microbial biodegradative activities have coevolved with the synthesis of natural organic matter. The relatively recent augmentation of the pool of organic matter with synthetic compounds, many of which are toxic and have few or no natural analogs, has taxed native microbial degradative systems. Microbial adaptation and evolution to degrade some synthetic aromatics that have been introduced in large quantities and/or that harbor novel substituents have in some cases resulted in inefficient removal from the environment. Phenol itself is a naturally occurring compound produced by microbial activities and the breakdown of plant material. Consequently, the persistence of phenol in the environment is not a particular problem (Howard et al., 1991). Today, however, more than 1.5×10^9 kg of phenol itself and vast quantities of its derivatives are produced annually in the United States alone. As with microbial catabolism of other toxic compounds, the efficiency with which phenolics can be metabolized is affected by variables such as concentration, availability of alternative carbon sources, and positions and nature of substituents on the phenol ring.

The potential applications of microbial aromatic catabolic activities, for example, (i) in bioremediation, (ii) for production of commercially valuable pathway intermediates and products of hybrid pathways, and (iii) in applications of the natural sensing (regulatory) systems of these bacteria in biosensor development, demand an understanding of the biological factors and constraints involved. Hence, these possibilities have stimulated the study of the genes and enzymes of individual isolates at the molecular level. Phenol is a relatively simple, unadorned, aromatic compound, and bacteria capable of degrading this substrate provide good model systems for addressing questions concerning limitations of the catabolic potential of bacteria.

Victoria Shingler • Department of Cell and Molecular Biology, Umeå University, 901 87 Umeå, Sweden.

GENETIC LOCATION AND BIOCHEMICAL ROUTE OF PHENOL CATABOLISM BY *PSEUDOMONAS* SP. STRAIN CF600

Many strains of *Pseudomonas* and related gram-negative bacteria are able to utilize aromatic compounds via pathways that are encoded in one or more functional operons of large, low-copy-number plasmids. The clustering of genes for the catabolic enzymes into functional metabolic units reflects the general bacterial strategy of channeling diverse compounds into a limited number of central pathways (reviewed by Williams and Sayers, 1994). Initial substrates are converted by distinct enzyme systems involving mono- and dioxygenases to a few key intermediates. These intermediates, usually catechols, contain two hydroxyl groups that destabilize the ring, making it amenable to cleavage by ring fission dioxygenases (reviewed by Dagley, 1986). The non-aromatic-ring cleavage products of catechol are subsequently transformed by one of two central pathways to substrates of mainstream metabolism, namely, pyruvate and acetyl-coenzyme A (CoA) by the *meta*-cleavage pathway and succinyl- and acetyl-CoA by the *ortho*-cleavage pathway.

Pseudomonas sp. strain CF600 can grow on phenol, monomethylated phenols (2-mp, 3-mp, and 4-mp), and 3,4-dimethylphenol (3,4-dmp) as sole carbon and energy sources by hydroxylation and a subsequent *meta*-cleavage pathway encoded by the *dmp* system. The genes of the *dmp* system are located on the IncP-2 megaplasmid pVI150 (Shingler et al., 1989). The results of the genetic dissection and nucleotide sequencing of 15 kb of pVI150-derived DNA involved in phenol catabolism and the locations of the 16 genes involved are summarized in Fig. 1A. The 15-gene *dmp* operon is one of the largest bacterial operons known; it encodes all the catabolic enzymes required for the nine biochemical steps of the pathway (Fig. 1B and Table 1). Tight regulation of transcription of the *dmp* operon is mediated by the closely linked, but divergently transcribed, *dmpR* gene product (Shingler et al., 1993).

PHENOL HYDROXYLASE: A NEW TYPE OF MULTICOMPONENT AROMATIC OXYGENASE

The phenol degradative pathway is initiated by hydroxylation of phenol to catechol. In *Pseudomonas* sp. strain CF600, a combination of nucleotide sequencing and polypeptide and deletion analyses identified six genes (*dmpKLMNOP*) and their corresponding gene products (P0, P1, P2, P3, P4, and P5) within the region coding for phenol hydroxylase. Furthermore, using growth on phenol as the assay and a series of plasmids lacking expression of each gene in turn, all six gene products were shown to be essential for conversion of phenol in intact bacteria (Nordlund et al., 1990). In vitro, however, purified P1 to P5 are sufficient to fully reconstitute the activity in the presence of Fe^{2+} and NAD(P)H (Powlowski and Shingler, 1990, 1994). Purification of P1 to P5 resolved these proteins into a P1-P3-P4 complex, a P2 component, and a P5 reductase component. The properties, homologies, and probable functions of these different components and a mechanistic comparison with methane monooxygenase have been reviewed in depth elsewhere (Powlowski and Shingler, 1994). In brief, P3 of the P1-P3-P4 complex contains ligands for a binuclear iron center, P2 has no obvious prosthetic groups, and P5 contains flavin adenine dinucleotide and a ferredoxin-like [2Fe-2S] center. The flavin of P5 is presumed

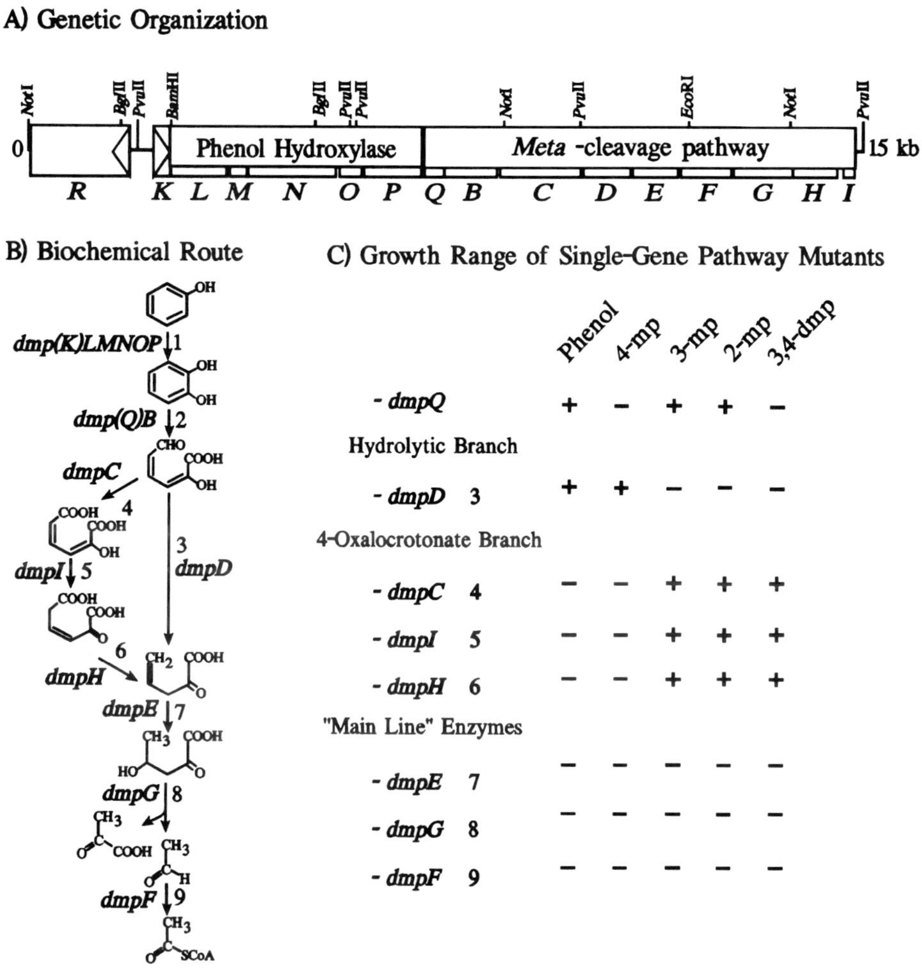

Figure 1. Phenol pathway encoded by a 15-kb region of the pVI150 catabolic plasmid of *Pseudomonas* sp. strain CF600. (A) Genetic organization. Arrowheads indicate divergent transcription of the *dmpR* regulatory gene and the *dmp* operon. (B) Biochemical route. Enzyme functions are as shown in Table 1. Both the hydrolytic (*dmpD*-encoded) and the 4-oxalocrotonate (*dmpC1H*-encoded) branches of the *meta*-cleavage pathway are shown. (C) Growth patterns of pathway mutants defective in single enzymes of the catabolic pathway (Powlowski and Shingler, 1994).

to accept electrons from the obligate two-electron donor NAD(P)H and pass them on one at a time to the oxygenase active site of the P1-P3-P4 complex via the [2Fe-2S] center. By analogy to methane monooxygenase, P2 might regulate regioselectivity of the oxygenase activity. The role of P0, whose primary sequence does not resemble that of any protein currently in the data bases, is as yet unclear. Its requirement in vivo but not in vitro, however, suggests a role in the correct assembly, synthesis, or stabilization of phenol hydroxylase or in the regulation of the activity of this enzyme.

Table 1. Summary of genes and gene products of the *dmp* operon and comparison with isofunctional enzymes

Gene	No. of residues (amino acids)	Product	Properties	Homologous or isofunctional proteins from other systems (% identity with *dmp* proteins)[a]
Phenol hydroxylase				
dmpK	92	P0	Unknown	PhhK (96), Phe A1 (100), PhlA (96)
dmpL	331	P1	Hydroxylase component	PhhL (99), Phe A2 (100), PhlB (99)
dmpM	90	P2	Unknown	PhhM (97), Phe A3 (100), PhlC (94)
dmpN	517	P3	Hydroxylase component	PhhN (96), Phe A4 (100), PhlD (98)
dmpO	119	P4	Hydroxylase component	PhhO (98), Phe A5 (100), PhlE (98)
dmpP	35	P5	Reductase component	PhhP (88), Phe A6 (99), PhlF (86)
***meta* Pathway**				
dmpO	112	DmpQ	Ferredoxin-like protein	XylT (64)
dmpB	307	C23O	Catechol 2,3-dioxygenase	XylE (84), TodE (22), BphC (22)
dmpC	486	HMSD	2-Hydroxymuconic semialdehyde dehydrogenase	XylG (84)
dmpD	283	HMSH	2-Hydroxymuconic semialdehyde hydrolase	XylF (75), TodF (64), BphD (43)
dmpE	261	OEH	2-Oxopent-4-dienoate hydratase	XylJ (89), TodG (41), BphE (43)
dmpF	312	ADA	Aldehyde dehydrogenase (acylating)	XylQ (90), TodI (75), BphG (78)
dmpG	345	HOA	4-Hydroxy-2-oxovalerate aldolase	XylK (87), TodH (78), BphF (81)
dmpH	264	4OD	4-Oxalocrotonate decarboxylase	XylI (89)
dmpI	63	4OI	4-Oxalocrotonate isomerase	XylH (78)

[a]Percent identity on the amino acid level is given. *dmp*, phenol-dimethylphenol pVI150-encoded pathway of *Pseudomonas sp.* strain CF600 (Bartilson and Shingler, 1989; Nordlund and Shingler, 1990; Nordlund et al., 1990; Shingler et al., 1992); Phh, chromosomally encoded phenol hydroxylase proteins of *P. putida* P35X (Ng et al., 1994); Phe, chromosomally encoded phenol hydroxylase proteins of *P. putida* BH (Takeo et al., 1995); Phl, pPGH1-encoded phenol hydroxylase proteins of *P. putida* H (Herrmann et al., 1995); Xyl, toluene-xylene pWW0-encoded *meta*-pathway genes (Nakai et al., 1983; Harayama et al., 1991; Harayama and Rekik, 1993; Horn et al., 1991; Chen et al., 1992); Tod, chromosomally encoded toluene pathway genes of *P. putida* F1 (Zylstra and Gibson, 1989; Menn et al., 1991; Lau et al., 1994); Bph, chromosomally encoded (chloro)biphenyl pathway of *Pseudomonas* sp. strain KKS102 (Kimbara et al., 1989; Kikuchi et al., 1994).

Several polypeptides of toluene-4-monooxygenase from *Pseudomonas mendocina* KR1 (Yen et al., 1991; Yen and Karl, 1992) and toluene-3-monooxygenase from *Pseudomonas pickettii* PKO1 (Byrne et al., 1995) share homology with the phenol hydroxylase of *Pseudomonas* sp. strain CF600. Oxygenation of electron-rich phenol should be a considerably easier task than oxygenation of unactivated compounds such as toluene and methane. Bacterial hydroxylations of compounds activated by the presence of an OH group are usually accomplished by using single-component flavoproteins. Indeed, this type of hydroxylation has been found to occur with phenol hydroxylase from *Pseudomonas* sp. strain EST1001 (Nurk et al., 1991), *P. pickettii* PKO1 (Kukor and Olsen, 1992), and *Bacillus stearothermophilus* BR219 (Kim and Oriel, 1995). The reason underlying the necessity for a multicomponent hydroxylase system such as that of CF600 thus remains an enigma. However, gene probing has revealed that DNA highly homologous to the DNA of *dmpKLMNOP* is associated with *meta*-cleavage pathway genes in the archetype phenol degrader *Pseudomonas putida* U (from the United States) and in gram-negative marine isolates collected off the Norwegian coast (Nordlund et al., 1993).

Moreover, recent nucleotide sequencing of chromosomally and plasmid-encoded phenol hydroxylase gene clusters associated with *meta*-cleavage pathways from four *P. putida* strains isolated in the United Kingdom, Germany, and Japan showed that the gene products share 86 to 100% identity with those of *dmpKLMNOP* (Table 1). Hence, some advantage appears to have conserved this complex multicomponent phenol hydroxylase during global dispersal of an ancestral strain.

THE *meta*-CLEAVAGE PATHWAY

The biochemical route of the *meta*-cleavage pathway is illustrated in Fig. 1B. The remaining nine genes of the *dmp* operon, *dmpQBCDEFGHI*, encode the *meta*-pathway enzymes that have isofunctional counterparts in other *meta*-cleavage pathways involved in catabolism of a variety of aromatic compounds (Table 1). All these gene products have been purified (reviewed by Powlowski and Shingler, 1994). With the exception of isofunctional genes homologous to *dmpB* and *dmpQ*, no other *meta*-pathway gene sequence had been published prior to work with the *dmp* system. Hence, functional assignments relied on correlation of individual gene expression with known enzymatic activities. Work with the phenol degrader *P. putida* U was responsible for much of the early progress in elucidating the steps of the *meta*-pathway (reviewed by Bayly and Barbour, 1984), resulting in the *meta* pathway being depicted as ending with pyruvate and acetaldehyde. Analysis of the *dmp* operon led to the discovery of a new *meta*-pathway enzyme, aldehyde dehydrogenase (acylating), encoded by *dmpF*. This enzyme further converts acetaldehyde to acetyl-CoA, providing an operon-controlled, energetically favorable mechanism for the metabolism of acetaldehyde (Shingler et al., 1992; Powlowski et al., 1993).

The sequence homologies and the implications for mechanistic studies of the *meta*-pathway enzymes were recently reviewed (Williams and Sayers, 1994; Powlowski and Shingler, 1994). The critical ring-opening step is catalyzed by catechol 2,3-dioxygenase. This enzyme is particularly sensitive to inactivation during turnover with 4-(*para*)-substituted catechol, probably by inadvertent oxidation of the active-site ferrous iron. Inactivation of the small ferredoxin-like proteins encoded by *xylT* (Polissi and Harayama, 1993) and *dmpQ* (Powlowski and Shingler, 1994) results in strains incapable of growth on substrates channeled via *para*-substituted methylcatechols (e.g., 4-mp and 3,4-dmp; Fig. 1C). XylT is involved in reactivating catechol 2,3-dioxygenase, thus expanding the substrate specificity of the *meta* pathway to include a compound metabolized via 4-methylcatechols (Polissi and Harayama, 1993). It is interesting that XylT homologs are encoded in the same position in many complete *meta*-pathway operons (reviewed by Williams and Sayers, 1994) but are absent in the abridged *tod* and *bph meta*-pathway operons, which lack the 4-oxalocrotonate branch (Table 1). Neither of these enzyme systems metabolizes compounds that would result in a *para*-substituted catechol intermediate.

2-Hydroxymuconic semialdehyde dehydrogenase (DmpC) and hydrolase (DmpD) act on the variably substituted products of ring cleavage. These enzymes initiate the two branches of the *meta* pathway that contribute to its metabolic versatility in the catabolism of alkylated substrates substituted at different positions on the aromatic ring. The role of the hydrolytic branch in dissimilating 3-methylcatechol and the 4-oxalocrotonate branch for unsubstituted and 4-methyl-substituted catechols was first described for *P. putida* U (Sala-Trepat et al., 1972; Bayly and Wigmore, 1973). These conclusions were validated and expanded for the *dmp meta* pathway by generating mutants defective in individual steps of the pathway (Fig. 1C). Hence, strains harboring defects in the *dmpCH1*-encoded 4-oxalocrotonate branch were incapable of growth on phenol and 4-methylphenol, which are dissimilated via catechol and 4-methylcatechol, while strains defective in the *dmpD*-encoded hydrolytic branch could not grow at the expense of 2- and 3-mp (via 3-methylcatechol) or on 3,4-dmp (via 3,4-dimethylcatechol).

One of the most interesting properties of the *meta* pathway, which has repercussions in terms of metabolic engineering, is the tight physical association of some of the pathway enzymes. The evolutionarily related decarboxylase and hydratase enzymes (DmpHE and XylIJ proteins [Powlowski and Shingler, 1994; Harayama et al., 1989]) copurify as a complex. Similarly, the unrelated aldolase and CoA-dependent dehydrogenase (DmpGF) [Powlowski et al., 1993]) form a bifunctional enzyme complex. Both of these enzyme pairs catalyze sequential steps within the pathway (Fig. 1B). Furthermore, the member of each pair that makes the substrate for its partner is apparently dependent on the presence of that partner for activity (Shingler et al., 1992; Harayama et al., 1989). In the case of the aldolase-CoA-dependent dehydrogenase pair, cross-regulation at the level of enzymatic activity is a possibility, since the activity of the aldolase is dependent on the presence of NAD^+, which is a cofactor required by the dehydrogenase (Powlowski et al., 1993). These two enzyme pairs raise the as yet unproven idea that metabolic channeling may be important for pathway efficiency. Copurification would only identify tight associations, and it may well be that other enzymes of the pathway are also associated, albeit more loosely.

DmpR AND THE σ^{54}-DEPENDENT FAMILY OF REGULATORS

Transcription of the *dmp* operon from the Po operon promoter is tightly regulated by the divergently transcribed *dmpR* gene product (Shingler et al., 1993). DmpR belongs to the extensive σ^{54}-dependent family of transcriptional activators that control expression of genes involved in a variety of physiological processes. The activities of these regulators are themselves modulated in response to a wide variety of environmental signals (reviewed by Shingler, 1996).

Members of the σ^{54}-dependent family of transcriptional activators act by binding to enhancer-like elements located 100 to 200 bp upstream from the promoters they regulate. These regulators act in concert with RNA polymerase utilizing the alternative sigma factor σ^{54} ($E\sigma^{54}$), which recognizes a distinct class of –24/–12 bacterial promoters that differ considerably from the more usual –35/–10 type of promoters that are recognized by $E\sigma^{70}$ utilizing the "housekeeping" sigma factor. Holoenzyme $E\sigma^{54}$ forms stable closed promoter complexes but, unlike $E\sigma^{70}$, is isomerization incompetent and therefore incapable of proceeding to form open transcriptional complexes in the absence of a positive regulator. Hence, all –24/–12 promoters are regulated by σ^{54}-dependent transcriptional activators that promote the isomerization process. ATP hydrolysis catalyzed by σ^{54}-dependent regulators is believed to provide the necessary energy for the isomerization process (Kustu et al., 1989). Close physical contact between the enhancer-bound regulator and the promoter-bound $E\sigma^{54}$ is facilitated by DNA-bending proteins such as integration host factor or intrinsic bends (reviewed by Pérez-Martin et al., 1994). However, the mechanism underlying the coupling of regulator-catalyzed ATP hydrolysis and the formation of open transcriptional complexes remains to be resolved.

Members of the σ^{54}-dependent family are composed of distinct functional domains involved in signal reception, transcriptional activation, and DNA binding (Fig. 2) (reviewed by Shingler, 1996). The highly conserved central C domain contains a nucleotide-binding motif, and the probable roles of this domain are interaction with σ^{54}-RNA polymerase and binding and hydrolysis of ATP. A region of variable length separates the C domain and the carboxy-terminal D domain, which contains a conserved helix-turn-helix DNA-binding motif found in a number of transcriptional activators and repressors. The B domain (Q linker) is a short hydrophobic region rich in Gln (Q) residues that serves as an interdomain linker between the C domain and the amino-terminal regulatory A domains.

MECHANISM OF AROMATIC ACTIVATION OF DmpR

The regulatory A domains of this family determine the activity of the regulator and fall into different subgroups that reflect the mechanism(s) of activation. Many members of the σ^{54}-dependent family are part of two-component regulatory systems composed of a sensory histidine protein kinase that activates the constitutively expressed transcriptional activator by transfer of a phosphate group to the regulatory A domain (reviewed by Parkinson, 1993). The A domain of DmpR (Shingler et al., 1993) and those of two other *Pseudomonas*-derived regulators of aromatic catabolism, XylR (Inouye et al., 1988)

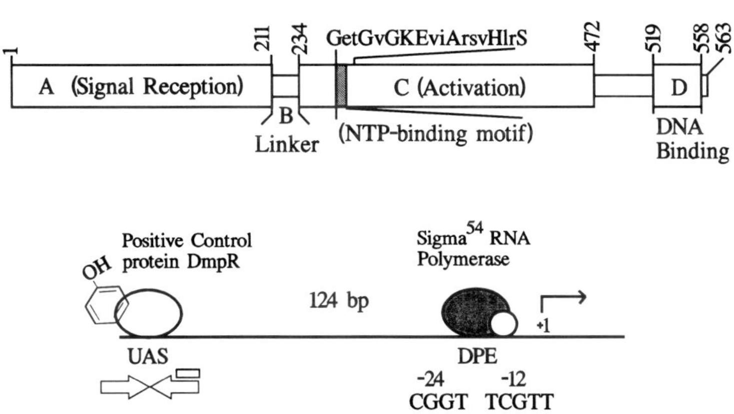

Figure 2. Schematic representation of the domain structure of DmpR (top) and the Po *dmp* operon promoter region (bottom). Shaded box represents the location of a motif (capital letters) implicated in ATP binding and hydrolysis. Open arrows indicate the location of the upstream activation sequence (UAS), which consists of a large inverted repeat implicated in DmpR binding. The location of an overlapping putative integration host factor binding site is indicated by an open bar below the UAS. The downstream –24/–12 promoter element (DPE) consensus sequence is also shown, along with the location of the +1 transcriptional start. NTP, nucleotide triphosphate.

and PhhR (Ng et al., 1995) share 62 to 86% identity on the amino acid level. In contrast to other σ^{54}-dependent activators, these three regulators do not require specific sensor proteins in order to respond to the presence of specific effector aromatic compounds in the growth medium. This specific activation is mediated by the A domains, as demonstrated with a chimeric DmpR-XylR protein in which only the A domain of DmpR has been exchanged for that of XylR. This hybrid responds to effectors of XylR but no longer to those of DmpR (Shingler and Moore, 1994). The isolation of effector specificity mutants of DmpR (Pavel et al., 1994; Shingler and Pavel, 1995) and XylR (Delgado and Ramos, 1994), which exhibit single amino acid changes in the A domains of the respective proteins, provides additional evidence that the specificity of effector activation of this group of regulators resides in the A domain. These observations suggest that the aromatic effectors may directly interact with the regulator. By using affinity-purified DmpR, aromatic effectors were recently shown to directly activate the ATPase activity of the regulator in vitro (Shingler and Pavel, 1995).

Effector-independent (semiconstitutive) DmpR and Xy1R derivatives that have alterations or single-amino-acid substitutions in their regulatory A domains, activation C domains, or the short flexible B-domains that link them have been isolated (Delgado and Ramos, 1995; Fernández et al., 1995; Shingler and Pavel, 1995). These mutants, which presumably partially mimic the activated state of the protein, gave the first indication that the A domains may serve a repressive function. Indeed, deletion derivatives of both DmpR and XylR lacking the regulatory domains have high effector-independent (constitutive) activity in vivo, and in the case of DmpR, the constitutive activity correlates with constitutive ATPase activity in vitro (Fernández et al., 1995; Shingler and Pavel, 1995). These observations led to a working model for regulation of the activities of DmpR and Xy1R (illustrated in Fig. 3) in which the A domain serves to repress the ATPase activity of the regulator in the absence of effector by occluding the ATP-binding and hydrolysis pocket of the C domain, while the presence of effectors relieves this repression. Evidence for specific interaction between residues of the A and C domains that would be

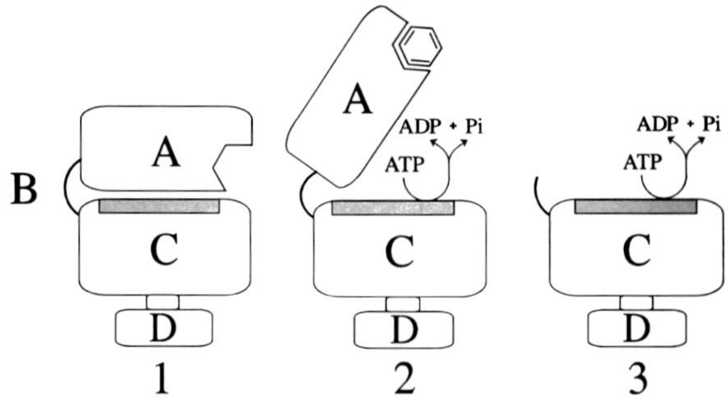

Figure 3. Model for the activation of DmpR by its specific effectors. Domain structures are indicated as boxes; their functions are discussed in the text. 1, The amino-terminal A domain, in the absence of effectors, blocks the ATP binding and hydrolysis surface (indicated by hatching) of the C domain. 2, In the presence of aromatic effectors, the repression mediated by the A domain is relieved. 3, Removal of the A domain results in a constitutively active, effector-independent regulator.

required for this repression model has recently been strengthened by two observations. First, in vivo overexpression of the A domain of XylR specifically represses the activities of A-domain-deleted derivatives of XylR and DmpR. Interestingly, however, this repression is not alleviated by the presence of effectors (Pérez-Martin and de Lorenzo, 1995). Second, compensatory mutations within the A domain of DmpR that suppress the constitutive phenotype mediated by a C-domain-located mutation and vice versa have been identified (Ng et al., 1996).

LIMITATIONS IMPOSED BY THE REGULATORY SYSTEM

For a given compound to support growth, it must serve as both an effector for the regulator DmpR and a substrate for the pathway enzymes. Activation of constitutively expressed DmpR by pathway substrates and some structural analogs not only depends on concentration but also is modulated by the nature and locations of the substituents on the aromatic ring (Shingler and Moore, 1994; Pavel et al., 1994). In the case of pathway substrates, the DmpR-mediated transcriptional response to *para*-substituted compounds (i.e., 4-mp and 3,4-dmp) is markedly poor, suggesting that the inefficient growth on these compounds might be due to low expression of the catabolic enzymes. Consistent with this idea is the finding that *Pseudomonas* strains carrying the *dmp* system at elevated copy numbers (16 to 20 copies per cell) have generation times 1.6- to 2.7-fold faster on *para*-substituted substrates than the wild-type system does (one or two copies per cell) (Pavel et al., 1994). However, this improved degrader was unable to grow on phenol and 2-mp, a phenomenon associated with hyperproduction of the multicomponent phenol hydroxylase at high copy number in response to the efficient effector properties of these compounds. This problem was overcome by isolation of an effector specificity mutant of DmpR that has an enhanced response to 4-mp and 3,4-dmp but retains its wild-type response to other pathway substrates. Introduction of the mutation into the wild-type *dmp* system resulted in a strain that showed enhanced catabolism of *para*-substituted substrates (1.6- to 2.6-fold) but was still capable of efficient growth on other pathway substrates (Pavel et al., 1994). These experiments demonstrate that aromatic effector activation of DmpR can be a major limiting factor in catabolic efficiency.

PhhR of *P. putida* P35X has extensive homology with DmpR, and the structural genes of the *phh* and *dmp* systems also share extensive homology (Ng et al., 1994, 1995). Despite the similarities, these two systems do not specify growth on the same range of compounds: while both mediate growth on phenol and monomethylated phenols, only the *dmp* system mediates growth on 3,4-dmp. The limitation of the *phh* system resides with the regulatory system rather than the catabolic enzymes. PhhR recognizes 3,4-dmp extremely poorly, and simple coexpression of DmpR is all that is required to expand the degradative capacity of *P. putida* P35X to include this substrate (Ng et al., 1995). Hence, effector specificity can also limit the range of compounds degraded by a phenol catabolic pathway.

CONCLUDING REMARKS

The applications of microbial aromatic catabolic activities have stimulated much interest in the constructions of strains with improved degradative abilities. With the possibility of such constructions in mind, the importance of a comprehensive knowledge of pathway genetics and biochemistry is apparent. The enzymes of the pathway are one obvious target for manipulation. For *Pseudomonas* sp. strain CF600, our attention initially focused on phenol hydroxylase, since hydroxylation has been implicated as the rate-limiting step in catabolism. However, we have been unable to test this possiblity as yet because of the growth-inhibitory effect of overexpression of this unusual multicomponent enzyme. A further hindrance to increased strain efficiency by brute force overexpression is suggested by the tight physical coupling of some of the pathway enzymes and the consequent interdependence of the associated enzymatic activities. These observations suggest that subtler modifications, such as specificity mutations that are known to be successful in enhancing efficiency via the specific regulator DmpR, are likely to be more fruitful.

REFERENCES

Bartilson, M., and V. Shingler. 1989. Nucleotide sequence and expression of the catechol 2,3-dioxygenase gene of phenol catabolizing *Pseudomonas* CF600. *Gene* **87:**233–238.

Bayly, R. C., and M. G. Barbour. 1984. The degradation of aromatic compounds, p. 253–294. *In* D. T. Gibson (ed.), *Microbial Degradation of Organic Compounds.* Marcel Dekker, New York.

Bayly, R. C., and G. J. Wigmore. 1973. Metabolism of phenol and cresols by mutants of *Pseudomonas putida. J. Bacteriol.* **113:**1112–1126.

Byrne, A. M., J. J. Kukor, and R. H. Olsen. 1995. Sequence analysis of the gene cluster encoding toluene-3-monooxygenase from *Pseudomonas pickettii* PKO1. *Gene* **154:**65–70.

Chen, L. H., G. L. Kenyon, F. Curtin, S. Harayama, M. E. Bembenek, G. Hajipour, and C. P. Whitman. 1992. 4-Oxalocrotonate tautomerase, an enzyme composed of 62 amino acid residues per monomer. *J. Biol. Chem.* **267:**17716–17721.

Dagley, S. 1986. Biochemistry of aromatic hydrocarbon degradation in *Pseudomonas,* p. 527–556. *In* J. R. Sokatch (ed.), *The Bacteria*, vol X. *The Biology of Pseudomonas.* Academic Press, London.

Delgado, A., and J.-L. Ramos. 1994. Genetic evidence for activation of the positive transcriptional regulator XylR, a member of the NtrC family of regulators, by effector binding. *J. Biol. Chem.* **269:**8059–8062.

Delgado, A., and J.-L. Ramos. 1995. Single amino acid changes in the signal receptor domain of Xy1R result in mutations that stimulate transcription in the absence of effectors. *J. Biol. Chem.* **270:**5144–5150.

Fernández, S., V. de Lorenzo, and J. Pérez-Martin. 1995. Activation of the transcriptional regulator XylR of *Pseudomonas putida* by release of repression between functional domains. *Mol. Microbiol.* **16:**205–213.

Harayama, S., A. Polissi, and M. Rekik. 1991. Divergent evolution of chloroplast-type ferredoxins. *FEBS Lett.* **285:**85–88.

Harayama, S., and M. Rekik. 1993. Comparison of the nucleotide sequence of the *meta*-cleavage pathway genes of TOL plasmid pWW0 from *Pseudomonas putida* with other *meta*-cleavage genes suggests that both single and multiple nucleotide substitutions contribute to enzyme evolution. *Mol. Gen. Genet.* **239:**81–89.

Harayama, S., M. Rekik, K.-I. Ngai, and L. N. Ornston. 1989. Physically associated enzymes produce and metabolize 2-hydroxy-2,4-dienoate, a chemically unstable intermediate formed in catechol metabolism via *meta*-cleavage in *Pseudomonas putida. J. Bacteriol.* **171:**6251–6258.

Herrmann, H., C. Müller, I. Schmidt, J. Mahnke, L. Petruchka, and K. Hahnke. 1995. Location and organisation of phenol degradation genes of *Pseudomonas putida* strain H. *Mol. Gen. Genet.* **247:**240–246.

Horn, J. A., S. Harayama, and K. N. Timmis. 1991. DNA sequence determination of the TOL plasmid *xylGFH* genes *Pseudomonas putida*; implications for the evolution of aromatic catabolism. *Mol. Microbiol.* **5:**2459–2474.

Howard, P. H., R. S. Boethling, W. F. Jarvis, W. M. Meylan, and E. M. Michalenko. 1991. *Handbook of Environmental Degradation Rates.* Lewis Publishers Inc., Chelsea, Mich.

Inouye, S., A. Nakazawa, and T. Nakazawa. 1988. Nucleotide sequence of the regulatory gene *xylR* of the TOL plasmid from *Pseudomonas putida. Gene* **66:**301–306.

Kikuchi, Y., Y. Yasukochi, Y. Nagata, M. Fukuda, and M. Takagi. 1994. Nucleotide sequence and functional analysis of the *meta*-cleavage pathway involved in biphenyl and polychlorinated biphenyl degradation in *Pseudomonas* sp. strain KKS102. *J. Bacteriol.* **176:**4269–4274.

Kim, I. C., and P. J. Oriel. 1995. Characterization of the *Bacillus stearothermophilus* BR219 phenol hydroxylase gene. *Appl. Environ. Microbiol.* **61:**1252–1256.

Kimbara, K., T. Hashimoto, M. Fukuda, T. Koana, M. Takagi, M. Oishi, and K. Yano. 1989. Cloning and sequencing of two tandem genes involved in degradation of 2,3-dihydroxybiphenol to benzoic acid in the polychlorinated biphenyl-degrading soil bacterium *Pseudomonas* sp. strain KKS102. *J. Bacteriol.* **171:**2740–2747.

Kukor, J. J., and R. H. Olsen. 1992. Complete nucleotide sequence of *tbuD*, the gene encoding phenol/cresol hydroxylase from *Pseudomonas pickettii* PKO1, and functional analysis of the encoded enzymes. *J. Bacteriol.* **174:**6518–6526.

Kustu, S., E. Santero, J. Keener, D. Popham, and D. Weiss. 1989. Expression of σ^{54} (*ntrA*)-dependent genes is probably united by a common mechanism. *Microbiol. Rev.* **53:**367–376.

Lau, P. C. K., H. Bergeron, D. Labbé, Y. Wang, R. Brousseau, and D. T. Gibson. 1994. Sequence and expression of the *todGIH* genes involved in the last three steps of toluene degradation by *Pseudomonas putida* F1. *Gene* **146:**7–13.

Menn, F.-M., G. J. Zylstra, and D. T. Gibson. 1991. Location and sequence of the *todF* gene encoding 2-hydroxy-6-oxohepta-2,4-dienoate hydrolase in *Pseudomonas putida* F1. *Gene* **104:**91–94.

Nakai, C., H. Kagamiyama, and M. Nozaki. 1983. Complete nucleotide sequence of the metapyrocatachase gene of the TOL plasmid of *Pseudomonas putida* mt-2. *J. Biol. Chem.* **258:**2923–2928.

Ng, L. C., E. O'Neill, and V. Shingler. Genetic evidence for inter-domain regulation of the phenol responsive σ^{54}-dependent activator DmpR. *J. Biol. Chem.*, in press.

Ng, L. C., C. L. Poh, and V. Shingler. 1995. Aromatic-effector activation of the NtrC-like transcriptional regulator, PhhR, limits the catabolic potential of the (methyl)phenol degradative pathway it controls. *J. Bacteriol.* **177:**1485–1490.

Ng, L. C., V. Shingler, C. C. Sze, and C. L. Poh. 1994. Cloning and nucleotide sequence of the first eight genes of the chromosomally-encoded (methyl)phenol pathway from *Pseudomonas putida* P35X. *Gene* **151:**29–36.

Nordlund, I., J. Powlowski, Å. Hagström, and V. Shingler. 1993. Conservation of regulatory and structural genes for a multicomponent phenol hydroxylase within phenol-catabolizing bacteria that utilize a *meta*-cleavage pathway. *J. Gen. Microbiol.* **139:**2695–2703.

Nordlund, I., J. Powlowski, and V. Shingler. 1990. Complete nucleotide sequence and polypeptide analysis of multicomponent phenol hydroxylase from *Pseudomonas* sp. strain CF600. *J. Bacteriol.* **172:**6826–6833.

Nordlund, I., and V. Shingler. 1990. Nucleotide sequences of the *meta*-cleavage pathway enzymes 2-hydroxymuconic semialdehyde dehydrogenase and 2-hydroxymuconic semialdehyde hydrolase from *Pseudomonas* CF600. *Biochim. Biophys. Acta* **1049:**227–230.

Nurk, A., L. Kasak, and M. Kivisaar. 1991. Sequence of the gene (*pheA*) encoding phenol monooxygenase from *Pseudomonas* EST1001: expression in *Escherichia coli* and *Pseudomonas putida*. *Gene* **102:**13–18.

Parkinson, J. S. 1993. Signal transduction schemes of bacteria. *Cell* **73:**857–871.

Pavel, H., M. Forsman, and V. Shingler. 1994. An aromatic effector specificity mutant of the transcriptional regulator DmpR overcomes the growth constraints of *Pseudomonas* sp. strain CF600 on *para*-substituted methylphenols. *J. Bacteriol.* **176:**7550–7557.

Pérez-Martin, J., and V. de Lorenzo. 1995. The N-terminal domain of the prokaryotic enhancer-binding protein XylR is a specific intramolecular repressor. *Proc. Natl. Acad. Sci. USA.* **92:** 9392–9396.

Pérez-Martin, J., F. Rojo, and V. de Lorenzo. 1994. Promoters responsive to DNA bending: a common theme in prokaryotic gene expression. *Microbiol. Rev.* **58:**268–290.

Polissi, A., and S. Harayama. 1993. *In vivo* reactivation of catechol 2,3-dioxygenase mediated by a chloroplast-type ferredoxin: a bacterial strategy to expand the substrate specificity of aromatic degradative pathways. *EMBO J.* **12:**3339–3347.

Powlowski, J., and V. Shingler. 1990. In vitro analysis of polypeptide requirement of multicomponent phenol hydroxylase from *Pseudomonas* sp. strain CF600. *J. Bacteriol.* **172:**6834–6840.

Powlowski, J., and V. Shingler. 1994. Genetics and biochemistry of phenol degradation by *Pseudomonas* sp. strain CF600. *Biodegradation* **5:**219–236.

Powlowski, J., V. Shingler, and L. Sahlman. 1993. Purification and properties of the physically associated *meta*-cleavage enzymes, 4-hydroxy-2-oxovalerate aldolase and acetaldehyde dehydrogenase (acylating), from *Pseudomonas* sp. strain CF600. *J. Bacteriol.* **175:**377–385.

Sala-Trepat, J. M., K. Murray, and P. A. Williams. 1972. The metabolic divergence in the *meta* cleavage of catechols by *Pseudomonas putida*. *Eur. J. Biochem.* **28:**347–356.

Shingler, V. 1996. Signal sensing by σ^{54}-dependent regulators: derepression as a control mechanism. *Mol. Microbiol.* **19:**409–416.

Shingler, V., M. Bartilson, and T. Moore. 1993. Cloning and nucleotide sequence of the positive regulator (DmpR) of the phenol catabolic pathway of pVI150 and identification as a member of the NtrC family of transcriptional activators. *J. Bacteriol.* **175:**377–385.

Shingler, V., F. C. H. Franklin, M. Tsuda, D. Holyroyd, and M. Bagdasarian. 1989. Molecular analysis of a plasmid-encoded phenol hydroxylase from *Pseudomonas* CF600. *J. Gen. Microbiol.* **135:**1083–1092.

Shingler, V., and T. Moore. 1994. Sensing of aromatic compounds by the DmpR transcriptional activator of phenol-catabolizing *Pseudomonas* sp. strain CF600. *J. Bacteriol.* **176:**1555–1560.

Shingler, V., and H. Pavel. 1995. Direct regulation of the ATPase activity of the transcriptional activator DmpR by aromatic compounds. *Mol. Microbiol.* **17:**505–513.

Shingler, V., J. Powlowski, and U. Marklund. 1992. Nucleotide sequence and functional analysis of the complete phenol/3,4-dimethylphenol catabolic pathway of *Pseudomonas* sp. strain CF600. *J. Bacteriol.* **174:**711–724.

Takeo, M., Y. Maeda, H. Okada, K. Miyama, K. Mori, M. Ike, and M. Fujita. 1995. Molecular cloning and sequencing of the phenol hydroxylase gene from *Pseudomonas putida* BH. *J. Ferment. Bioeng.* **79:**485–488.

Williams, P. A., and J. R. Sayers. 1994. The evolution of pathways for aromatic hydrocarbon oxidation in *Pseudomonas*. *Biodegradation* **5:**195–217.

Yen, K.-M., and M. R. Karl. 1992. Identification of a new gene, *tmoF*, in the *Pseudomonas mendocina* KR1 gene cluster encoding toluene-4-monooxygenase. *J. Bacteriol.* **174:**7253–7261.

Yen, K.-M., M. R. Karl, L. M. Blatt, M. J. Simon, R. B. Winter, P. R. Fausset, H. S. Lu, A. A. Harcourt, and K. K. Chen. 1991. Cloning and characterization of a *Pseudomonas mendocina* KR1 gene cluster encoding toluene-4-monooxygenase. *J. Bacteriol.* **173:**5315–5327.

Zylstra, G. J., and D. T. Gibson. 1989. Toluene degradation by *Pseudomonas* F1: nucleotide sequence of the *todC1C2BADE* genes and their expression in *Escherichia coli*. *J. Biol. Chem.* **264:**14940–14946.

Molecular Biology of Pseudomonads
Edited by T. Nakazawa et al.

Chapter 13

Specificity and Promiscuity of Catabolic Promoters of *Pseudomonas* spp.

Silvia Fernández, José Pérez-Martín, and Víctor de Lorenzo

Pathways for catabolism of the recalcitrant compounds that are frequently found in *Pseudomonas* spp. and related bacteria provide excellent experimental systems for addressing central questions on the molecular mechanisms of adaptation during evolution. The success of a particular biodegradative pathway depends on two major steps that bacteria must overcome to respond adequately to the selective pressure imposed by the presence of novel chemical species as carbon sources. On the one hand, the right complement of genes for catabolic enzymes must be recruited to express an optimal chain of sequential transformations leading to mineralization of the compound. Then, however, only those operons that come under efficient transcriptional control have a reasonable chance to prosper. Regulated promoters are the key element that permit catabolic operons to be transcribed only when required and at levels sufficient to guarantee an adequate metabolic return when there is enough concentration of the substrate. Although constitutively expressed pathways may succeed temporarily, when the unusual C source is not available, nonregulated expression of the catabolic genes may endow the host bacteria with an energetic burden that will ultimately lead to instability of the biodegradation phenotype.

The acquisition of adequate transcriptional control is not at all a trivial matter: as discussed below, comparative studies of the regulation of some biodegradative pathways of *Pseudomonas* spp. bring up very puzzling questions on how regulatory circuits evolve. Many strains of *Pseudomonas* are able to use as carbon sources a variety of unusual aromatic chemicals, including various xenobiotic compounds such as chloroaromatics (Chaudhry and Chapalamadugu, 1991). Analysis of DNA and the protein sequences of the enzymes that form catabolic pathways reveals that, as a rule, isoenzymes that catalyze similar steps within catabolic pathways tend to be highly homologous even when the initial substrates of the pathway are very different (van der Meer et al., 1992; Harayama et al., 1992). These homologies suggest a common evolutionary origin for the enzymes

Silvia Fernández, José Pérez-Martín, and Víctor de Lorenzo • Department of Microbial Biotechnology, Centro Nacional de Biotecnología, Campus de Cantoblanco, 28049 Madrid, Spain.

and even for different portions of the pathways, which may be recruited at a given time to respond to a novel substrate (Yeh and Ornston, 1980).

TRANSCRIPTIONAL CONTROL OF BIODEGRADATIVE PATHWAYS EVOLVES SEPARATELY FROM THEIR CATABOLIC GENES

In sharp contrast to the homology among enzymes that utilize the same or similar substrates in different pathways, transcriptional regulators of catabolic operons may be extremely different. For example, the *meta*-NAH pathway, which is induced by salicylate, uses transcriptional control based on the NahR protein, which belongs to the LysR family of regulators (Schell and Sukordhaman, 1989). In contrast, the *meta*-TOL pathway is regulated by an activator, XylS, of the AraC family (Marqués and Ramos, 1993). Each of the two families of proteins activates transcription through a totally different constellation of protein-protein and protein-DNA contacts at the cognate promoter regions. Since XylS mutants that respond to salicylate can easily be found (Ramos et al., 1990), the question arises as to why bacteria evolved a totally different transcriptional control for degradation of salicylate based on NahR when it would have been easy to produce an equally effective XylS variety.

In fact, we also wonder why in some pathways, the inducer of the corresponding regulator is the actual substrate to be used as a carbon source, while in other cases, the inducer is an intermediate compound produced. A good example of the former is the induction by toluene and *m*- and *p*-xylene of the upper TOL pathway (Marqués and Ramos, 1993), while one of the most remarkable cases of the latter is, again, the induction by salicylate of the upper NAH operon for biodegradation of naphthalene. In this case, one could speculate that induction by an intermediate should occur when the initial substrate is too hydrophobic to act as a protein effector. This is not true, however, since naphthalene is perfectly able to illegitimately activate the XylR regulator of the TOL plasmid (S. Fernández and V. de Lorenzo, unpublished data).

Similarly, the *meta*-cleavage pathway for the degradation of phenol and methylphenols of *Pseudomonas* plasmid pVI150 is driven by a promoter named Po. This promoter belongs to the class that requires the RNA polymerase to contain the alternative sigma factor named σ^{54}. Po also requires the concourse of a cognate activator, DmpR (dimethylphenol regulator). This regulator belongs to the so-called NtrC family of proteins (Shingler et al., 1993), which share a very particular modular structure resembling the structures of eukaryotic transcription factors. Given the enzymatic similarity between this pathway and the *meta*-TOL pathway (Shingler et al., 1992), one would expect the regulation to be organized the same, i.e., through a regulator of the AraC family like XylS, but such is not the case, and responsiveness to phenol has been raised in a different class of activators. Amazingly, in an alternative pathway for its biodegradation, phenol activates its own catabolism by sneaking into the regulation of the catechol pathway of *Pseudomonas* spp. (Parsek et al., 1995). In this case, the promoter for the *pheBA* gene cluster, which encodes a phenol monooxygense (the product of whose activity on phenol is catechol) and a catechol 1,2-dioxygenase, has acquired a binding site for the activator protein CatR, which itself controls expression of the catechol-degrading *cat* system and is effected by *cis,cis*-muconate, the result of *ortho* cleavage of the catechol ring (Parsek et al., 1995).

The corollary of these observations is that very different transcriptional control systems can be assembled around virtually identical signals (i.e., chemical species), and therefore, the specific regulation of biodegradative operons seems to have evolved independently of catabolic genes.

THE REGULATORY NOISE HYPOTHESIS

A detailed examination of the control of expression of the TOL promoters has given rise to the so-called regulatory noise hypothesis, which states that new catabolic operons can evolve transcriptional control systems because of the leakiness of preexisting promoters. As discussed below, this notion has been developed mostly on the basis of the regulation of the σ^{54}-dependent Pu and Ps promoters of the TOL plasmid pWW0. As summarized in Fig. 1 and described in detail elsewhere (Salto et al., this volume), in the presence of *m*-xylene, these promoters are activated at a distance by the prokaryotic enhancer-binding protein XylR of the NtrC family of transcriptional regulators (Inouye et al., 1988; Inouye et al., 1990).

Activation of TOL Promoters by XylR

Like other regulators of the family, the XylR protein (63.7 kDa) has a modular structure (Fig. 2A). While the central activating (C) domain and the DNA-binding (D) domain of XylR are functionally similar to those of other related regulators of the NtrC family (Inouye et al., 1988; Morett and Segovia, 1993; North et al., 1993), the receiver A domain of XylR interacts directly with the aromatic effector of the TOL system, i.e., *m*-xylene (Delgado and Ramos,

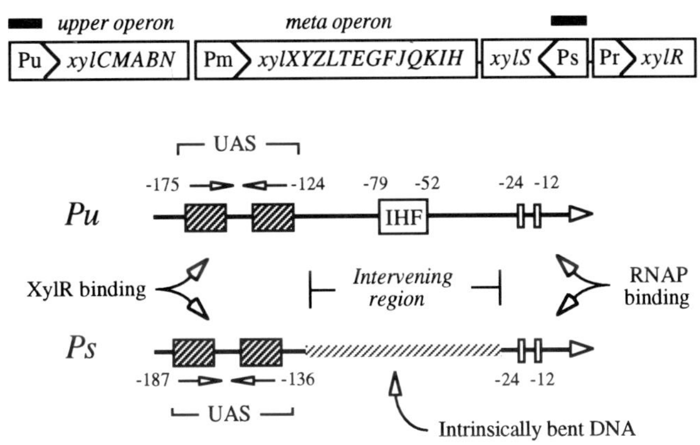

Figure 1. Organization of *xyl* genes in the TOL plasmid pWW0 and its σ^{54}-dependent promoters Pu and Ps. The TOL system for degradation of toluene, *m*-xylene, and *p*-xylene includes two gene clusters and two regulatory genes, *xylS* and *xylR*, as shown at the top. The system also has two σ^{54}-dependent promoters, namely Pu and Ps (indicated by solid bars at the top), that are activated by the cognate activator XylR in the presence of pathway substrates. Below the scheme of the operons, the Pu and Ps promoter regions are expanded to show the locations of relevant features. These features include the UAS for XylR, the −12/−24 motif recognized by σ^{54}-RNA polymerase (RNAP), and the IHF binding site or intrinsic DNA bends located at the intervening regions of Pu or Ps, respectively.

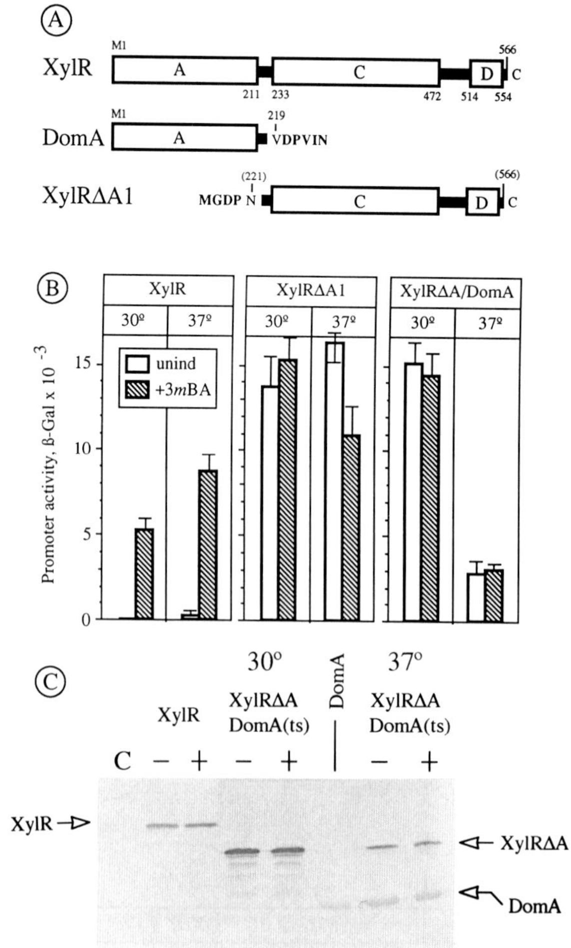

Figure 2. Repression in *trans* of the constitutive activity of XylRΔA by the isolated signal-sensing A domain. (A) Truncated proteins employed in the experiment. XylRΔA1 is an N-terminal-truncated XylR derivative that spans only amino acids 221 to 566 of the XylR sequence (Fernández et al., 1995). DomA, on the other hand, spans the leading 219 amino acids of the XylR protein and is followed by a short sequence (in boldface letters) that is inherited. (B) Δ*lac E. coli* S90C was cotransformed with the reporter Pu-*lacZ* plasmid pFH32 and either *xylR*⁺ plasmid pCKXylR or *xylRΔA*⁺ plasmid pTTΔA along with a third plasmid (pFH9) that conditionally expresses DomA in a temperature-dependent fashion through a T7-polymerase-based system. Each strain was then grown at 30°C to an optical density at 600 nm of 0.5 in Luria-Bertani medium supplemented with adequate antibiotics. At that point, the temperature was shifted to 37°C, and the cultures were exposed for 5 h to saturating vapors of 3-methylbenzyl alcohol (3mBA). The graph shows levels of β-galactosidase (β-Gal) for each strain under various conditions. unind, uninduced. (C) Conditional expression of the A domain of XylR. The protein extracts of *E. coli* cells from relevant cultures used in the experiment described above were run in a denaturing 8% polyacrylamide gel and subjected to a Western blot (immunoblot) analysis with polyclonal rabbit anti-XylR serum. Expression of XylR was not affected by exposure to inducer. Lane C is a control devoid of any XylR. The position of each of the truncated proteins is indicated. Note the production of the A domain only at 37°C and the lack of effect of inducer presence (+) or absence (–). Lane DomA is a control sample from cells transformed only with pFH9 (*domA*⁺) and grown at 37°C.

1994), an event that is finally translated into activation of the cognate promoters Pu and Ps. The fact that an N-terminal deletion of XylR causes the activator to be fully constitutive (Fernández et al., 1995) suggests that the N-terminal portion of the protein downregulates the activity of the whole system. Furthermore, disruptive amino acid changes at the interdomain B region (Q linker) result in a semiconstitutive phenotype (Fernández et al., 1995). The sequence of events leading to the activation of XylR seems, therefore, to involve the offsetting of the A domain from a protein surface that is required for activation and that is otherwise masked by the receiver module of the regulator.

Acquisition of Effector Responsiveness by XylR: the A Domain Is a Specific Intramolecular Repressor

One hypothesis to explain the evolution of the ability of the TOL promoters to respond to the presence of toluene and xylenes in the medium is that a precursor activator protein spanning only domains C and D later acquired an aromatic-responsive repressor module with the ability to inhibit the activity of the otherwise fully active regulator. Should this be true, it might be possible to produce the repressor module and the constitutive truncated protein separately and to reproduce the inhibition between proteins in *trans*.

We previously showed that a truncated XylR derivative with the whole N-terminal domain deleted, i.e., the region spanning former amino acid positions 226 to 566, was produced as a stable and constitutively active regulator (Fernández et al., 1995). Similarly, we sought to produce the A domain as an isolated peptide. For this, we constructed an expression plasmid in which the polypeptide spanning amino acid positions 1 to 219 of the XylR sequence was expressed through a thermosensitive promoter system. Prior to its use, we confirmed that the resulting product was synthesized in vivo as a full-size protein (Fig. 2C) with no indications of instability or proteolytic degradation. To examine the potential activity of the isolated A domain on the truncated and constitutive XylRΔA1 protein, we set up the system explained in the legend to Fig. 2. In this assay, expression of the truncated XylRΔA1 protein takes place at both 30 and 37°C, while expression of the A domain occurs only at 37°C. As shown in Fig. 2B and C, coexpression in *trans* of the A domain along with the C and D portions of the protein resulted in ≥80% inhibition of the otherwise constitutive activity of the XylRΔA1 protein. Under equivalent conditions, expression of the isolated A domain of XylR had no effect on activation of a *PnifH-lacZ* fusion by its cognate regulator NifA, of the σ^{54}-dependent class (not shown), thus ruling out that the inhibition of Pu could be due to somewhat nonspecific effect on σ^{54}-dependent systems. In fact, the inhibition of XylRΔA1 activity by the A domain appeared to reproduce part of its predicted role as an intramolecular repressor, yet the presence of the XylR effector 3-methylbenzyl alcohol did not restore the inducibility of the system to aromatic effectors, thus suggesting that the activation process may require an intact hinge connecting the N-terminal portion with the rest of the protein. An alternative approach to substantiating these points was reported by Pérez-Martín and de Lorenzo (1995b).

Cross-Activation of Pu by DmpR

The Po promoter of plasmid pVI150 controls expression of an operon of *Pseudomonas* sp. strain CF600 that is required for the complete catabolism of phenol and cresols

(Shingler et al., 1993). This promoter, which belongs to the σ^{54}-dependent class, is regulated by its cognate activator, DmpR. XylR and DmpR share a remarkable degree of similarity, and both require aromatic compounds as effector molecules for the activity. However, these two proteins respond to very different profiles of aromatic compounds (Shingler and Moore, 1994). We found that the two activators can functionally substitute for each other in the regulation of their corresponding promoters (Fernández et al., 1994). In fact, XylR and DmpR seem to recognize DNA sequences located within the same region of the Pu promoter and, most likely, within the Po promoter as well. The mutual interchange for the activation of each other's cognate promoter is not just residual cross-talk but is a physiologically significant cross-activation, since the two regulators effect the promoters at comparable levels in vivo. Surprisingly, XylR stimulates the production of the catabolic enzymes for degradation of phenol in response to *m*-xylene to higher levels than those afforded by the native DmpR regulator of the system. These results support the notion that the regulators of the NtrC family (such as DmpR and XylR) have the potential to coevolve along with their target sequences as "regulatory cassettes" that can eventually be recruited by very different operons. Perhaps the basic unit includes the activator gene constitutively and divergently expressed from the σ^{54}-dependent promoter that it regulates, as is the case with Ps (Fig. 1) and Po. Other gene clusters could then come under the same regulatory control by simple acquisition of a properly positioned upstream activating sequence (UAS).

DNA-Bending Specificity of Pu and Ps

As shown in Fig. 1, the DNA segment between the UAS and the segments encoding RNA polymerase binding at Pu contains an integration host factor (IHF) attachment site, which is required for full transcriptional activity (de Lorenzo et al., 1991; Abril et al., 1991). IHF is a small protein (20 kDa) known to participate in a variety of cellular processes that, upon binding to its target DNA sequence, causes a sharp bend (~140°) in the DNA. The predominant role of IHF in Pu and other σ^{54}-dependent promoters is that of providing a structural aid to improve contacts between the σ^{54}-RNA polymerase bound to the −12/−24 positions and the activator protein attached to the UAS (Pérez-Martín et al., 1994). However, the other σ^{54}-dependent promoter of the TOL system (Ps) does not bear functional IHF sites (although it does carry potential IHF binding sites [Holtel et al., 1992]). The question that then arises is why one of the two TOL σ^{54}-dependent promoters requires IHF, while the other, regulated by the same activator, does not. Except for the presence of the functional IHF site, Pu and Ps display the same arrangement of their core elements (UAS for XylR binding and −12/−24 sequence for attachment of σ^{54}-RNA polymerase; Fig. 1). We (Pérez-Martín and de Lorenzo, 1995a) and others (Gomada et al., 1994) reported the presence of a static DNA bend at the intervening region of Ps that may be used as the guiding element by the histone-like protein HU to assist in the formation of a productive DNA loop when IHF is not available (Pérez-Martín and de Lorenzo, 1995a).

One major difference between IHF and HU in σ^{54}-dependent promoters lies in the ability of IHF to maintain the low basal activity of Pu in the absence of XylR-mediated induction (Pérez-Martín and de Lorenzo, in press b). Although IHF provides a scaffold for a loop that brings the two proteins into close proximity (thus increasing transcription efficiency), such an effect may, at the same time, restrict the flexibility of the region. The rigid conformation that DNA may adopt upon IHF binding increases activation specificity by preventing access to heterologous NtrC-like activators other than that properly bound and positioned in the UAS. It seems, therefore, that the role of IHF in Pu is not only that of coactivator (Pérez-Martín et al., 1994) but also that of suppressor of cross regulation. We coined the term "restrictor" (graphically explained in Fig. 3) to operatively describe this specificity-enhancing function assigned to protein-induced or static bends.

To test directly the concept that σ^{54}-dependent promoters devoid of sharply bent DNA sequences can be activated by other regulators of the NtrC family of proteins, the effect of the NifA protein of *Klebsiella pneumoniae* on the activity of the Ps promoter was studied. NifA is a convenient regulator for this purpose, since it is active in *Escherichia coli,* does not require any inducer (Drummond et al., 1990), and stimulates transcription even in the absence of DNA binding (Drummond et al., 1990; Cannon and Buck, 1992). In one experiment, we produced wild-type NifA in isogenic IHF$^+$ and IHF$^-$ strains harboring a *lacZ* fusion to Ps. The results shown in Fig. 4 indicate that NifA could activate Ps regardless of the presence or absence of IHF. In other experiments reported elsewhere (Pérez-Martín and de Lorenzo, 1995c), we observed that Pu could be activated by NifA only when IHF was lacking. A similar assay was repeated with a truncated NifA protein (instead of wild-type NifA), which maintains its central activating domain but is unable to bind DNA (Berger et al., 1994). The results shown in Fig. 4 rule out the presence of a cryptic UAS for NifA at the corresponding promoter region and show that the activation

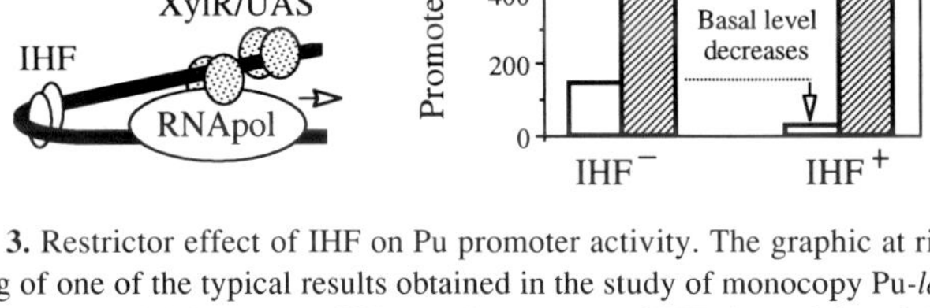

Figure 3. Restrictor effect of IHF on Pu promoter activity. The graphic at right is a redrawing of one of the typical results obtained in the study of monocopy Pu-*lacZ* fusions (Pérez-Martín and de Lorenzo, 1995c). In the absence of IHF, the activity of the promoter is lower and the basal level is higher than when the cell contains IHF. Since the increase in basal promoter activity is independent of XylR but still dependent on *rpoN* (encoding σ^{54}), IHF not only assists XylR-RNA polymerase interactions (Abril et al., 1991; de Lorenzo et al., 1991) but also prevents promiscuous cross-activation by other activators of the same family, as sketched at left. The result of this effect is the in vivo selection of a certain window of activity of the promoter from the whole potential available in the system (Pérez-Martín and de Lorenzo, 1995c). Unind, uninduced; *m*-xyl, *m*-xylene; β-gal, β-galactosidase.

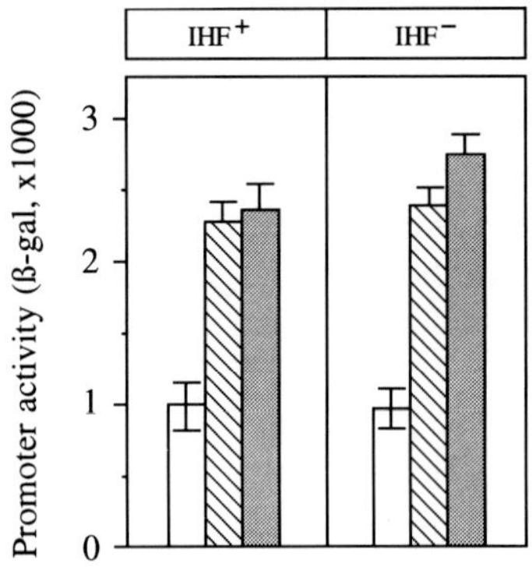

Figure 4. Cross-activation of Ps by NifA. Δ*lac E. coli* S90C and its isogenic derivative *E. coli* DBP102 *himA* (IHF^-) were cotransformed with pACYC184 (open bars; control, devoid of *nifA*), pMC71A (hatched bars; $nifA^+$) or pNifAΔC (shaded bars; expresses the activating central domain of NifA, is unable to bind DNA under a P_{tac}=$lacI^q$ system) along with pRSPs, a compatible plasmid bearing a transcriptional *lacZ* fusion to the Ps promoter. Cotransformants were grown overnight at 30°C in liquid medium (plus 0.1 mM isopropyl-β-D-thiogalactopyranoside in the case of cells carrying pNifAΔC). Accumulation of β-galactosidase (β-Gal) by cells is shown.

of Ps does not require binding of the heterologous regulator to DNA sequences at the promoter region.

Why Are IHF-Dependent and -Independent Promoters in the Same System?

Restrictor elements may provide an additional level of control to σ^{54}-dependent promoters for fine-tuning their physiological activity. The TOL plasmid of *P. putida* determines a catabolic pathway for the degradation of *m*-xylene. This occurs in two major steps, each being determined by the products of two cognate operons, that are regulated coordinately in response to pathway substrates (reviewed by Marqués and Ramos, 1993). Pu drives expression of the so-called upper operon, which mediates the conversion of *m*-xylene to *m*-toluate, while Ps transcribes the gene for the regulator of the *meta* operon (called XylS), which determines the stepwise degradation of *m*-toluate to pyruvate and acetaldehyde. Both Pu and Ps are positively regulated by XylR, but the requirements for the products they transcribe are different: in the absence of *m*-xylene, the restrictor-containing Pu promoter remains totally silent, while the restrictorless Ps promoter still has a considerable level of basal activity. This allows growth on *m*-xylene through transcription of the upper and *meta* operons because of the XylR-dependent activities of Pu and Ps. Also, cells can grow on *m*-toluate alone through the activity of the *meta* pathway permitted by the XylR-independent transcription of XylS from Ps, while the upper pathway remains totally silent. At least in the TOL system, the presence or absence of a restrictor element therefore seems to displace the responsiveness of each promoter toward either specificity or promiscuity for the sake of a proper physiological balance.

CONCLUSIONS

The transcriptional control of the catabolic TOL plasmid pWW0 of *Pseudomonas putida* for toluene biodegradation is a paradigm of the complexity of the regulation of gene expression in prokaryotes (reviewed by Marqués and Ramos, 1993, and also by Salto et al., in this volume). Various features of such a complex regulation have shed some light on the mechanisms by which biodegradative operons have acquired through evolution conditionally active promoters that permit the corresponding genes to be transcribed only when required. The regulatory noise hypothesis proposes that new catabolic operons can evolve transcriptional control systems because of the leakiness of preexisting promoters. Such leakiness is displayed at many levels and finds its best example in the regulation of the σ^{54}-dependent promoters and the TOL plasmid: XylR can recognize as effectors a whole variety of aromatic structures quite different from those that are the substrates of the pathway (Abril et al., 1989). Also, Pu can be efficiently cross regulated by DmpR, the regulator of a different catabolic pathway (Fernández et al., 1995). Finally, Ps and Pu (in the absence of IHF) can be residually activated by heterologous proteins such as NifA (Pérez-Martín and de Lorenzo, in press b). Such illegitimate activation may not require the binding of the second regulators to DNA and is suppressed by bent DNA structures, either static or protein induced, between the promoter core elements (UAS and RNA polymerase recognition sequence).

The phenomenon of cross-activation between regulators and promoters of different pathways has been found in other biodegradative operons of *Pseudomonas* spp. besides the TOL system (Parsek et al., 1994). It therefore seems that in general, catabolic promoters may possess a remarkable level of unspecificity regarding the signals to which they respond. We believe that it is this feature that allows them to evolve and to be eligible for recruitment in front of novel pathways that may improve their evolutionary success by introducing a certain degree of regulation which, over time, may itself evolve toward specificity. All the data reviewed in this article support these notions.

Acknowledgments. The participation of V. Shingler (University of Umeå, Umeå, Sweden) in some of the experiments referred to in this article is gratefully acknowledged. This research was financed by Comisión Interministerial de Ciencia y Tecnología (BIO92-1018-CO2-01), Agencia del Medio Ambiente de la Comunidad Autónoma de Madrid, and BIOTECH contract BIO2-CT92-0084 of the European Union.

REFERENCES

Abril, M. A., M. Buck, and J. L. Ramson. 1991. Activation of the *Pseudomonas* TOL plasmid *upper* pathway operon: identification of binding sites for the positive regulator XylR and for integration host factor protein. *J. Biol. Chem.* **266:**5832–5838.

Abril, M. A., C. Michan, K. N. Timmis, and J. L. Ramson. 1989. Regulator and enzyme specificities of the TOL plasmid-encoded upper pathway for degradation of aromatic hydrocarbons and expansion of the substrate range of the pathway. *J. Bacteriol.* **171:**6782–6790.

Berger, K. D., F. Narberhaus, and S. Kustu. 1994. The isolated catalytic domain of NIFA, a bacterial enhancer-binding protein, activates transcription in vitro: activation is inhibited by NIFL. *Proc. Natl. Acad. Sci. USA* **91:**103–107.

Cannon, W., and M. Buck. 1992. Central domain of the positive control protein NifA and its role in transcriptional activation. *J. Mol. Biol.* **225:**271–286.

Chaudhry, G. R., and S. Chapalamadugu. 1991. Biodegradation of halogenated aromatic compounds. *Microbiol. Rev.* **55:**59–79.

Delgado, A., and J. L. Ramos. 1994. Genetic evidence for activation of the positive transcriptional regulator XylR, a member of the NtrC family of regulators, by effector binding. *J. Biol. Chem.* **269:**8059–8062.

de Lorenzo, V., M. Herrero, M. Metzke, and K. N. Timmis. 1991. An upstream XylR-and IHF-induced nucleoprotein complex regulates the σ^{54}-dependent *Pu* promoter of TOL plasmid. *EMBO J.* **10:**1159–1167.

Drummond, M. H., A. Contreras, and L. A. Mitchenall. 1990. The function of isolated domains and chimaeric proteins constructed from the transcriptional activators NifA and NtrC of *Klebsiella pneumoniae*. *Mol. Microbiol.* **4:**29–37.

Fernández, S., V. de Lorenzo, and J. Pérez-Martín. 1995. Activation of the transcriptional regulator XylR of *Pseudomonas putida* by release of repression between functional domains. *Mol. Microbiol.* **16:**205–213.

Fernández, S., V. Shingler, and V. de Lorenzo. 1994. Cross-regulation by XylR and DmpR activators of *Pseudomonas putida* suggests that transcriptional control of biodegradative operons evolves independently of catabolic genes. *J. Bacteriol.* **176:**5052–5058.

Gomada, M., H. Imaishi, K. Miura, S. Inouye, T. Nakazawa, and A. Nakazawa. 1994. Analysis of DNA bend structure of promoter regulatory regions of xylene-metabolizing genes on the *Pseudomonas* TOL plasmid. *J. Biochem.* **116:**1096–1104.

Harayama, S., M. Kok, and E. L. Niedle. 1992. Functional and evolutionary relationships between diverse oxygenases. *Annu. Rev. Microbiol.* **46:**565–601.

Holtel, A., K. N. Timmis, and J. L. Ramos. 1992. Upstream binding sequences of the XylR activator protein and integration host factor in the *xylS* gene promoter region of *Pseudomonas* TOL plasmid. *Nucleic Acids Res.* **20:**1755–1762.

Inouye, S., M. Gomada, U. M. X. Sangodkar, A. Nakazawa, and T. Nakazawa. 1990. Upstream regulatory sequences for transcriptional activator XylR in the first operon of xylene metabolism of the TOL plasmid. *J. Mol. Biol.* **216:**251–260.

Inouye, S., A. Nakazawa, and T. Nakazawa. 1988. Nucleotide sequence of the regulatory gene *xylR* of the TOL plasmid from *Pseudomonas putida*. *Gene* **66:**301–306.

Marqués, S., and J. L. Ramos. 1993. Transcriptional control of the *Pseudomonas putida* TOL plasmid catabolic pathways. *Mol. Microbiol.* **9:**923–929.

Morett, E., and L. Segovia. 1993. The σ^{54} bacterial enchancer-binding protein family: mechanism of action and phylogenetic relationship of their functional domains. *J. Bacteriol.* **178:**6067–6074.

North, A., K. E. Klose, K. M. Stedman, and S. Kustu. 1993. Prokaryotic enhancer-binding proteins reflect eukaryote-like modularity: the puzzle of nitrogen regulatory protein C. *J. Bacteriol.* **175:**4267–4273.

Parsek, M. R., M. Kivisaar, and A. M. Chakrabarty. 1995. Differential DNA bending introduced by the *Pseudomonas putida* LysR-type regulator, CatR, at the plasmid-borne *pheBA* and chromosomal *catBC* promoters. *Mol. Microbiol.* **15:**819–828.

Parsek, M. R., S. McFall, D. Shinabarger, and A. M. Chakrabarty. 1994. Interaction of two LysR-type regulatory proteins CatR and ClcR with heterologous promoters: functional and evolutionary implications. *Proc. Natl. Acad. Sci. USA* **91:**12393–12397.

Pérez-Martín, J., and V. de Lorenzo. 1995a. The σ^{54}-dependent promoter Ps of the TOL plasmid of *Pseudomonas putida* requires HU for transcriptional activation in vivo by XylR. *J. Bacteriol.* **177:**3758–3763.

Pérez-Martín, J., and V. de Lorenzo. 1995b. The N-terminal domain of the prokaryotic enhancer-binding protein XylR is a specific intramolecular repressor. *Proc. Natl. Acad. Sci. USA* **92:**9392–9396.

Pérez-Martín, J., and V. de Lorenzo. 1995c. Integration host factor (IHF) suppresses promiscuous activation of the σ^{54}-dependent promoter *Pu* of *Pseudomonas putida*. *Proc. Natl. Acad. Sci. USA* **92:**7277–7281.

Pérez-Martín, J., K. N. Timmis, and V. de Lorenzo. 1994. Co-regulation by bent DNA: functional substitutions of the IHF site at the σ^{54}-dependent promoter *Pu* of the *upper*-TOL operon by intrinsically curved sequences. *J. Biol. Chem.* **269:**22657–22662.

Ramos, J. L., C. Michán, F. Rojo, D. Dwyer, and K. N. Timmis. 1990. Signal-regulator interactions. Genetic analysis of the effector binding site of XylS, the benzoate-activated positive regulator of *Pseudomonas* TOL plasmid *meta*-cleavage pathway operon. *J. Mol. Biol.* **211:**373–382.

Schell, M., and M. Sukordhaman. 1989. Evidence that the transcription activator encoded by the *Pseudomonas putida nahR* gene is evolutionarily related to the transcription activators encoded by the *Rhizobium nodD* genes. *J. Bacteriol.* **171:**1952–1959.

Shingler, V., M. Bartilson, and T. Moore. 1993. Cloning and nucleotide sequence of the gene encoding the positive regulator (DmpR) of the phenol catabolic pathway encoded by pVI150 and identification of DmpR as a member of the NtrC family of transcriptional activators. *J. Bacteriol.* **175:**1596–1604.

Shingler, V., and T. Moore. 1994. Sensing aromatic compounds by the DmpR transcriptional activator of phenol-catabolizing *Pseudomonas* sp. strain CF600. *J. Bacteriol.* **176:**1555–1560.

Shingler, V., J. Powlowski, and U. Marklund. 1992. Nucleotide sequence and functional analysis of the complete phenol/3,4-dimethylphenol catabolic pathway of *Pseudomonas* sp. strain CF600. *J. Bacteriol.* **174:**711–724.

van der Meer, J. R., W. H. de Vos, S. Harayama, and A. J. B. Zehnder. 1992. Molecular mechanisms of genetic adaptation to xenobiotic compounds. *Microbiol. Rev.* **56:**677–694.

Yeh, W. K., and L. N. Ornston. 1980. Origins of metabolic diversity: substitutions for homologous sequences into genes for enzymes with different catalytic activities. *Proc. Natl. Acad. Sci. USA* **143:**5365–5369.

Molecular Biology of Pseudomonads
Edited by T. Nakazawa et al.

Chapter 14

Two-Component Signal Transduction Systems Regulating Toluene and Biphenyl–Polychlorinated-Biphenyl Degradations in a Soil Pseudomonad and an Actinomycete

Peter C. K. Lau, Ying Wang, Diane Labbé, Hélène Bergeron, and James Garnon

For a successful bioremediation scheme in which microbes are the workhorses and enzymes are the underlying entities for the degradation or detoxification of environmental pollutants, there is little or no doubt that knowledge of the limitations and the driving forces in an optimal performance of a biodegradation pathway are invaluable in sustained development of the technology. Fundamental to addressing these issues are the needs to obtain detailed information on the gene structure and organization of the degradative pathways and to seek sequence information in order to facilitate studies of regulators, inducers, and environmental factors that could modulate or otherwise affect the expression of the degradative operons.

PATHWAYS AND CONTROLLING FAMILIES

A number of vigorous studies of degradative pathways, such as those for naphthalene, toluene-xylene, phenol, and biphenyl (BP)-polychlorinated BP (PCB; for a review, see van der Meer et al., 1992), make it evident that different pathways have evolved to degrade the same chemical (e.g., toluene can be aerobically degraded five ways; for a review, see Zylstra and Gibson, 1991) or that similar pathways have been assembled to degrade what appear to be very different chemical substrates (e.g., toluene and BP-PCB; for a review, see Furukawa, 1994). At one extreme, a few amino acid changes in a critical enzyme, namely, the large subunit of the BP dioxygenase in *Pseudomonas* sp. strain LB400 and *Pseudomonas pseudoalcaligenes* KF707, can lead to dramatic differences in the PCB substrate ranges and specificities of these enzymes (Gibson et al., 1993; Erickson and Mondello, 1993).

Peter C. K. Lau, Ying Wang, Diane Labbé, Hélène Bergeron, and James Garnon • Biotechnology Research Institute, National Research Council Canada, 6100 Royalmount Avenue, Montreal, Quebec H4P 2R2, Canada.

On the regulation front, different transcriptional control systems have evolved to regulate the expression of similar catabolic pathways and phenotypes. Until this study, regulators of aromatic hydrocarbon metabolism have been considered to belong to one of three families (Table 1). The majority so far belong to the LysR family of transcriptional regulators (LTTR; Schell, 1993). The 300-residue NahR of the NAH7 plasmid-encoded naphthalene and salicylate degradation pathways in *Pseudomonas putida* G7 (Schell, 1993) is one of the well-characterized LTTRs. It has functional domains that consist of

Table 1. Regulators of aromatic catabolic pathways

Family and proteins	Strain	Catabolic function[a]	Reference(s)
LysR family			
BphR[b]	*P. pseudoalcaligenes* KF707	BP-PCB	Labbé et al., unpublished data
CatM	*Acinetobacter calcoaceticus*	Catechol	Niedle et al., 1989[c]
CatR	*P. putida*	Catechol	Rothmel et al., 1990[c]
ClcR	Plasmid pAC25	Chlorocatechol	Coco et al., 1993[c]
	Plasmid pAC27 in *P. putida*	Chlorocatechol	
NahR	NAH7 plasmid of *P. putida* G7	Naphthalene-salicylate	Schell and Sukordhaman, 1989[c]
TcbR	*Pseudomonas* sp. strain P51	Chlorocatechol	van der Meer et al., 1991[c]
TfdR	*A. eutrophus* plasmid JP4	2,4-Dichlorophenyl acetate, *tfdB*, 2,4-D hydroxylase	Matrubutham and Harker, 1994 You and Ghosal, 1995
TfdS	*A. eutrophus* plasmid JP4	2,4-D (*tfdA* oxygenase)	Kaphammer et al., 1990[c] You and Ghosal, 1995
TodR[b]	*P. putida* F1	Toluene	Wang et al., 1995b
NtrC family (σ^{54} dependent)			
DmpR	*Pseudomonas* sp. strain CF600	(Dimethyl)phenol	Shingler et al., 1993[d]
DmpR-like	*P. putida* U	(Dimethyl)phenol	Nordlund et al., 1993[d]
PphR	*P. putida* P35X	(Methyl)phenol	Ng et al., 1995
TbuT	*P. pickettii* PX01	Toluene	Byrne et al., 1995
TomR	*P. cepacia* G4	Toluene (*ortho*-monooxygenase pathway)	Francesconi et al., 1995
XylR	*P. putida* mt-2 (pWW0)	Toluene-xylene	Inouye et al., 1988
	P. putida pWW53	Toluene-xylene	Williams et al., 1992
AraC family			
XylS	*P. putida* (pWW0)	Toluene (*meta* pathway)	Inouye et al., 1988; Gallegos et al., 1993
XylS1	*P. putida* pWW53	Toluene (*meta* pathway)	Williams et al., 1992
XylS2			
XylS3			
XylS	*P. putida* pDR1	Toluene (*meta* pathway)	
Two-component signal transduction family			
TodS-TodT	*P. putida* F1	Toluene (dioxygenase pathway)	Lau et al., 1994a; this study
BpdS-BpdT	*Rhodococcus* sp. strain M5	BP-PCB	Lau et al., 1994b; this study

[a] 2,4-D, 2,4-dichlorophenoxyacetic acid.
[b] Appears cryptic in function.
[c] Reference cited in Schell (1993).
[d] Reference cited in Powlowski and Shingler (1994).

an amino-terminal DNA-binding region, coinducer recognition and response regions, and a conserved carboxy-terminal region. Recently classified members of the "aromatic" LTTRs are TfdR of 2,4-dichlorophenoxy acetate catabolism in *Alcaligenes eutrophus* plasmid JP4 (You and Ghosal, 1995) and BphR of KF707, a near-identical homolog of NahR that appears to be functionally cryptic (D. Labbé et al., unpublished data). TodR, recently found in *P. putida* F1, is the first example of a truncated LTTR: it has only 100 amino acids, which represent the putative DNA-binding domain of this group of proteins (Wang et al., 1995b). Lacking other domains typically found in LTTRs, it may not be a surprise that *todR* insertion inactivation experiments show that *P. putida* F1 is not involved in the regulation of the *tod* operon. The NtrC family (σ^{54} dependent) is exemplified by XylR of the TOL plasmid pWW0 of *P. putida* mt-2, which participates in the control of the upper *xyl* operon for the oxidation of xylene-toluene to benzoate-toluate (reviewed by Nakazawa et al., 1992, and Marqués and Ramos, 1993). DmpR, the sole regulator of the phenol-dimethylphenol operon of *Pseudomonas* sp. strain CF600 (Powlowski and Shingler, 1994), is another well-characterized protein of this family. These proteins act by binding to eukaryotic enhancer-like elements and regulating transcription from a distinct set of promoters recognized by σ^{54} RNA polymerase (hence, σ^{54} dependent). The functional domains of XylR or DmpR include a C-terminal helix-turn-helix DNA-binding region and a conserved central domain that interacts with RNA polymerase. In the control of the *meta*-cleavage pathway operon of the TOL plasmid and related systems (Williams et al., 1992), a 36-kDa XylS protein belonging to the AraC family of regulators is operative (Gallegos et al., 1993). In this family of regulators, the nonhomologous N-terminal and central regions of the proteins contain binding sites for activator molecules that confer specificity, whereas the homologous C terminus contains a helix-turn-helix DNA-binding motif.

In TOL, the *xylS* and *xylR* genes are transcribed from divergent promoters and are located adjacent to each other at the 3′ ends of the 12 *meta*-cleavage genes. In plasmid NAH7, *nahR* is divergently transcribed from a site 60 bp upstream of the salicylate operon transcription start site, but the *nahA* promoter is 17 kbp upstream (Schell, 1993). In the phenol-dimethylphenol system, *dmpR* is divergently transcribed from the downstream 15-gene operon that encodes the phenol hydroxylase and the *meta*-cleavage enzymes, many of which are common and are conserved among the aromatic hydrocarbon degradative systems (Powlowski and Shingler, 1994; Lau et al., 1994a).

Clearly, regulation of the expression of catabolic operons can be extremely different even when inducers of the particular pathways are structurally similar or identical. The regulation of toluene degradation in *P. putida* F1 and of BP-PCB degradation in a soil nocardioform actinomycete by the two-component family of signal transduction proteins is a new example of regulation diversity among aromatic degradation pathways. This new, yet familiar, family of transcriptional regulators is elaborated below.

TWO-COMPONENT FAMILY OF SIGNAL TRANSDUCTION PROTEINS

Until 1993, the two-component signal transduction system was exclusive to the prokaryotic world (Parkinson and Kofoid, 1992), but now it is not far from the madding eukaryotic crowd, since similar systems have been found in yeasts and plants (reviewed by Koshland, 1993, and Swanson et al., 1994) and perhaps in mammalian cells (Crovello et al., 1995). Processes governed by the two-component systems are far-ranging; they include chemotaxis, osmoregulation, cell competence, sporulation, virulence, etc. The core of this system rests on two proteins that work interactively: a histidine kinase (sensor) that uses ATP to autophosphorylate at a specific histidine residue in response to an environmental stimulus, and a response regulator containing a conserved aspartate that receives the phosphate, which then mediates changes in gene expression (mostly activation) or interacts with a protein machinery (as in chemotaxis) in response to sensor signals. Most commonly, the response regulator domain (~120 amino acids) is found at the N terminus of a composite protein that also encodes a DNA-binding (helix-turn-helix) domain. On the other hand, the histidine kinase domain spans ~240 amino acids at the C terminus of a composite protein that is either cytoplasmic or membrane bound. However, "hybrid kinase-regulators" exist; in them, the histidine kinase and the response regulator domains are part of the same protein (Fig. 1). These hybrid kinase systems contain, in addition, a separate response regulator protein. An example of the "simple" two-component system is FixJ-FixL in *Rhizobium meliloti,* a system that responds to oxygen limitation (Lois et al., 1993). A hybrid kinase regulator is exemplified by ArcB, a component that together with ArcA regulates gene expression in response to the redox environment in *Escherichia coli* (Iuchi and Lin, 1993). The action of ArcB, complicated as it is (Iuchi, 1993), was recently shown to involve a second histidine that can act as an alternative phosphodonor (Ishige et al., 1994). This activity made ArcB a possible dual

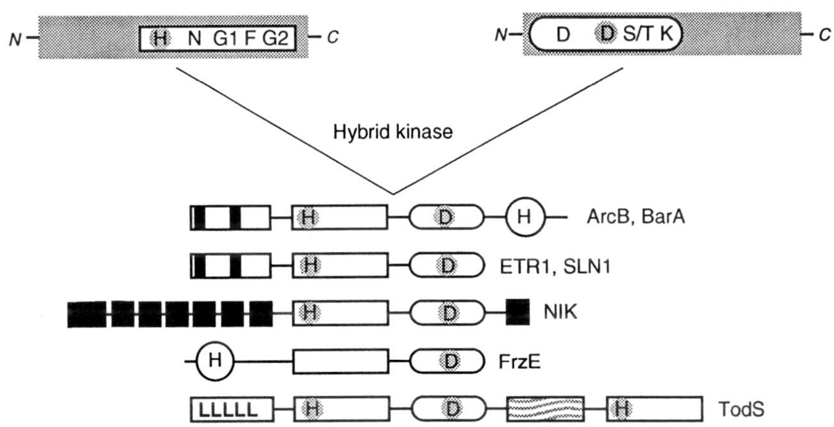

Figure 1. Schematic representations of some hybrid kinase regulators of two-component systems. This figure is modified from Swanson et al. (1994) and references therein. The block including H, N, G1, F, and G2 and that including D, D, S/T, and K are conserved amino acid blocks characteristic of histidine kinases and response regulators, respectively, as analyzed by Parkinson and Kofoid (1992) and Volz (1993). Shaded H and D, phosphorylated residues; circled H, unorthodox kinase site (Ishige et al., 1994); vertical black bars, membrane-spanning regions; other shaded regions, domains other than the regulator or kinase domains (may not represent the same function); ArcB and BarA, *E. coli* response to osmolarity and redox changes; ETR1, ethylene response in plant; SLN1, osmosensor in yeasts; NIK, sensor of unknown function in *Neurospora crassa;* FrzE, formation of fruiting body in *Myxococcus* spp.; TodS, response to toluene in *P. putida* F1 (LLLLL, bZIP; wavy block, possible oxygen sensing [this study]).

sensory device that can propagate as yet undefined dual, if not multiple, input and output signals.

TodS AND TodT: A DISTINCTIVE PAIR OF THE TWO-COMPONENT SYSTEM

More than 60 two-component systems in more than 40 bacterial species have been reported (Stock and Shinagawa, 1994), but none of the histidine kinase components, including those recently found in eukaryotes (Swanson et al., 1994), has so complicated a structure and is so novel as that of TodS (Fig. 1), a 109-kDa protein encoded by *todS* downstream of the *tod* operon (Fig. 2) (Lau et al., 1994b; Lau et al., submitted). The predicted primary structure of TodS consists of at least five domains: an N-terminal basic leucine zipper (bZIP; characterized by a heptad repeat of leucine preceded by some charged residues); a histidine kinase domain (by virtue of conserved amino acid blocks His, Asn, Gly-1, Phe, and Gly-2; Parkinson and Kofoid, 1992); a response regulator domain (characterized by conserved amino acid blocks, Asp, Asp, Ser, and Lys); a putative oxygen-sensing domain similar in sequence to a well-characterized oxygen-sensing, heme-binding domain of *R. meliloti* FixL protein (Lois et al., 1993); and a duplicated histidine kinase domain at the C terminus. A fully duplicated histidine kinase domain within a single polypeptide is novel among known histidine kinases. Although ArcB of *E. coli* was recently found to contain an alternative histidine capable of autophosphorylation, the remaining characteristic amino acid blocks are not present (Ishige et al., 1994). Another notable feature of TodS is the presence of the bZIP motif, which is essentially a eukaryotic feature common among transcriptional factors such as yeast GCN4 and oncogene products Fos and Jun (Kerppola and Curran, 1991). In these systems, the bZIP domain is known to mediate protein dimerization and to bind DNA in a sequence-specific manner. Thus, a series of questions comes to mind. Does TodS act by dimerization via its bZIP motif? Is the synthesis of TodS self-regulated? Is DNA binding affected by the state of phosphorylation? Answers to these questions await further investigations, and the questions will undoubtedly provide the basis of investigations for many years to come.

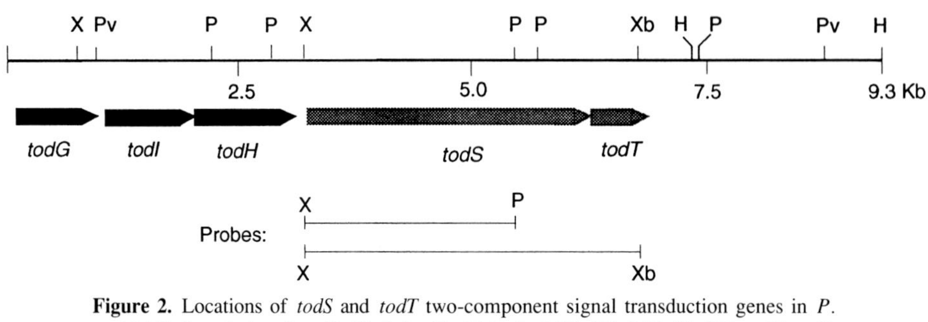

Figure 2. Locations of *todS* and *todT* two-component signal transduction genes in *P. putida* F1. Restriction sites: X, *Xho*I; Pv, *Pvu*II; P, *Pst*I; Xb, *Xba*I; H, *Hin*dIII. *todG, todI,* and *todH* code for 2-hydroxy-penta-2,4-dienoate hydratase, 4-hydroxy-2-oxovalerate aldolase, and acylating aldehyde dehydrogenase, respectively (Lau et al., 1994a). These enzymes catalyze the last three steps of toluene degradation. The *Xho*I-*Pst*I and *Xho*I-*Xba*I fragments are probes used in a *todST* specificity study (Fig. 3 and Table 2).

Overlapping the termination codon (TGA) of *todS* is the initiator codon (ATG) of *todT* (Fig. 2), which codes for a 206-amino-acid protein (TodT) that is designated the cognate response regulator of TodS. The diagnostic amino acids are Asp-13, Asp-56, Ser-84, and Lys-106. The amino acid sequence of TodT is most closely related (46% identity) to NodW, the response regulator of the two-component system NodVW in *Bradyrhizobium japonicum* (Gottfert et al., 1990). Similarities to known systems (Volz, 1993) indicate that Asp-56 in TodT (and Asp-500 in TodS) is the predicted site of phosphorylation. His-190 and His-760 in TodS are presumably the phosphodonors. Whether both of these histidines undergo simultaneous phosphorylation in response to the same signal or respond to different signals is under investigation. Finding a domain with sequence similarity to the oxygen-sensing domain of FixL may not be fortuitous, since the initial dioxygenase step and the third dehydrogenation step of the *tod* pathway are oxygen dependent.

That TodS and TodT are involved in the regulation of the *tod* operon has been supported by a kanamycin gene disruption at a specific site in either *todS* or *todT* that leads to mutants unable to grow on toluene as a sole carbon source. These mutants impart an indigo-minus (toluene dioxygenase-minus) phenotype (Lau et al., submitted). Indigo production from indole is characteristic of a functional toluene dioxygenase (Ensley et al., 1988), which is encoded by *todC1C2BA* (the initial genes of the *tod* operon that consists of *todXFC1C2BADEGIH*) (Lau et al., 1994a; Wang et al., 1995b). TodT has been overexpressed as a fusion protein in *E. coli,* and the affinity-purified protein was shown to bind to the *todRX* intergenic region (unpublished data).

TodST SYSTEM APPEARS TO BE STRAIN SPECIFIC

Several bacterial strains of the genera *Pseudomonas, Sphingomonas, Rhodococcus,* and *Comamonas* were screened for the presence of genes homologous to the *todS* and *todT* genes of *P. putida* F1 (Table 2). The majority of these strains degrade aromatic hydrocarbons such as toluene, ethylbenzene, naphthalene, BP-PCB, nitrophenol, and polycyclic aromatic hydrocarbons, e.g., fluoranthene. Even under low-stringency conditions, however, the 2.3-kb *todS*-specific probe hybridizes only to the control DNAs; the ~7-kb *Pvu*II fragment and the 2.6-kb *Pst*I fragment (Fig. 3) can be accounted for by a known restriction map of *P. putida* F1 DNA (Fig. 2). The source of the weak *Pvu*II fragment is not known. The long *Xho*I-*Xba*I probe, which includes *todT* (Fig. 2), does not hybridize to candidates other than *P. putida* F1 (not shown). In *P. putida* F1, a 1.6-kb *Pst*I fragment is also detected (not shown), as was expected from the known restriction map (Fig. 2).

DNA hybridization, even under low-stringency conditions, may not be sensitive enough to pick up otherwise functionally related sequences. This failure is expected of the two-component family, since sequence homology between these systems has been reported to be generally low; e.g., as little as 6% identity and an average of 23% are found among some 64 response regulators (Volz, 1993). That DNA sequencing is a more sensitive technique and would yield more fruitful results is illustrated below in a discussion of the discovery of the BpdS and BpdT system in *Rhodococcus* sp. strain M5.

Table 2. Specificity of *todST* gene of *P. putida* F1[a]

Microorganism	DNA-DNA hybridization[b]	Reference or laboratory source
Pseudomonas spp.		
P. putida F1	+	This study
P. putida G1	–	ATCC 17453
P. putida G7	–	D. Gibson
P. putida mt-2	–	ATCC 33015
P. putida JS150	–	J. Spain
P. putida PRS2000	–	C. Harwood
P. putida Idaho (NRRL B-18435)	–	Agricultural Research Service Culture Collection, Peoria, Ill.
P. pseudoalcaligenes KF707	–	K. Furukawa via C. Greer
P. cepacia G4	–	J. Mueller
P. stutzeri KC	–	C. Criddle
Pseudomonas sp. strain X1	–	C. Criddle
Pseudomonas sp. strain LB400	–	D. Gibson
Sphingomonas spp.		
S. yanoikuyae sp. strain B1[c]	–	Wang and Lau, 1996
S. yanoikuyae sp. strain Q1[d]	–	Wang and Lau, 1996
S. paucimobilis EPA505	–	J. Mueller
Sphingomonas sp. strain YB3-3a	–	C. Greer
Rhodococcus spp.		
R. erythropolis BD2	–	Dabrock et al., 1994
R. zopfii	–	Stoecker et al., 1994
Rhodococcus sp. strain M5[e]	–	Wang et al., 1995a
Comamonas testosteroni B356	–	M. Sylvestre

[a]DNA probes are defined in the legend to Fig. 2.
[b]Positive hybridization results are shown in Fig. 3.
[c]Formerly *Beijerinckia* sp. strain B1.
[d]Formerly *S. (Pseudomonas) paucimobilis* Q1.
[e]Formerly *Arthrobacter* sp. strain M5.

BpdS AND BpdT: A TWO-COMPONENT SYSTEM REGULATING BP-PCB DEGRADATION IN *RHODOCOCCUS* SP. STRAIN M5

Formerly known as *Arthrobacter* sp. strain M5 (Furukawa and Chakrabarty, 1982), *Rhodococcus* sp. strain M5 is a nocardioform actinomycete and one of the few gram-positive microorganisms that has been studied at the molecular level in terms of the BP-PCB degradation pathway (Wang et al., 1995a). Like the BP degradation system in KF707 (Furukawa, 1994), the M5 BP degradation genes (*bpd*) for the conversion of BP to benzoic acid and 2-hydroxy-penta-2,4-dienoate are not contiguous (Fig. 4); the *bpdC1C2BADE* genes, which encode enzymes for the first three steps of BP-PCB degradation (Wang et al., 1995a), are separated from the downstream 2-hydroxy-6-oxo-6-phenylhexa-2,4-dienoate hydrolase-encoding gene (*bpdF*) by 5.4 kb (Lau et al., in press). However, unlike KF707, the *bpdE* and *bpdF* genes are separated by two regulatory genes, designated *bpdS* and *bpdT* (Fig. 4). *bpdS* codes for a 1,576-amino-acid residue protein that is predicted to be a transmembrane histidine kinase and that contains sequence fea-

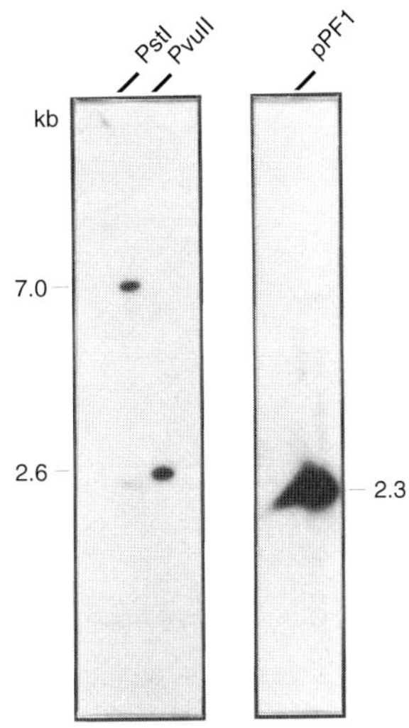

Figure 3. Southern hybridization of *todS* probe to *P. putida* F1 DNA. Negative results obtained with bacterial strains listed in Table 2 are not shown. For each genome, two single restriction digests with *Pvu*II and *Pst*I were carried out. DNAs were alkaline transferred to Hybond-N membranes (Amersham). Hybridization was carried out at 50°C overnight in 3× SSC (1× SSC is 0.15 M NaCl plus 0.015 M sodium citrate)–10× Denhardt's solution–0.1% sodium dodecyl sulfate (SDS). Washes were carried out consecutively in 3× SSC–0.1% SDS at room temperature, 1× SSC–0.1% SDS at 50°C, and 0.5× SSC–0.1% SDS at 50°C. pPF1, a 2.3-kb *Xho*I-*Pst*I fragment containing a partial *tod*S gene (Fig. 2), serves as a positive marker. The *todS* probe was ^{32}P-labeled and random primed using Boehringer Mannheim's DNA Labelling Kit.

tures such as a region resembling the eukaryotic serine/threonine or tyrosine protein kinases and a Walker-type A consensus nucleotide-binding site (GXXGXGKS; Walker et al., 1982). Near the middle of BpdS is a heptad repeat of leucine. However, its function as a leucine zipper, in contrast to bZIP in TodS, is unlikely, since prolines are present within the repeating heptad.

The molecular mass of BpdS (170 kDa) has been verified by expression in the *E. coli* T7 system (unpublished data). Hence, BpdS is by far the largest known histidine kinase. It is second only to sensor ChvG of *Agrobacterium tumefaciens* (Charles and Nester, 1993), which also has an ATP-binding consensus sequence. That BpdS is involved in regulation of the BP degradation pathway is so far supported by chromosomal disruption at the 3′ end of *bpdS* by a kanamycin gene cassette. M5(*bpdS*::Km) mutants are unable to use BP as sole carbon source for growth. These mutants also do not produce the yellow cleavage products that the parent M5 produces when BP crystals are provided.

BpdT is a 209-residue protein (23 kDa) that has a typical response regulator domain, indicated by the presence of conserved aspartates (positions 9 and 54), serine (position 82), and lysine (position 104) (Fig. 4). By sequence homology, BpdT belongs to the UhpA subfamily of response regulators (Volz, 1993). Like most response regulators, BpdT has a low sequence identity (22%) with TodT, which explains the lack of hybridization in Southern experiments (not shown).

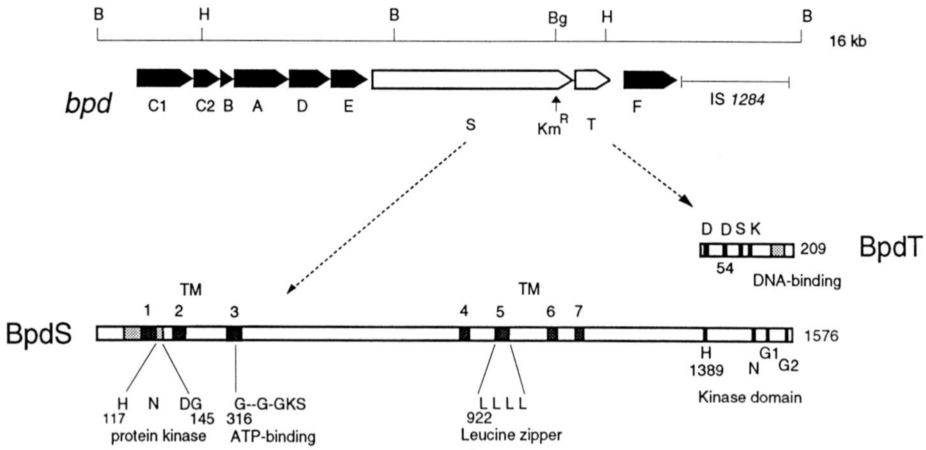

Figure 4. Gene location of BP-PCB receptor histidine kinase (*bpdS*) and its cognate response regulator (*bpdT*) in *Rhodococcus* sp. strain M5. The *bpdC1C2BADE* gene cluster codes for the first three enzymes of BP degradation (Wang et al., 1995a), and *bpdF*, a hydrolase-encoding gene, completes the conversion of BP to benzoate and 2-hydroxypenta-2,4-dienoate (Lau et al., in press). IS*1284*, insertion sequence element (unpublished data); B, H, and Bg, *Bam*HI, *Hin*dIII, and *Bgl*II restriction sites, respectively; Km^R, site of kanamycin resistance gene insertion that caused inactivation of the *bpd* operon. The predicted amino acid sequences of BpdS and BpdT revealed several motifs: H, N, D, and G are conserved His, Asn, Asp, and Gly among eukaryotic protein kinases in the domains designated VIA, VIB, and VII (Lindberg et al., 1992); G--G-GKS signifies an ATP-binding sequence; LLLL is an alternating leucine heptad repeat; H, N, G1, and G2 and D, D, S, and K are invariant residues defined in the legend to Fig. 1. The positions of some of these amino acids are numbered. As in other histidine kinases (Parkinson and Kofoid, 1992), the F block is missing in BpdS. A possible helix-turn-helix (DNA-binding) motif is indicated in BpdT. TM, seven possible transmembrane segments predicted by the Rao and Argos program.

By analogy with known systems, His-1389 is predicted to be the autophosphorylation site and Asp-54 is predicted to be the acceptor of the phosphate. BpdT has been overproduced in an *E. coli* expression vector system (unpublished data) to make phosphorylation assays and protein-DNA-binding experiments possible. An intriguing possibility is that by virtue of the ATP-binding domain, the BpdST signal transduction process might be coupled to transport.

CONCLUDING REMARKS

The two-component system is the most common positive regulator in prokaryotes, and for the first time, this family of signal transduction proteins, exemplified by TodS and TodT in *P. putida* F1 degradation of toluene and by BpdS and BpdT in *Rhodococcus* sp. strain M5 degradation of BP-PCB, is added to the list of aromatic regulators. Although details of the signal transduction pathway in either *P. putida* F1 or *Rhodococcus* sp. strain M5 have yet to be worked out, the actions of TodS-TodT and BpdS-BpdT are reminiscent of dioxin action in eukaryotes (reviewed by Whitlock, 1994). Dioxin undergoes protein kinase C-dependent phosphorylation mediated by a large ligand-activated transcription factor (~175 kDa) commonly known as AHR (aryl hydrocarbon receptor). AHR is a member of the basic helix-loop-helix superfamily of DNA-binding proteins and is activated by ligand binding and by dimerization with the AHR nuclear translocator. Whereas dioxin induces the microsomal aryl hydrocarbon hydroxylase catalyzed by the cytochrome P-450A1 enzyme, BP-PCB in M5 or toluene in *P. putida* F1 induces the initial BP or toluene dioxygenase complex in the respective degradation pathway. Hence, analogies between dioxin action in eukaryotes and toluene or BP-PCB action in two diverse kingdoms are noteworthy.

Judging from the sequence motifs and domain structures of TodS or BpdS, these systems are undoubtedly more complex than previously known systems. Answers to many obvious questions must come from studies both at the cellular level and in vitro with purified components of the regulatory system. Such experiments are in progress. Finally, the involvement of the two-component regulatory system in the regulation of pollutant-degradative pathways in bacteria may be underestimated if assessed based on hybridization data alone. A genomic sequencing approach would likely yield more fruitful results.

Acknowledgments. P.L. thanks David Gibson for his hospitality and mentorship during a subbatical stay at the University of Iowa. We thank A. Patel for a careful reading of the manuscript. A. Patel and Y. Hasegawa (visiting professor from Kansai University, Osaka, Japan) have recently begun a detailed study of TodS. This publication is issued as NRCC no. 34488.

REFERENCES

Byrne, A. M., J. Kukor, and R. H. Olson. 1995. Cascade regulation of the *Pseudomonas pickettii* PKO1 toluene-3-monooxygenase operon abstract Q-221, p. 438. *Abstracts of the 95th General Meeting of the American Society for Microbiology, 1995.*

Charles, T. C., and E. W. Nester. 1993. A chromosomally encoded two-component sensory transduction system is required for virulence of *Agrobacterium tumefaciens*. *J. Bacteriol.* **175:**6614–6625.

Crovello, C. S., B. C. Furie, and B. Furie. 1995. Histidine phosphorylation of P-selectin upon stimulation of human platelets: a novel pathway for activation-dependent signal transduction. *Cell* **82:**279–286.

Dabrock, B., M. Kebeler, B. Averhoff, and G. Gottschalk. 1994. Identification and characterization of a transmissible linear plasmid from *Rhodococcus erythropolis* BD2 that encodes isopropylbenzene and trichloroethene catabolism. *Appl. Environ. Microbiol.* **60:**853–860.

Ensley, B. D., B. J. Ratzkin, T. D. Osslund, M. J. Simon, L. P. Wackett, and D. T. Gibson. 1988. Expression of naphthalene oxidation genes in *Escherichia coli* results in the biosynthesis of indigo. *Science* **222:**167–169.

Erickson, B. D., and F. J. Mondello. 1993. Enhanced biodegradation of polychlorinated biphenyls after site-directed mutagenesis of a biphenyl dioxygenase gene. *Appl. Environ. Microbiol.* **59:**3858–3862.

Francesconi, S. C., A. C. Blake, and M. S. Shields. 1995. Nucleotide sequence, organization, and regulation of the toluene *ortho*-monooxygenase (Tom) operon of *Pseudomonas cepacia* G4 and its constitutive variants, abstract K-198, p. 570. *Abstracts of the 95th General Meeting of the American Society for Microbiology, 1995.*

Furukawa, K. 1994. Molecular genetics and evolutionary relationship of PCB-degrading bacteria. *Biodegradation* **5:**289–300.

Furukawa, K., and A. M. Chakrabarty. 1982. Involvement of plasmids in total degradation of chlorinated biphenyls. *Appl. Environ. Microbiol.* **44:**619–626.

Gallegos, M.-T., C. Michan, and J. L. Ramos. 1993. The XylS/AraC family of regulators. *Nucleic Acids Res.* **21:**807–810.

Gibson, D. T., D. L. Cruden, J. D. Haddock, G. J. Zylstra, and J. M. Brand. 1993. Oxidation of polychlorinated biphenyls by *Pseudomonas* sp. strain LB400 and *Pseudomonas pseudoalcaligenes* KF707. *J. Bacteriol.* **175:**4561–4564.

Gottfert, M., P. Grob, and H. Hennecke. 1990. Proposed regulatory pathway encoded by the *nodV* and *nodW* genes, determinants of host specificity in *Bradyrhizobium japonicum*. *Proc. Natl. Acad. Sci. USA* **87:**2680–2684.

Inouye, S., A. Nakazawa, and T. Nakazawa. 1988. Nucleotide sequence of the regulatory gene *xylR* of the TOL plasmid from *Pseudomonas putida*. *Gene* **66:**301–306.

Ishige, K., S. Nagasawa, S.-I. Tokishita, and T. Mizuno. 1994. A novel device of bacterial signal transducers. *EMBO J.* **13:**5195–5202.

Iuchi, S. 1993. Phosphorylation/dephosphorylation of the receiver module at the conserved aspartate residue controls transphosphorylation activity of histidine kinase in sensor protein ArcB of *Escherichia coli*. *J. Biol. Chem.* **268:**23972–23980.

Iuchi, S., and E. C. C. Lin. 1993. Adaptation of *Escherichia coli* to redox environments by gene expression. *Mol. Microbiol.* **9:**9–15.

Kerppola, T. K., and T. Curran. 1991. Transcription factor interactions: basics on zippers. *Curr. Opin. Struct. Biol.* **1:**71–79.

Koshland, D., Jr. 1993. The two-component pathway comes to eukaryotes. *Science* **262:**532.

Lau, P. C. K., H. Bergeron, D. Labbé, Y. Wang, R. Brousseau, and D. T. Gibson. 1994a. Sequence and expression of the *todGIH* genes involved in the last three steps of toluene degradation by *Pseudomonas putida* F1. *Gene* **146:**7–13.

Lau, P. C. K., J. Garnon, D. Labbé, and Y. Wang. Location and sequence analysis of a 2-hydroxy-6-oxo-6-phenylhexa-2,4-dienoate hydrolase-encoding gene (*bpdF*) of the biphenyl/polychlorinated biphenyl degradation pathway in *Rhodococcus* sp. M5. *Gene*, in press.

Lau, P. C. K., Y. Wang, J. Garnon, D. Labbé, H. Bergeron, R. Brousseau, and D. T. Gibson. 1994b. Regulation of toluene and PCB degradations by novel members of the two-component system, abstr. Q395, p. 458. *Abstracts of the 94th General Meeting of the American Society for Microbiology, 1994*.

Lau, P. C. K., Y. Wang, A. Patel, D. Labbé, H. Bergeron, R. Brousseau, Y. Konishi, and M. Rawlings. A bacterial bZIP histidine kinase regulating toluene degradation. Submitted for publication.

Lindberg, R. A., A. M. Quinn, and T. Hunter. 1992. Dual-specificity protein kinases: will any hydroxyl do? *Trends Biol. Sci.* **17:**114–119.

Lois, A. F., G. S. Ditta, and D. R. Helinski. 1993. The oxygen sensor FixL of *Rhizobium meliloti* is a membrane protein containing four possible transmembrane segments. *J. Bacteriol.* **175:**1103–1109.

Marqués, S., and J. L. Ramos. 1993. Transcriptional control of the *Pseudomonas putida* TOL plasmid catabolic pathways. *Mol. Microbiol.* **9:**923–929.

Matrubutham, U., and A. Harker. 1994. Analysis of duplicated gene sequences associated with *tfdR* and *tfdS* in *Alcaligenes eutrophus* JMP134. *J. Bacteriol.* **176:**2348–2353.

Nakazawa, A., S. Inouye, M. Gomada, H. Imaishi, and T. Nakazawa. 1992. Upstream regulatory sequence for transcriptional activation of catabolic genes on the TOL plasmid, p. 353–357. *In* E. Galli, S. Silver, and B. Witholt (ed.), *Pseudomonas: Molecular Biology and Biotechnology*. American Society for Microbiology, Washington, D.C.

Ng, L. C., C. L. Poh, and V. Shingler. 1995. Aromatic effector activation of the NtrC-like transcriptional regulator PhhR limits the catabolic potential of the (methyl)phenol degradative pathway it controls. *J. Bacteriol.* **177:**1485–1490.

Parkinson, J. S., and E. C. Kofoid. 1992. Communication modules in bacterial signaling proteins. *Annu. Rev. Genet.* **26:**71–112.

Powlowski, J., and V. Shingler. 1994. Genetics and biochemistry of phenol degradation of *Pseudomonas* sp. CF600. *Biodegradation* **5:**219–236.

Schell, M. A. 1993. Molecular biology of the LysR family of transcriptional regulators. *Annu. Rev. Microbiol.* **47:**597–626.

Stock, A. M., and H. Shinagawa. 1994. Signal transduction and phosphoproteins, p. 282–284. *In* A. Torriani-Gorini, E. Yagil, and S. Silver (ed.), *Phosphates in Microorganisms: Cellular and Molecular Biology*. American Society for Microbiology, Washington, D.C.

Stoecker, M. A., R. P. Herwig, and J. T. Staley. 1994. *Rhodococcus zopfii* sp. nov., a toxicant-degrading bacterium. *Int. J. Syst. Bacteriol.* **44:**106–110.

Swanson, R. V., L. A. Alex, and M. I. Simon. 1994. Histidine and aspartate phosphorylation: two component systems and the limits of homology. *Trends Biol. Sci.* **19:**485–490.

van der Meer, J. R., W. M. De Vos, S. Harayama, and A. J. B. Zehnder. 1992. Molecular mechanisms of genetic adaptation to xenobiotic compounds. *Microbiol. Rev.* **56:**677–694.

Volz, K. 1993. Structural conservation in the CheY superfamily. *Biochemistry* **32:**11741–11753.

Walker, J. E., M. Sarste, M. J. Runswick, and N. J. Gay. 1982. Distantly related sequences in the a- and b-subunits of ATP synthase, myosin, kinases, and other ATP-requiring enzymes and a common nucleotide binding fold. *EMBO J.* **1:**945–951.

Wang, Y., J. Garnon, D. Labbé, H. Bergeron, and P. C. K. Lau. 1995a. Sequence and expression of the *bpdC1C2BADE* genes involved in the initial steps of biphenyl/chlorobiphenyl degradation by *Rhodococcus* sp. M5. *Gene* **164:**117–122.

Wang, Y., and P. C. K. Lau. 1996. Sequence and expression of an isocitrate dehydrogenase-encoding gene from a polycyclic aromatic hydrocarbon oxidizer, *Sphingomonas yanoikuyae* B1. *Gene* **168:**15–21.

Wang, Y., M. Rawlings, D. T. Gibson, D. Labbé, H. Bergeron, R. Brousseau, and P. C. K. Lau. 1995b. Identification of a membrane protein and a truncated LysR-type regulator associated with the toluene degradative pathway in *Pseudomonas putida* F1. *Mol. Gen. Genet.* **246:**570–579.

Whitlock, J. P., Jr. 1994. The aromatic hydrocarbon receptor, dioxin action, and endocrine homeostasis. *Trends Endocrinol. Metabol.* **5:**183–188.

Williams, P. A., S. J. Assinder, P. de Marco, K. J. O'Donnell, C. L. Poh, L. E. Shaw, and M. K. Winson. 1992. Catabolic gene duplications in TOL plasmid, p. 341–352. *In* E. Galli, S. Silver, and B. Witholt (ed.), *Pseudomonas: Molecular Biology and Biotechnology.* American Society for Microbiology, Washington, D.C.

You, I.-S., and D. Ghosal. 1995. Genetic and molecular analysis of a regulatory region of the herbicide, 2,4-dichlorophenoxyacetate catabolic plasmid pJP4. *Mol. Microbiol.* **16:**321–331.

Zylstra, G. J., and D. T. Gibson. 1991. Aromatic hydrocarbon degradation: a molecular approach, p. 183–203. *In* J. K. Setlow (ed.), *Genetic Engineering: Principles and Methods,* vol. 13. Plenum Press, New York.

Molecular Biology of Pseudomonads
Edited by T. Nakazawa et al.

Chapter 15

Chemotactic Signal Transduction Network in *Pseudomonas aeruginosa*

Hisao Ohtake, Junichi Kato, Akio Kuroda, Kazunori Taguchi, and Yukihiro Sakai

Chemotaxis is the movement of an organism toward chemical attractants and away from chemical repellents (Adler, 1966). Bacterial chemotaxis can be viewed as an important prelude to metabolism, prey-predator relationships, symbiosis, and other ecological interactions in microbial communities (Chet and Mitchell, 1979). *Pseudomonas aeruginosa* is attracted to 20 commonly occurring L-amino acids (Craven and Montie, 1985) and is less strongly responsive to sugars and organic acids (Moulton and Montie, 1979). *P. aeruginosa* is also repelled by thiocyanic and isothiocyanic esters, including ethyl thiocyanate and methyl isothiocyanate (Ohga et al., 1993). Several lines of evidence suggest the presence of regulatory mechanisms underlying chemotaxis in *P. aeruginosa*. For example, the taxis toward several L-amino acids is subject to control by nitrogen availability in a manner similar to the control of various enzymes of nitrogen metabolism (Craven and Montie, 1985). The strength of chemotactic responses to glucose and citrate is also dependent on prior growth of the cells on those carbon sources (Moulton and Montie, 1979). In addition, *P. aeruginosa* is known to show taxis toward P_i when the cells are starved for P_i (Kato et al., 1992). However, these regulatory mechanisms are still poorly understood at the molecular level. In this review, we summarize present knowledge about the genetics of *P. aeruginosa* chemotaxis.

REGULATION OF P_i TAXIS

Since P_i is an essential constituent in bacteria, P_i taxis presumably gives bacteria a selective advantage in microbial communities. However, bacterial chemotaxis toward P_i has been reported only with *P. aeruginosa* (Kato et al., 1992). Enteric bacteria such as *Escherichia coli* and *Salmonella typhimurium* do not exhibit P_i taxis even under conditions of P_i limitation (Kato et al., 1994a). In *P. aeruginosa,* P_i limitation results in the synthesis of several protein species, including alkaline phosphatase (AP), an outer-mem-

Hisao Ohtake, Junichi Kato, Akio Kuroda, Kazunori Taguchi, and Yukihiro Sakai • Department of Fermentation Technology, Hiroshima University, Higashi-Hiroshima, Hiroshima 739, Japan.

brane channel-forming protein (protein P), a binding protein for P_i, and a hemolytic and a nonhemolytic phospholipase C (Hancock et al., 1982; Ostroff and Vasil, 1987; Poole and Hancock, 1984). As in *E. coli,* some of these gene promoters are regulated by two proteins, PhoB and PhoR, and have a common consensus sequence, the Pho box (Anba et al., 1990). To investigate the regulation of P_i taxis, chromosomal *phoB* and *phoR* mutants were constructed by inserting a kanamycin resistance (Km^r) gene cassette into wild-type genes. The chromosomal mutants, designated PHOB1 and PHOR1, did not induce AP synthesis under conditions of P_i limitation but still exhibited inducible P_i taxis, showing that P_i taxis is not regulated by the PhoB and PhoR proteins (Kato et al., 1994b).

AP constitutive *P. aeruginosa* mutants were constructed by *N*-methyl-*N'*-nitro-*N*-nitrosoguanidine (NTG) mutagenesis and selected by the procedure of Poole and Hancock (1984). An AP constitutive mutant, designated APC1, showed P_i taxis regardless of whether the cells were starved for P_i. A genomic library was prepared from PAO1 chromosomal DNA for use in transforming APC1. A single clone, designated pPT06, complemented the mutation of APC1 (Fig. 1). Subcloning and sequence analysis revealed that the *P. aeruginosa phoU* gene is required for the negative regulation of P_i taxis. To further confirm that regulation of P_i taxis requires PhoU but is independent of PhoB and PhoR, a *phoB* mutation was constructed on the chromosome of APC1 in the same way as in PHOB1. The *phoB* mutant, designated APC1.1, no longer showed detectable AP activi-

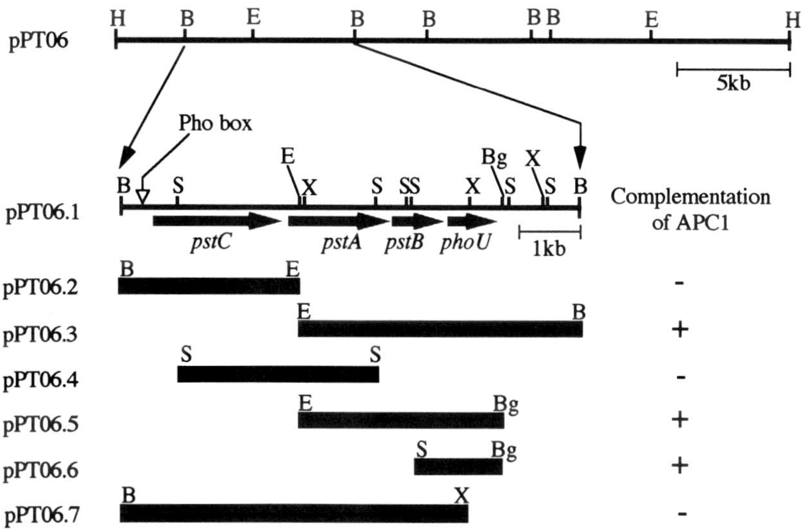

Figure 1. Restriction maps of plasmid pPT06, which contains the 29.5-kb *Hin*dIII fragment from *P. aeruginosa* chromosomal DNA, and its subclones. Restriction sites: B, *Bam*HI; Bg, *Bgl*II; E, *Eco*RI; H, *Hin*dIII; S, *Sal*I; X, *Xho*I. The locations and orientations of *pstC*, *pstA*, *pstB*, and *phoU* are indicated by horizontal arrows below the restriction map of pPT06.1. Closed bars show *P. aeruginosa* chromosomal DNA fragments subcloned into vector pCP19. The abilities of recombinant plasmids to complement the mutation of APC1 are indicated on the right. Chemotaxis assays were performed by the method of Nikata et al. (1992).

ties but still exhibited constitutive P_i taxis. Furthermore, plasmid pPT06.6, which contains the entire *phoU* gene, restored the ability of APC1.1 to repress P_i taxis under conditions of P_i excess.

The *P. aeruginosa pstC, pstA,* and *pstB* genes, which are required for P_i specific transport, were found immediately upstream of the *phoU* gene (Fig. 1). These genes, together with the *phoU* gene, form the *P. aeruginosa pst* operon. A well-conserved Pho box sequence exists in the promoter region (Nikata et al., in press). However, in contrast to the known *E. coli pst* operon, this operon lacked the *pstS* gene encoding a periplasmic P_i-binding protein. Moreover, the integral membrane components PstC and PstA had only sparse homology to their *E. coli* counterparts. A chromosomal deletion in the entire *pst* operon rendered *P. aeruginosa* unable to repress P_i taxis under conditions of P_i excess. Complementation analysis revealed that the cytoplasmic components PstB and PhoU are essential for exerting negative control of P_i taxis. However, mutants lacking either PstC or PstA protein still showed inducible P_i taxis. At present, it is not known whether a positive regulator exists for P_i taxis.

P. aeruginosa possesses a P_i-binding protein that exists as the major protein in the periplasm under conditions of P_i limitation (Poole and Hancock, 1984). The periplasmic P_i-binding protein is probably a candidate for the role of P_i chemoreceptor in *P. aeruginosa,* even though a similar protein in *E. coli* does not show P_i taxis (Kato et al., 1994a). The fact that the periplasmic glucose-binding protein has been identified as the glucose chemoreceptor of *P. aeruginosa* led to this hypothesis. To answer the question of whether the periplasmic protein is the P_i chemoreceptor, we need to determine whether *P. aeruginosa* mutants lacking the P_i-binding protein are defective in P_i taxis.

P. AERUGINOSA che GENES

To date, little is known about chemotaxis genes in species belonging to the genus *Pseudomonas.* Three *P. aeruginosa* chemotaxis mutants, designated PC1, PC2, and PC3, were selected by the swarm plate method after NTG mutagenesis (Armstrong et al., 1973). PC1 and PC2 were fully motile but rarely reversed swimming directions, while PC3 changed its swimming direction much more frequently than did the wild-type PAO1 (Masduki et al., 1995). All of the mutants grew as well as the parent strain PAO1, confirming that the impaired swarming ability was not due to a metabolic defect. PC1 was transformed with a genomic library from *P. aeruginosa* PAO1. A cosmid, pPT07, which complemented the mutation of PC1, was selected (Fig. 2). Subsequent analysis revealed that the 2.0-kb *Xho*I fragment of pPT07.6 could complement PC1 and PC2. Nucleotide sequence analysis of the 2.0-kb *Xho*I fragment showed the presence of two open reading frames, ORF1 and ORF2. Computer analysis showed that ORF1 encodes the *P. aeruginosa* homolog of the enterobacterial *cheY* gene, which had been already reported (Starnbach and Lory, 1992). The putative polypeptide encoded by ORF2 shared 39% identical amino acid residues with the product of the *E. coli cheZ* gene. The *P. aeruginosa cheZ*-like gene encoded a polypeptide comprising 227 amino acid residues with a molecular weight of 25,738. The mutation of PC1 was partially complemented by the *S. typhimurium cheY* gene (Stock et al., 1987). To characterize the *cheZ*-like gene, a mutation of the chromosomal gene was constructed by inserting a Km^r gene cassette into the wild-type gene. The chromosomal mutant, designated CHEZ1, was fully motile but changed swimming

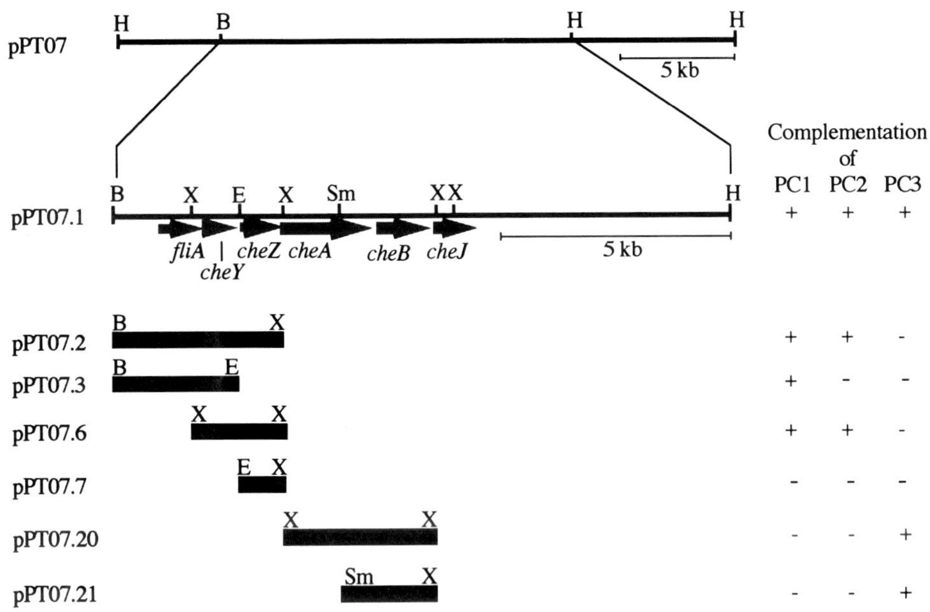

Figure 2. Restriction maps of plasmid pPT07, which contains two *Hin*dIII fragments of 7 and 20 kb from *P. aeruginosa* chromosomal DNA, and its subclones. The locations and orientations of *fliA*, *cheY*, *cheZ*, *cheA*, *cheB*, and *cheJ* are indicated by horizontal arrows below the restriction map of pPT07.1. Closed bars indicate *P. aeruginosa* chromosomal DNA fragments subcloned into vector plasmids. The abilities of recombinant plasmids to complement the mutations of PC1, PC2, and PC3 are indicated on the right. Sm, *Sma*I. See the legend to Fig. 1 for abbreviations of other restriction sites.

direction much more frequently than did the wild-type strain PAO1. The mutation of CHEZ1 was partially complemented by the *S. typhimurium cheZ* gene. Therefore, ORF1 and ORF2 were termed *cheY* and *cheZ*, respectively.

Further sequence analysis of the *cheY-cheZ* region revealed three additional open reading frames immediately downstream of the *cheZ* gene. The predicted translation product of the first gene consisted of 753 amino acids with a molecular weight of 79,733. This putative protein had overall 30% identity with the histidine-kinase CheA of *Rhizobium meliloti* (Greck et al., 1995). The second gene encoded a putative polypeptide of 368 amino acids with a molecular weight of 39,016. Overall, this protein was 41% identical to the methyl esterase CheB protein of *R. meliloti*. Insertional inactivation of the *cheA*-like gene rendered *P. aeruginosa* defective in chemotaxis. A recombinant plasmid carrying the entire *cheB*-like gene complemented the mutation of PC3. Consequently, these two genes were termed *cheA* and *cheB*, respectively. The third gene encoded a putative polypeptide of 246 amino acids with a molecular weight of 25,958. The putative protein had no significant homology to any known protein sequences. Insertional inactivation of the third gene rendered *P. aeruginosa* defective in chemotaxis. This chromosomal mutant is fully motile, indicating that the third gene product is not a component of the flagellar apparatus. We tentatively termed the third gene *cheJ*. CheJ may play an unexpected role in the chemotactic signal transduction pathway in *P. aeruginosa*.

CHEMOTACTIC TRANSDUCER GENES

The methyl-accepting chemotaxis proteins (MCPs) are the best-characterized signal transducers of the chemosensory apparatus (Boyd et al., 1983). Craven and Montie (1983) reported that *P. aeruginosa* possesses approximately 73-kDa proteins that are labeled with L-[methyl-^{3}H]methionine in response to L-serine. To clone the chemotactic transducer gene, we selected another *P. aeruginosa* mutant that was defective in taxis toward L-serine but normal toward peptone. This mutant, designated PCT1, failed to exhibit chemotactic responses to glycine, L-serine, L-threonine, and L-valine (Kuroda et al., 1995). PCT1 also showed weaker responses to other commonly occurring L-amino acids than did the wild-type strain PAO1. PCT1 was transformed with a genomic library from *P. aeruginosa* PAO1. Then a recombinant cosmid, designated pPT08, was found to complement the mutation of PCT1 (Fig. 3). Subcloning and complementation analysis showed that a 2.2-kb *Hin*dIII-*Sal*I fragment in pPT08.4 was necessary for complementing the mutation of PCT1.

Nucleotide sequence analysis revealed the presence of a 1,890-bp open reading frame, designated *pctA*, that encodes a putative protein of 629 amino acids with a molecular weight of 68,042. Computer analysis revealed that the *pctA* gene product is homologous to a large group of proteins known as MCPs (Dahl et al., 1989). Overall, PctA showed 30% identity with *E. coli* Tsr. The strongest homology was found in the region referred to as the "highly conserved domain." The hydropathy plot of PctA suggests the presence of two hydrophobic regions (TM1 and TM2) at the N-terminal and central regions of PctA. To further characterize the *pctA* gene, a chromosomal *pctA* mutant was constructed by inserting a Km^r gene cassette into the wild-type gene. The chromosomal *pctA* mutant, designated PCTA1, showed the same observed deficiency in taxis toward L-amino acids as PCT1. The calculated molecular weight of PctA (68,042) agreed with the electro-

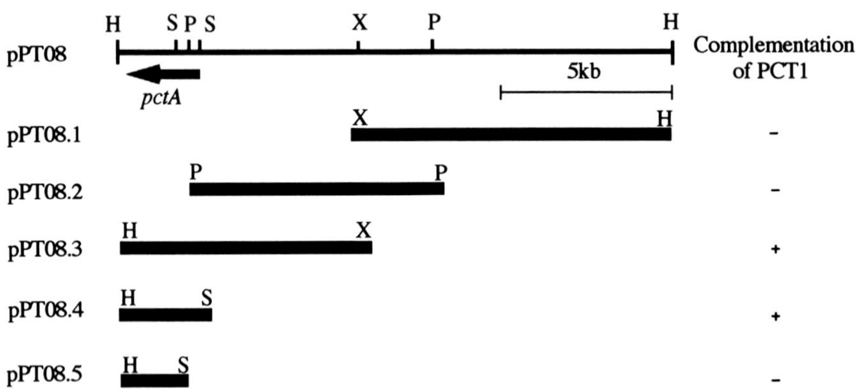

Figure 3. Restriction maps of plasmid pPT08, which contains the 17-kb *Hin*dIII fragment from *P. aeruginosa* chromosomal DNA, and its subclones. The location and orientation of *pctA* are indicated by the horizontal arrow below the restriction map of pPT08. Closed bars indicate *P. aeruginosa* chromosomal DNA fragments subcloned into vector plasmids. The abilities of recombinant plasmids to complement the mutation of PCT1 are indicated on the right. P, *Pst*I. See the legend to Fig. 1 for abbreviations of other restriction sites.

phoretic mobility of the MCPs reported by Craven and Montie (1983). The chromosomal *pctA* mutant showed normal chemotaxis toward P_i. Further sequence analysis of the *pctA* region revealed two additional genes, *pctB* and *pctC*, encoding MCP-like proteins (A. Kuroda et al., unpublished data).

CONCLUSIONS

P. aeruginosa is attracted toward P_i when the cells are starved for P_i. Regulation of P_i taxis is not dependent on PhoB and PhoR but requires PhoU. The *P. aeruginosa pst* gene products, which are required for P_i-specific transport, are also involved in the negative regulation of P_i taxis. However, whether a positive regulator exists for P_i taxis is not known. Nothing is known about the P_i chemoreceptor. Five chemotaxis genes, including *cheY, cheZ, cheA, cheB*, and *cheJ*, have been identified in a large gene cluster in *P. aeruginosa*. The predicted proteins of the first four genes resemble known *E. coli* Che proteins. However, the CheJ protein has no significant homology to any known protein sequences. This putative protein may play an unexpected role in the chemotactic signal transduction pathway in *P. aeruginosa*. Three possible chemotactic transducer genes, *pctA, pctB*, and *pctC*, have also been cloned and sequenced. The gene products have structural homology to the enteric MCPs. Our future work on the chemotaxis of *P. aeruginosa* will be directed at (i) identifying the P_i chemoreceptor, (ii) seeking additional chemotaxis genes, and (iii) cloning chemotactic transducer genes that remain to be identified.

REFERENCES

Adler, J. 1966. Chemotaxis in bacteria. *Science* **153:**708–716.

Anba, J., M. Bidaud, M. L. Vasil, and A. Lazdunski. 1990. Nucleotide sequence of the *Pseudomonas aeruginosa phoB* gene, the regulatory gene for the phosphate regulon. *J. Bacteriol.* **172:**4685–4689.

Armstrong, J. B., J. Adler, and M. M. Dahl. 1973. Nonchemotactic mutants of *Escherichia coli. J. Bacteriol.* **93:**390–398.

Boyd, A., K. Kendall, and M. I. Simon. 1983. Structure of the serine chemoreceptor in *Escherichia coli. Nature* (London) **301:**623–626.

Chet, I., and R. Mitchell. 1979. Ecological aspects of microbial chemotactic behavior. *Annu. Rev. Microbiol.* **30:**221–239.

Craven, R. C., and T. C. Montie. 1983. Chemotaxis of *Pseudomonas aeruginosa:* involvement of methylation. *J. Bacteriol.* **154:**780–786.

Craven, R. C., and T. C. Montie. 1985. Regulation of *Pseudomonas aeruginosa* chemotaxis by the nitrogen source. *J. Bacteriol.* **164:**544–549.

Dahl, M. K., W. Boos, and M. D. Manson. 1989. Evolution of chemotactic-signal transducers in enteric bacteria. *J. Bacteriol.* **171:**2361–2371.

Greck, M., J. Platzer, V. Sourjik, and R. Schmitt. 1995. Analysis of a chemotaxis operon in *Rhizobium meliloti. Mol. Microbiol.* **15:**989–1000.

Hancock, R. E. W., K. Poole, and R. Benz. 1982. Outer membrane protein P of *Pseudomonas aeruginosa:* regulation by phosphate deficiency and formation of small anion-specific channels in lipid bilayer membranes. *J. Bacteriol.* **150:**730–738.

Kato, J., A. Ito, T. Nikata, and H. Ohtake. 1992. Phosphate taxis in *Pseudomonas aeruginosa. J. Bacteriol.* **174:**5149–5151.

Kato, J., Y. Sakai, T. Nikata, A. Masduki, and H. Ohtake. 1994a. Phosphate taxis and its regulation in *Pseudomonas aeruginosa*, p. 315–317. *In* A. Torriani-Gorini, E. Yagil, and S. Silver (ed.), *Phosphate in Microorganisms: Cellular and Molecular Biology.* American Society for Microbiology, Washington, D.C.

Kato, J., Y. Sakai, T. Nikata, and H. Ohtake. 1994b. Cloning and characterization of a *Pseudomonas aeruginosa* gene involved in the negative regulation of phosphate taxis. *J. Bacteriol.* **176:**5874–5877.

Kuroda, A., T. Kumano, K. Taguchi, T. Nikata, J. Kato, and H. Ohtake. 1995. Molecular cloning and characterization of a chemotactic transducer gene in *Pseudomonas aeruginosa. J. Bacteriol.* **177:**7019–7025.

Masduki, A., J. Nakamura, T. Ohga, R. Umezaki, J. Kato, and H. Ohtake. 1995. Isolation and characterization of chemotaxis mutants and genes of *Pseudomonas aeruginosa. J. Bacteriol.* **177:**948–952.

Moulton, R. C., and T. C. Montie. 1979. Chemotaxis by *Pseudomonas aeruginosa. J. Bacteriol.* **137:**274–280.

Nikata, T., Y. Sakai, K. Shibata, J. Kato, A. Kuroda, and H. Ohtake. Molecular analysis of the phosphate-specific transport (*pst*) operon of *Pseudomonas aeruginosa. Mol. Gen. Genet.*, in press.

Nikata, T., K. Sumida, J. Kato, and H. Ohtake. 1992. Rapid method for analyzing bacterial behavioral responses to chemical stimuli. *Appl. Environ. Microbiol.* **58:**2250–2254.

Ohga, T., A. Masduki, J. Kato, and H. Ohtake. 1993. Chemotaxis away from thiocyanic and isothiocyanic esters in *Pseudomonas aeruginosa. FEMS Microbiol. Lett.* **113:**63–66.

Ostroff, R. M., and M. L. Vasil. 1987. Identification of a new phospholipase C activity by analysis of an insertional mutation in the hemolytic phospholipase C structural gene of *Pseudomonas aeruginosa. J. Bacteriol.* **169:**4597–4601.

Poole, K., and R. E. W. Hancock. 1984. Phosphate transport in *Pseudomonas aeruginosa:* involvement of a periplasmic phosphate-binding protein. *Eur. J. Biochem.* **144:**607–612.

Starnbach, M. N., and S. Lory. 1992. The *fliA* (*rpoF*) gene of *Pseudomonas aeruginosa* encodes an alternative sigma factor required for flagellin synthesis. *Mol. Microbiol.* **6:**459–469.

Stock, A., J. Mottonen, T. Chen, and J. Stock. 1987. Identification of a possible nucleotide binding site in CheW, a protein required for sensory transduction in bacterial chemotaxis. *J. Biol. Chem.* **262:**535–537.

Molecular Biology of Pseudomonads
Edited by T. Nakazawa et al.

Chapter 16

Signal Transduction through Quorum Sensing in *Pseudomonas aeruginosa*

Paul Williams, Gordon S. A. B. Stewart, Miguel Camara, Michael K. Winson, Siri Ram Chhabra, George P. C. Salmond, and Barrie W. Bycroft

By transducing sensory information, bacteria readily adapt to changes in their prevailing growth environment. Two-component histidine protein kinase response regulator systems that relay information via phosphoryl transfer appear to be ubiquitous in bacteria. Such sensor-regulator circuits characteristically operate intracellularly, and as microbiologists, we rarely consider the possibility of bacterial intercellular cooperativity. The few notable exceptions are the swarming motility exhibited by bacteria, e.g., *Proteus mirabilis*; the peptide "sex" pheromones of *Enterococcus faecalis*; and the bioluminescence (*lux*) phenotype of marine bacteria, e.g., *Vibrio* (*Photobacterium*) *fischeri*. It is now apparent that the sensory mechanism by which light emission is regulated in *V. fischeri* is common to diverse gram-negative bacteria and constitutes an intercellular communication device through which an organism can recognize "self" and coordinate a "multicellular" response. This chapter reviews our current understanding of cell density-dependent regulation of gene expression through quorum sensing in *Pseudomonas aeruginosa*.

QUORUM SENSING AND BIOLUMINESCENCE

Although *V. fischeri* emits light only at high cell densities, Nealson et al. (1970) noted that the organism produces an extracellular substance that could induce bioluminescence in cultures of low cell density. This molecule, termed an "autoinducer" or "pheromone," was identified as *N*-(3-oxohexanoyl) homoserine lactone (OHHL; Fig. 1; Eberhard

Paul Williams, Miguel Camara, Siri Ram Chhabra, and Barrie W. Bycroft • Department of Pharmaceutical Sciences, University of Nottingham, Nottingham NG7 2RD, United Kingdom. ***Gordon S. A. B. Stewart and Michael K. Winson*** • Department of Applied Biochemistry and Food Science, University of Nottingham, Sutton Bonington Campus, Loughborough LE12 5RD, United Kingdom. ***George P. C. Salmond*** • Department of Biological Sciences, University of Warwick, Coventry CV4 7AL, United Kingdom.

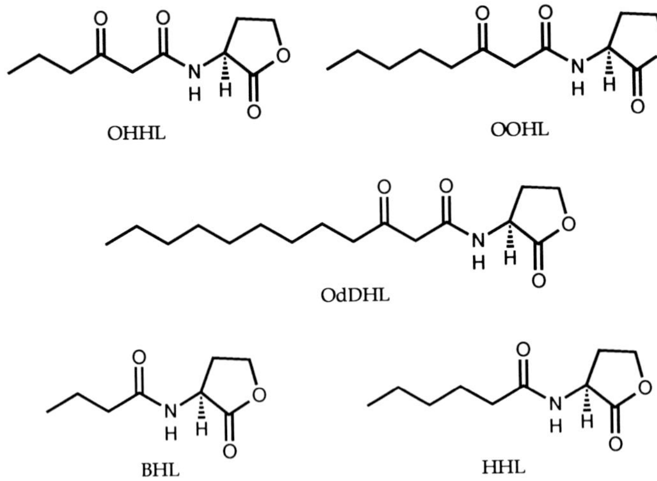

Figure 1. Structures of some *N*-acyl-L-homoserine lactones. OHHL, *N*-(3-oxohexanoyl)-L-homoserine lactone; OOHL, *N*-(3-oxooctanoyl)-L-homoserine lactone; OdDHL, *N*-(3-oxododecanoyl-L-homoserine lactone; BHL, *N*-butanoyl-L-homoserine lactone; HHL, *N*-hexanoyl-L-homoserine lactone.

et al., 1981). As *V. fischeri* multiplies, OHHL accumulates in the growth medium until it reaches a critical threshold concentration, whereupon bioluminescence is induced. The fact that OHHL freely diffuses across cell membranes (Kaplan and Greenberg, 1985) suggests a mechanism by which a strong coordinated response can be achieved in a population of bacterial cells; i.e., OHHL represents a cell-cell communication device. In *V. fischeri,* the *luxI* gene product directs the synthesis of OHHL, which interacts with the positive transcriptional activator LuxR to stimulate transcription of the *lux* structural genes (*luxICDABE*). The fact that *luxI* is the first gene in this operon leads to increased levels of LuxI and thus more OHHL, which further activates LuxR, setting up an autoinduction cascade and the characteristic cell density-dependent induction of bioluminescence (Meighen, 1991).

Until 1992, OHHL was exclusively associated with the regulation of bioluminescence in *V. fischeri* and a few closely related marine bacteria. However, while working on the biosynthesis of the simple β-lactam antibiotic carbapen-2-em-3-carboxylic acid in the plant pathogen *Erwinia carotovora*, we discovered that antibiotic production was regulated in a cell density-dependent manner by OHHL (Bainton et al., 1992a; Bainton et al., 1992b). This finding suggested that OHHL production might be much more widespread than was previously supposed. To pursue this possibility experimentally, we constructed a recombinant OHHL sensor plasmid that contains *V. fischeri luxR, luxAB*, and the *lux* promoter region. Since this construct lacks *luxI, Escherichia coli* transformed with this plasmid is dark unless supplied with exogenous OHHL and a long-chain aliphatic aldehyde (as a substrate for the luciferase-driven liberation of blue-green light). The induction of bioluminescence following incubation of this sensor strain with spent bacterial culture supernatants therefore indicates the presence of OHHL or a closely related *N*-acylhomoserine lactone. Using this strategy, we demonstrated that *P. aeruginosa* and many other gram-negative bacteria produce substances capable of eliciting bioluminescence (Bainton et al., 1992a; Bainton et al., 1992b; Swift et al., 1993). Since then, it has become apparent that many gram-negative bacteria possess homologs of LuxR and LuxI and employ *N*-acylhomoserine lactones to facilitate the induction of genetic regulons when a significant population of cells has accumulated (Williams et al., 1992; Fuqua et al., 1994; Swift et al., 1994; Salmond et al., 1995). This cell density-dependent intercellular communication mechanism has become known as quorum sensing (Fuqua et al., 1994). In *Pseudomonas* spp., the expression of many virulence determinants and secondary metabolites is regulated through quorum sensing.

PSEUDOMONADS MAKE *N*-ACYLHOMOSERINE LACTONES: REGULATION OF ELASTASE PRODUCTION IN *P. AERUGINOSA*

When incubated with the *E. coli lux* sensor, supernatants from several *Pseudomonas* spp., including *P. aeruginosa, P. fluorescens, P. putida, P. aureofaciens,* and *P. (Burkholderia) cepacia,* induce bioluminescence. In *P. aeruginosa* PAO1, the first *N*-acylhomoserine lactone to be isolated and purified from spent culture supernatants and chemically characterized was OHHL (Bainton et al., 1992a). Finding OHHL raised questions as to the nature of the operon(s) regulated by such a signal molecule. Two observations suggested that OHHL may be involved in the regulation of elastase production. First, the appearance of elastase in the culture supernatant had long been associated with the late logarithmic and early stationary phases of growth (Whooley et al., 1983). Second, Gambello and Iglewski (1991) described a homolog of LuxR, termed LasR, that was required for transcriptional activation of the elastase structural gene *lasB*. On the basis of this information, we sought an elastase-negative PAO1 mutant in which elastase synthesis could be restored by adding exogenous OHHL. By using chemical mutagenesis, we obtained a mutant, PAN067, in which production of the 33-kDa *lasB* gene product could be partially restored by OHHL (Jones et al., 1993). We therefore presumed that PAN067 contained a mutation in a regulatory gene, the primary candidate being a *P. aeruginosa luxI* homolog. While our work was in progress, such a gene was identified downstream of *lasR* and termed *lasI* (Passador et al., 1993). When introduced into *E. coli* on a multicopy plasmid, *lasI* directs the synthesis of predominantly *N*-(3-oxododecanyl-L-homoserine lactone (OdDHL; Fig. 1) with small amounts of molecules exhibiting the same high-pressure liquid chromatography retention times as OHHL and *N*-(3-oxooctanoyl)-L-homoserine lactone (OOHL; Fig. 1; Pearson et al., 1994). Subsequently, Gray et al. (1994) reported that in the presence of LasR, OdDHL but not OHHL could activate a *lasB-lacZ* promoter fusion in an *E. coli* genetic background. However, PAN067 had responded, albeit partially, to the addition of exogenous OHHL but not of OdDHL (Latifi et al., 1995). Since OdDHL failed to stimulate elastase synthesis in PAN067, the mutation was unlikely to be in *lasI*. Further examination of PAN067 revealed that this strain is highly pleiotropic, has an altered colonial morphology, and is defective in the production of alkaline protease, hemolysin, pyocyanin, hydrogen cyanide, and chitinase (Latifi et al., 1995; Winson et al., 1995) and in staphylolytic activity (unpublished data). These data suggest that PAN067 must contain a mutation in a global regulatory locus. From a cosmid library of PAO1 chromosomal DNA, we identified a cosmid (pAX27) capable of restoring colonial morphology, autoinducer synthesis, and exoproduct production (Latifi et al., 1995).

P. AERUGINOSA PAO1 POSSESSES MULTIPLE HOMOLOGS OF *luxR* AND *luxI*

To identify the genetic locus on pAX27 that is capable of complementing PAN067, we employed the strategy first described by Swift et al. (1993) for cloning homologs of *luxI*. Because of the low levels of DNA sequence homology, DNA hybridization cannot generally be used to identify the genes that encode *luxI* homologs. An alternative approach is to employ the *E. coli lux* sensor; the introduction of *luxI* or a *luxI* homolog in *trans* on a compatible plasmid should result in the in vivo production of an *N*-acylhomoserine lactone and, consequently, a bioluminescence phenotype. Since LuxR shows some molecular specificity, this method does have limitations; for example, the sensor would not detect OdDHL. Nevertheless, we identified highly bioluminescent transformants containing subclones of pAX27. Spent, cell-free culture supernatants from one of these transformants activated the *lux* sensor, suggesting that we had cloned a locus capable of directing autoinducer synthesis. Further analysis of this clone indicated that it contained a 2-kb fragment of PAO1 DNA encoding two genes, the predicted translation products of which were identified as homologs of LuxR and LuxI (Latifi et al., 1995). These homologs are distinct from LasR and LasI and are termed VsmR and VsmI to indicate their role in regulating both virulence determinants and secondary metabolites. Two almost identical genes, termed *rhlR* and *rhlI* because of their association with the regulation of rhamnolipid biosurfactant synthesis, have also been identified in another *P. aeruginosa* strain, DSM2659 (Ochsner et al., 1994; Ochsner and Reiser, 1995). Disruption of *rhlR* or *rhlI* resulted in a rhamnolipid-deficient mutant that also lacked elastolytic activity.

VsmR and RhlR are clearly members of the LuxR family and show around 30% identity with LuxR and LasR as well as with the *P. aureofaciens* homolog PhzR (Pierson et al., 1994). This family of transcriptional activators can be considered modular proteins: the C-terminal region of the protein contains a classical helix-turn-helix DNA-binding motif, while the N-terminal two-thirds of the protein, at least in LuxR, appears to constitute the autoinducer-binding site (Choi and Greenberg, 1992; Stevens et al., 1994). Indeed, Hanzelka and Greenberg (1995) showed that in whole *E. coli* cells, the LuxR N-terminal domain can fold into a polypeptide capable of binding ^{3}H-labeled OHHL in the absence of the C-terminal domain. Therefore, it is perhaps not very surprising to find that the most highly conserved amino acid sequence stretches in the LuxR homologs encompass the DNA- and autoinducer-binding regions. One interesting feature to emerge from sequence comparisons with VsmR is that VsmR is >50% identical to the *E. coli* LuxR homolog SdiA, which is known to act as a transcriptional *trans*-activator of cell division genes in the *ftsQAZ* locus (Wang et al., 1991). As yet, no *E. coli* equivalent of LuxI or an *N*-acylhomoserine lactone has been found.

vsmI DIRECTS SYNTHESIS OF TWO *N*-ACYLHOMOSERINE LACTONES

In *P. aeruginosa* PAO1, *vsmI* is located downstream of *vsmR*. VsmI is almost identical to RhlI and is more closely related to the *P. aureofaciens* LuxI homolog PhzI (Wood and Pierson, 1995) than to LasI (Fig. 2). Phylogenetic analyses of the LuxI homologs currently deposited in databases suggest that those from enteric bacteria such as *Erwinia, Yersinia, Serratia,* and *Enterobacter* spp. form a group distinct from those of *Pseudomonas, Agrobacterium,* and *Vibrio* spp. Despite the relatively large number of LuxI homologs now known, the precise contribution of this polypeptide to the synthesis of *N*-acylhomoserine lactones remains to be elucidated.

When introduced into *E. coli,* LasI directs the synthesis of OdDHL and also apparently that of OHHL and OOHL, though to a much lesser extent (Pearson et al., 1994). On this basis, we assumed that VsmI must direct the synthesis of another *N*-acylhomoserine lactone(s) that would probably be responsible for activating VsmR. To explore this possibility, we developed a novel bioassay employing the autoinducer-negative *Chromobacterium violaceum* mutant CV026. This transposon-insertion mutant is white and responds to a range of exogenous *N*-acylhomoserine lactones by producing the violet pigment violacein (Winson et al., 1994). Since PAO1 induced pigmentation but neither PAN067 nor OdDHL did, we realized that CV026 could usefully be exploited in the testing of crude extracts and fractions collected from chromatographic separations derived from cell-free culture supernatants. Using this approach, we purified two active compounds from supernatants of *E. coli* transformed with the *vsmRI* locus (Winson et al., 1995). Their structures were deduced from high-resolution mass and nuclear magnetic resonance spectra and confirmed by chemical synthesis. The major compound was identified as *N*-butanoyl-L-homoserine lactone (BHL; Fig. 1); the minor compound was identified as *N*-hexanoyl-L-homoserine lactone (HHL; Fig. 1). Neither compound is made by PAN067, and in PAO1, the two autoinducers are made at a ratio (BHL/HHL) of approximately 15:1 (Winson et al., 1995). These data clearly demonstrate that *P. aeruginosa* produces signal molecules that have either 3-oxo-substituted (OHHL and OdDHL) or unsubstituted (BHL and HHL) *N*-acyl side chains. HHL was also recently identified in *Yersinia enterocolitica* (Throup et al., 1995) and *V. fischeri* (Kuo et al., 1994). Interestingly, neither of these bacteria makes BHL, and in *Y. enterocolitica,* the LuxI homolog YenI directs the synthesis of OHHL and HHL in an approximately 1:1 ratio (Throup et al., 1995). This information is all the more remarkable because it is clear that when introduced into *E. coli, luxI, lasI, yenI,* and *vsmI* each direct synthesis of the correct *N*-acylhomoserine lactone molecules in the same proportions as those found in the parent organism (Kuo et al., 1994; Pearson et al., 1994; Throup et al., 1995; Winson et al., 1995). This must mean that *E. coli* possesses all of the necessary substrates and accessory proteins. The fact that these signal molecules differ only in the structures of their *N*-acyl side chains presumably reflects the capacity of LuxI homologs to "lock into" fatty acid metabolism at different stages to sequester specific *N*-acyl side chains that are enzymatically linked to the homoserine lactone. Why or how a single LuxI homolog directs the synthesis of one or more *N*-acylhomoserine lactones remains to be elucidated.

ACTIVATION OF VsmR

A region of dyad symmetry, termed the *lux* box, that centers on residue –40 from the *luxI* transcriptional start site appears to act as the target site for LuxR in *V. fischeri.* Related sequences have been found upstream of the *P. aeruginosa lasB*

	Sequence	
1	M I E F L S E S L E G L S A A M I A E L	VSMI
1	M I E L L S E S L E G L S A A M I A E L	RHLI
1	M H - M E E H T L N Q M S D E L K L M L	PHZI
1	M I V Q I G R R - E E F D K K L L G E M	LASI
1	M T I M I K K S - D F L A I P S E E Y K	LUXI
21	G R Y R H Q V F I E K L G W D V V S T S	VSMI
21	G R Y R H Q V F I E K L G W D V V S T S	RHLI
20	G R F R H E Q F V E K L G W R L P A H P	PHZI
20	H K L R A Q V F K E R K G W D V S V I D	LASI
20	G I L S L R Y Q V F K Q R L E W D L V V	LUXI
41	R V R D Q E F D Q F D H P Q T R Y I V A	VSMI
41	R V R D Q E F D Q F D H P Q T R Y I V A	RHLI
40	S Q A G C E W D Q Y D T E H A R Y L L A	PHZI
40	- E M E I D G Y D A L S P Y Y M L I Q E	LASI
40	- E N N L E S D E Y D N S N A E Y I Y A	LUXI
61	M G R Q - G I C G C A R L L P T T D A Y	VSMI
61	M G R Q - G I C G C A R L L P T T D A Y	RHLI
60	F N E D R A I V G C A R L I P T T F P N	PHZI
59	D T P E A Q V F G C W R I L D T T G P Y	LASI
59	C D D T E N V S G C W R L X P T T G D Y	LUXI
80	L L K E V F A - Y L C S E T P P S D P S	VSMI
80	L L K E V F A - Y L C S E T P P S D P S	RHLI
80	L L E G V F G - H T C A G A P P K H P A	PHZI
79	M L K N T F P E L L H G K E A P C S P H	LASI
79	M L K S V F P E L L G Q Q S A P K D P N	LUXI
99	V W E L S R Y A A S A A D D P Q L A M K	VSMI
99	V W E L S R Y A A S A A D D P Q L A M K	RHLI
99	I W E M T R F T T R - - - E P Q L A M P	PHZI
99	I W E L S R F A I - N S G Q K G S L G F	LASI
99	I V E L S R F A V G K N S S K I N N S A	LUXI
119	I F W S S L Q C A W Y L G A S S V V A V	VSMI
119	I F W S S L Q C A W Y L G A S S V V A V	RHLI
116	L F W R S L K T A S L A G A D A I V G I	PHZI
118	S D C T L E A M R A L A R Y S L Q N D I	LASI
119	S E I T M K L F E A I Y K H A V S Q G I	LUXI
139	T T T A M E R Y F V R N G V I L Q R L G	VSMI
139	T T T A M E R Y F V R N G V I L Q R L G	RHLI
136	V N S T M E R Y Y K I N G V H Y E R L G	PHZI
138	Q T L V T V T T V G V E K M M I R A G L	LASI
139	T E Y V T V T S T A I E R F L K R I K V	LUXI
159	P P Q K V K G E T L V A I S F P A Y Q E	VSMI
159	P P Q K V K G E T L V A I S F P A Y Q E	RHLI
156	P V T V H Q N E K I L A I K L S A H R E	PHZI
158	D V S R F G P H L K I G I E R A V A L R	LASI
159	P C H R I G D K E I H V L G D T K S - -	LUXI
179	R G L E M L L R Y H P E W L Q R T - L S	VSMI
179	R G L E M L L R Y H P E W L Q G V P L S	RHLI
176	H H R S A V A - - P S A F M S D T L L R	PHZI
178	I E L N A K T Q I A L Y G G V L V E Q R	LASI
177	- - - - - - V V L S M P I N E Q F K K A	LUXI
198	M A V □	VSMI
199	M A V □	RHLI
194	E T A □	PHZI
198	L A V S	LASI
191	V L N □	LUXI

Figure 2. Amino acid sequence similarity between the LuxI homologs of *P. aeruginosa* (VsmI, RhlI, and LasI), *P. aureofaciens* (PhzI), and *V. fischeri* (LuxI). Boxed regions highlight identical amino acid residues in VsmI and other LuxI homologs. The DNA sequences for *vsmI* (accession no. U15644), *rhlI* (accession no. U11811), and *phzI* (accession no. L33724) are in the EMBL nucleotide sequence data library.

gene as well as upstream of the *Agrobacterium tumefaciens traA* and *traI* genes (Fuqua et al., 1994). We also identified a putative *lux* box element between *vsmR* and *vsmI* that is very similar to that of *lasB* (Latifi et al., 1995). This provided an opportunity to determine whether VsmR was activated by BHL or OdDHL and to define in more detail the structural requirements for the activation of VsmR by *N*-acylhomoserine lactones. To achieve this, we constructed a bioluminescent reporter in which *vsmR* together with the *vsmI* promoter-operator region was linked to the *Photorhabdus luminescens lux* structural operon. Unlike the *lux* reporter described previously, which employed *V. fischeri lux* genes, this new reporter construct, when introduced into *E. coli*, does not require the addition of exogenous long-chain aldehyde and functions at temperatures up to 37°C. Using this assay, we observed that BHL and HHL activate this bioluminescent reporter similarly: around 1 μM BHL or HHL is required to generate a half-maximal response (Winson et al., 1995). Extension of the side chain to the 8-carbon *N*-octanoyl-L-homoserine lactone reduced activity by over 50%, while the 12-C analog *N*-dodecanoyl-L-homoserine lactone was inactive. Introduction of an oxygen at the C-3 position of BHL to give *N*-(3-oxobutanoyl)-L-homoserine lactone (OBHL) also reduced activity to around the same level as that observed with OHHL, i.e., to about half that obtained with BHL and HHL. OdDHL was slightly active but was much less efficient at inducing light emission than any of the other analogs examined (Winson et al., 1995). This structure-activity analysis makes clear that optimal activation of VsmR requires a short *N*-acyl side chain without a 3-oxo substituent. In contrast, the 3-oxo substituent and a C_{12} *N*-acyl side chain have been reported to be essential for the optimal activation of LasR (Passador et al., 1994). For other LuxR homologs such as LuxR and CarR (from *Erwinia carotovora*), which, like VsmR, depend on short-chain *N*-acyl homoserine lactones for activation, the 3-oxo substituent is critical. In *Erwinia carotovora*, carbapenem biosynthesis depends on the activation of CarR by OHHL (Bainton et al., 1992a; Bainton et al., 1992b; McGowan et al., 1995); compounds such as HHL and *N*-(3-hydroxybutanoyl)-L-homoserine lactone (the *Vibrio harveyi* autoinducer; Fig. 1) exhibit less than 1% of the activity of OHHL; BHL, *N*-(3-hydroxyhexanoyl)-L-homoserine lactone, and OBHL show less than 0.15% of the activity of OHHL (Chhabra et al., 1993). In *V. fischeri*, HHL has around 10% the activity of OHHL (Eberhard et al., 1981). Thus, although the pattern of substrate specificity emerging for the LuxR homologs indicates high specificity, the homologs show a degree of flexibility in their recognition of *N*-acyl homoserine lactones.

RESTORATION OF EXOPRODUCT SYNTHESIS IN PAN067 BY BHL AND HHL

Since transformation of PAN067 with a multicopy plasmid carrying the *vsm* locus restored production of multiple exoproducts and since this mutant had responded to the addition of exogenous OHHL, we added either BHL or HHL to the PAN067 growth medium. Figure 3 shows that both autoinducers restored elastase production and that BHL is more effective than HHL. Further analysis indicated that both chitinase and cyanide synthesis had also been restored. However, the concentration of exogenous autoinducer required to restore all three phenotypes to around 50% of that of the parent

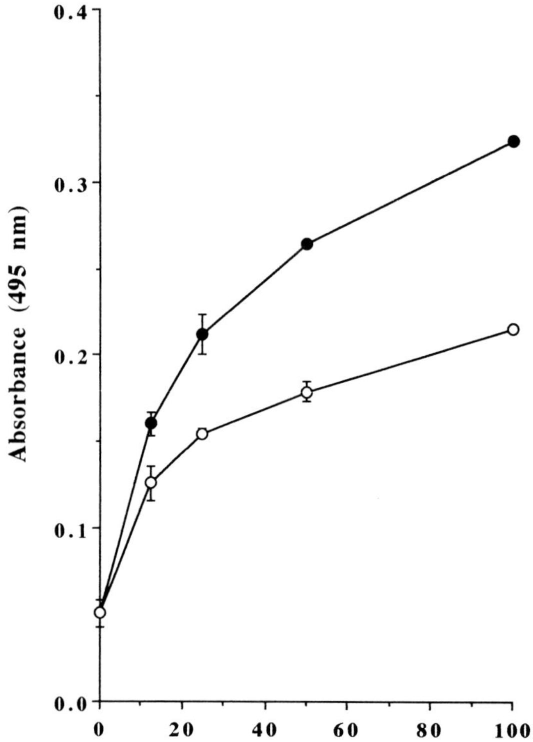

Figure 3. Restoration of elastase production in PAN067 by BHL (●) or HHL (○) added to the growth medium immediately prior to inoculation. After overnight growth, cell-free culture supernatants were assayed for elastolytic activity (recorded as absorbance at 495 nm) by using elastin-Congo red as substrate, as described by Gambello and Iglewski (1991). At 100 μM BHL, elastase synthesis is restored to around 50% of that observed in the parent strain PAO1.

PAO1 was far greater (100 μM) than that required for activation of the *vsmR vsmI*::*lux* reporter (1 μM; Winson et al., 1995). While this difference may reflect the greater sensitivity of the *vsmI* promoter, it also highlights the unknown nature of the mutation in PAN067. Although PAN067 can be complemented by plasmid-borne copies of *vsmRI*, the strain has wild-type *vsmRI* genes.

In *P. aeruginosa* PG201, Ochsner and Reiser (1995) constructed an *rhlI* (*vsmI*) mutant in which restoration of rhamnolipid synthesis requires the addition of 0.5 μM BHL to achieve a half-maximal response; a similar response with OHHL requires 10 μM BHL. This information clearly resolves the apparent contradictions in the literature with regard to the regulation of elastase expression by OdDHL and OHHL (Jones et al., 1993; Gray et al., 1994). In particular, the inability of OHHL to activate a reporter system in *E. coli* containing *lasR* and a *lasB*::*lacZ* fusion (Gray et al., 1994) while being able to induce elastase production in a *P. aeruginosa* genetic background (Jones et al., 1993) can now be explained, given the characterization of the *vsm* (*rhl*) locus and the identification of BHL and HHL. Although OHHL is unable to activate LasR (Gray et al., 1994), it is clearly capable of activating VsmR (RhlR) (Winson et al., 1995; Ochsner and Reiser, 1995).

A HIERARCHICAL AUTOINDUCTION CASCADE REGULATES PRODUCTION OF VIRULENCE DETERMINANTS AND SECONDARY METABOLITES IN *P. AERUGINOSA*

Thus far, two LuxR homologs (LasR and VsmR [RhlR]) and two LuxI homologs (LasI and VsmI [RhlI]) have been described in *P. aeruginosa* PAO1, and their cognate signal molecules have been chemically characterized. Both regulatory loci are involved in the expression of alkaline protease and elastase, whereas exotoxin A (Latifi et al., 1995) and rhamnolipids (Ochsner and Reiser, 1995) each appear to be regulated by only one system, LasR-OdDHL or VsmR-BHL, respectively. LasR-OdDHL and VsmR-BHL thus represent two arms of a complex regulatory circuit involved in the control of multiple physiological traits. With regard to *lasB* expression, a picture of the interrelationship between the two quorum-sensing circuits is beginning to emerge. Pearson et al. (1995) recently reported that although OdDHL is able to activate a *lasB*::*lacZ* fusion in a *P. aeruginosa lasR* mutant containing a plasmid with *lasR* under the control of the *lac* promoter, it does not activate the reporter when *lasR* is placed under the control of its natural promoter. In fact, BHL was reported to be necessary for the expression of *lasR* in *P. aeruginosa* (Pearson et al., 1995). Whether this BHL-mediated activation of *lasR* requires VsmR was not reported. However, in collaboration with A. Lazdunski's group (Centre National de la Recherche Scientifique, Marseille, France), we obtained evidence to indicate that LasR-OdDHL is required for activation of *vsmR* and that VsmR (in the presence or absence of BHL) has a negative effect on the expression of *lasR*. Thus, two interdependent quorum-sensing circuits have emerged, and although additional work is required to dissect in detail the nature of the interrelationship between the LasRI-OdDHL and VsmRI-BHL circuits, elastase synthesis clearly depends on both systems. Our current understanding of this hierarchical autoinducer-dependent regulatory cascade with regard to *lasB* expression is illustrated by Fig. 4. LasR activates *lasI* such that OdDHL is produced, setting up the first autoinduction cascade (Seed et al., 1995). LasR-OdDHL activates expression of *vsmR* such that VsmR induces *vsmI* expression such that BHL (and HHL) is produced (Winson et al., 1995). Since *vsmR* (*rhlR*) mutants are elastase negative (Ochsner and Reiser, 1995) and since VsmR-BHL activates *vsmI* via a *lux* box almost identical to that located within the *lasB* promoter (Latifi et al., 1995; Winson et al., 1995), we presume that, physiologically, VsmR-BHL is responsible for *lasB* activation in *P. aeruginosa*. However, Gray et al. (1994) provided evidence that LasR-OdDHL directly activates *lasB*. Thus, although the model presented offers an explanation of why mutations in either *lasR* or *vsmR* lead to the loss of elastase production, it is not yet clear why LasR-OdDHL does not activate the *lasB* promoter directly in a *vsmR* (*rhlR*)-negative background. Clearly, many additional layers of regulatory complexity in *P. aeruginosa* remain to be eluci-

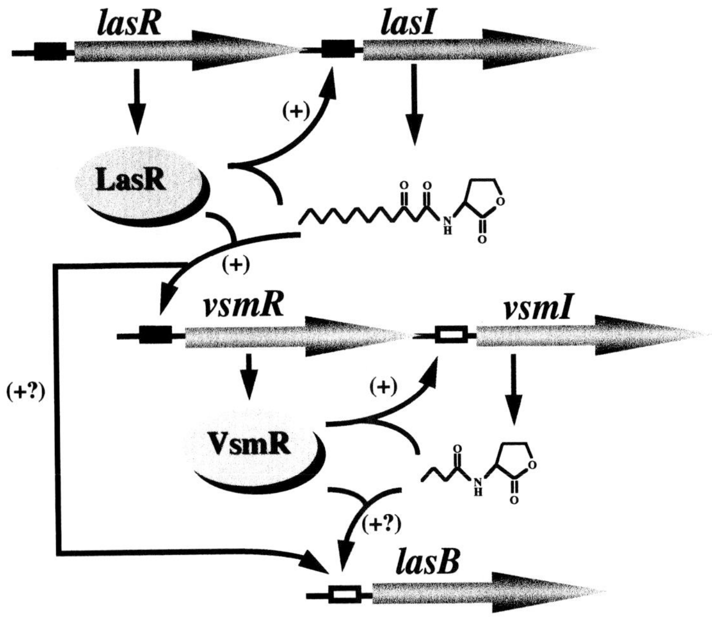

Figure 4. Model for regulation of the elastase structural gene, *lasB*. Boxes between *vsmR* and *vsmI*, between *lasR* and *lasI*, and in front of *lasR* and *lasB* represent promoter-operator regions. *lux* box-like elements have been found upstream of *vsmI* and *lasB* only. For clarity, the *vsmI* and *lasI* gene products have been omitted, and only the *N*-acylhomoserine lactones BHL and OdDHL, for whose synthesis VsmI and LasI, respectively, are responsible, are shown (see text for a full description of the model). Promoter activation is indicated by (+).

dated. Nevertheless, recognition of the phenomenon of cell-cell communication is beginning to offer new insights into the physiology and molecular biology of *Pseudomonas* spp.

Acknowledgments. We thank Andrée Lazdunski, Amel Latifi, Maryline Foglino, Virginia Chapon, and Marc Bally for their collaboration and contribution to work described in this chapter. We are also indebted to Derek Wood, Sandy Pierson, and Urs Ochsner for providing us with material prior to publication.

REFERENCES

Bainton, N. J., B. W. Bycroft, S. R. Chhabra, P. Stead, L. Gledhill, P. J. Hill, C. E. D. Rees, M. K. Winson, G. P. C. Salmond, G. S. A. B. Stewart, and P. Williams. 1992a. A general role for the *lux* autoinducer in bacterial cell signalling: control of antibiotic synthesis in *Erwinia*. *Gene* **116:**87–91.

Bainton, N. J., P. Stead, S. R. Chhabra, B. W. Bycroft, G. P. C. Salmond, G. S. A. B. Stewart, and P. Williams. 1992b. *N*-(3-Oxohexanoyl)-L-homoserine lactone regulates carbapenem antibiotic production in *Erwinia carotovora*. *Biochem. J.* **288:**997–1004.

Chhabra, S. R., P. Stead, N. J. Bainton, G. P. C. Salmond, G. S. A. B. Stewart, P. Williams, and B. W. Bycroft. 1993. Autoregulation of carbapenem biosynthesis in *Erwinia carotovora* by analogues of *N*-(3-oxohexanoyl)-L-homoserine lactone. *J. Antibiot.* **46:**441–449.

Choi, S. H., and E. P. Greenberg. 1992. Genetic dissection of DNA-binding and luminescence gene activation by the *Vibrio fischeri* LuxR protein. *J. Bacteriol.* **174:**4064–4069.

Eberhard, A., A. L. Burlingame, G. L. Kenyon, K. H. Nealson, and N. J. Oppenheimer. 1981. Structural identification of the autoinducer of *Photobacterium fischeri* luciferase. *Biochemistry* **20:**2444–2449.

Eberhard, A., C. A. Widrig, P. McBath, and J. B. Schineller. 1986. Analogs of the autoinducer of bioluminescence in *Vibrio fischeri. Arch. Microbiol.* **146:**35–40.

Fuqua, W. C., S. C. Winans, and E. P. Greenberg. 1994. Quorum sensing in bacteria: the LuxR-LuxI family of cell density responsive transcriptional regulators. *J. Bacteriol.* **176:**269–275.

Gambello, M. J., and B. H. Iglewski. 1991. Cloning and characterization of *Pseudomonas aeruginosa lasR* gene, a transcriptional activator of elastase expression. *J. Bacteriol.* **173:**3000–3009.

Gray, K. M., L. Passador, B. H. Iglewski, and E. P. Greenberg. 1994. Interchangeability and specificity of components from the quorum-sensing regulatory systems of *Vibrio fischeri* and *Pseudomonas aeruginosa. J. Bacteriol.* **176:**3076–3080.

Hanzelka, B. L., and E. P. Greenberg. 1995. Evidence that the N-terminal region of the *Vibrio fischeri* LuxR protein constitutes an autoinducer-binding domain. *J. Bacteriol.* **177:**815–817.

Jones, S., B. Yu, N. J. Bainton, M. Birdsall, B. W. Bycroft, S. R. Chhabra, A. J. R. Cox, P. Golby, P. J. Reeves, S. Stephens, M. K. Winson, G. P. C. Salmond, G. S. A. B. Stewart, and P. Williams. 1993. The *lux* autoinducer regulates the production of exoenzyme virulence determinants in *Erwinia carotovora* and *Pseudomonas aeruginosa. EMBO J.* **12:**2477–2482.

Kaplan, H. B., and E. P. Greenberg. 1985. Diffusion of autoinducer is involved in regulation of the *Vibrio fischeri* luminescence system. *J. Bacteriol.* **163:**1210–1214.

Kuo, A., N. V. Blough, and P. V. Dunlap. 1994. Multiple *N*-acyl-L-homoserine lactone autoinducers of luminescence in the marine symbiotic bacterium *Vibrio fischeri. J. Bacteriol.* **176:**7558–7565.

Latifi, A., M. K. Winson, M. Foglino, B. W. Bycroft, G. S. A. B. Stewart, A. Lazdunski, and P. Williams. 1995. Multiple homologues of LuxR and LuxI control expression of virulence determinants and secondary metabolites through quorum sensing in *Pseudomonas aeruginosa* PAO1. *Mol. Microbiol.* **17:**333–343.

McGowan, S., M. Sebaihia, S. Jones, B. Yu, N. J. Bainton, P. F. Chan, B. W. Bycroft, G. S. A. B. Stewart, P. Williams, and G. P. C. Salmond. 1995. Carbapenem antibiotic production in *Erwinia carotovora* is regulated by CarR, a homologue of the LuxR transcriptional activator. *Microbiology* **141:**541–550.

Meighen, E. A. 1991. Molecular biology of bacterial bioluminescence. *Microbiol. Rev.* **55:**123–142.

Nealson, K. H., T. Platt, and J. W. Hastings. 1970. Cellular control of synthesis and activity of the bacterial bioluminescence system. *J. Bacteriol.* **104:**313–322.

Ochsner, U. A., A. K. Koch, A. Fiechter, and J. Reiser. 1994. Isolation and characterization of a regulatory gene affecting rhamnolipid biosurfactant synthesis in *Pseudomonas aeruginosa. J. Bacteriol.* **176:**2044–2054.

Ochsner, U. A., and J. Reiser. 1995. Autoinducer-mediated regulation of rhamnolipid biosurfactant synthesis in *Pseudomonas aeruginosa. Proc. Natl. Acad. Sci. USA* **92:**6424–6428.

Passador, L., J. M. Cook, M. J. Gambello, L. Rust, and B. H. Iglewski. 1993. Expression of *Pseudomonas aeruginosa* virulence genes requires cell-to-cell communication. *Science* **260:**1127–1130.

Passador, L., J. P. Pearson, K. M. Gray, K. Guertin, A. S. Kende, E. P. Greenberg, and B. H. Iglewski. 1994. Use of structural analogs to determine critical features of *Pseudomonas aeruginosa* autoinducer, abstr. D-84, p. 111. *Abstracts of the 94th Annual Meeting of the American Society of Microbiology 1994.*

Pearson, J. P., K. M. Gray, L. Passador, K. D. Tucker, A. Eberhard, B. H. Iglewski, and E. P. Greenberg. 1994. Structure of the autoinducer required for expression of *Pseudomonas aeruginosa* virulence genes. *Proc. Natl. Acad. Sci. USA* **91:**197–201.

Pearson, J. P., L. Passador, B. H. Iglewski, and E. P. Greenberg. 1995. A second *N*-acylhomoserine lactone signal produced by *Pseudomonas aeruginosa. Proc. Natl. Acad. Sci. USA* **92:**1490–1494.

Pierson, L. S., V. D. Keppenne, and D. W. Wood. 1994. Phenazine antibiotic biosynthesis in *Pseudomonas aureofaciens* 30-84 is regulated by PhzR in response to cell density. *J. Bacteriol.* **176:**3966–3974.

Salmond, G. P. C., B. W. Bycroft, G. S. A. B. Stewart, and P. Williams. 1995. The bacterial 'enigma' cracking the code of cell-cell communication. *Mol. Microbiol.* **16:**615–624.

Seed, P. C., L. Passador, and B. H. Iglewski. 1995. Activation of the *Pseudomonas aeruginosa lasI* gene by LasR and the *Pseudomonas* autoinducer PAI: an autoinduction regulatory hierarchy. *J. Bacteriol.* **177:**654–659.

Stevens, A. M., K. M. Dolan, and E. P. Greenberg. 1994. Synergistic binding of the *Vibrio fischeri* LuxR transcriptional activator domain and RNA polymerase to the *lux* promoter region. *Proc. Natl. Acad. Sci. USA* **91:**12619–12623.

Swift, S., N. J. Bainton, and M. K. Winson. 1994. Gram negative bacterial communication by *N*-acyl homoserine lactones: a universal language? *Trends Microbiol.* **2:**193–198.

Swift, S., M. K. Winson, P. F. Chan, N. J. Bainton, M. Birdsall, P. J. Reeves, C. E. D. Rees, S. R. Chhabra, P. J. Hill, J. P. Throup, B. W. Bycroft, G. P. C. Salmond, P. Williams, and G. S. A. B. Stewart. 1993. A novel strategy for the isolation of *luxI* homologues: evidence for the widespread distribution of a LuxR:LuxI superfamily in enteric bacteria. *Mol. Microbiol.* **10:**511–520.

Throup, J., M. Camara, G. S. Briggs, M. K. Winson, S. R. Chhabra, B. W. Bycroft, P. Williams, and G. S. A. B. Stewart. 1995. Characterization of the *yenI/yenR* locus from *Yersinia enterocolitica* mediating the synthesis of two *N*-acylhomoserine lactone signal molecules. *Mol. Microbiol.* **17:**345–356.

Wang, X., P. A. J. de Boer, and L. I. Rothfield. 1991. A factor that positively regulates cell division by activating transcription of the major cluster of essential cell division genes of *Escherichia coli. EMBO J.* **10:**3363–3372.

Whooley, M. A., J. A. O'Callaghan, and A. J. McLoughlin. 1983. Effect of substrate on the regulation of exoprotease production by *Pseudomonas aeruginosa* ATCC 10145. *J. Gen. Microbiol.* **129:**981–988.

Williams, P., N. J. Bainton, S. Swift, M. K. Winson, S. R. Chhabra, G. S. A. B. Stewart, G. P. C. Salmond, and B. W. Bycroft. 1992. Small molecule mediated density dependent control of gene expression in prokaryotes: bioluminescence and the biosynthesis of carbapenem antibiotics. *FEMS Microbiol. Lett.* **100:**161–168.

Winson, M. K., N. J. Bainton, S. R. Chhabra, B. W. Bycroft, G. P. C. Salmond, P. Williams, and G. S. A. B. Stewart. 1994. Control of *N*-acyl homoserine lactone-regulated expression of multiple phenotypes in *Chromobacterium violaceum,* abstr. H-71, p. 212. *Abstracts of the 94th Annual Meeting of the American Society of Microbiology 1994.*

Winson, M. K., M. Camara, A. Latifi, M. Foglino, S. R. Chhabra, M. Daykin, M. Bally, V. Chapon, G. P. C. Salmond, B. W. Bycroft, A. Lazdunski, G. S. A. B. Stewart, and P. Williams. 1995. Multiple *N*-acyl-L-homoserine lactone signal molecules regulate production of virulence determinants and secondary metabolites in *Pseudomonas aeruginosa. Proc. Natl. Acad. Sci. USA* **92:**9427–9431.

Wood, D. W., and L. S. Pierson. 1995. The *phzI* gene of *Pseudomonas aureofaciens* is responsible for the production of a diffusible signal required for phenazine antibiotic production. *Gene* **168:**49–53.

Molecular Biology of Pseudomonads
Edited by T. Nakazawa et al.

Chapter 17

Fine Control of Expression of the Catabolic Pathways of TOL Plasmid of *Pseudomonas putida* for Mineralization of Aromatic Hydrocarbons

Rafael Salto, Asunción Delgado, Maria-Trinidad Gallegos, Maximino Manzanera, Silvia Marqués, and Juan L. Ramos

THE TOL PLASMID AND ITS REGULATION

The TOL plasmid pWW0 of *Pseudomonas putida* encodes the catabolic pathways for the metabolism of toluene and related compounds (Williams and Murray, 1974). The lateral methyl group of these hydrocarbons is first oxidized to the corresponding carboxylic acid derivatives by a set of reactions known as the upper pathway (Worsey and Williams, 1975). The corresponding benzoates are then oxidized to Krebs cycle intermediates in a set of reactions known as the *meta*-cleavage pathway (Fig. 1).

The genetic information for the upper pathway (genes *xylCMABN*) is located in the upper operon (Harayama et al., 1989), whereas information for the *meta*-cleavage pathway is encoded by a separate operon (Franklin et al., 1981; Harayama et al., 1984). This latter operon comprises 13 genes extending over 11 kb and is thus one of the largest operons in prokaryotes (Harayama and Rekik, 1990). In addition to the catabolic operons, two regulatory genes, called *xylS* and *xylR*, are involved in transcriptional control; these genes are located 3′ of the *meta* operon (Fig. 1). These regulatory genes are transcribed from physically close but functionally divergent promoters (Inouye et al., 1987a; Ramos et al., 1987). In this review, the promoters for the upper operon, *meta* operon, and *xylS* and x*ylR* genes are called Pu, Pm, Ps, and Pr, respectively.

As a result of the isolation of nitrosoguanidine- and Tn5-induced mutants, it was proposed that XylS is involved in control of the *meta*-cleavage pathway and that XylR is involved in activation of transcription from the upper pathway (Franklin et al., 1983; Inouye et al., 1981; Worsey et al., 1978). Because of the induction pattern of the pathway enzymes, it was also proposed that XylR and XylS act in concert to activate transcription from the *meta* operon when cells are growing on a substrate of the upper path-

---

Rafael Salto, Asunción Delgado, Maria-Trinidad Gallegos, Maximino Manzanera, Silvia Marqués, and Juan L. Ramos • Department of Biochemistry, Molecular and Cellular Biology of Plants, Consejo Superior de Investigaciones Científicas, Apdo 419, E-18008 Granada, Spain.

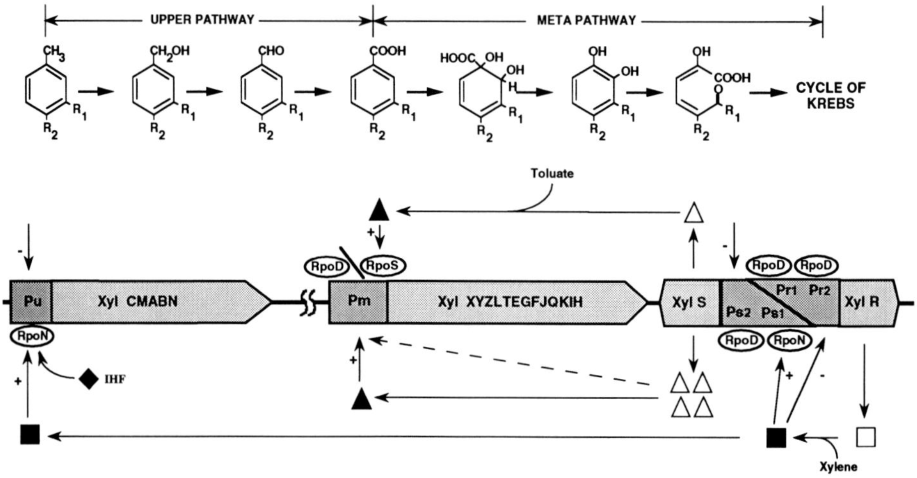

Figure 1. Regulatory elements that control expression of TOL plasmid pWW0. Symbols: box, XylR; triangle, XylS; diamond, IHF. Open symbols correspond to transcriptional regulator forms unable to stimulate transcription; closed symbols correspond to forms able to stimulate transcription.

way. By making deletions and insertions in Pm, the promoter of the *meta* operon, it is possible to demonstrate that as soon as activation from Pm by XylS is lost, activation by the XylR-XylS pair is also lost, and therefore the only activator of the Pm promoter is XylS (Ramos et al., 1987). When the rate of synthesis of *xylS* mRNA was studied, it was found that the *xylS* gene is expressed at low levels in cells growing on glucose or *m*-toluate but that *xylS* mRNA levels can be as high as 0.3% of the total RNA synthesis when cells are grown in the presence of *m*-xylene (Inouye et al., 1987a; Ramos et al., 1987). Therefore, the model of TOL plasmid regulation proposes that the XylR protein activated by toluene or other hydrocarbon effectors stimulates transcription from both Pu and Ps. Overexpression of the *xylS* gene yields high levels of XylS protein, which even in the absence of benzoate is able to stimulate transcription from Pm (Inouye et al., 1987b; Mermod et al., 1987; Ramos et al., 1987). This model is confirmed if the rate of mRNA synthesis is studied in *Pseudomonas* spp. *P. putida* cells were grown on glucose and transferred to toluene, and at different times, RNA was extracted and analyzed by using different primers for *xylR, xylS,* Pu, and Ps. It was found that *xylR* mRNA is made from two overlapping promoters in cells growing on glucose or in toluene (Pr1 and Pr2 in Fig. 1) (Inouye et al., 1988; Marqués et al., 1994). Before toluene was added, no mRNA from Pm, Pu, or Ps was detected. Two minutes after the addition of toluene, the level of Pu was high, and mRNA from *xylS* was detected, although it took about 10 min for maximal levels to be reached. The Pm message required about 5 min to be detected, which probably represents the time required for activation of transcription from Ps, synthesis of *xylS* mRNA, and synthesis and accumulation of the XylS protein (Marqués et al., 1994).

STRUCTURE OF THE TOL PLASMID PROMOTERS

The XylR protein positively controls expression from the *P. putida* TOL plasmid upper pathway operon promoter (Pu) and the *xylS* gene promoter (Ps). The XylR regulator needs to be activated by effectors for expression from Pu and from Ps.

Sequence alignment of Pu and Ps revealed that the two promoters regulated by XylR exhibit a modular structure composed of three elements (Abril and Ramos, 1993; Abril et al., 1991; Inouye et al., 1984a; Inouye et al., 1987a; Inouye et al., 1990; de Lorenzo et al., 1991). The two promoters share homologies at three regions, namely at −12/−24, −40/−60, and −120/−180. The −12/−24 region of Pu and Ps contains the sequence 5′-TGGCN$_7$TTGCTA-3′ (Inouye et al., 1984a; Inouye et al., 1987a; Ramos et al., 1987), which is typical of RpoN-dependent promoters (Buck et al., 1986). Furthermore, in an RpoN-null background of *P. putida*, no induction of the upper or *meta*-cleavage pathway enzymes takes place in response to the addition of toluene. These results were confirmed when the Pu and Ps promoters were fused to reporter genes such as *′lacZ* and β-galactosidase activity was determined in *Escherichia coli* and in *P. putida* with and without RpoN.

The −40/−70 region of both Pu and Ps is rich in A and T. The −55/−67 segment of Pu and the −35/−47 segment of Ps show homology to the consensus motif for the binding of integration host factor (IHF), a protein involved in bending DNA (Holtel et al., 1990). This protein is involved in transcription from Pu. In an IHF-minus background, the level of transcription is around 10 to 20% of the level achieved in an IHF-plus background. Furthermore, disruption of the IHF site leads to loss of activation in an IHF-plus background (Abril et al., 1991). IHF binds to Pu and retards DNA in gel retardation assays (de Lorenzo et al., 1991). Also (Pérez-Martin et al., 1994), insertions of intrinsically curved DNA can substitute for the IHF binding domain of Pu; these altered promoters display 40 to 100% of the activity of Pu and are independent of IHF. Therefore, it has been proposed that IHF coregulates expression from Pu by bending the DNA rather than by interacting directly with the RNA polymerase. Furthermore, Pérez-Martín and de Lorenzo (in press) suggested that IHF may prevent cross-talk by other members of the XylR family such as NtrC and NifA.

In addition to the −35/−47 segment homologous to the IHF binding site, another IHF binding site is recognized in Ps by DNA homology at −137/−156 (Holtel et al., 1992; Holtel et al., 1995). A high concentration of IHF specifically retards Ps DNA in gel retardation assays, and the farthest site from the transcription initiation point is clearly protected in vitro from DNase digestion (Holtel et al., 1995). However, in an IHF-minus background, activation from Ps is as high as that in an IHF-plus background (Holtel et al., 1992). Recently, Pérez-Martín and de Lorenzo (1995) showed that in vivo, the histone-like HU protein may be involved in transcription stimulation from the Ps promoter.

The −120/−180 region of Pu and Ps is the target for the XylR regulator. Fine deletions in Pu (Abril et al., 1991; Inouye et al., 1990) and Ps (Holtel et al., 1992) define a large segment required for XylR-dependent transcription stimulation. In vivo (Abril et al., 1991) and in vitro footprinting experiments in the Pu promoter region (de Lorenzo et al., 1991) revealed that XylR recognizes a 5′ motif, which appears twice in inverted orientation. These upstream activator sequence (UAS) were identified in the −160 (UAS1) and −130 (UAS2) regions; deletion of one or both of these motifs abolishes transcription activation by the wild-type XylR regulator (Abril et al., 1991; Holtel et al., 1990; Inouye et al., 1990). In vivo footprinting experiments revealed that the −140 and −180 regions exhibit different patterns of protection-methylation depending upon the presence of effectors. Densitometric analysis of the footprints clearly showed that XylR is always bound to the target sequences but that contacts are different in the presence and the absence of effectors (Abril et al., 1991). Inouye et al. (1990) showed that the XylR-binding sequences can be moved between 20 bp and 1 kb in the Pu promoter, and Gomada et al. (1992) reported that these sequences remain active when moved about 1.2 kb in the Ps promoter.

Planar projections of binding sites in Pu showed that RpoN and XylR binding sites are located on the same DNA face, wherease the IHF binding site is located on the opposite face (de Lorenzo et al., 1991). The introduction of a half helix turn between the IHF binding domain and the XylR binding site decreases transcription stimulation by 90% (Abril and Ramos, 1993). In contrast, the introduction of one full helix turn does not alter transcription stimulation from Pu. According to the proposed mechanism of activation, as in other RpoN promoters, XylR needs to form a loop to contact the RNA polymerase at the transcription site. The mechanism of activation by the RpoN-RNA polymerase complex requires that the regulator make contact with the RpoN-RNA polymerase complex bound at the promoter site (Buck et al., 1986). The intervening DNA sequences may loop out to allow interactions (Buck et al., 1986). The role of IHF in the Pu promoter is probably to assist in loop formation, although it may also assist in the formation and stabilization of the complex (Collado-Vides et al., 1991).

A feature not explained by *xylS* expression from a single RpoN-regulated promoter is that in an RpoN-null background, *P. putida* (pWWO) can grow on *m*-toluate, though at a low growth rate (Köhler et al., 1989). This effect is not due to cross-talk by a functionally analogous XylS protein but rather to expression of the *xylS* gene from an RpoD-dependent promoter, which is located about 100 bp downstream of the RpoN-regulated promoter (Gallegos et al., 1996). Furthermore, given that the mRNA initiated from the RpoN promoter is undetectable when cells are growing on *m*-toluate, perhaps a small amount of XylS protein in these cells is made from a constitutive promoter. In Fig. 1, the RpoD-dependent promoter is called Ps2, and the RpoN-XylR-dependent promoter is called Ps1.

The genes coding for *meta*-cleavage fission of products from the upper pathway are organized in a single operon that is transcribed from the operon promoter Pm (Inouye et al., 1984b; Marqués et al., 1993; Mermod et al., 1984). A single main transcription initiation point is located on this operon (Inouye et al., 1984b; Marqués et al., 1993), and about 85 bp upstream from the main transcription initiation point is needed to stimulate transcription from Pm (Kessler et al., 1993; Ramos et al., 1987). Within this region, DNA sequences show no significant homology to typical promoters; however, the nucleotide sequence around −10 is rich in A and T. The −35 region shows no homology to the −35 region of constitutive promoters in *E. coli*, as is the case for many positively regulated RpoD-dependent promoters in *E. coli* (Collado-Vides et al., 1991). Insertions and deletions in the intervening sequence (−25 to −30 region) decrease transcription stimulation from Pm (Ramos et al., 1987). In the −40 to −70 region, an almost perfect direct repeat motif rich in A has been suggested to constitute part of the motif recognized by the XylS regulator. Mutations in the direct repeats and the introduction of a half-helix turn between the repeats decrease transcription stimulation from Pm, whereas mutations outside the direct repeats have no effect on the ability to induce transcription (Kessler et al., 1993).

An interesting feature of *m*-toluate–XylS-dependent expression from the Pm promoter is that transcription from this promoter is high regardless of the growth phase. To shed light on this feature, transcription from Pm was analyzed in different sigma backgrounds. In RpoD-plus and RpoS-plus backgrounds, transcription from Pm is high regardless of the growth phase. However, in an RpoS-deficient background, transcription from Pm is high only in the early logarithmic phase and decreases thereafter. These results were confirmed at the mRNA level, which showed that the main transcription initiation point was the same (Marqués et al., 1995). Transcription from the *xylS* gene Ps promoter is RpoS independent, and participation of RpoS should therefore be assigned to the Pm promoter (Gallegos et al., unpublished data). The requirement of RpoS for expression from certain Pm mutants can be suppressed by certain XylS mutations (see below), which suggests, but does not prove, that XylS interacts with the transcriptional machinery (Marqués et al., 1995).

The XylR protein controls its own synthesis; this regulator is constitutively transcribed from two RpoD tandem promoters called Pr1 and Pr2 (Fig. 1). Transcription of *xylR* is divergent from that of the nearby Ps promoters (Inouye et al., 1987a; Marqués et al., 1994; Ramos et al., 1987). Furthermore, both UASs of the *xylS* gene promoter, which constitute the target for binding of XylR and the RpoN-dependent *xylS* promoter, overlap the two *xylR* gene promoters (Holtel et al., 1992). This seems to be the basis for the autoregulation of XylR expression, since XylR, when bound to both UASs of Ps, may reduce the access of RNA polymerase to the Pr promoters. In agreement with the fact that XylR is always bound to its target sequences (even in the absence of effectors) is the finding that the regulation of its own expression from Pr is the same in the absence and presence of effectors (Marqués et al., 1994). Finally, the Ps-Pr region is extremely complex, since four promoters are located within 300 bp, a segment that also includes IHF and HU binding sites (Gomada et al., 1992; Holtel et al., 1992; Inouye et al., 1987a; Marqués et al., 1993; Marqués et al., 1994; Pérez-Martín and de Lorenzo, 1995).

THE XylR TRANSCRIPTIONAL REGULATOR

As mentioned above, the XylR protein is expressed constitutively (Inouye et al., 1987a; Inouye et al., 1988; Abril et al., 1989; Marqués et al., 1994) but stimulates transcription from Pu and Ps only in the presence of pathway substrates or effectors, including a wide variety of toluenes, benzyl alcohols, and *p*-chlorobenzaldehyde (Abril et al., 1989).

The XylR protein belongs to the NtrC family of positive regulators and exhibits four domains, three of which are highly conserved among members of this family (North et al., 1993). Carboxy-terminal domain D contains an α-helix–turn–α-helix DNA-binding motif. Central domain C, the best conserved region in the family, seems to be involved in interactions with RNA polymerase and ATP hydrolysis to allow the formation of open transcriptional complexes. The B domain (Q linker) is a short hydrophilic region whose role is probably to serve as a linker between the C and A domains.

The NtrC family of prokaryotic enhancer-like positive regulators becomes activated either by phosphorylation of an aspartyl residue at NH_2-terminal domain A (Ninfa and Magasanik, 1986), as in NtrC, or through the binding of effectors, as in XylR and DmpR

(Abril et al., 1989; Abril et al., 1991; Delgado and Ramos, 1994; Shingler et al., 1993; Shingler and Moore, 1994). The domain involved in signal reception in this family is the nonhomologous NH_2-terminal domain A, which is about 120 to 200 amino acids long (North et al., 1993). This can be deduced from the following facts: (i) the Asp-54 residue is the phosphorylated residue in NtrC (North et al., 1993); (ii) the mutation Glu-172→Lys in XylR results in a mutant regulator with altered effector specificity, which allows the regulator to recognize *m*-nitrotoluene as an effector, in contrast to the wild-type (Delgado and Ramos, 1994); and (iii) when the sensing module of DmpR is replaced with that of XylR, the chimeric protein responds to XylR effectors (Shingler and Moore, 1994).

To further elucidate the mechanism of positive regulation by XylR of RpoN-dependent Pu and Ps promoters, XylR mutants that constitutively mediate transcription from Pu and Ps were isolated after nitrosoguanidine mutagenesis (Delgado et al., 1995). We isolated two constitutive mutants that exhibit a unique point mutation at the NH_2-terminal domain that resulted in substitution of Asn for Asp-135 and Pro for Ser-85, which suggests that these substitutions in XylR partially mimic the effector requirement.

Another interesting feature of the XylRD135N mutant is its ability to mediate transcription from modified Pu promoters lacking one of the UASs. This ability is probably due to an increased affinity for the target DNA that is induced by a conformational change in the regulator caused by the point mutation in the sensing domain. Analyses of the autoregulation of expression of Pr confirmed that affinity of the mutant regulator for its DNA-binding sequences is increased: expression from the Pr promoter is more effectively repressed by the mutant XylRD135N than by the wild-type regulator.

The constitutive character conferred on XylR by the change Asp-135→Asn is abolished by the Glu-172→Lys mutation, since the XylRD135N-E172K double mutant loses the constitutive character (Delgado et al., 1995). This loss suggests that binding of the effector to XylR induces conformational changes that are probably transmitted to the DNA-binding and central domains to stimulate transcription and that alteration of this chain of signal transmission may have important consequences for the transcriptional activity of the regulator.

Therefore, an attractive hypothesis is that the NH_2-terminal domain A of this regulator exerts inhibitory effects on DNA binding and ATPase activity of the COOH-terminal and central domains. This effect may then be eliminated by the binding of effectors or through mutations in the NH_2-terminal domain. This hypothesis is supported by the fact that removal of the NH_2-terminal domain of XylR results in a truncated protein that activates transcription constitutively (Fernández et al., 1995).

THE XylS TRANSCRIPTIONAL REGULATOR

The XylS protein is 321 amino acid residues long (Inouye et al., 1986; Mermod et al., 1987; Spooner et al., 1986) and belongs to the XylS-AraC family of transcriptional regulators (Gallegos et al., 1993). The COOH-terminal end of XylS is highly homologous to the COOH-terminal ends of members of this family of proteins. Within this conserved region, an α-helix–turn–α-helix motif, comprising residues 230 to 250 of XylS, is probably involved in DNA binding. Mutations adjacent to this motif (Ser-229→ILe) result in mutants that mediate high basal transcription levels from Pm in the absence of effectors (Zhou et al., 1990), whereas a mutation within the motif (Phe-248→Cys) results in a mutant unable to stimulate transcription from Pm (Gallegos et al., unpublished data).

Studies on the effector profile of XylS through the activation of transcription from Pm::′*lacZ* fusions (Ramos et al., 1986; Ramos et al., 1990) and through the isolation of mutants with altered effector specificities (Michán et al., 1992; Ramos et al., 1990) show that the XylS regulator interacts with benzoate effectors. Clusters of mutations located at positions 37 to 45, 88 to 92, and 151 to 155 and mutations at residues 256 and 288 result in regulators with altered specificities or impaired effector recognition. Equally important is the observation that XylS mutants at the NH_2-terminal region (Gly-44→Ser and Pro-37→Leu) mediate transcription from Pm in the absence of effectors, which suggests that these changes mimic effector-regulator interactions (Michán et al., 1992). The mutant regulator XylSGly-44→Ser was able to bypass the requirement for RpoS in the late log phase, as high levels of transcripts generated from mutant Pm5 promoter were observed in the stationary phase (Marqués et al., 1995).

Other interesting features of the XylS transcriptional activator are that it is able to stimulate transcription not only in the presence of effectors but also in the absence of effector when the protein is overexpressed because of induction of the Ps promoter by XylR (Inouye et al., 1987a; Ramos et al., 1987) or when the protein is expressed at high levels from exogenous constitutive promoters (Inouye et al., 1987b; Mermod et al., 1987). An important issue yet to be resolved is whether the overproduced form of XylS and the effector-activated form of XylS are equivalent in terms of transcriptional activity.

INTEGRATION OF TOL REGULATION IN GLOBAL CELL METABOLISM

Pu and Ps, the two promoters that are activated by XylR, are also subjected to repression under a number of growth conditions. Holtel et al. (1994) reported that in cells growing on high concentrations of glucose (1.5%, wt/vol), the metabolism of upper pathway substrates is inhibited. This inhibition is due to the absence of promoter activity from both Pu and Ps, measured as mRNA synthesis in wild-type *P. putida* (pWW0). Repression was further confirmed with promoter-′*lacZ* fusions in *E. coli* (Holtel et al., 1994). Marqués et al. (1994) showed that although activation of Pu and Ps promoters occurs immediately after pathway effector is added to cells growing on minimal medium, a delay of several hours is observed with cells growing on Luria-Bertani medium. This absence of induction is thought to be due to the repressive effect of amino acids in the medium.

In continuous culture, where cells can be maintained for many generations in a steady state, both promoters are strongly repressed during nonlimiting growth on succinate in the presence of inducer (6 mM excess succinate concentration) (Duetz et al., 1994). This set of results shows that repression is not the consequence of the presence of one particular carbon source but rather that a number of compounds related to carbohydrate metabolism are able to impair the degradation of aromatics by the TOL plasmid. This finding points to a hypothetical mechanism in which the energy status of the cell and/or the presence of an additional carbon source seems to negatively regulate the expression of the XylR-dependent promoters. XylS-dependent expression from the Pm promoter was not repressed.

Acknowledgments. Work in our laboratory was supported by grants from the CICYT (AMB1O38-CO2-01) and the EC programs BIOTECH (CT92-0084) and ENVIRONMENT (CT94-0539).

REFERENCES

Abril, M. A., M. Buck, and J. L. Ramos. 1991. Activation of the *Pseudomonas* TOL plasmid upper pathway operon: identification of binding sites for the positive regulator XylR and for integration host factor protein. *J. Biol. Chem.* **266:**15832–15838.

Abril, M. A., C., Michán, K. N. Timmis, and J. L. Ramos. 1989. Regulator and enzyme specificities of the TOL-plasmid-encoded upper pathway for degradation of aromatic hydrocarbons and expansion of the substrate range of the pathway. *J. Bacteriol.* **171:**4326–4333.

Abril, M. A., and J. L. Ramos. 1993. Physical organization of the *Pseudomonas* TOL plasmid upper pathway operon promoter. Sequence and positional requirements for XylR-dependent activation of transcription. *Mol. Gen. Genet.* **239:**281–288.

Buck, M., S. Miller, and R. Dixon. 1986. Upstream activators are present in the promoters of nitrogen fixation genes. *Nature* (London) **320:**374–378.

Collado-Vides, J., B. Magasanik, and J. D. Gralla. 1991. Control site location and transcriptional regulation in *Escherichia coli*. *Microbiol. Rev.* **55:**371–394.

Delgado, A., and J. L. Ramos. 1994. Genetic evidence for activation of the positive transcriptional regulator XylR, a member of the NtrC family of regulators, by effector binding. *J. Biol. Chem.* **266:**8059–8062.

Delgado, A., R. Salto, S. Marqués, and J. L. Ramos. 1995. Single amino acid changes in the signal receptor domain of XylR resulted in mutants that stimulate transcription in the absence of effectors. *J. Biol. Chem.* **270:**5144–5150.

de Lorenzo, V., M. Herrero, M. Metzke, and K. N. Timmis. 1991. An upstream *xylR* and IHF induced nucleoprotein complex regulates the sigma-54 dependent Pu promoter of TOL plasmid. *EMBO J.* **10:**1159–1167.

Duetz, W. A., S. Marqués, C. de Jong, J. L. Ramos, and J. G. van Andel. 1994. Inducibility of the TOL catabolic pathway in *Pseudomonas putida* (pWW0) growing on succinate in continuous culture: evidence of carbon catabolite repression control. *J. Bacteriol.* **176:**2354–2361.

Fernández, S., J. Pérez-Martín, and V. de Lorenzo. 1995. Activation of the transcriptional regulator XylR of *Pseudomonas putida* by release of intramolecular repression between functional domains. *Mol. Microbiol.* **16:**205–213.

Franklin, F. C. H., M. Bagdasarian, M. M. Bagdasarian, and K. N. Timmis. 1981. Molecular and functional analysis of the TOL plasmid pWW0 from *Pseudomonas putida* and cloning of genes for the entire regulated aromatic ring *meta*-cleavage pathway. *Proc. Natl. Acad. Sci. USA* **78:**7458–7462.

Franklin, F. C. H., P. R. Lehrbach, R. Lurz, B. Rueckert, M. Bagdasarian, and K. N. Timmis. 1983. Localization and functional analysis of transposon mutations in regulatory genes of the TOL catabolic pathway. *J. Bacteriol.* **154:**676–685.

Gallegos, M. T., S. Marqués, and J. L. Ramos. 1996. Expression of the TOL plasmid *xyRS* gene in *Pseudomonas putida* occurs from a σ^{70}-dependent promoter or from σ^{70}- and σ^{54}-dependent tandem promoters according to the compound used for growth. *J. Bacteriol.* **178:**2356–2361.

Gallegos, M. T., C. Michán, and J. L. Ramos. 1993. The XylS/AraC family of regulators. *Nucleic Acids Res.* **21:**807–810.

Gomada, M., S. Inouye, H. Imanishi, A. Nakazawa, and T. Nakazawa. 1992. Analysis of an upstream regulatory sequence required for activation of the regulatory gene *xylS* in xylene metabolism directed by the TOL plasmid of *Pseudomonas putida*. *Mol. Gen. Genet.* **233:**419–426.

Harayama, S., P. R. Lehrbach, and K. N. Timmis. 1984. Transposon mutagenesis analysis of the *meta*-cleavage pathway operon genes of the TOL plasmid of *Pseudomonas putida* mt-2. *J. Bacteriol.* **160:**251–255.

Harayama, S., and M. Rekik. 1990. The *meta* cleavage operon of TOL degradative plasmid pWW0 comprises 13 genes. *Mol. Gen. Genet.* **221:**113–120.

Harayama, S., M. Rekik, M. Wubbolts, K. Rose, R. A. Leppik, and K. N. Timmis. 1989. Characterization of five genes in the upper-pathway operon of TOL plasmid of pWW0 from *Pseudomonas putida* and identification of the gene products. *J. Bacteriol.* **171:**5048–5055.

Holtel, A., M. A. Abril, S. Marqués, K. N. Timmis, and J. L. Ramos. 1990. Promoter-upstream activator sequences are required for expression of the *xylS* gene and upper-pathway operon on the *Pseudomonas* TOL plasmid. *Mol. Microbiol.* **4:**1551–1556.

Holtel, A., D. Goldenberg, H. Giladi, A. B. Oppennheim, and K. N. Timmis. 1995. Involvement of IHF protein in expression of the Ps promoter of the *Pseudomonas putida* TOL plasmid. *J. Bacteriol.* **177:**331–335.

Holtel, A., S. Marqués, I. Möhler, U. Jakubzik, and K. N. Timmis. 1994. Carbon source-dependent inhibition of *xyl* operon expression of the *Pseudomonas putida* TOL plasmid. *J. Bacteriol.* **176:**1773–1776.

Holtel, A., K. N. Timmis, and J. L. Ramos. 1992. Upstream binding sequences of the XylR activator protein and integration host factor in the *xylS* gene promoter region of the *Pseudomonas* TOL plasmid. *Nucleic Acids Res.* **20:**1755–1762.

Inouye, S., Y. Ebina, A. Nakazawa, and T. Nakazawa. 1984a. Nucleotide sequence surrounding transcription initiation site of *xylABC* operon on TOL plasmid of *Pseudomonas putida. Proc. Natl. Acad. Sci. USA* **81:**1688–1691.

Inouye, S., M. Gomada, U. M. X. Sangodkar, A. Nakazawa, and T. Nakazawa. 1990. Upstream regulatory sequence for transcriptional activator *xylR* in the first operon of xylene metabolism on the TOL plasmid. *J. Mol. Biol.* **216:**251–260.

Inouye, S., A. Nakazawa, and T. Nakazawa. 1981. Molecular cloning of *xylS* gene of the TOL plasmid: evidence for positive regulation of the *xylDEGF* operon by *xylS*. *J. Bacteriol.* **148:**413–418.

Inouye, S., A. Nakazawa, and T. Nakazawa. 1984b. Nucleotide sequence of the promoter region of the *xylDEFG* operon on TOL plasmid of *Pseudomonas putida. Gene* **29:**323–330.

Inouye, S., A. Nakazawa, and T. Nakazawa. 1986. Nucleotide sequence of the regulatory gene *xylS* on the *Pseudomonas putida* TOL plasmid and identification of the protein product. *Gene* **44:**235–242.

Inouye, S., A. Nakazawa, and T. Nakazawa. 1987a. Expression of the regulatory gene *xylS* on the TOL plasmid is positively controlled by the *xylR* gene product. *Proc. Natl. Acad. Sci. USA* **84:**5182–5186.

Inouye, S., A. Nakazawa, and T. Nakazawa. 1987b. Overproduction of the *xylS* gene product and activation of the *xylDLEGF* operon on the TOL plasmid. *J. Bacteriol.* **169:**3587–3592.

Inouye, S., A. Nakazawa, and T. Nakazawa. 1988. Nucleotide sequence of the regulatory gene *xylR* of the TOL plasmid from *Pseudomonas putida. Gene* **66:**301–306.

Kessler, B., V. De Lorenzo, and K. N. Timmis. 1993. Identification of a *cis*-acting sequence within the Pm promoter of the TOL plasmid which confers XylS-mediated responsiveness to substituted benzoates. *J. Mol. Biol.* **230:**699–703.

Köhler, T., S. Harayama, J. L. Ramos, and K. N. Timmis. 1989. Involvement of *Pseudomonas putida* rpoN sigma factor in regulation of various metabolic functions. *J. Bacteriol.* **171:**4326–4333.

Marqués, S., M. T. Gallegos, and J. L. Ramos. 1995. Role of sigma-S in transcription stimulation from the positively controlled Pm promoter of the TOL plasmid of *Pseudomonas putida. Mol. Microbiol.* **18:**851–857.

Marqués, S., A. Holtel, K. N. Timmis, and J. L. Ramos. 1994. Transcriptional pathways of the TOL plasmid pWW0 of *Pseudomonas putida* for metabolism of aromatics. *J. Bacteriol.* **176:**2517–2524.

Marqués, S., J. L. Ramos, and K. N. Timmis. 1993. Analysis of the mRNA structure of the *Pseudomonas putida* TOL *meta* fission pathway operon around the transcription initiation point at the *xylE* gene. Evidence for endonucleolytic cleavage. *Biochim. Biophys. Acta* **1216:**227–236.

Mermod, M., P. R. Lehrbach, W. Reineke, and K. N. Timmis. 1984. Transcription of the TOL plasmid toluate catabolic pathway operon of *Pseudomonas putida* is determined by a pair of co-ordinately and positively regulated overlapping promoters. *EMBO J.* **3:**2461–2466.

Mermod, N., J. L. Ramos, A. Bairoch, and K. N. Timmis. 1987. The *xylS* gene positive regulator of TOL plasmid pWW0: identification, sequence analysis and overproduction leading to constitutive expression of the *meta* cleavage operon. *Mol. Gen. Genet.* **235:**406–412.

Michán, C., L. Zhou, M. T. Gallegos, K. N. Timmis, and J. L. Ramos. 1992. Identification of critical amino-terminal regions of XylS: the positive regulator encoded by the TOL plasmid. *J. Biol. Chem.* **267:**22897–22901.

Ninfa, A. J., and B. Magasanik. 1986. Covalent modification of the *glnG* product NRI, by the *glnL* product, NRII, regulates the transcription of the *glnALG* operon in *Escherichia coli. Proc. Natl. Acad. Sci. USA* **83:**5909–5913.

North, A., K. E. Klose, K. M. Stedman, and S. Kustu. 1993. Prokaryotic-enhancer-binding proteins reflect eukaryotic-like modularity: the puzzle of nitrogen regulatory protein NtrC. *J. Bacteriol.* **175:**4267–4273.

Pérez-Martín, J., and V. de Lorenzo. Integration host factor suppresses promiscuous activation in the σ^{54}-dependent promoter Pu of *Pseudomonas putida. Proc. Natl. Acad. Sci. USA*, in press.

Pérez-Martín, J., and V. de Lorenzo. 1995. The σ^{54}-dependent promoter Ps of the TOL plasmid of *Pseudomonas putida* requires HU for transcriptional activation in vivo by XylR. *J. Bacteriol.* **177:**3758–3763.

Pérez-Martín, J., K. N. Timmis, and V. de Lorenzo. 1994. Co-regulation by bent DNA. Functional substitutions of the integration host factor site at σ^{54}-dependent promoter Pu of the upper-TOL operon by intrinsically curved sequences. *J. Biol. Chem.* **269:**22657–22662.

Ramos, J. L., N. Mermod, and K. N. Timmis. 1987. Regulatory circuits controlling transcription of TOL plasmid operon encoding *meta*-cleavage pathway for degradation of alkylbenzoates by *Pseudomonas. Mol. Microbiol.* **1:**293–300.

Ramos, J. L. C. Michán, F. Rojo, D. Dwyer, and K. N. Timmis. 1990. Signal-regulator interactions. Genetic analysis of the effector binding site of *xylS*, the benzoate-activated positive regulator of *Pseudomonas* TOL plasmid *meta*-cleavage pathway operon. *J. Mol. Biol.* **211:**373–382.

Ramos, J. L., A. Stolz, W. Reineke, and K. N. Timmis. 1986. Altered effector specificities in regulators of gene expression: TOL plasmid XylS mutants and their use to engineer expansion of the range of aromatics degraded by bacteria. *Proc. Natl. Acad. Sci. USA* **83:**8467–8471.

Shingler, V., M. Bartilson, and T. Moore. 1993. Cloning and nucleotide sequence of the positive regulator, DmpR, of the phenol catabolic pathway of pVI150: a member of the NtrC family of transcriptional activators. *J. Bacteriol.* **175:**1596–1604.

Shingler, V., and T. Moore. 1994. Sensing of aromatic compounds by the DmpR transcriptional activator of phenol-catabolizing *Pseudomonas* sp. strain CF600. *J. Bacteriol.* **176:**1555–1560.

Spooner, R. A., K. Lindsay, and F. C. H. Franklin. 1986. Genetic, functional and sequence analysis of the *xylR* and *xylS* regulatory genes of the TOL plasmid pWW0. *J. Gen. Microbiol.* **132:**1347–1358.

Williams, P. A., and K. Murray. 1974. Metabolism of benzoate and the methylbenzoates by *Pseudomonas putida (arvilla)* mt-2: evidence for the existence of a TOL plasmid. *J. Bacteriol.* **120:**416–423.

Worsey, M. J., F. C. H. Franklin, and P. A. Williams. 1978. Regulation of the degradative pathway enzymes coded for by the TOL plasmid (pWW0) from *Pseudomonas putida* mt-2. *J. Bacteriol.* **134:**757–764.

Worsey, M. J., and P. A. Williams. 1975. Metabolism of toluene and xylenes by *Pseudomonas putida (arvilla)* mt-2: evidence for a new function of the TOL plasmid. *J. Bacteriol.* **124:**7–13.

Zhou, L., K. N. Timmis, and J. L. Ramos. 1990. Mutations leading to constitutive expression from the TOL plasmid *meta*-cleavage pathway operon are located at the C-terminal end of the positive regulator protein XylS. *J. Bacteriol.* **172:**3707–3710.

Section IV

DYNAMIC FEATURES OF PSEUDOMONADS

Molecular Biology of Pseudomonads
Edited by T. Nakazawa et al.

Chapter 18

Catabolic Transposons in Pseudomonads

Masataka Tsuda

Pseudomonads and their relatives are known for their powerful catabolism of a number of natural and xenobiotic organic compounds. Extensive biochemical and genetic studies of many catabolic pathways for various aromatics have illustrated the flexibility of these pathways at the level of gene clusters (Chaudhry and Chapalamadugu, 1991; Harayama et al., 1992; van der Meer et al., 1992; Williams and Sayers, 1994). Very similar catabolic gene clusters are widely distributed on a variety of plasmids and on the chromosomes of different bacterial species, implying that these catabolic gene clusters, which presumably have common origins, must have become broadly disseminated in the natural environment (Assinder and Williams, 1990; Boronin, 1992; Yen and Serdar, 1988). Such catabolic gene clusters can also undergo various types of genetic rearrangements, including deletion, duplication, inversion, or insertion into other replicons. These rearrangement events are easily detected at high frequencies during the bacterial adaptive response by which organisms acquire novel catabolic activities (van der Meer et al., 1992), and such rearrangements may have played important roles in the evolution of catabolic pathways. I have been focusing my studies on insertion events of the catabolic gene clusters of three plasmids from *Pseudomonas putida*.

CLASS II TRANSPOSONS

Insertions of bacterial genes and gene clusters into other replicons are often mediated by transposons, which are discrete DNA segments able to move even in the absence of genetic homology between the donor and target sites (Berg and Howe, 1989). Many bacterial transposons belong to the class II (Tn*3*-like) transposons, and they commonly (i) lead to a 5-bp duplication of the target sequence after transposition, (ii) carry short (<50-bp) terminal inverted repeats (IRs) and an *res* region that is required during transposition, and (iii) transpose by a two-step process (Fig. 1A; Grinsted et al., 1990). In the first step of transposition, the transposase (TnpA) recognizes the IRs and catalyzes formation of the cointegrate of the donor and target DNA molecules connected by two directly repeated copies of the transposon, one at each junction. In the second step, the

Masataka Tsuda • Department of Biology, Faculty of Science, Okayama University, Okayama 700, Japan.

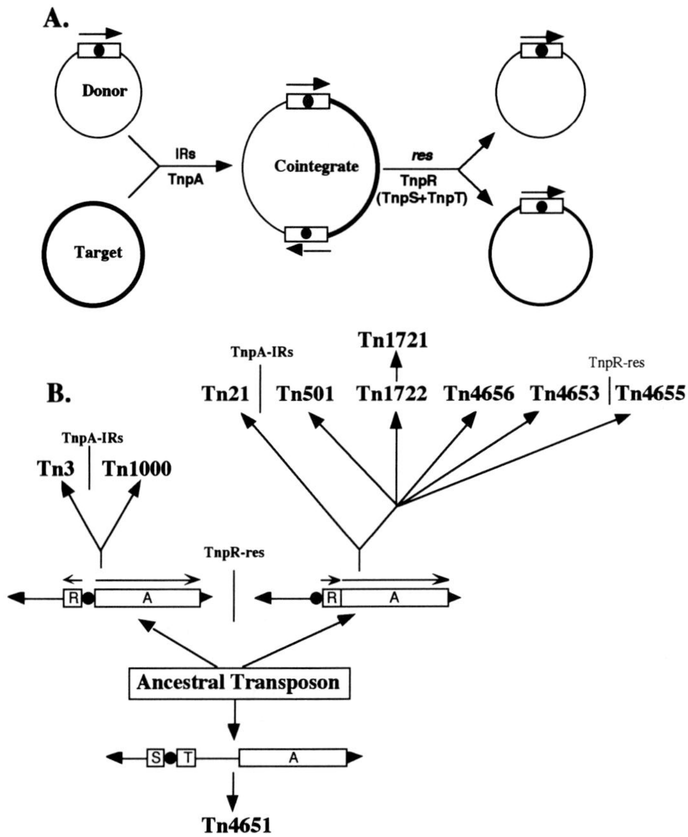

Figure 1. Basic transposition mechanism of class II transposons (A) and their phylogenetic tree, with an emphasis on catabolic transposons (B). Boxes in panel A denote transposons, and their orientations on the replicons are shown by arrows. The basis of categorization of the class II transposons in panel B is indicated above the vertical bar. ●, *res* region; A, *tnpA;* R, S, and T, genes for resolution. Tn*501* and Tn*1721* encode the resistance determinants for mercuric ion and tetracycline, respectively (Fig. 3; Grinsted et al., 1990).

resolvase (TnpR) catalyzes the site-specific resolution of the cointegrate between the two *res* regions. The class II transposons can be divided into several subgroups that are to some extent related to one another. Members of each subgroup share highly conserved structures in the genes and sites required for transposition and show interchangeability in their transposition functions. These properties allow one to draw a phylogenetic tree for class II transposons (Fig. 1B).

TRANSPOSONS ON PLASMID pWW0

Among the TOL plasmids responsible for catabolism of toluene, pWW0 from *P. putida* mt-2 has been most extensively characterized (van der Meer et al., 1992).

This 117-kb plasmid is transmissible and belongs to a broad-host-range incompatibility (IncP-9) group of plasmids. The toluene-degrading (*xyl*) genes on pWW0 are clustered into two operons: the upper pathway operon for conversion of toluene to benzoate and the *meta*-pathway operon for channeling benzoate through catechol to the tricarboxylic acid cycle (Fig. 2). Expression of both operons is controlled positively by the two regulatory gene products XylR and XylS. Many groups have recorded the insertion of the *xyl* gene cluster into other replicons, leading to the proposal that this *xyl* gene cluster must be on one or more transposons. This proposal has not been proven, since (i) the *xyl* inserts vary in length from 56 to 104 kb, and (ii) strains in which these insertions are detected are *recA*$^+$.

Our use of *Escherichia coli recA* mutant strains provided definite evidence to support the proposal just outlined (Tsuda and Iino, 1987, 1988; Tsuda et al., 1989). All of the *xyl* genes on pWW0 are located in a 56-kb transposon, Tn*4651*, that is included within another 70-kb transposon, Tn*4653* (Fig. 3 and Table 1). The two transposons can apparently move independently and have properties that are characteristic of class II transposons. Tn*4651* carries a complete set of transposition functions that are not interchangeable with those of other class II transposons. The Tn*4651*-encoded resolution system is markedly different from those of the usual class II transposons. The 2.2-kb DNA segment containing the *res* region is located 48 kb away from the *tnpA* gene and encodes the two uncharacterized products TnpS and TnpT, both of which are required for resolution. On the basis of these properties, Tn*4651* is considered to belong to a novel subgroup of the class II transposons (Grinsted et al., 1990).

Tn*4653* encodes its own transposase, which is not interchangeable with the Tn*4651* transposase, ensuring independent cointegration of the two transposons. The Tn*4653* transposase is instead interchangeable with those of the Tn*1722* subgroup transposons (Fig. 1B). Consistent with this, the structures of the IRs of Tn*4653* and other Tn*1722* subgroup transposons are highly conserved (Allmeier et al., 1992). Upstream of its *tnpA* gene, Tn*4653* carries a functional *tnpR* gene that is able to complement the *tnpR* muta-

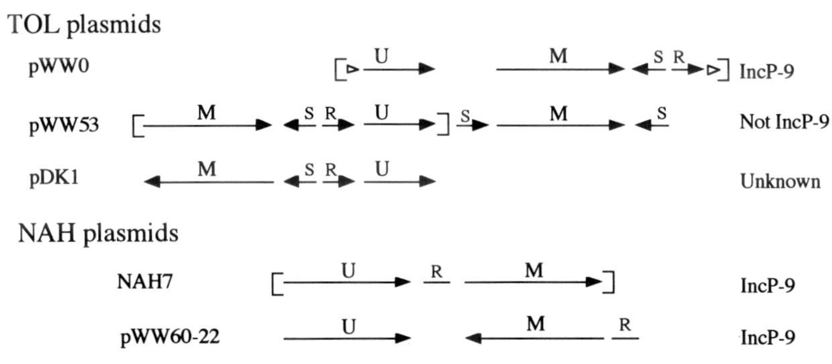

Figure 2. Various TOL and NAH plasmids. U, upper pathway operon; M, *meta*-pathway operon; R, *xylR* for TOL plasmids and *nahR* for NAH plasmids; S, *xylS;* open arrowhead, IS*1246*. The gene cluster in a transposon is bracketed by parentheses. The incompatibility group of the plasmid is shown at the right of each map (Assinder and Williams, 1988; Boronin, 1992; Williams et al., 1992).

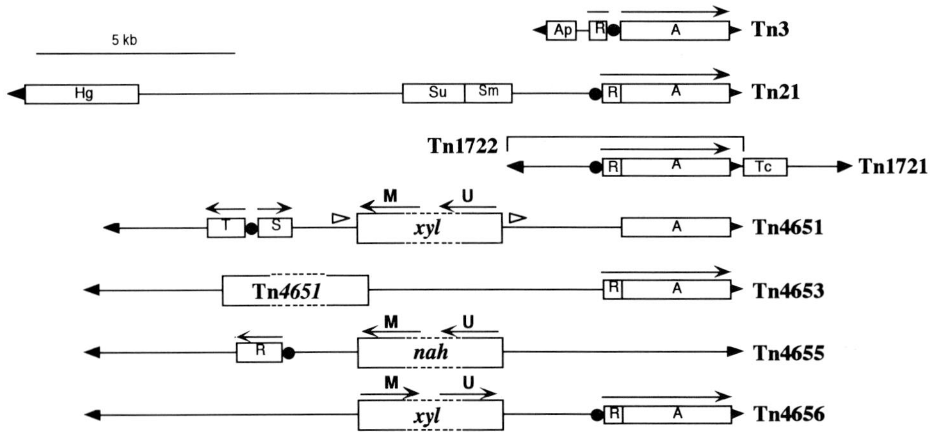

Figure 3. Structures of class II transposons with emphasis on catabolic transposons. Resistance determinants: Ap, ampicillin; Hg, mercuric ion; Sm, streptomycin; Su, sulfonamide; Tc, tetracycline. Other abbreviations and symbols are the same as those in Fig. 1 and 2.

tions in Tn*1722*, and the Tn*4653* and Tn*1722* resolvases are identical in amino acid sequence (Grinsted et al., 1990). Resolution of the Tn*4653*-mediated cointegrate, however, depends on the Tn*4651*-specified resolution system. The inability of the Tn*4653* resolvase to participate in resolution is caused by a defect in the *res* region that is located upstream of the *tnpR* gene. The Tn*4653 res* region lacks a 30-bp sequence (site I) that contains the crossover site absolutely required for resolution of the cointegrate (Allmeier et al., 1992).

A specific 39-kb fragment containing the *xyl* gene cluster in Tn*4651* is lost at a high frequency (Fig. 2; Assinder and Williams, 1990). This deletion is mediated by reciprocal recombination between the directly repeated copies of an identical 1,275-bp sequence (Reddy et al., 1994). This sequence is related to some insertion sequence (IS) elements and is thus termed IS*1246*. The deleted region does not carry additional genes or sites for transposition of Tn*4651* or Tn*4653*.

Table 1. Toluene and naphthalene transposons

Transposon	Plasmid	Marker	Size (kb)	Size of IRs (bp)	Cointegration[a]	Resolution[a]	Remarks
Tn*4651*	pWW0	Toluene	56	46	*tnpA*[b]	*tnpS-res-tnpT*[b]	Within Tn*4653*
Tn*4653*	pWW0	Toluene	70	38	*tnpA* (Tn*1722*)	*tnpR* (Tn*1722*)	Defect in *res*
Tn*4656*	pWW53	Toluene	39	38	*tnpA* (Tn*1722*)	*res-tnpR* (Tn*1722*)	DNA rearrangement?
Tn*4655*	NAH7	Naphthalene	38	38	None (Tn*1722*)	*res-tnpR*[b]	Defect in *tnpA* Site-specific integrase

[a]Transposons whose transposition functions are exchangeable are indicated in parentheses. See text for details.
[b]Novel transposon-specific function.

Transposition of Tn*4651* or Tn*4653* explains most of the recorded insertions of the *xyl* gene cluster into various chromosomes and into other resistance and catabolic plasmids (Assinder and Williams, 1990; Jahnke et al., 1993; Sinclair et al., 1986; Sinclair and Holloway, 1991; Wyndham et al., 1994). Two other *xyl*-containing regions on pWW0 have been reported to be inserted into resistance plasmids (Lehrbach et al., 1982). One endpoint of each insert appears to be identical to the *tnpA*-proximal end of Tn*4651* or Tn*4653*, and these two insertion events may have resulted from "imprecise" transposition (Grinsted et al., 1990) with involvement of the Tn*4651*- or Tn*4653*-encoded transposition machinery.

TRANSPOSON ON PLASMID NAH7

A transmissible 83-kb plasmid, NAH7, from *P. putida* PpG7 is involved in naphthalene catabolism (Fig. 2; Yen and Serdar, 1988). The *nah* genes for naphthalene catabolism are organized into two operons: the upper pathway operon for conversion of naphthalene to salicylate and the *meta*-pathway operon for channeling salicylate through catechol to the tricarboxylic acid cycle. A positive regulatory gene, *nahR*, is required for expression of both operons. NAH7 is closely related to pWW0: (i) it has a highly conserved organization of the gene clusters for catabolism of catechol, (ii) it belongs to the IncP-9 group of plasmids, and (iii) it shows a high degree of DNA homology in the regions encoding replication and transfer functions (Lehrbach et al., 1983; Yen and Serdar, 1988).

Analysis in *E. coli recA* mutants demonstrated that the *nah* gene cluster on NAH7 resides on a 38-kb class II transposon, Tn*4655* (Fig. 3 and Table 1; Tsuda and Iino, 1990). Tn*4655* is defective in the cointegration step and is able to move only in the presence of a complementing transposase from other Tn*1722* subgroup transposons (Fig. 1). The Tn*4655* IRs share extensive sequence similarity with the IRs of Tn*4653* and Tn*1722*, and the sequence conservation between the left ends of Tn*4655* and Tn*4653* continues for more than 600 bp. Sequence conservation at their right ends is limited to a 49-bp stretch, and Tn*4655* lacks the DNA fragment homologous to the *res-tnpR-tnpA* cluster of Tn*4653*. Tn*4655* instead encodes its own resolution function that is not interchangeable with those encoded by other class II transposons. Sequence analysis (M. Tsuda, unpublished data) clearly places the Tn*4655* TnpR protein into the integrase family of site-specific recombinases but not the resolvase family (Berg and Howe, 1989; Abremski and Hoess, 1992). Distinct from the resolvase family, the integrase family is able to catalyze both integration and resolution reactions. The Tn*4655* TnpR protein has been demonstrated experimentally to have site-specific integrase activity (Tsuda, unpublished data).

Plasmid SAL1 from another *P. putida* strain carries a set of salicylate-degrading (*sal*) genes (Chakrabarty et al., 1978). Since SAL1 is considered to be a mutant of NAH7 bearing a substitution of a small DNA fragment in the upper pathway operon (Lehrbach et al., 1983; Yen and Serdar, 1988), it seems most likely that the *sal* gene cluster also resides on a transposon closely related to Tn*4655*. This situation easily accounts for insertion of the *sal* gene cluster into a resistance plasmid with a Tn*4653* insert. The Tn*4653* transposase must have helped the defective Tn*4655*-like element to transpose onto this resistance plasmid.

TRANSPOSON DERIVED FROM PLASMID pWW53

A 107-kb plasmid, pWW53, is a nontransmissible TOL plasmid residing in a *P. putida* strain, MT53 (Fig. 2; Assinder and Williams, 1990; Williams et al., 1992). The four types of the *xyl* transcriptional units are highly conserved between pWW53 and pWW0. pWW53 is different from pWW0 in the copy numbers of the four transcriptional units as well as in their relative order and orientation. There are two nearly identical copies of the *meta*-pathway operon and three copies of the *xylS* homolog on pWW53.

Keil et al. (1985) isolated pWW53-4, a resistance plasmid that had received the four *xyl* transcriptional units of pWW53. We demonstrated that a 39-kb insert in pWW53-4 is a Tn*1722* subgroup transposon, Tn*4656* (Fig. 3 and Table 1; Tsuda, unpublished data). The pWW53 genome carries a single contiguous piece of DNA that corresponds to the 35-kb portion of Tn*4656* to the left of its *res* region. However, the remaining 4-kb segment of Tn*4656* carrying the *res-tnpR-tnpA*-IR cluster was not present at its expected position on pWW53, that is, at the position between the upper pathway operon and the second *meta*-pathway operon not incorporated into Tn*4656* (Fig. 2). One attractive hypothesis to explain this paradox is in vivo assembly of the pWW53-derived *xyl* gene cluster with a 4-kb segment that exists elsewhere in MT53. Our preliminary result indicates the presence of an *res*-like sequence at the right end of the 35-kb segment on pWW53, suggesting involvement of site-specific recombination in assembly of the two physically separated segments (Tsuda, unpublished data). Investigation of the original location of the 4-kb segment in MT53 will shed light on the mechanism that gave rise to Tn*4656*.

EVOLUTION OF CATABOLIC TRANSPOSONS

Our assignment of Tn*4653* and Tn*4655* to the Tn*1722* subgroup suggests that the two catabolic transposons have evolved from a common ancestor. Both transposons are present on IncP-9 plasmids, and indistinguishable replication and transfer functions are specified by the 45- to 47-kb "backbone" regions of pWW0 and NAH7 that are outside of Tn*4653* and Tn*4655*, respectively. These backbone regions also have considerable structural conservation (Lehrbach et al., 1983). A common primordial IncP-9 plasmid may have been the target replicon for insertion of Tn*4653* and Tn*4655*, both of which might have been established in other replicons. Alternatively, the ancestral transposon inserted on the original IncP-9 plasmid may have evolved divergently to form the current structures of pWW0 and NAH7. In either of these plausible situations, it is most probable that the ancestral transposon underwent different types of DNA rearrangements. Evolution to form Tn*4655* possibly involved (i) removal of the *res-tnpR-tnpA* cluster from the ancestral transposon, (ii) insertion of a novel resolution system having an integrase activity, and (iii) incorporation of the *nah* gene cluster, while formation of Tn*4653* could have been associated with removal of part of the *res* region in the ancestral transposon and insertion of another unrelated class II transposon, Tn*4651*, or its ancestral transposon.

The *xyl* gene cluster in Tn*4651* is, as described above, flanked by the direct repeats of IS*1246*. One copy of IS*1246*, fortuitously present on the ancestral transposon, may have provided the homologous sequence to permit acquisition of another copy of IS*1246* along with its adjacent *xyl* gene cluster. Dehò et al. (1995) compared the organization of the pWW0-encoded, toluene-degrading genes with that of the genes encoded by the chromosome of *P. putida* TMB, and they proposed that the replicative transposition of IS*1246* might have been involved in incorporation of the *xyl* gene cluster into the ancestral transposon of Tn*4651*. Unfortunately, no experimental evidence has yet been obtained for transposition of IS*1246* or transposition of the *xyl* gene cluster flanked by the two copies of IS*1246*.

To date, a number of TOL and NAH plasmids that belong to different incompatibility groups have been reported, and several plasmids, including pWW53, differ from pWW0 and NAH7 in their copy numbers and the relative orientations of the three to four transcriptional units of the *xyl* and *nah* operons (Fig. 2; Assinder and Williams, 1990; Boronin, 1992; Williams et al., 1992; Williams and Sayers, 1994; Yen and Serdar, 1988). Some *Pseudomonas* strains in which the upper and *meta*-pathway operons are separately encoded on different replicons, one on the chromosome and the other on a plasmid, have also been isolated. On the basis of these observations, it has been proposed that the current state in each replicon of the gene cluster for complete catabolism of toluene or naphthalene must have been established after successive assembly of the three or four separate catabolic DNA modules (the upper pathway operon, the *meta*-pathway operon, and the block of regulatory gene[s]) in an unknown order (van der Meer et al., 1992; Williams and Sayers, 1994). Comparison of various resistance plasmids led to identification of a group of mobile DNA elements, termed integrons (Hall and Collis, 1995). These mobile elements are responsible for the site-specific integration of defined gene cassettes into other specific regions, thus contributing to wide variation in the resistance markers associated with different plasmids. Movement of these integrons is mediated by the site-specific recombinases belonging to the integrase family. Since the Tn*4655* resolvase is a member of the integrase family, it is of interest to establish whether an integron is involved in the insertion events of the presumptive catabolic DNA modules to form Tn*4655*.

Some other catabolic genes were recently demonstrated to reside on transposons (Table 2; Wyndham et al., 1994). The chlorobenzoate transposon (Tn*5271*) and the chlorobenzene transposon (Tn*5280*) carry only parts of the catabolic pathway genes, and complete catabolism of the initial substrates therefore requires additional genes located outside of these transposons (Nakatsu et al. 1991; van der Meer et al., 1991). These two transposons are distinct from the toluene and naphthalene transposons in that the former two are the composite transposons flanked by two identical copies of IS elements. Fortuitous insertion of two copies of an IS element may have given rise to each composite transposon (Berg and Howe, 1989). The genes for catabolism of nylon oligomers and halogenated alkanoates are located on such IS-composite-type transposon structures, although their transposition activity has not yet been proven (Kato et al., 1994; Kawasaki et al., 1992).

A number of catabolic genes that exhibit the properties of transposons have been recorded but not yet characterized sufficiently (van der Meer et al., 1992; Yen and Serdar, 1988; Williams et al., 1992; Williams and Sayers, 1994; Wyndham et al., 1994), and many more catabolic transposons may well be identified in the near future. The combination of transposons with plasmids plays a major role in the rapid dissemination and evolution of antibiotic and heavy-metal resistance markers in the clinical environment (Amábile-Cuevas and Chicurel, 1992), and catabolic genes would play that role in the natural environment. The dynamic adaptability of catabolic gene clusters is also medi-

Table 2. Other catabolic transposons

Transposon	Size (kb)	Marker	Genus	Location	Class	Remarks	References
Known class							
Tn*951*	16.6	Lactose	*Yersinia*	Plasmid	II	Defect in *tnpA*	Michiels et al., 1987
Tn*3411*	7.4	Citrate	*Escherichia*	Plasmid	I[a]	IS*3411* (1.3 kb, direct)	Ishiguro and Sato, 1988
Tn*5271*	17	Chlorobenzoate	*Alcaligenes*	Plasmid	I[a]	IS*1071* (3.2 kb, direct)	Nakatsu et al., 1991
Tn*5280*	5.1	Chlorobenzene	*Pseudomonas*	Plasmid	I[a]	IS*1066* (1.1 kb, direct)	van der Meer et al., 1991
Tn*5276*	70	Sucrose	*Lactococcus*	Chromosome	Conjugative		Rauch and de Vos, 1992
Unknown class							
Tn*5272*	ND[b]	Chlorobenzoate	*Pseudomonas*	Plasmid		Covering Tn*5271*	Wyndham et al., 1994
Tn*4371*	60	Chlorobiphenyl	*Alcaligenes*	Chromosome			Springael et al., 1993
Tn*4372*	60	Chlorobiphenyl	*Alcaligenes*	Chromosome			Springael et al., 1994

[a] IS composite transposon.
[b] Not described.

ated by (i) accumulation of point mutations followed by gene conversion and (ii) duplication of a gene cluster followed by acquisition of mutations in one of the copies (van der Meer et al., 1992; Williams et al., 1992; Williams and Sayers, 1994). In the natural environment, all of these mechanisms presumably act in concert and contribute to the dynamic rearrangement and evolution of catabolic genes in pseudomonads and their relatives.

REFERENCES

Abremski, K. E., and R. H. Hoess. 1992. Evidence for a second conserved arginine residue in the integrase family of recombination proteins. *Protein Eng.* **5:**87–91.

Allmeier, H., B. Cresnar, M. Greck, and R. Schmitt. 1992. Complete nucleotide sequence of Tn*1721*: gene organization and a novel gene product with features of a chemotaxis protein. *Gene* **111:**11–20.

Amábile-Cuevas, C. F., and M. E. Chicurel. 1992. Bacterial plasmids and gene flux. *Cell* **70:**189–199.

Assinder, S. J., and P. A. Williams. 1988. Comparison of the *meta* pathway operons on NAH plasmid pWW60-22 and TOL plasmid pWW53-4 and its evolutionary significance. *J. Gen. Microbiol.* **134:**2769–2778.

Assinder, S. J., and P. A. Williams. 1990. The TOL plasmids: determinants of the catabolism of toluene and the xylenes. *Adv. Microb. Physiol.* **31:**1–69.

Berg, D. E., and M. M. Howe (ed.). 1989. *Mobile DNA*. American Society for Microbiology, Washington, D.C.

Boronin, A. M. 1992. Diversity and relationships of *Pseudomonas* plasmids, p. 329–340. *In* E. Galli, S. Silver, and B. Witholt (ed.), *Pseudomonas: Molecular Biology and Biotechnology*. American Society for Microbiology, Washington, D.C.

Chakrabarty, A. M., D. A. Friello, and L. H. Bopp. 1978. Transposition of plasmid DNA segments specifying hydrocarbon degradation and their expression in various microorganisms. *Proc. Natl. Acad. Sci. USA* **75:**3109–3112.

Chaudhry, G. R., and S. Chapalamadugu. 1991. Biodegradation of halogenated organic compounds. *Microbiol. Rev.* **55:**59–79.

Dehò, G., C. Bernasconi, N. Passini, R. Favaro, M. L. Giorello, P. Castelli, G. Bestetti, and E. Gali. 1995. Gene organization and control of a catabolic operon in *Pseudomonas putida* TMB, p. 116. *Abstr. 5th Int. Symp. Pseudomonas.*

Grinsted, J., F. de la Cruz, and R. Schmitt. 1990. The Tn*21* subgroup of bacterial transposable elements. *Plasmid* **24:**163–189.

Hall, R. M., and C. M. Collis. 1995. Mobile gene cassettes and integrons: capture and spread of genes by site-specific recombination. *Mol. Microbiol.* **15:**593–600.

Harayama, S., M. Kok, and E. L. Neidle. 1992. Functional and evolutionary relationships among diverse oxygenases. *Annu. Rev. Microbiol.* **46:**565–601.

Ishiguro, N., and G. Sato. 1988. Nucleotide sequence of insertion sequence IS*3411*, which flanks the citrate utilization determinant of transposon Tn*3411*. *J. Bacteriol.* **170:**1902–1906.

Jahnke, M., F. Lehmann, A. Schoebel, and G. Auling. 1993. Transposition of the TOL catabolic genes (Tn*4651*) into the degradative plasmid pSAH of *Alcaligenes* sp. O-1 ensures simultaneous mineralization of sulpho- and methyl-substituted aromatics. *J. Gen. Microbiol.* **139:**1959–1966.

Kato, K., K. Ohtsuki, H. Mitsuda, T. Yomo, S. Negoro, and I. Urabe. 1994. Insertion sequence IS*6100* on plasmid pOAD2, which degrades nylon oligomers. *J. Bacteriol.* **176:**1197–1200.

Kawasaki, H., K. Tsuda, I. Matsushita, and K. Tonomura. 1992. Lack of homology between two haloacetate dehalogenase genes encoded on a plasmid from *Moraxella* sp. strain B. *J. Gen. Microbiol.* **138:**1317–1323.

Keil, H., S. Keil, R. W. Pickup, and P. A. Williams. 1985. Evolutionary conservation of genes coding for *meta* pathway enzymes within TOL plasmids pWW0 and pWW53. *J. Bacteriol.* **164:**887–895.

Lehrbach, P. R., I. McGregor, J. M. Ward, and P. Broda. 1983. Molecular relationships between *Pseudomonas* IncP-9 plasmids TOL, NAH, and SAL. *Plasmid* **10:**164–174.

Lehrbach, P. R., J. Ward, P. Meulien, and P. Broda. 1982. Physical mapping of TOL plasmids pWW0 and pND2 and various R plasmid-TOL derivatives from *Pseudomonas* spp. *J. Bacteriol.* **152:**1280–1283.

Michiels, T., G. Cornelis, K. Ellis, and J. Grinsted. 1987. Tn*2501*, a component of the lactose transposon Tn*951*, is an example of a new category of class II transposable elements. *J. Bacteriol.* **169:**624–631.

Nakatsu, C., J. Ng, R. Singh, N. Straus, and C. Wyndham. 1991. Chlorobenzoate catabolic transposon Tn*5271* is a composite class I element with flanking class II insertion sequences. *Proc. Natl. Acad. Sci. USA* **88:**8312–8316.

Rauch, P. J. G., and W. M. de Vos. 1992. Characterization of the novel nisin-sucrose conjugative transposon Tn*5276* and its insertion in *Lactococcus lactis. J. Bacteriol.* **170:**1907–1912.

Reddy, B. R., L. E. Shaw, J. R. Sayers, and P. A. Williams. 1994. Two identical copies of IS*1246,* a 1275 base pair sequence related to other bacterial insertion sequences, enclose the *xyl* genes on TOL plasmid pWW0. *Microbiology* **140:**2305–2307.

Sinclair, M. I., and B. W. Holloway. 1991. Chromosomal insertion of TOL transposons in *Pseudomonas aeruginosa* PAO. *J. Gen. Microbiol.* **137:**1111–1120.

Sinclair, M. I., P. C. Max, B. R. Lyon, and B. W. Holloway. 1986. Chromosomal location of TOL plasmid DNA in *Pseudomonas putida. J. Bacteriol.* **168:**1302–1308.

Springael, D., L. Diels, and M. Mergeay. 1994. Transfer of PCB-degrading genes into heavy metal resistant *Alcaligenes eutrophus* strains. *Biodegradation* **5:**343–357.

Springael, D., S. Kreps, and M. Mergeay. 1993. Identification of a catabolic transposon, Tn*4371,* carrying biphenyl and 4-chlorobiphenyl degradation genes in *Alcaligenes eutrophus* A5. *J. Bacteriol.* **175:**1674–1681.

Tsuda, M., and T. Iino. 1987. Genetic analysis of a transposon carrying toluene degrading genes on a TOL plasmid pWW0. *Mol. Gen. Genet.* **210:**270–276.

Tsuda, M., and T. Iino. 1988. Identification and characterization of Tn*4653,* a transposon covering the toluene transposon Tn*4651* on TOL plasmid pWW0. *Mol. Gen. Genet.* **213:**72–77.

Tsuda, M., and T. Iino. 1990. Naphthalene degrading genes on plasmid NAH7 are on a defective transposon. *Mol. Gen. Genet.* **223:**33–39.

Tsuda, M., K.-I. Minegishi, and T. Iino. 1989. Toluene transposons Tn*4651* and Tn*4653* are class II transposons. *J. Bacteriol.* **171:**1386–1393.

van der Meer, J. R., W. M. de Vos, S. Harayama, and A. J. B. Zehnder. 1992. Molecular mechanisms of genetic adaptation to xenobiotic compounds. *Microbiol. Rev.* **56:**677–694.

van der Meer, J. R., A. J. B. Zehnder, and W. M. de Vos. 1991. Identification of a novel composite transposable element, Tn*5280,* carrying chlorobenzene dioxygenase genes of *Pseudomonas* sp. strain P51. *J. Bacteriol.* **173:**7077–7083.

Williams, P. A., S. J. Assinder, P. De Marco, K. J. O'Donnell, C. L. Poh, L. E. Shaw, and M. K. Winson. 1992. Catabolic gene duplications in TOL plasmids, p. 341–352. *In* E. Galli, S. Silver, and B. Witholt (ed.), *Pseudomonas: Molecular Biology and Biotechnology.* American Society for Microbiology, Washington, D.C.

Williams, P. A., and J. R. Sayers. 1994. The evolution of pathways for aromatic hydrocarbon oxidation in *Pseudomonas. Biodegradation* **5:**195–217.

Wyndham, R. C., A. E. Cashore, C. H. Nakatsu, and M. C. Peel. 1994. Catabolic transposons. *Biodegradation* **5:**323–342.

Yen, K.-M., and C. M. Serdar. 1988. Genetics of naphthalene catabolism in pseudomonads. *Crit. Rev. Microbiol.* **15:**247–268.

Molecular Biology of Pseudomonads
Edited by T. Nakazawa et al.

Chapter 19

Improved Methods for Gene Analysis and Expression in *Pseudomonas* spp.

Herbert P. Schweizer, Tanya Klassen, and Tung Hoang

Until recently, direct molecular and genetic analyses of many agriculturally, industrially, and medically important *Pseudomonas* species were hampered by the limited number of suitable tools. Initially, many broad-host-range vectors that became available were rather large and often lacked versatile selectable markers, and some did not allow for convenient characterization of the cloned DNA segments. Our general approach to developing and improving useful, widely applicable tools was to adapt well-characterized *Escherichia coli* genetic systems for use in other bacteria, especially the pseudomonads. Some of the resulting tools include broad-host-range cloning and fusion vectors (Schweizer, 1991a, 1991b; West et al., 1994), gene replacement vectors (Schweizer, 1992; Schweizer and Hoang, 1995), and various gene cassettes that facilitate mutational analyses directly in the respective bacterial hosts (Schweizer, 1993a, 1993b). In this chapter, we present an overview of the methods for gene analysis and expression developed in our laboratory, and we also describe our most recent efforts aimed at continually improving these systems and expanding their use.

THE pUCP FAMILY OF BROAD-HOST-RANGE CLONING AND EXPRESSION VECTORS

The pUCP family of general-purpose cloning and expression vectors is based on the well-characterized and popular pUC18/19 vectors (Yanisch-Perron et al., 1985) and contains the broad-host-range replicon from pRO1600 (ori_{1600}), which was originally isolated as a cryptic plasmid from *Pseudomonas aeruginosa* (Olsen et al., 1982). This family of vectors was constructed with the objective of preserving all the features of the pUC18/19 vectors while expanding their host range (Schweizer, 1991a). Their features include (i) a versatile multiple cloning site, (ii) direct screening for recombinants, (iii) use as sequencing and PCR amplification vectors, and (iv) regulated expression from the

Herbert P. Schweizer • Department of Microbiology, Colorado State University, Fort Collins, Colorado 80523. ***Tanya Klassen and Tung Hoang*** • Department of Microbiology and Infectious Diseases, University of Calgary, Calgary, Alberta T2N 4N1, Canada.

lac promoter. Genetic engineering of host strains for blue/white screening and regulated expression was facilitated by construction of selectable, transposon-based expression and regulation modules that contain the *E. coli lacZ*ΔM15 and *lacI*^{q} genes (Karkhoff-Schweizer and Schweizer, 1994; Schweizer, 1994). As previously described (Schweizer, 1991a), recombinants can also be identified as white colonies on MacConkey lactose indicator medium (Miller, 1992). This property offers an added advantage over other similar expression vectors, since in *lacI*$^{q+}$ strains, screening on this medium avoids the need for induction with the gratuitous inducer isopropyl-β-D-thiogalactopyranoside (IPTG), a situation that can result in selective loss or even inviability of certain recombinants. In recombinants, insertions within *lacZ*α of pUC(P) abolish α complementation, and there is no active β-galactosidase when the insertions are present. Hence, on MacConkey lactose medium, no inducer (allolactose) is formed, and no induction occurs. An overview of some of the most important physical properties and features of the pUCP family of vectors is presented in Table 1.

A detailed molecular analysis of the pRO1600-derived replicon revealed that it is different from other hitherto identified replicons, although its replication protein shares significant homology with other Rep proteins (West et al., 1994; Jansons et al., 1994). Although some rather circumstantial evidence initially suggested that this replicon might belong to the IncP group (Olsen et al., 1982), to our knowledge, no systematic analysis substantiating this suggestion has been conducted. IncP replicons rely on a complex network of replication functions (Pansegrau et al., 1994). Hence, it is unlikely that pRO1600 could have evolved from an IncP plasmid. Nucleotide sequence analysis allowed compilation of the pUCP vector sequences and deletion of unnecessary DNA sequences and facilitated substitution of the resident *bla* gene with alternative selectable markers for use when this marker is not applicable (West et al., 1994). Although originally derived for use in *P. aeruginosa,* the pRO1600-derived replicon present on the various pUCP vectors functions in other *Pseudomonas* species (Table 2).

The physical map of pUCP28T (Fig. 1) represents an example of the newest generation of pUCP plasmids and illustrates our most recent efforts, which are geared to further

Table 1. Physical and genetic properties of the pUCP family of vectors

Vector[a]	Size (bp)	GenBank no.	Selectable marker(s)[b]	Mobilizable	Reference
pUCP18	4,557	U07164	Carbenicillin	No	Schweizer, 1991a
pUCP20	3,897	U07165	Carbenicillin	No	West et al., 1994
pUCP22	4,728	U07166	Carbenicillin, gentamicin	No	West et al., 1994
pUCP24	4,035	U07167	Gentamicin	No	West et al., 1994
pUCP26	4,976	U07168	Tetracycline	No	West et al., 1994
pUCP20T	4,174	U33750	Carbenicillin	Yes	This study
pUCP28T	4,080	U33751	Trimethoprim	Yes	This study
pUCP30T	4,303	U33752	Gentamicin	Yes	This study

[a]These vectors contain the pUC18 (Yanisch-Perron et al., 1985) polylinker in the orientation *Eco*RI-*Sac*I-*Kpn*I-*Sma*I-*Bam*HI-*Xba*I-*Sal*I-*Pst*I-*Sph*I-*Hin*dIII (all sites are unique). Corresponding vectors containing the polylinker in the opposite orientation are also available (they are designated pUCP19 through pUCP31T, respectively).

[b]The concentrations of antibiotics used in selective media are as follows: in *E. coli,* ampicillin (instead of carbenicillin), 100 μg/ml; gentamicin, 10 μg/ml; tetracycline, 10 μg/ml; trimethoprim, 100 μg/ml. In *P. aeruginosa,* carbenicillin, 500 μg/ml; gentamicin, 300 μg/ml; tetracycline, 100 μg/ml; trimethoprim, 100 μg/ml. In other *Pseudomonas* species, these concentrations are similar (see Table 2), but they should be determined empirically for each individual strain.

Table 2. Maintenance of selected members of the pUCP family of vectors in various pseudomonads

Strain	Vector	Medium and antibiotic (per ml)[a]	Method of plasmid transfer
Pseudomonas aeruginosa PAO1	pUCP20T	PIA + 500 μg of Cb	Conjugation with SM10 (Schweizer, 1992)
Pseudomonas aeruginosa PAO1	pUCP20	LB + 500 μg of Cb	Transformation (Visca et al., 1994)
Burkholderia (Pseudomonas) cepacia 715i	pUCP28T	PIA + 100 μg of Tp	Conjugation with SM10
Burkholderia (Pseudomonas) cepacia K30-6	pUCP28T	PIA + 100 μg of Tp	Conjugation with SM10
Burkholderia (Pseudomonas) pseudomallei subsp.	pUCP28T	LB + 200 μg of Gm + 100 μg of Tp	Conjugation with SM10
Pseudomonas putida PPG1	pUCP30T	PIA + 300 μg of Gm	Conjugation with SM10
Pseudomonas putida PPG1	pUCP18	LB + 750 μg of Cb	Electroporation (Diver et al., 1990)
Pseudomonas fluorescens PSFB63	pUCP30T	PIA + 300 μg of Gm	Conjugation with SM10
Pseudomonas fluorescens spp.	pUCP18	LB + 750 μg of Cb	Electroporation

[a]Abbreviations: Cb, carbenicillin; Gm, gentamicin; LB, Luria broth (Miller, 1992); PIA, *Pseudomonas* isolation agar (Difco, Detroit, Mich.); Tp, trimethoprim.

expanding the applications of the pUCP vectors. Insertion of a small RK2-derived *oriT* segment facilitates efficient conjugal transfer of the vectors from *E. coli* SM10 (Schweizer, 1992) into pseudomonads for which no efficient transformation and/or electroporation methods exist. The small trimethoprim-resistant dihydrofolate reductase (*dhfR*II) marker (Zolg and Hanggi, 1981) is of use in some pseudomonads, e.g., *Burkholderia* (formerly *Pseudomonas*) *pseudomallei* and *Burkholderia* (formerly *Pseudomonas*) *cepacia,* which are resistant to most other commonly used antibiotics. Since these elements are inserted into nonessential regions of the vector, the other useful features of the pUCP vectors described above are preserved. Table 1 also describes two other vectors, pUCP20T and pUCP30T, which are mobilizable derivatives of the originally described pUCP20 and pUCP24, encoding carbenicillin and gentamicin resistance, respectively (West et al., 1994).

Although the *lac* promoter-driven expression of genes cloned in the pUCP vectors can efficiently be regulated in genetically engineered *P. aeruginosa* PAO-LAC hosts containing the chromosomally integrated *lacI*$^{q+}$ gene (Karkhoff-Schweizer and Schweizer, 1994), such regulated expression has not yet been achieved in other *Pseudomonas* species. To overcome this problem, we are currently completing construction of an expression vector with the following features: (i) the *ori*$_{1600}$-*oriT* broad-host-range cassette from pSF2 (Fig. 2A); (ii) expression of cloned genes from the strong *trc* promoter (Brosius et al., 1985), whose transcript is efficiently terminated by the *E. coli* 5S rRNA gene-derived double transcriptional terminators, thus providing increased plasmid stability (Brosius, 1989); (iii) a unique *Nco*I site at the ATG start codon of the β-galactosidase α peptide that allows in-frame cloning and strong expression of appropriately engineered coding sequences and, with the unique re-

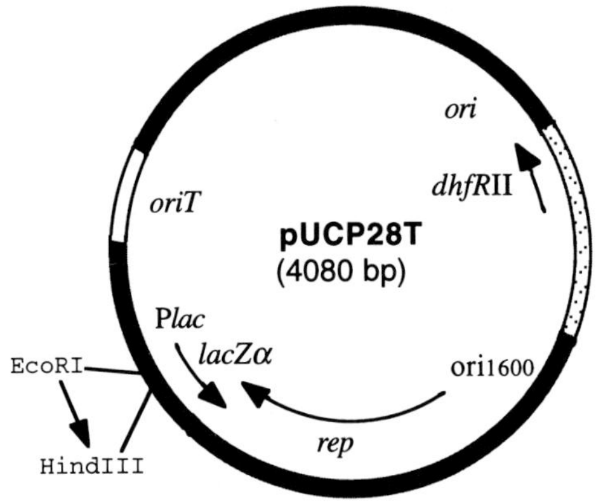

Figure 1. Physical map of pUCP28T. Origins of DNA segments are as follows: pUC18 (Yanisch-Perron et al., 1985), black bar; pRO1600 (Olsen et al., 1982), gray bar; RK2 via PCR amplification from pVW9962 (Waters and Guiney, 1993), white bar; R388 (Zolg and Hanggi, 1981), stippled bar. Abbreviations: *dhfR*II, trimethoprim-resistant dihydrofolate reductase II gene; *lacZ*α, β-galactosidase α-peptide-encoding gene; P*lac*, *E. coli lac* operon promoter; *ori*, pMB1-derived origin of replication; *ori*1600, pRO1600-derived *ori*; *rep*, Rep protein from pRO1600. EcoRI→HindIII, *Eco*RI-*Sac*I-*Kpn*I-*Sma*I-*Bam*HI-*Xba*I-*Sal*I-*Pst*I-*Sph*I-*Hin*dIII (all sites are unique). Vector pUCP29T is identical to pUCP28T except that it contains the polylinker sites in inverted orientation. The other pUCP vectors listed in Table 1 basically share the same architecture but contain different antibiotic resistance markers (all in the same transcriptional orientation), lack *oriT*, or contain additional pRO1600-derived sequences.

striction sites located within the *lacZ*α-encoding sequences, allows for easy construction and identification of recombinants by blue/white screening; and (iv) the presence of the regulatory gene *lacI*^{q} on the same plasmid. Similar, less versatile constructs have been described elsewhere (Morales et al., 1990; De Lorenzo et al., 1993; Franklin and Ohman, 1993).

A BROAD-HOST-REPLICON *oriT* "ADAPTER" CASSETTE

Before the broad-host-range ori_{1600} replicon was utilized by us (Schweizer, 1991a, 1991b; West et al., 1994) and others (Farinha and Kropinski, 1989; Ronald et al., 1990) for construction of versatile general-purpose cloning and gene fusion vectors, various other laboratories had shown that a 1,894-bp *Pst*I fragment from pRO1614 (Olsen et al., 1982) could be utilized to stabilize *E. coli* vectors containing the ColE1 (or pMB1)-derived origin of replication for use in *P. aeruginosa*. Thus, in the literature, this fragment is often referred to as the "stabilizing fragment." To examine its utility for the construction of broad-host-range plasmids based on known *E. coli* vectors, pMB1-based pBR322 (Balbas et al., 1986) and p15A-based pACYC177 (Chang and Cohen, 1978) were equipped with the 1.9-kb ori_{1600}-containing fragment. Transformation of *P. aeruginosa* PAO1 (Olsen et al., 1982) yielded, on average, between 5×10^3 and 1×10^4 transformants per μg of *E. coli*-derived plasmid DNA. In contrast and for unknown rea-

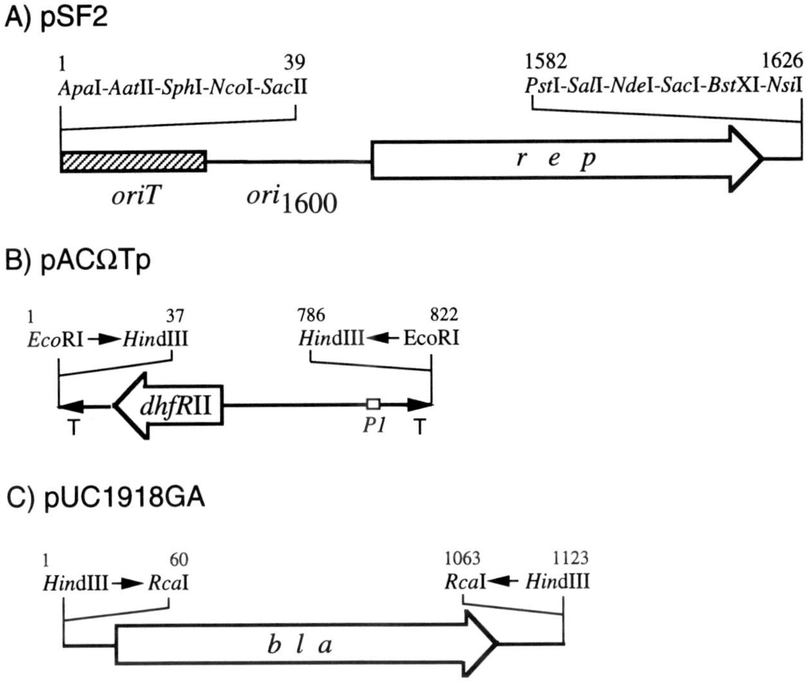

Figure 2. Structures of selected gene cassettes (drawn to scale). (A) pRO1600-derived broad-host-range replicon and *oriT* cassette contained on pSF2 (based on pGEM-T [Promega, Madison, Wis.]). For abbreviations and origins of individual segments, see the legend to Fig. 1. (B) Trimethoprim resistance-encoding cassette contained on pACYC184ΔAse (Schweizer and Hoang, 1995). Abbreviations: *P1*, *dhfR*II promoter (Levesque et al., 1994); T and *Eco*RI→*Hin*dIII, T4 transcription–translation terminators and *Eco*RI-*Sma*I-*Bam*HI-*Hin*dIII polylinker, respectively, from Ω (Prentki and Krisch, 1984). (C) pUC1918GA ampicillin resistance-encoding cassette. The *bla* gene is derived from pUC19 (Yanisch-Perron et al., 1985). *Hin*dIII→*Rca*I, *Hin*dIII-*Sph*I-*Pst*I-*Sal*I-*Xba*I-*Bam*HI-*Sma*I-*Kpn*I-*Sac*I-*Eco*RI-*Rca*I (the *Eco*RI site is missing from the left polylinker region).

sons, no transformants were obtained when the ori_{p15A}- and ori_{1600}-containing pACYC177 derivative was used (H. P. Schweizer and C. Po, unpublished results).

Since subsequent nucleotide sequence analysis indicated that the 1.9-kb fragment contained redundant sequences, including the 3′ end of *bla* and its flanking Tn*3*-like terminal repeat (West et al., 1994; Jansons et al., 1994), a more useful ori_{1600}-containing cassette was constructed (Fig. 3A). The cassette includes the minimal ori_{1600} sequences, *rep*, and RK2-derived *oriT*. The cassette can conveniently be isolated by digestion with a combination of restriction enzymes and has proven useful for broad-host-range vector construction. In principle, this cassette should be very useful for adapting any existing *E. coli* plasmids with ori_{pMB1} and cloned *Pseudomonas* genes for transfer, maintenance, and expression of the cloned sequences into various pseudomonads.

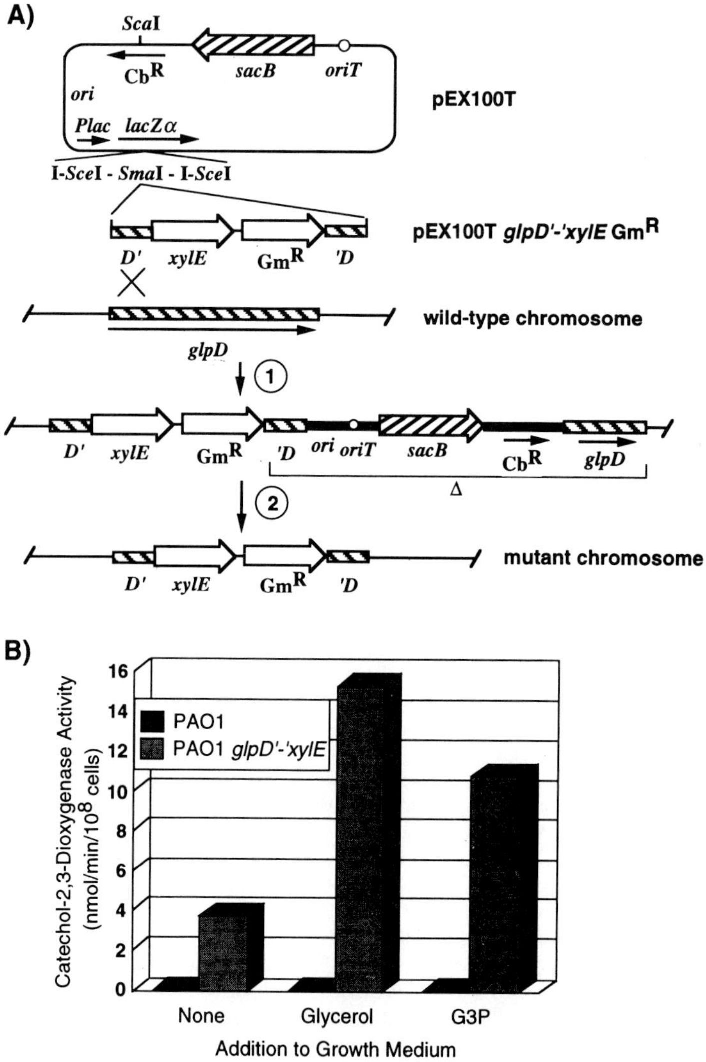

Figure 3. Gene replacement utilizing the *sacB* counterselectable marker. (A) Integration of a *glpD′-′xylE* fusion at the *glpD* locus (Schweizer and Po, 1994) of the *P. aeruginosa* PAO1 chromosome. Plasmid pEX100T *glpD′-′xylE* Gm^R was constructed by cloning the insertionally inactivated *glpD* fragment into the unique *Sma*I site of the polylinker of pEX100T (Schweizer and Hoang, 1995). Step 1 illustrates the formation of a merodiploid strain by integration of the conjugally transferred pEX100T-based *glpD′-′xylE* fusion plasmid into the homologous *glpD* region of the chromosome (selection is for gentamicin resistance). Step 2 depicts the excision of plasmid sequences and wild-type *glpD* promoted by selection of sucrose resistance in the presence of gentamicin, resulting in a strain containing a transcriptional *glpD′-′xylE* fusion. Abbreviations: Cb^R, β-lactamase-encoded carbenicillin resistance; *lacZ*α, β-galactosidase α-peptide-encoding gene; *ori*, pMB1-derived origin of replication; *oriT*, origin of transfer; *Plac*, *E. coli lac* operon promoter, *sacB*, levansucrase-encoding gene from *Bacillus subtilis;* I-*Sce*I-*Sma*I-I-*Sce*I, polylinker cloning site. The unique *Sca*I site located within the Cb^r-encoding gene can be utilized to equip pEX100T with different selectable markers. (B) Activity of a chromosomal *glpD′-′xylE* fusion. Cells were grown in minimal-Casamino Acids medium with the indicated additions, and catechol-2,3-dioxygenase activity was assayed (Schweizer and Hoang, 1995). The *glpD′-′xylE*-encoded catechol-2,3-dioxygenase activity shows the same induction pattern as *glpD* (Schweizer and Po, 1994), and no activity is observed in PAO1 cells. G3P, glycerol 3-phosphate.

GENE CASSETTES FOR VECTOR CONSTRUCTION AND MUTATIONAL ANALYSIS

To facilitate vector construction and mutational analysis of cloned DNA sequences, we previously described the development of several cassettes containing various antibiotic resistance markers (Schweizer, 1993b; Schweizer and Hoang, 1995) as well as of screenable and selectable *lacZ* and *xylE* cassettes for gene fusion analyses (Schweizer, 1993a; Schweizer and Hoang, 1995). Figures 2B and C show the schematic physical maps of two newly developed cassettes. One cassette contains a trimethoprim resistance-encoding Ω element that can conveniently be excised by utilizing various unique restriction sites. This element can be used for mutational analysis when other markers are not functional or have already been utilized. In addition, it serves as a convenient source for the trimethoprim resistance marker for use in plasmid constructions, as described above for pUCP28T. Since the trimethoprim-resistant dihydrofolate reductase *dhfR*II is originally derived from R388 (Zolg and Hanggi, 1981), it is expressed in a wide spectrum of bacteria. The second cassette contains the ampicillin resistance-encoding *bla* gene from pUC19 (Yanisch-Perron et al., 1985). This small element has successfully been used for mutagenesis of *sodB* in *P. aeruginosa* (Hassett et al., 1995) and is useful when other antibiotic markers have already been used in previous mutagenesis experiments. Traditionally, *bla* has not widely been used for insertional mutagenesis, mainly because of (i) the availability of so few suitable cassettes (Fellay et al., 1987) and (ii) its interference with subsequent complementation experiments, since many cloning vectors contain the ampicillin resistance selectable marker. However, with the development of the more user-friendly *bla* cassette described above and the availability of cloning vectors with alternative selectable markers, its use in carbenicillin-susceptible *Pseudomonas* spp. should become more widespread.

GENE REPLACEMENT SYSTEMS FOR *P. AERUGINOSA*

Our laboratory was the first to describe a gene replacement system for *P. aeruginosa* that allowed positive selections for all steps involved in the gene replacement process (Schweizer, 1992). The most significant improvement was the inclusion of the *Bacillus subtilis sacB* gene as a counterselectable marker. Including this marker allows for positive selection of the segregation of true mutants from the more frequently occurring merodiploids on medium containing 5% sucrose. This selection process greatly facilitates the genetic exchange not only of selectable markers but also of screenable markers, e.g., *lacZ*- or *xylE*-based gene fusions. Although the originally described version of the replacement system proved extremely useful, it suffers from some drawbacks, mostly in the multiple cloning steps that involve specialized vectors as previously detailed (Schweizer, 1992). For even greater flexibility of the *sacB*-based gene replacement system, a gene replacement vector, pEX100T (Schweizer and Hoang, 1995), that was genetically engineered to facilitate the cloning and genetic manipulation of virtually any DNA fragment was developed. This flexibility was achieved by incorporating into a single vector (i) the counterselectable *sacB* marker, (ii) a *lacZ*α allele for blue/white screening, (iii) an *oriT* for conjugation-mediated plasmid transfer, and (iv) unique cloning sites for *Sma*I and the rare-cutting meganuclease I-*Sce*I. By site-specific mutagenesis and subcloning, most restriction sites within the replacement vector were eliminated to give greater access to restriction sites within the cloned fragment, thus facilitating the construction of marked or unmarked insertions, deletions, and frameshifts. The ampicillin resistance-encoding marker contained on this plasmid can easily be replaced by cloning other antibiotic resistance-encoding gene cassettes into a unique *Sca*I site within *bla,* which should make this system adaptable to other pseudomonads, although this possibility has not been explored to date.

The use of this vector for construction of a glycerol-inducible, single-copy chromosomal *glpD'-'xylE* fusion is illustrated in Fig. 3. The *glpD* gene of *P. aeruginosa* encodes glycerol-3-phosphate dehydrogenase (Schweizer and Hoang, 1995).

Acknowledgments. The work described in this chapter was supported by a grant from the Canadian Cystic Fibrosis Foundation and, in part, by the Medical Research Council of Canada (MRC), an MRC Medical Scholarship, and the Canadian Bacterial Diseases Network. We thank P. Sokol, University of Calgary, for *Pseudomonas* strains; D. DeShazer, University of Calgary, for the trimethoprim-resistant *dhfR* clone p34E-Tp; and A. Kropinski, Queen's University, for the gift of the PCR-amplified *oriT* fragment.

REFERENCES

Balbas, P., X. Soberon, E. Merino, M. Zurita, Z. Lomeli, F. Valle, N. Flores, and F. Bolivar. 1986. Plasmid vector pBR322 and its special purpose derivatives—a review. *Gene* **50:**3–40.

Brosius, J. 1989. Superpolylinkers in cloning and expression vectors. *DNA* **8:**759–777.

Brosius, J., M. Erfle, and J. Storella. 1985. Spacing of the −10 and −35 regions in the *tac* promoter. *J. Biol. Chem.* **260:**3539–3541.

Chang, A. C. Y., and S. N. Cohen. 1978. Construction and characterization of amplifiable multicopy DNA cloning vehicles derived from the P15A cryptic miniplasmid. *J. Bacteriol.* **134:**1141–1156.

De Lorenzo, V., L. Eltis, B. Kessler, and K. N. Timmis. 1993. Analysis of *Pseudomonas* gene products using *lacI*^{q}/*Ptrp-lac* plasmids and transposons that confer conditional phenotypes. *Gene* **123:**17–24.

Diver, J. M., L. E. Bryan, and P. A. Sokol. 1990. Transformation of *Pseudomonas aeruginosa* by electroporation. *Anal. Biochem.* **189:**75–79.

Farinha, M. A., and A. M. Kropinski. 1989. Construction of broad-host-range vectors for general cloning and promoter selection in *Pseudomonas* and *Escherichia coli. Gene* **77:**205–210.

Fellay, R., J. Frey, and H. Krisch. 1987. Interposon mutagenesis of soil and water bacteria: a family of DNA fragments designed for in vitro insertional mutagenesis of Gram-negative bacteria. *Gene* **52:**147–152.

Franklin, M. J., and D. E. Ohman. 1993. Identification of *algF* in the alginate biosynthetic gene cluster of *Pseudomonas aeruginosa* which is required for alginate acetylation. *J. Bacteriol.* **175:**5057–5065.

Hassett, D. J., H. P. Schweizer, and D. E. Ohman. 1995. *Pseudomonas aeruginosa sodA* and *sodB* mutants defective in manganese- and iron-cofactored superoxide dismutase activity demonstrate the importance of the iron-cofactored form in aerobic metabolism. *J. Bacteriol.* **177:**6330–6337.

Jansons, I., G. Touchie, R. Sharp, K. Almquist, M. A. Farinha, J. S. Lam, and A. Kropinski. 1994. Deletion and transposon mutagenesis and sequence analysis of the pRO1600 OriR region found in the broad-host-range plasmids of the pQF series. *Plasmid* **31:**265–274.

Karkhoff-Schweizer, R. R., and H. P. Schweizer. 1994. Utilization of mini-D*lac* transposable element to create an α-complementation and regulated expression system for molecular cloning in *Pseudomonas aeruginosa. Gene* **140:**7–15.

Levesque, C., S. Brassard, J. Lapointe, and P. Roy. 1994. Diversity and relative strength of tandem promoters for the antibiotic resistance genes of several integrons. *Gene* **142:**49–54.

Miller, J. H. 1992. *A Short Course in Bacterial Genetics.* Cold Spring Harbor Laboratory Press, Cold Spring Harbor, N.Y.

Morales, V., M. M. Bagdasarian, and M. Bagdasarian. 1990. Promiscuous plasmids of the IncQ group: mode of replication and use for gene cloning in gram-negative bacteria, p. 229–241. *In* S. Silver, A. M.

Chakrabarty, B. Iglewski, and S. Kaplan (ed.), *Pseudomonas: Biotransformations, Pathogenesis, and Evolving Biotechnology*. American Society for Microbiology, Washington, D.C.

Olsen, R. H., G. DeBusscher, and W. R. McCombie. 1982. Development of broad-host-range vectors and gene banks: self-cloning of the *Pseudomonas aeruginosa* PAO chromosome. *J. Bacteriol.* **150:**60–69.

Pansegrau, W., E. Lanka, P. T. Barth, D. H. Figurski, D. G. Guiney, D. Haas, D. R. Helinski, H. Schwab, V. A. Stanisich, and C. M. Thomas. 1994. Complete nucleotide sequence of Birmingham IncP alpha plasmids. Compilation and comparative analysis. *J. Mol. Biol.* **239:**623–663.

Prentki, P., and H. Krisch. 1984. *In vitro* insertional mutagenesis with a selectable DNA fragment. *Gene* **29:**303–313.

Ronald, S. L., A. M. Kropinski, and M. A. Farinha. 1990. Construction of broad-host-range vectors for the selection of divergent promoters. *Gene* **90:**145–148.

Schweizer, H. P. 1991a. *Escherichia-Pseudomonas* shuttle vectors derived from pUC18/19. *Gene* **97:**109–112.

Schweizer, H. P. 1991b. Improved broad-host-range *lac*-based plasmid vectors for the isolation and characterization of protein fusions in *Pseudomonas aeruginosa. Gene* **103:**87–92.

Schweizer, H. P. 1992. Allelic exchange in *Pseudomonas aeruginosa* using novel ColE1-type vectors and a family of cassettes containing a portable *oriT* and the counter-selectable *Bacillus subtilis sacB* marker. *Mol. Microbiol.* **6:**1195–1204.

Schweizer, H. P. 1993a. Two plasmids, X1918 and Z1918, for easy recovery of the *xylE* and *lacZ* reporter genes. *Gene* **134:**89–91.

Schweizer, H. P. 1993b. Small broad-host-range gentamycin resistance cassettes for site-specific insertion and deletion mutagenesis. *BioTechniques* **15:**831–833.

Schweizer, H. P. 1994. A method for construction of bacterial hosts for *lac*-based cloning and expression vectors: α complementation and regulated expression. *BioTechniques* **17:**452–456.

Schweizer, H. P., and T. Hoang. 1995. An improved system for gene replacement and *xylE* fusion analysis in *Pseudomonas aeruginosa. Gene* **158:**15–22.

Schweizer, H. P., and C. Po. 1994. Cloning and nucleotide sequence of the *glpD* gene encoding *sn*-glycerol-3-phosphate dehydrogenase from *Pseudomonas aeruginosa. J. Bacteriol.* **176:**2184–2193.

Visca, P., A. Ciervo, and N. Orsi. 1994. Cloning and nucleotide sequence of the *pvdA* gene encoding the pyoverdin biosynthetic enzyme L-ornithine N^5-oxygenase in *Pseudomonas aeruginosa. J. Bacteriol.* **176:**1128–1140.

Waters, V. L., and D. G. Guiney. 1993. Processes at the nick region link conjugation, T-DNA transfer and rolling circle replication. *Mol. Microbiol.* **9:**1123–1130.

West, S. E. H., H. P. Schweizer, C. Dall, A. K. Sample, and L. J. Runyen-Janecky. 1994. Construction of improved *Escherichia-Pseudomonas* shuttle vectors derived from pUC18/19 and the sequence of the region required for their replication in *Pseudomonas aeruginosa. Gene* **148:**81–86.

Yanisch-Perron, C., J. Vieira, and J. Messing. 1985. Improved M13 cloning vectors and host strains: nucleotide sequences of the M13mp18 and pUC19 vectors. *Gene* **33:**103–119.

Zolg, J. W., and U. J. Hanggi. 1981. Characterization of R-plasmid associated, trimethoprim-resistant dihydrofolate reductase and determination of the nucleotide sequence of the reductase gene. *Nucleic Acids Res.* **9:**697–710.

Molecular Biology of Pseudomonads
Edited by T. Nakazawa et al.

Chapter 20

Insertion Sequence IS*21*: Related Insertion Sequence Elements, Transpositional Mechanisms, and Application to Linker Insertion Mutagenesis

Dieter Haas, Bernard Berger, Sergio Schmid, Thomas Seitz, and Cornelia Reimmann

When classical genetic and physical experiments established that the chromosome of *Escherichia coli* is a single, circular, double-stranded DNA molecule (Hayes, 1964), it was expected that other bacteria would also contain a circular chromosome; the presence of a linear chromosome or two circular chromosomes in some bacteria was recognized much later (Cole and Saint Girons, 1994). In *Pseudomonas aeruginosa,* chromosomal markers could initially be located on a major linkage group by classical genetics. Although several chromosome-mobilizing plasmids (FP2, FP5, FP39, and others) and generalized transducing bacteriophages were available, the *P. aeruginosa* PAO chromosome map remained linear throughout the 1970s (Holloway et al., 1979). Since plasmids FP2 and FP5 mobilize chromosomal genes from similar sites in strain PAO, there was a need for a new sex plasmid that could promote chromosome transfer from other, preferably random chromosomal regions. The broad-host-range IncP plasmid R68.45 meets these requirements (Haas and Holloway, 1976, 1978). R68.45 is a derivative of R68, a plasmid originally isolated from a carbenicillin-resistant clinical strain of *P. aeruginosa* (Holloway and Richmond, 1973). R68 carries a single copy of the insertion sequence (IS) IS*21*. A spontaneous tandem duplication of IS*21* occurred in the laboratory, producing R68.45. The IS*21* tandem repeat [designated $(IS21)_2$] is necessary for chromosome mobilization ability (Willetts et al., 1981; Currier and Morgan, 1982; Haas and Riess, 1983). Using conjugational linkage in matings with R68.45 donors, Royle et al. (1981) established genetic circularity of strain PAO, confirming Pemberton's (1974) earlier physical data. R68.45 also helped demonstrate circular chromosomes in *Agrobacterium* and *Rhizobium* spp. Moreover, R68.45-mediated chromosome mobilization has been reported in about 30 species of gram-negative bacteria, including organisms in genera as

Dieter Haas, Bernard Berger, Thomas Seitz, and Cornelia Reimmann • Laboratoire de Biologie Microbienne, Université de Lausanne, CH-1015 Lausanne, Switzerland. ***Sergio Schmid*** • Ingenieurschule Wallis, CH-1950 Sion, Switzerland.

diverse as *Ancylobacter, Azospirillum, Azotobacter, Bordetella, Erwinia, Escherichia, Hyphomicrobium, Klebsiella, Legionella, Methylobacterium, Methylophilus, Paracoccus, Rhodobacter, Thiobacillus, Vibrio, Xanthomonas,* and *Zymomonas* (reviewed by Reimmann and Haas, 1993; Gliesche and Hirsch, 1992). This wide host range reflects the versatility of the IncP replication and conjugation systems on the one hand and the high transpositional activity of (IS*21*)$_2$ on the other hand.

TRANSPOSITION PATHWAYS OF IS*21*

The principal transposition pathways of IS*21* can be summarized as follows. (i) IS*21* can give simple insertions (Fig. 1A; Reimmann and Haas, 1986). When the IS*21* transposition functions are overexpressed by genetic manipulation, the frequency of IS*21* simple insertion is ca. 10^{-4} (our unpublished results). (ii) The formation of (IS*21*)$_2$ from IS*21* may involve transposition of an IS*21* element to a site immediately adjacent to another IS*21* element in an inter- or intraplasmidic reaction (Fig. 1B, a and b). In natu-

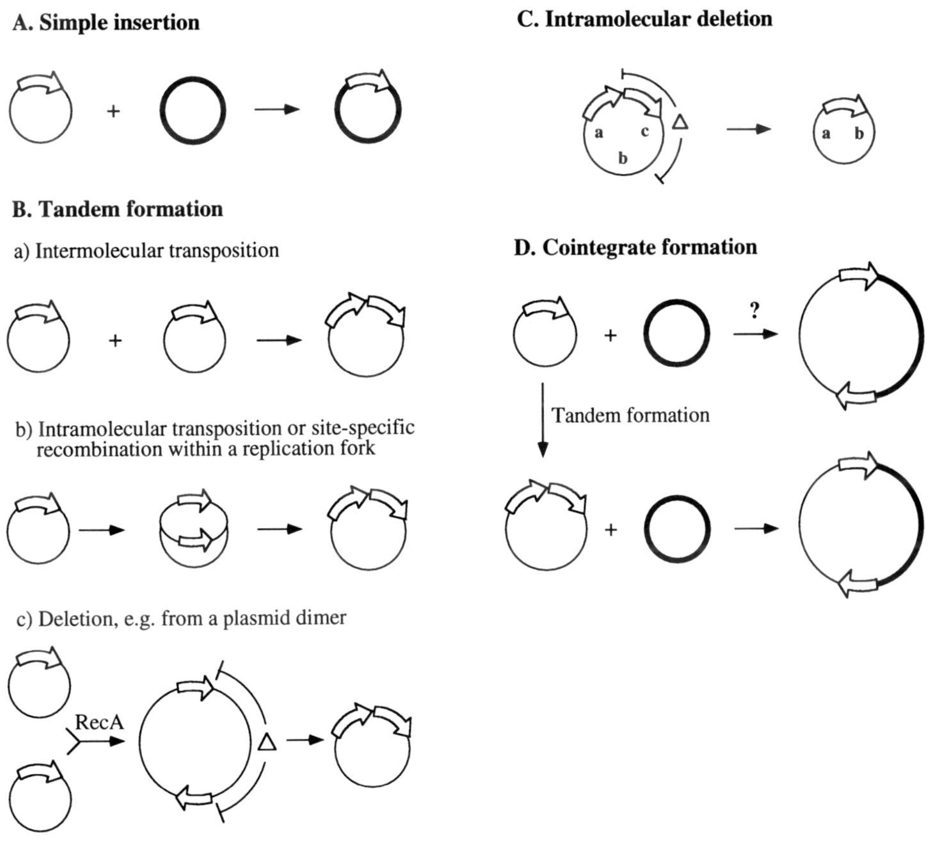

Figure 1. Model for transposition pathways of IS*21*. See text for explanation of details. ⇨, IS*21*; —, donor replicon; **—**, target replicon; Δ, deletion.

rally occurring IS*21* tandems, the IS*21* elements are separated by a variable junction sequence of 2 or 3 bp (Reimmann et al., 1989). The frequency of tandem formation in *P. aeruginosa* has been estimated to be $\leq 10^{-4}$ (Reimmann and Haas, 1993), but direct measurements are not available. When a plasmid carries two widely separated copies of IS*21* in the same orientation, a spontaneous deletion can remove the DNA segment between the IS elements (Reimmann and Haas, 1987). Assuming RecA-dependent dimerization of a plasmid carrying a single IS*21* element, this type of deletion could also account for the formation of $(IS\mathit{21})_2$ (Fig. 1B, c). (iii) Plasmids carrying $(IS\mathit{21})_2$, such as R68.45, are somewhat unstable in $RecA^+$ and $RecA^-$ strains, especially following conjugation to a new host. Instability can manifest itself in two ways: loss of one IS*21* element plus flanking DNA, presumably due to intramolecular transposition, leading to a deletion plasmid (Fig. 1C; Currier and Morgan, 1982; Haas and Riess, 1983), or loss of one IS*21* element with regeneration of R68 (not shown). Despite this intrinsic instability in the percent range, R68.45 donor strains can be maintained for more than 20 generations in many bacterial species. (iv) The formation of cointegrates between an $(IS\mathit{21})_2$ plasmid and a target replicon (i.e., another plasmid or a chromosome) is very efficient (approaching 10^{-1} in *E. coli* under optimal conditions) and presumably proceeds via a nonreplicative cut-and-paste mechanism (Reimmann and Haas, 1987, 1990). Plasmids carrying a single IS*21* element rarely ($<10^{-6}$) form cointegrates. Whether this reaction involves replicative IS*21* transposition or $(IS\mathit{21})_2$ formation followed by nonreplicative cointegration is not known (Fig. 1D; Reimmann and Haas, 1987).

These pathways are not unique to IS*21*. *E. coli* IS*30* shows a series of very similar reactions and, in particular, the formation of reactive IS*30* tandems (Olasz et al., 1993). One major difference, however, is apparent: $(IS\mathit{30})_2$ structures are very unstable intermediates and are difficult to isolate (Olasz et al., 1993). Tandem repeats of IS*3*, which might be intermediates during IS*3*-dependent cointegrate formation, have been constructed artificially but could not be isolated because of instability (Spielmann-Ryser et al., 1991). Finally, IS*911*, an element related to IS*3*, provokes replicon fusions that are mediated by an active junction composed of an IS*911* end and, in inverted orientation, a sequence resembling the IS*911* terminal repeat (Polard et al., 1992). This replicon fusion pathway closely resembles cointegrate formation by $(IS\mathit{21})_2$ plasmids (Fig. 1D).

GENES OF IS*21* AND RELATED IS ELEMENTS

The 2,131-bp nucleotide sequence of IS*21* includes two genes, *istA* and *istB*, apparently organized as an operon. The ends of IS*21* contain 11-bp inverted repeats. However, similarities in the terminal sequences continue toward the interior of the element for some additional 40 bp (Reimmann et al., 1989). Both *istA* and *istB* are required for faithful transpositional activity of IS*21*, which is characterized by target duplications of 4 bp (occasionally 5 bp) (Reimmann et al., 1989; Reimmann and Haas, 1990). In mating-out assays measuring cointegrate formation, an *istA* mutant is completely inactive, whereas an *istB* mutant has 1,000-fold-reduced activity and produces aberrant target duplications (our unpublished results). The IstA protein shares typical structural features with transposases and integrases (see below). IstB might help capture and align the target DNA. Similar roles have been established for the MuB protein of bacteriophage Mu and the TnsC protein of transposon Tn*7* (Mizuuchi, 1992; Gamas and Craig, 1992).

IS*21* is the prototype element of a family of insertion sequences found in a variety of gram-negative and gram-positive bacteria (Fig. 2). All members of this family have *istA*- and *istB*-like open reading frames (Fig. 3). IS*5376* of *Bacillus stearothermophilus,* which creates 5-bp target duplications, resembles IS*21* most in terms of sequence similarities (Xu et al., 1993). IS*100,* an IS element occurring on a 9.5-kb plasmid of *Yersinia pestis* (Fig. 2), is flanked by a 5-bp target duplication. This IS element might modulate the expression of virulence phenotypes (Podladchikova et al., 1994). IS*232* of an endotoxin-producing strain of *Bacillus thuringiensis* (Fig. 2) transposes in *E. coli* with low efficiency and gives 4- or 5-bp target duplications (Menou et al., 1990). In *Bacteroides fragilis* isolates that produce high levels of cephalosporinase encoded by the *cepA* gene, Rogers et al. (1994) repeatedly found a specific type of insertion upstream of *cepA*. These insertions (IS-RBF103) have significant homology with IS*21* (Fig. 2); whether they are transposable elements has not been tested. Two IS*21*-like elements have also been detected in *Pseudomonas* spp.: IS*1162,* an IS element that transposes infrequently in *E. coli,* occurs in *Pseudomonas fluorescens,* and IS*408* occurs in *Burkholderia cepacia* (formerly *Pseudomonas cepacia*) (Fig. 2; Solinas et al., 1995; Byrne and Lessie, 1994). Fragmentary sequence data indicate that IS*640* of *Shigella sonnei* (Matsutani et al., 1987) and IS*53* of *Pseudomonas syringae* pv. *savastanoi* (Soby et al., 1993) may also be related to IS*21*.

A comparison of IstA from IS*21* with its homologs (Fig. 3A) reveals two typical motifs. First, the N-terminal regions of all deduced IstA-like proteins contain sequences that have a high probability of forming a helix-turn-helix configuration capable of DNA binding (Dodd and Egan, 1990; Solinas et al., 1995). Several transposases of bacterial IS elements have an N-terminal DNA binding domain (reviewed by Polard and Chandler,

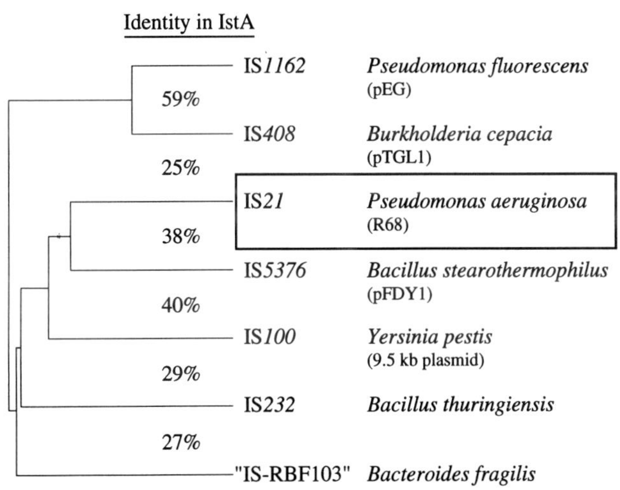

Figure 2. The IS*21* family. The relatedness of the IS elements shown was calculated by the Pileup and Gap programs (Genetics Computer Group, University of Wisconsin, Madison). Percent identities refer to the amino acid sequences between each pair of the deduced IstA-like proteins. A similar tree was constructed using the identities of the IstB proteins, the only difference being exchanged positions of IS*100* and IS*232* (not shown).

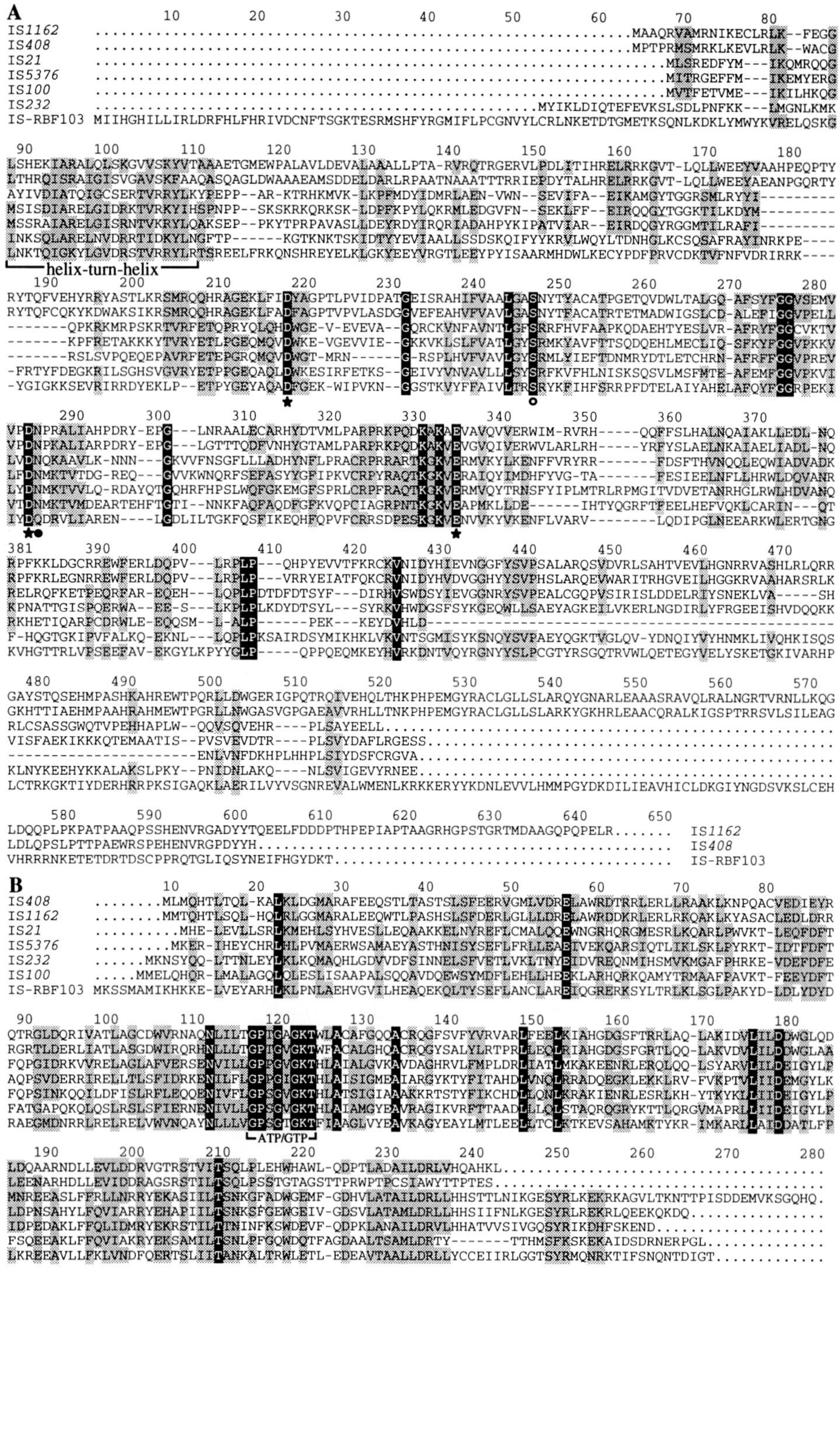
A
IS1162
IS408
IS21
IS5376
IS100
IS232
IS-RBF103
helix-turn-helix
B
IS408
IS1162
IS21
IS5376
IS232
IS100
IS-RBF103
ATP/GTP

1995). One might speculate that as a first step in transposition (or cointegration), the IstA protein could bind to the inverted repeats of IS*21* and that this recognition process could involve the N-terminal part of IstA and specific nucleotides in the inverted repeats. When an IS*21*-IS*21* junction on a linearized plasmid was incubated with IstA protein in a crude extract, stretches of about 30 nucleotides in the inverted repeats were protected from nuclease attack (Reimmann and Haas, 1990), suggesting a possible zone of interaction. The second motif in IstA that stands out is the DDE triad (indicated by asterisks in Fig. 3A). Integrases of retroviruses and retrotransposons as well as transposases of many bacterial transposable elements are characterized by a DDE motif in their catalytic domains (Katz and Skalka, 1994). All *istA*-like open reading frames in the IS*21* family (Fig. 3A) and all putative transposases of the IS*3* family (Polard and Chandler, 1995) contain the DDE motif; the distances between the conserved aspartate and glutamate residues vary. The second aspartate in retroviral integrases and IS*3* family transposases is typically followed by an asparagine or glutamine residue (Polard and Chandler, 1995); so is the second aspartate in the IS*21* family (Fig. 3A). The importance of the DDE residues for catalysis is supported by site-directed mutagenesis of retroviral integrases and of the MuA transposase (Katz and Skalka, 1994; Polard and Chandler, 1995; Kim et al., 1995). The crystal structures of dimeric human immunodeficiency virus type 1 integrase and the MuA core domain reveal that the conserved DDE residues are close to each other within the enzyme monomer, as expected for a catalytic domain (Dyda et al., 1994; Rice and Mizuuchi, 1995; Grindley and Leschziner, 1995).

Retroviral integrases and putative transposases of the IstA type (Fig. 3A) also each contain a highly conserved serine residue located midway between the essential aspartate residues. Mutations that change this serine to alanine or glycine affect retroviral integrase activity, possibly by interfering with correct folding of the enzyme (Katz et al., 1992; van Gent et al., 1992).

The dinucleotide 5′-CA-3′ is typically found at the termini of retroviruses, the IS*3* family, bacteriophage Mu, and Tn*7*. Processing cuts by integrase or transposase create a 3′-OH group at the terminal A; this reaction initiates strand transfer (Mizuuchi and Adzuma, 1991; Engelman et al., 1991; Polard and Chandler, 1995). IS*21* and at least four other members of the same family (IS*100*, IS*408*, IS*1162*, and IS*5376*) also contain terminal 5′-CA-3′ nucleotides. (The ends of IS*232* and IS-RBF103 have not been defined with sufficient precision.) In vitro, the IstA protein processes an IS*21*-IS*21* junction by cutting at the 3′ end of the CA dinucleotide (cf. Fig. 4) (Reimmann and Haas, 1990). Mutational A→T changes in the IS*21* termini totally abolish cointegrate formation, confirming the essential function of the terminal A (our unpublished data).

IstA of IS*21* needs a helper protein, IstB, for transposition and cointegration. Open reading frames resembling *istB* are typical components of all members of the IS*21* fam-

Figure 3. Alignment of the proteins deduced from nucleotide sequences in the IS*21* family. References to the sequences shown are given in the text. ■, identical amino acid residues in all elements; ░, similar or partially conserved (in five or more of seven sequences) residues. The 3′ end of IS*408* has not been sequenced. The alignment was carried out by the Pileup program and manually adjusted. Residues within the following groups were considered similar: G, A, S, T, P; L, I, V, M; F, Y, W; D, E, N, Q; K, R, H. (A) IstA and related proteins. ★, DDE motif; ● and ○, conserved residues referred to in the text. (B) IstB and related proteins.

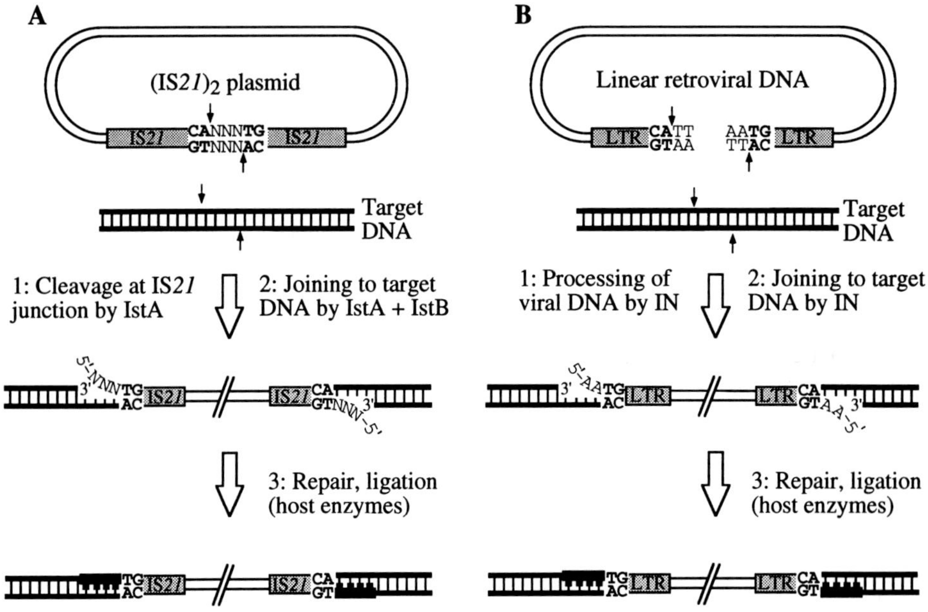

Figure 4. Analogies between IS*21*-mediated cointegration (A) and retroviral insertion (B). Details of the IS*21* pathway have been established with plasmids (Reimmann and Haas, 1987, 1990; Reimmann et al., 1989) or with a bacterial chromosome as the target (Reimmann et al., 1988). Retroviral insertion has been reviewed by Goff (1992) and Katz and Skalka (1994). Vertical arrows indicate processing cuts. ▬, 4-bp target duplications formed by repair enzymes of the host; IN, unspecified nucleotide; LTR, long terminal repeat.

ily (Fig. 3B). A potential ATP-GTP binding motif is strongly conserved in the IstB protein family and is reminiscent of similar motifs in the DnaA and DnaC proteins (Koonin, 1992). Like MuB of phage Mu and TnsC of Tn*7* (Mizuuchi, 1992; Gamas and Craig, 1992), IstB might be an ATP-dependent DNA binding protein.

COINTEGRATION PATHWAY OF (IS*21*)$_2$ PLASMIDS

Cointegrate formation by (IS*21*)$_2$ plasmids (Fig. 1D) is one of the most active transpositional pathways in prokaryotes. In single IS*21* copies, the *istAB* genes are normally expressed at low levels for lack of good promoter activity in IS*21*. In contrast, tandem duplication of IS*21* creates a promoter at the IS*21*-IS*21* junction that drives expression of the *istAB* genes in the downstream element. The –35 promoter sequence is located at the 3′ end of the upstream element, whereas the –10 region lies in the downstream element, with appropriate 17- or 18-bp spacing (Reimmann et al., 1989).

Some structural analogies between the transposition functions of retroviruses and IS*21* have already been pointed out above. Functional analogies are also apparent (Fig. 4). The processing cuts are made at analogous positions in IS*21*-IS*21* junction plasmids and at the long terminal repeats of linear retroviruses. Strand transfer of processed donor ends to target DNA is known to involve a transesterification mechanism in retroviruses: 4- to 6-bp staggered cleavage of target DNA is coupled to ligation of the 5′-CA_{OH}-3′ ends of the donor DNA. The processing and joining activities of integrase are both due to the DDE catalytic domain (Goff, 1992; Katz and Skalka, 1994). In the case of IS*21,* IstA is required for donor cleavage and, with IstB, for joining to the target (Fig. 4). Cleavage, but not joining, has been demonstrated in vitro (Reimmann and Haas, 1990). The subsequent steps, i.e., repair and ligation by host enzymes, create 4- to 6-bp target duplications that flank the integrated retroviruses, IS*21* (Fig. 4), IS*5376, IS232,* and IS*100.* Target selection by retroviruses and IS*21* is (almost) random, implying that integrases and the IstAB proteins have little sequence specificity for target DNA. Integrases appear to tolerate many mutational changes in the terminal sequences of the donor DNA except in the last 5′-CA-3′ dinucleotide, which has to be conserved for good processing and joining activities (Goff, 1992; Katz and Skalka, 1994). Interestingly, cointegrate formation of $(IS21)_2$ plasmids also appears to be rather insensitive to mutational alterations of the IS*21* inverted repeats, with the exception of the CA pairs at the inner 3′ ends (our unpublished results).

An interesting specialization of transposition functions occurs in IS*21*. The *istA* gene has two translational starts in the same reading frame. The full-length IstA protein has a molecular mass of ca. 46 kDa. Its eight N-terminal amino acids are missing in the smaller IstA protein of ca. 45 kDa. Both proteins can be produced by the wild-type IS*21* element (Reimmann et al., 1989). We recently constructed mutants expressing either IstA(P46) or IstA(P45) alone. IstA(P46) promoted simple insertion and cointegration with similar efficiencies (ca. 10^{-3}) in *E. coli* and was named transposase. Compared to IstA(P46), IstA(P45) is 100-fold more active in cointegration but 100-fold less effective in simple insertion. For this reason, IstA(P45) is called cointegrase (Reimmann and Haas, 1993). The high activity of cointegrase may be facilitated by the fact that the active IS*21* ends are covalently linked to each other by 2- or 3-bp junction sequences in $(IS21)_2$ plasmids. In contrast, transposases and retroviral integrases must bring together the active ends (which are usually separated by more than 1 kb) in a synaptic process before productive interaction with the target can occur.

IS*21*-BASED LINKER INSERTION MUTAGENESIS

Site-directed mutagenesis of selected codons is a powerful technique allowing the study of structure-function relationships in a protein whenever the protein can be expressed from a cloned gene and a fair amount of structural information is available. When the information on functional domains and the three-dimensional structure of a protein is scarce, linker insertion mutagenesis can be an effective tool (Barany, 1985; Zebala and Barany, 1991; Goff and Prasad, 1991). In this technique, short palindromic oligonucleotides each containing a restriction site are inserted into various sites of a cloned gene. The oligonucleotides used typically consist of 6, 9, or 12 bp; their introduction into an open reading frame produces in-frame insertion mutations of 2, 3, or 4 codons. The effects of these mutations are often confined to local parts of the proteins and may result in modification rather than complete loss of biological activity. A major limitation of various protocols of in vitro linker insertion mutagenesis is the fact that the insertion sites are not random (Barany, 1985; Goff and Prasad, 1991; Kegler-Ebo et al., 1994). A transpositional mode of linker insertion, based on a transposable element showing little target specificity, may provide a solution to the problem. Here, we briefly describe the principle of a transpositional linker insertion mutagenesis that takes advantage of the (IS*21*)$_2$-mediated cointegration reaction.

The *istA*(P45) and *istB* genes were placed downstream of the *tac* promoter and integrated into the chromosome of *E. coli* (ECOLIST; Fig. 5). A cloned gene (*xyz*) of interest carried by a multicopy plasmid such as pBluescript (Stratagene) is introduced into this host. If pBluescript is used, its *lac* promoter can serve to drive the expression of the cloned gene. A suicide plasmid derived from an R6K replicon (Penfold and Pemberton, 1992) is introduced next. This plasmid (pME5) contains a synthetic IS*21*-IS*21* junction region of about 120 bp that has strategically located artificial *Sal*I and *Bgl*II sites in the 11-bp inverted repeats. These sites do not interfere with the cointegration reaction promoted by IstA(P45) and IstB. Selection for the kanamycin resistance marker of pME5 in

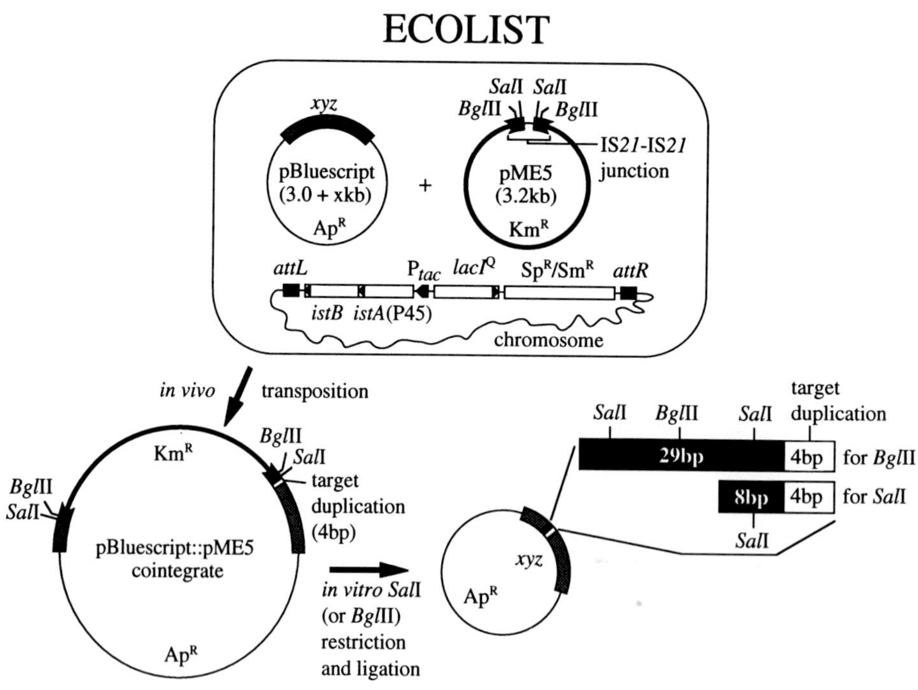

Figure 5. Outline of IS*21*-based linker insertion mutagenesis. The *E. coli* host strain (ECOLIST) contains the *istA*(P45) and *istB* genes of IS*21* in the λ attachment site *attL*/*attR*. Expression of *istAB* can be controlled by the *lacI*^{q} repressor and the *tac* promoter system. The target plasmid (e.g., pBluescript with cloned gene *xyz*) and the suicide plasmid containing a reactive IS*21*-IS*21* junction region of 123 bp plus a selectable marker (e.g., pME5) are introduced successively. Note that the target plasmid should not contain *Sal*I or *Bgl*II sites. Resolution of the pBluescript::pME5 cointegrates formed in vivo is carried out in vitro with *Sal*I or *Bgl*II and ligase, creating 12- or 33-bp insertions in the target gene. pME5 insertions in the vector moiety are discarded.

the *E. coli* host results in the recovery of cointegrates consisting of pBluescript::pME5 (frequent) or chromosome::pME5 (rare). The conditions of antibiotic selection used (50 μg of kanamycin per ml) appear to favor the isolation of plasmid cointegrates, which have more copies of the kanamycin resistance determinant than the chromosomal insertions of pME5 have. The plasmid cointegrates are extracted; those containing pME5 in gene *xyz* are digested by *Sal*I or *Bgl*II and religated (Fig. 5). In this way, most of pME5 is excised, and insertions of 12 bp with a *Sal*I site or 33 bp with a *Bgl*II site (flanked by two *Sal*I sites) are created, thus producing a series of in-frame insertions in the gene of interest (Fig. 5). A 4-bp target duplication in gene *xyz* that is formed during transposition is an integral part of the insertions and ensures that any codon at the insertion site will remain unaltered.

We are testing our novel IS*21*-based method with the *arcB* gene of *P. aeruginosa* as the target. The *arcB* gene encodes catabolic ornithine carbamoyltransferase, an allosteric enzyme involved in anaerobic arginine degradation (Baur et al., 1987; Tricot et al., 1993). Expression of the *arcB* gene cloned downstream of the pBluescript *lac* promoter is very efficient in *E. coli,* allowing direct analysis of the *arcB* product in this host. Of some 30 linker insertions in *arcB* analyzed thus far, two insertions are not in frame because of target duplications of 5 or 6 bp. The remaining in-frame mutations are well distributed in *arcB*. Of the mutant proteins, 45% retain enzymatic activity; the remainder are inactive. Interestingly, two active enzymes have novel properties: one is insensitive to the allosteric activator AMP, and one is hypercooperative for the substrate carbamoylphosphate (V. T. Nguyen, B. Berger, C. Tricot, V. Stalon, and D. Haas, unpublished data). Minor clustering of insertions has been noticed in *arcB,* but no target sequence specificity can be deduced. Perhaps DNA secondary structure plays a role in target site selection (Davies and Hutchison, 1995).

In conclusion, the method outlined here should be broadly applicable to the analysis of structure-function relationships in proteins. Moreover, since insertions are marked by *Sal*I or *Bgl*II restriction sites, these sites can be further exploited for epitope mapping (Charbit et al., 1986) by insertion of an oligonucleotide specifying an antigenic determinant.

Acknowledgments. This research was supported by grants from the Swiss National Foundation for Scientific Research (project 31-28570.90), the Roche Research Foundation, the Internationale Brachet Stiftung, and the Eidgenössische Technische Hochschule Zürich.

REFERENCES

Barany, F. 1985. Single-stranded hexameric linkers: a system for in-phase insertion mutagenesis and protein engineering. *Gene* **37:**111–123.

Baur, H., V. Stalon, P. Falmagne, E. Lüthi, and D. Haas. 1987. Primary and quaternary structure of the catabolic ornithine carbamoyltransferase from *Pseudomonas aeruginosa. Eur. J. Biochem* **166:**111–117.

Byrne, A. M., and T. G. Lessie. 1994. Characteristics of IS*401*, a new member of the IS*3* family implicated in plasmid rearrangements in *Pseudomonas cepacia. Plasmid* **31:**138–147.

Charbit, A., J. C. Boulain, A. Ryter, and M. Hofnung. 1986. Probing the topology of a bacterial membrane protein by genetic insertion of a foreign epitope; expression at the cell surface. *EMBO J.* **5:**3029–3037.

Cole, S. T., and I. Saint Girons. 1994. Bacterial genomics. *FEMS Microbiol. Rev.* **14:**139–160.

Currier, T. C., and M. K. Morgan. 1982. Direct DNA repeat in plasmid R68.45 is associated with deletion formation and concomitant loss of chromosome mobilization ability. *J. Bacteriol.* **150:**251–259.

Davies, C. J., and C. A. Hutchison III. 1995. Insertion site specificity of the transposon Tn*3*. *Nucleic Acids Res.* **23:**507–514.

Dodd, I. B., and J. B. Egan. 1990. Improved detection of helix-turn-helix DNA-binding motifs in protein sequences. *Nucleic Acids Res.* **18:**5019–5026.

Dyda, F., A. B. Hickman, T. M. Jenkins, A. Engelman, R. Craigie, and D. R. Davies. 1994. Crystal structure of the catalytic domain of HIV-1 integrase: similarity to other polynucleotidyl transferases. *Science* **266:** 1981–1986.

Engelman, A., K. Mizuuchi, and R. Craigie. 1991. HIV-1 DNA integration: mechanism of viral DNA cleavage and DNA strand transfer. *Cell* **67:**1211–1221.

Gamas, G., and L. Craig. 1992. Purification and characterization of TnsC, a Tn*7* transposition protein that binds ATP and DNA. *Nucleic Acids Res.* **20:**2525–2532.

Gliesche, C. G., and P. Hirsch. 1992. Mutagenesis and chromosome mobilization in *Hyphomicrobium facilis* B-522. *Can. J. Microbiol.* **38:**1167–1174.

Goff, S. P. 1992. Genetics of retroviral integration. *Annu. Rev. Genet.* **26:**527–544.

Goff, S. P., and V. R. Prasad. 1991. Linker insertion mutagenesis as probe of structure-function relationships. *Methods Enzymol.* **208:**586–603.

Grindley, N. D. F., and A. E. Leschziner. 1995. DNA transposition: from a black box to a color monitor. *Cell* **83:**1063–1066.

Haas, D., and B. W. Holloway. 1976. R factor variants with enhanced sex factor activity in *Pseudomonas aeruginosa*. *Mol. Gen. Genet.* **144:**243–251.

Haas, D., and B. W. Holloway. 1978. Chromosome mobilization by the R plasmid R68.45: a tool in *Pseudomonas* genetics. *Mol. Gen. Genet.* **158:**229–237.

Haas, D., and G. Riess. 1983. Spontaneous deletions of the chromosome-mobilizing plasmid R68.45 in *Pseudomonas aeruginosa* PAO. *Plasmid* **9:**42–52.

Hayes, W. 1964. *The Genetics of Bacteria and Their Viruses.* Blackwell Scientific Publications, Oxford.

Holloway, B. W., V. Krishnapillai, and A. F. Morgan. 1979. Chromosomal genetics of *Pseudomonas*. *Microbiol. Rev.* **43:**73–102.

Holloway, B. W., and M. H. Richmond. 1973. R-factors used for genetic studies in strains of *Pseudomonas aeruginosa* and their origin. *Genet. Res.* **21:**103–105.

Katz, R. A., J. P. G. Mack, G. Merkel, J. Kulkosky, and Z. Ge. 1992. Requirement for a conserved serine in both processing and joining activities of retroviral integrase. *Proc. Natl. Acad. Sci. USA* **89:**6741–6745.

Katz, R. A., and A. M. Skalka. 1994. The retroviral enzymes. *Annu. Rev. Biochem.* **63:**133–173.

Kegler-Ebo, D. M., C. M. Docktor, and D. DiMaio. 1994. Codon cassette mutagenesis: a general method to insert or replace individual codons by using universal mutagenic cassettes. *Nucleic Acids Res.* **22:**1593–1599.

Kim, K., S.-Y. Namgoong, M. Jayaram, and R. M. Harshey. 1995. Step-arrest mutants of phage Mu transposase. *J. Biol. Chem.* **270:**1472–1479.

Koonin, E. V. 1992. DnaC protein contains a modified ATP-binding motif and belongs to a novel family of ATPases including also DnaA. *Nucleic Acids Res.* **20:**1997.

Matsutani, S., H. Ohtsubo, Y. Maeda, and E. Ohtsubo. 1987. Isolation and characterization of IS elements repeated in the bacterial chromosome. *J. Mol. Biol.* **196:**445–455.

Menou, G., J. Mahillon, M. M. Lecadet, and D. Lereclus. 1990. Structural and genetic organization of IS*232*, a new insertion sequence of *Bacillus thuringiensis*. *J. Bacteriol.* **172:**6689-6696.

Mizuuchi, K. 1992. Transpositional recombination: mechanistic insights from studies of Mu and other elements. *Annu. Rev. Biochem.* **61:**1011–1051.

Mizuuchi, K., and K. Adzuma. 1991. Inversion of the phosphate chirality at the target site of Mu DNA strand transfer: evidence for a one-step transesterification mechanism. *Cell* **66:**129–140.

Olasz, F., R. Stalder, and W. Arber. 1993. Formation of the tandem repeat (IS*30*)$_2$ and its role in IS*30*-mediated transpositional DNA rearrangements. *Mol. Gen. Genet.* **239:**177–187.

Pemberton, J. M. 1974. Size of the chromosome of *Pseudomonas aeruginosa* PAO. *J. Bacteriol.* **119:**748–752.

Penfold, R. J., and J. M. Pemberton. 1992. An improved suicide vector for construction of chromosomal insertion mutations in bacteria. *Gene* **118:**145–146.

Podladchikova, O. N., G. G. Dikhanov, A. V. Rakin, and J. Heesemann. 1994. Nucleotide sequence and structural organization of *Yersinia pestis* insertion sequence IS*100*. *FEMS Microbiol. Lett.* **121:**269–274.

Polard, P., and M. Chandler. 1995. Bacterial transposases and retroviral integrases. *Mol. Microbiol.* **15:**13–23.

Polard, P., M. F. Prère, O. Fayet, and M. Chandler. 1992. Transposase-induced excision and circularization of the bacterial insertion sequence IS*911*. *EMBO J.* **11:**5079–5090.

Reimmann, C., and D. Haas. 1986. IS*21* insertion in the *trfA* replication control gene of chromosomally integrated plasmid RP1: a property of stable *Pseudomonas aeruginosa* Hfr strains. *Mol. Gen. Genet.* **203:**511–519.

Reimmann, C., and D. Haas. 1987. Mode of replicon fusion mediated by the duplicated insertion sequence IS*21* in *Escherichia coli. Genetics* **115:**619–625.

Reimmann, C., and D. Haas. 1990. The *istA* gene of insertion sequence IS*21* is essential for cleavage at the inner 3′ ends of tandemly repeated IS*21* elements *in vitro. EMBO J.* **9:**4055–4063.

Reimmann, C., and D. Haas. 1993 Mobilization of chromosomes and nonconjugative plasmids by cointegrative mechanisms, p. 137–188. *In* D. B. Clewell (ed.), *Bacterial Conjugation.* Plenum Press, New York.

Reimmann, C., R. Moore, S. Little, A. Savioz, N. S. Willetts, and D. Haas. 1989. Genetic structure, function and regulation of the transposable element IS*21*. *Mol. Gen. Genet.* **215:**416–424.

Reimmann, C., M. Rella, and D. Haas. 1988. Integration of replication-defective R68.45-like plasmids into the *Pseudomonas aeruginosa* chromosome. *J. Gen. Microbiol.* **134:**1515–1523.

Rice, P., and K. Mizuuchi. 1995. Structure of the bacteriophage Mu transposase core: a common structural motif for DNA transposition and retroviral integration. *Cell* **82:**209–220.

Rogers, M. B., T. K. Bennett, C. M. Payne, and C. J. Smith. 1994. Insertional activation of *cepA* leads to high-level β-lactamase expression in *Bacteroides fragilis* clinical isolates. *J. Bacteriol.* **176:**4376–4384.

Royle, P. L., H. Matsumoto, and B. W. Holloway. 1981. Genetic circularity of the *Pseudomonas aeruginosa* PAO chromosome. *J. Bacteriol.* **145:**145–155.

Soby, S., B. Kirkpatrick, and T. Kosuge. 1993. Characterization of an insertion sequence (IS*53*) located within IS*51* on the *iaa*-containing plasmid of *Pseudomonas syringae* pv. *savastanoi. Plasmid* **29:**135–141.

Solinas, F., A. M. Marconi, M. Ruzzi, and E. Zennaro. 1995. Characterization and sequence of a novel insertion sequence. IS*1162*, from *Pseudomonas fluorescens. Gene* **155:**77–82.

Spielmann-Ryser, J., M. Moser, P. Kast, and H. Weber. 1991. Factors determining the frequency of plasmid cointegrate formation mediated by insertion sequence IS*3* from *Escherichia coli. Mol. Gen. Genet.* **226:**441–448.

Tricot, C., V. T. Nguyen, and V. Stalon. 1993. Steady-state kinetics and analysis of pH dependence on wild-type and a modified allosteric *Pseudomonas aeruginosa* ornithine carbamoyltransferase containing the replacement of glutamate 105 by alanine. *Eur. J. Biochem.* **215:**833–839.

Van Gent, D. C., A. A. M. Oude Groeneger, and R. H. A. Plasterk. 1992. Mutational analysis of the integrase protein of human immunodeficiency virus type 2. *Proc. Natl. Acad. Sci. USA* **89:**9598–9602.

Willetts, N. S., C. Crowther, and B. W. Holloway. 1981. The insertion sequence IS*21* of R68.45 and the molecular basis for mobilization of the bacterial chromosome. *Plasmid* **6:**30–52.

Xu, K., Z. Q. He, Y. M. Mao, R. Q. Sheng, and Z. J. Sheng. 1993. On two transposable elements from *Bacillus stearothermophilus. Plasmid* **29:**1–9.

Zebala, J., and F. Barany. 1991. Mapping catalytically important regions of an enzyme using two-codon insertion mutagenesis: a case study correlating β-lactamase mutants with the three-dimensional structure. *Gene* **100:**51–57.

Molecular Biology of Pseudomonads
Edited by T. Nakazawa et al.

Chapter 21

Phylogenetic Identification of *Pseudomonas* Strains Based on a Comparison of *gyrB* and *rpoD* Sequences

Shigeaki Harayama and Satoshi Yamamoto

Pseudomonas strains are well known for their widespread occurrence in natural habitats and their ability to utilize a great variety of organic compounds. Some species are animal or plant pathogens. In classical taxonomy, the pseudomonads constitute a group of gram-negative, rod-shaped, non-spore-forming, polar-flagellated bacteria whose G+C content is higher than 50%. Molecular studies show that the pseudomonads do not form a homogeneous entity but consist of phylogenetically unrelated genera (Palleroni, 1993).

rRNA homology was used to deduce the phylogenetic relationships between different *Pseudomonas* isolates, and these isolates were classified into five RNA homology groups (Palleroni, 1992). Molecular taxonomy based on 16S rRNA sequences placed the majority of gram-negative bacteria into the alpha, beta, gamma, and delta subdivisions of the family *Proteobacteria* (Stackebrandt et al., 1988). DNA-rRNA hybridization and analysis of the 16S rRNA sequences of *Pseudomonas* strains revealed that the bacteria in different rRNA groups are distantly related and belong to the alpha, beta, or gamma subdivision (de Vos et al., 1989; Olsen et al., 1994; Woese et al., 1985). At present, only rRNA group I, which contains the type species, *Pseudomonas aeruginosa*, is called *Pseudomonas;* the other groups have been reclassified into newly created genera (Table 1). However, the criteria for creating new genera are not uniform, and some genera may still contain species that are only distantly related. Although the authentic (group I) *Pseudomonas* genus consists of more than 100 species (Schroth et al., 1992), these species may be reclassified into a much smaller number of species if genetic diversity between them is reinvestigated by using molecular taxonomy.

The molecular monitoring of microbial ecosystems has recently received increasing attention as a way of understanding, for example, the fate of microorganisms introduced into natural environments and the effect of inocula on indigenous microbial populations. DNA probes in combination with PCR technology have been used to detect specific bacteria in various habitats with or without cell cultivation (Amann et al., 1995). However, the application of molecular techniques in the study of microbial ecology is still

Shigeaki Harayama and Satoshi Yamamoto • Marine Biotechnology Institute, Kamaishi Laboratories, 3-75-1 Heita, Kamaishi City, 026 Iwate, Japan.

Table 1. Examples of reclassified pseudomonads

Previous name	New name	Subclass	Reference
Group I *Pseudomonas*	*Pseudomonas*	Gamma	Woese et al., 1985
P. acidovorans	*Comamonas acidovorans*	Beta	Tamaoka et al., 1987
P. aminovorans	*Aminobacter aminovorans*	Alpha	Urakami et al., 1992
P. betle	*Stenotrophomonas maltophilia*	Gamma	Palleroni and Bradbury, 1993
P. carboxidovorans	*Oligotropha carboxidovorans*	Alpha	Meyer, 1993
P. cepacia	*Burkholderia cepacia*	Beta	Yabuuchi et al., 1992
P. compransoris	*Zavarzinia compransoris*	Alpha	Meyer et al., 1993
P. diminuta	*Brevundimonas diminuta*	Alpha	Segers et al., 1994
P. facilis	*Acidovorax facilis*	Beta	Willems et al., 1990
P. flava	*Hydrogenophaga flava*	Beta	Willems et al., 1989
P. gardneri	*Xanthomonas campestris*	Gamma	Holt et al., 1993
P. maltophilia	*Stenotrophomonas maltophilia*	Gamma	Palleroni and Bradbury, 1993
P. marina	*Deleya marina*	Gamma	Holt et al., 1993
P. mesophilica	*Methylobacterium mesophilicum*	Alpha	Holt et al., 1993
P. mixta	*Telluria mixta*	Beta	Bowman et al., 1993
P. paucimobilis	*Sphingomonas paucimobilis*	Alpha	Yabuuchi et al., 1990
P. ruhlandii	*Alcaligenes xylosoxidans*	Beta	
P. vesicularis	*Brevundimonas vesicularis*	Alpha	Segers et al., 1994
Pseudomonas sp. strain K172^{T}	*Thauera aromatica*	Beta	Anders et al., 1995
Pseudomonas sp. strain KB740^{T}	*Azoarcus evansii*	Beta	Anders et al., 1995

limited because of the difficulty in developing probes that are highly specific to each type of bacterium.

We were thus interested in developing a new molecular method for detecting and identifying bacteria (Yamamoto and Harayama, 1995). For this purpose, we used *gyrB* genes that encode the subunit B protein of DNA gyrase. DNA gyrase regulates the supercoiling of double-stranded DNA and is indispensable for DNA replication (McMacken et al., 1987). We describe here (i) a set of PCR primers that allow the amplification and sequencing of *gyrB* genes from a great variety of bacteria and (ii) PCR primers that amplify the *gyrB* genes from specific sets of *Pseudomonas putida* strains.

DESIGN OF UNIVERSAL PRIMERS FOR THE PCR AMPLIFICATION OF *gyrB*

Degenerate PCR primers for the amplification of *gyrB* genes were designed from two conserved regions of the amino acid sequences of the DNA gyrase subunit B proteins of *Escherichia coli* (GYRB_ECOLI in the SWISS-PROT database), *P. putida* (GYRB_PSEPU), and *Bacillus subtilis* (GYRB_BACSU). The two conserved amino acid sequences were reverse-translated, and a 41-nucleotide-long N-terminal PCR primer (NP) and a 44-nucleotide-long C-terminal PCR primer (CP) were synthesized accordingly (Fig. 1). The nucleotide sequences of the first 23 residues at the 5′ ends of both primers are not degenerate and therefore are not necessarily complementary to the target *gyrB* sequences. These 23 residues, however, can be used as hybridization sites of the sequencing primers, NS and CS (Fig. 1). The remaining 18 and 21

```
Sense Primers:

N-aa              E  V  I  M  T  V  L  H  A  G  G  K  F  D
N-na       5'  GARGTNATHATGACNGTNYTNCAYGCNGGNGGNAARTTYGAY 3'
PRIMER NP  5'  GAAGTCATCATGACCGTTCTGCAYGCNGGNGGNAARTTYGA 3'
PRIMER NS  5'  GAAGTCATCATGACCGTTCTGCA 3'

Antisense Primers:

C-aa              M  T  D  A  D  V  D  G  S  H  I  R  T  L  L
C-na       5'  ATGACNGAYGCNGAYGTNGAYGGNWSNCAYATHMGNACNYTNYTN 3'
PRIMER CP  3'  TACTGNCTRCGNCTRCANCTRCCGAGCGTGTAGGCATGGGACGA 5'
PRIMER CS                            3'  CCGAGCGTGTAGGCATGGGACGA 5'
```

Figure 1. Nucleotide sequences of the PCR primers (NP and CP) and sequencing primers (NS and CS). The 3′ region of each PCR primer is the degenerate region containing all possible combinations of nucleotide bases, while the 5′ region of each primer comprises the unique sequence among all possible nucleotide bases. The sequencing primers possess the unique sequences of the PCR primers. N-aa, conserved N-terminal amino acid sequence; N-na, nucleotide sequence encoding the conserved N-terminal amino acid sequence; C-aa, conserved C-terminal amino acid sequence; C-na, nucleotide sequence encoding the conserved C-terminal amino acid sequence; H = A, C, or T; M = A or C; N = A, C, G, or T; R = A or G; S = C or G; W = A or T; Y = C or T.

nucleotides of the N-terminal and C-terminal primers, respectively, are degenerate, and each of them makes 512 variations.

PCR amplification of *gyrB* was carried out by using DNA from bacteria of different taxonomic groups, and PCR products with sizes predicted from the known *gyrB* sequences (1.2 kb) were amplified from the strains listed in Table 2. Thus, by using the set of primers presented in Fig. 1, it was possible to amplify the *gyrB* genes from a broad range of bacteria: the alpha, beta, and gamma subdivisions of *Proteobacteria*; the *Cytophaga-Flexibacter-Bacteroides* group; and low- and high-G+C gram-positive bacteria (Olsen et al., 1994). Consequently, the primer set appears to be able to amplify the *gyrB* sequences of most gram-negative bacteria and some gram-positive bacteria.

SEQUENCING OF *gyrB* AND 16S rDNA OF *P. putida* STRAINS

Sixteen *P. putida* strains were used for further analysis. DNA from these strains was isolated, and the *gyrB* genes were amplified and sequenced by using the primer sets NP-CP and NS-CS, respectively, by the method of Yamamoto and Harayama (1995). The sequences of 16S rDNAs (DNA coding for rRNA) from these strains were also determined as described previously (Edwards et al., 1989). The frequency of base substitutions in 16S rDNA was lower than that in *gyrB*. For example, in *P. putida* JCM 6156 and IFO 14164^{T}, 92 base substitutions were observed in the 1,167-bp-long *gyrB* sequences, but only 14 base substitutions were observed in the 1,329-bp-long 16S rDNA sequences. Similarly, in JCM 6156 and PB4, 28 base substitutions were found in the *gyrB* sequences, but only 2 base substitutions were found in the 16S rDNA sequences. Most of the base

Table 2. Bacteria in which the *gyrB* gene is amplified by universal primers

Acinetobacter calcoaceticus (ATCC 31012 and ATCC 33308)
Acinetobacter sp. (many strains)
Alcaligenes faecalis (ATCC 8750)
Alteromonas espejiana (ATCC 29659)
Alteromonas haloplanktis (ATCC 14393)
Alteromonas macleodii (ATCC 27126)
Bacillus subtilis 222 (Marburg strain, ATCC 6051)
Chromatium vinosum (ATCC 12472)
Chromobacterium violaceum (ATCC 12472)
Comamonas acidovorans (IFO 13582)
Cytophaga aprica (ATCC 23126)
Cytophaga marinoflava (IFO 14170)
Cytophaga uliginosa (ATCC 14397)
Erythrobacter longus (IFO 14126)
Escherichia coli (many natural isolates)
Escherichia coli K-12 (ATCC 10798)
Flavobacterium breve (IFO 14943)
Flavobacterium odoratum (IFO 14945)
Flavobacterium sp. (many strains)
Flexibacter maritimus (ATCC 43398)
Flexibacter sp. (PJSA17)
Gardnerella vaginalis (ATCC 14018)
Lactobacillus sp. (144L, TQ3)
Pseudomonas aeruginosa (ATCC 15692 and many other strains; see Fig. 2)
Pseudomonas alkanolytica (IFO 12319)
Pseudomonas atlantica (ATCC 19262 and ATCC 43667)
Pseudomonas doudoroffii (ATCC 27123 and two other strains)
Pseudomonas fluorescens (DSM 50108)
Pseudomonas nautica (ATCC 27132)
Pseudomonas piscicida (ATCC 15057)
Pseudomonas putida (IFO 14164^{T} and many other strains; see Fig. 2)
Pseudomonas stutzeri (IFO 14165)
Rhodobacter sphaeroides 2.4.1 (ATCC 17023)
Salmonella typhimurium (ATCC 19585)
Shewanella bathycetes (ATCC 23597)
Sphingomonas adhaesiva (IFO 15099)
Sphingomonas asaccharolytica (IFO 15499)
Sphingomonas capsulata (IFO 12533)
Sphingomonas macrogoltabidus (IFO 15033)
Sphingomonas mali (IFO 15500)
Sphingomonas paucimobilis (IFO 13935)
Sphingomonas pruni (IFO 15498)
Sphingomonas sp. (many strains)
Sphingomonas terrae (IFO 15103)
Sphingomonas yanoikuyae (IFO 15102)
Sphingomonas parapaucimobilis (IFO 15100)
Streptococcus salivarius (ATCC 13419)
Xanthomonas maltophilia (ATCC 13637)

substitutions in the *gyrB* genes occurred at synonymous positions. For example, only 4 of 92 base substitutions caused amino acid substitutions in JCM 6156 and IFO 14164^T.

Thus, in *P. putida*, the base substitution frequency in *gyrB* was much higher than that in 16S rDNA. The base substitutions of 16S rDNA may be restricted by the fact that a large part of the primary and secondary structures of 16S rRNA are important for its functions (Gutell et al., 1994). The primary constraint for the molecular evolution of *gyrB* genes is the conservation of amino acid sequence in order to maintain the functions of the gene, and synonymous base substitutions that do not provoke amino acid substitutions are generally accepted. The difference in the base substitution frequency in 16S rDNA and *gyrB* may thus be due to the difference in the number of sites available for neutral base substitutions.

PHYLOGENETIC RELATIONSHIPS AMONG *P. putida* STRAINS

The phylogenetic tree based on *gyrB* nucleotide sequences is shown in Fig. 2 (middle). Previous studies divided *P. putida* strains into two subgroups, biotypes A and B (Stanier et al., 1966). In agreement with the division, biotype A strains (ATCC 17485, ATCC 23973, ATCC 11172, and IFO 14164^T) and biotype B strains (ATCC 17484 and ATCC 17522) were separately clustered in the two major branches of the phylogenetic tree. The first branch was further divided into three lineages. The first lineage contained five strains: KD23 and PB4 isolated from seawater around Kuwait and Palau, respectively; and

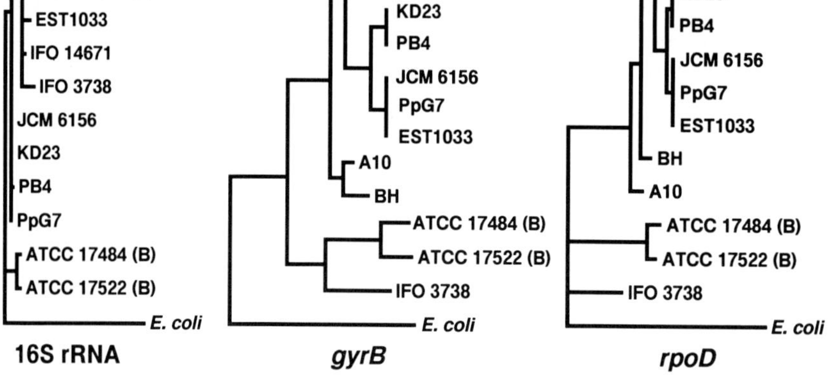

Figure 2. *P. putida* strain phylogenetic trees based on the nucleotide sequences of 16S rDNA (left), *gyrB* (middle), and *rpoD* (right). The tree was constructed by the maximum parsimony method. (A) and (B) after strain numbers indicate biotypes A and B, respectively.

EST1033, JCM 6156 (= *P. putida* mt-2 containing the TOL pWW0 plasmid), and PpG7 isolated from soils in Italy, Japan, and the United States, respectively. The second lineage contains strains FK715 and IFO 14671 in addition to biotype A strains, and the third lineage contained A10 and BH, both isolated in Japan as mandelate- and phenol-degrading bacteria, respectively. Strain IFO 3738 (= ATCC 8209) was located in the second major branch with biotype B strains.

Comparison of the topology of the *gyrB*-based phylogenetic tree with that based on 16S rDNA sequences (Fig. 2, left) shows that the two are quite different from each other. In the 16S rDNA-based tree, typical representatives of biotype A are resolved from those of biotype B, but IFO 3738 and EST1033 are grouped with IFO 14671. In the analysis of 16S rDNA, the numbers of substitutions in compared sequences were low, and statistical errors due to these low numbers may be the cause of the aberrant structure of the 16S rDNA-based phylogenetic tree. If this is the case, then 16S rDNA analysis may not be appropriate for deducing phylogenetic relationships among closely related bacteria.

To substantiate this hypothesis, we amplified and sequenced the *rpoD* genes (the structural genes for the major sigma factor of RNA polymerase) of these *P. putida* strains by using specific primers designed from the consensus sequences of RpoD from *E. coli* (RP70_ECOLI) and *P. aeruginosa* (RP70_PSEAE) (S. Yamamoto and S. Harayama, manuscript in preparation). When the topology of the *rpoD*-based phylogenetic tree (Fig. 2, right) is compared with those of the *gyrB*- and 16S rRNA-based trees, it is apparent that the *rpoD*-based tree resembles the *gyrB*-based tree but differs from the 16S rDNA-based tree.

In modern bacterial taxonomy, rRNA sequence analysis is the standard method for investigating phylogenetic relationships (Olsen et al., 1994). However, the results of rDNA sequence analysis sometimes disagree with the results of classical taxonomy (Christensen et al., 1994) or with those of DNA hybridization, which is also considered a standard measure of relatedness (Fox et al., 1992; Rainey et al., 1994; Stackebrandt and Goebel, 1994). When the numbers of substituted bases in compared rDNAs are small (as happens when bacteria are closely related), it is advisable not to use rDNA results but to rely on a gene determining a protein (e.g., *gyrB* sequence) for comparison in order to establish the phylogenetic relationships of the bacteria examined.

DEVELOPMENT OF PCR PRIMERS FOR DETECTING SPECIFIC STRAINS OF *P. putida*

Three sets of PCR primers were developed to amplify the *gyrB* genes of specific *P. putida* strains. A set of primers (set A) was designed from the consensus *gyrB* sequences of *P. putida* strains located in the first major branch of the *gyrB*-based tree (Fig. 2, middle). The second set of primers (set B) was designed from the *gyrB* sequence specific to the second cluster of the first branch (JCM 6156 and PB4), and the third set of primers (set C) was designed from a specific sequence of PB4. The results of PCR amplification when these primers are used are shown in Fig. 3. Primer set A amplified the *gyrB* sequences of all the *P. putida* strains but did not amplify those of the other *Pseudomonas* strains tested (*P. stutzeri*, *P. alkanolytica*, *P. fluorescens*, and *P. aeruginosa*). Primer set B promoted amplification of the *gyrB* sequences of JCM 6156 and PB4 but not of IFO 14164^{T}, while primer set C promoted amplification of the *gyrB* sequence of PB4 only. It was thus possible to differentially amplify the *gyrB* fragments of *P. putida* strains.

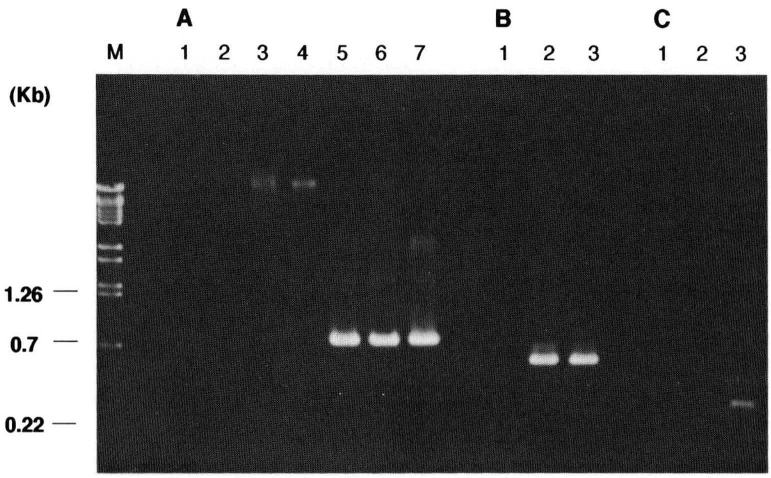

Figure 3. PCR amplification of *gyrB* of *P. putida* using specific primers. (A) PCR amplification with primer set A (specific to *P. putida*). Lanes: M, *Bst*EII-digested lambda DNA; 1, *P. stutzeri*; 2, *P. alkanolytica*; 3, *P. fluorescens*; 4, *P. aeruginosa*; 5, *P. putida* IFO 14164^T; 6, *P. putida* JCM 6156; 7, *P. putida* PB4. (B) PCR amplification with primer set B (specific to JCM 6156 and PB4). Lanes: 1, *P. putida* IFO 14164^T; 2, *P. putida* JCM 6156; 3, *P. putida* PB4. (C) PCR amplification with primer set C (specific to PB4). Lanes: 1, *P. putida* IFO 14164^T; 2, *P. putida* JCM 6156; 3, *P. putida* PB4. Sets A, B, and C correspond to the combinations of primers P734 and P1455r, P895 and P1455r, and P895 and P1213r, respectively, as described by Yamamoto and Harayama (1995).

CONCLUSIONS

Sequence analysis of *gyrB* is a rapid and effective method for identifying bacterial species and examining their phylogenetic relationships. In principle, any protein-coding sequences can be used for phylogenetic analysis. However, many genes, especially those for catabolism, are known to spread horizontally among different bacterial species, and they cannot be used to trace the evolutionary record of host bacteria. Criteria for selecting appropriate taxonomic marker genes may be that (i) they are essential for housekeeping activities such as DNA replication, transcription, and translation; (ii) they exist as a single copy on each genome; and (iii) at least two regions in their amino acid sequences should be conserved for the production of a set of PCR primers. We searched for such genes, and we conclude that *gyrB* is ideal for such a purpose.

Acknowledgments. We are grateful to Ikuko Hiramatsu for technical assistance. This work was supported by New Energy and Industrial Technology Development Organization.

REFERENCES

Amann, R. I., W. Ludwig, and K.-H. Schleifer. 1995. Phylogenetic identification and *in situ* detection of individual microbial cells without cultivation. *Microbiol. Rev.* **59:**143–169.

Anders, H.-J., A. Kaetzke, P. Kämpfer, W. Ludwig, and G. Fuchs. 1995. Taxonomic position of aromatic-degrading denitrifying pseudomonad strains K 172 and KB 740 and their description as new members of the genera *Thauera*, as *Thauera aromatica* sp. nov., and *Azoarcus*, as *Azoarcus evansii* sp. nov., respectively, members of the beta subclass of the *Proteobacteria*. *Int. J. Syst. Bacteriol.* **45:**327–333.

Bowman, J. P., L. I. Sly, A. C. Hayward, Y. Spiegel, and E. Stackebrandt. 1993. *Telluria mixta (Pseudomonas mixta* Bowman, Sly, and Hayward 1988) gen. nov., comb. nov., and *Telluria chitinolytica* sp. nov., soil-dwelling organisms which actively degrade polysaccharides. *Int. J. Syst. Bacteriol.* **43:**120–124.

Christensen, H., M. Boye, L. K. Poulsen, and O. F. Rasmussen. 1994. Analysis of fluorescent pseudomonads based on 23S ribosomal DNA sequences. *Appl. Environ. Microbiol.* **60:**2196–2199.

De Vos, P., A. van Landschoot, P. Segers, R. Tytgat, M. Gillis, M. Bauwens, R. Rossau, M. Goor, B. Pot, K. Kersters, P. Lizzaraga, and J. de Ley. 1989. Genotypic relationships and taxonomic localization of unclassified *Pseudomonas* and *Pseudomonas*-like strains by deoxyribonucleic acid:ribosomal ribonucleic acid hybridizations. *Int. J. Syst. Bacteriol.* **39:**35–49.

Edwards, U., T. Rogall, H. Blocker, M. Emde, and E. C. Bottger. 1989. Isolation and direct complete nucleotide determination of entire genes. Characterization of a gene coding for 16S ribosomal RNA. *Nucleic Acids Res.* **17:**7843–7853.

Fox, G. E., J. D. Wisotzkey, and P. J. Jurtshuk. 1992. How close is close:16S rRNA sequence identity may not be sufficient to guarantee species identity. *Int. J. Syst. Bacteriol.* **42:**166–170.

Gutell, R. R., H. Larsen, and C. R. Woese. 1994. Lessons from an evolving rRNA: 16S and 23S rRNA structures from a comparative perspective. *Microbiol. Rev.* **58:**10–26.

Holt, J. G., N. R. Krieg, P. H. A. Sneath, J. T. Staley, and S. T. Williams. 1993. *Bergey's Manual of Determinative Bacteriology*, 9th ed. The Williams & Wilkins Co., Baltimore.

McMacken, R., L. Silver, and C. Georgopoulos. 1987. DNA replication, p. 578–580. *In* F. C. Neidhardt, J. L. Ingraham, K. B. Low, B. Magasanik, M. Schaechter, and H. E. Umbarger (ed.), *Escherichia coli and Salmonella typhimurium: Cellular and Molecular Biology*. American Society for Microbiology, Washington, D.C.

Meyer, O., E. Stackebrandt, and G. Auling. 1993. Reclassification of ubiquinone Q-10 containing carboxidotrophic bacteria: transfer of "*[Pseudomonas] carboxydovorans*" OM5^T to *Oligotropha*, gen. nov., as *Oligotropha carboxidovorans*, comb. nov., transfer of "*[Alcaligenes] carboxydus*" DSM 1086^T to *Carbophilus*, gen. nov., *as Carbophilus carboxidus*, comb. nov., transfer of "*[Pseudomonas] compransoris*" DSM 1231^T to *Zavarzinia*, gen. nov., as *Zavarzinia compransoris*, comb. nov., and amended descriptions of the new genera. *Syst. Appl. Microbiol.* **16:**390–395.

Olsen, G. J., C. R. Woese, and R. Overbeek. 1994. The winds of (evolutionary) change: breathing new life into microbiology. *J. Bacteriol.* **176:**1–6.

Palleroni, N. J. 1992. Present situation of the taxonomy of the aerobic pseudomonads, p. 105–115. *In* E. Galli, S. Silver, and B. Witholt (ed.*), Pseudomonas: Molecular Biology and Biotechnology*. American Society for Microbiology, Washington, D.C.

Palleroni, N. J. 1993. *Pseudomonas* classification. A new case history in the taxonomy of Gram-negative bacteria. *Antonie van Leeuwenhoek* **64:**231–251.

Palleroni, N. J., and J. F. Bradbury. 1993. *Stenotrophomonas*, a new bacterial genus for *Xanthomonas maltophilia* (Hugh 1980) Swings et al., 1983. *Int. J. Syst. Bacteriol.* **43:**606–609.

Rainey, F. A., E. Lang, and E. Stackebrandt. 1994. The phylogenetic structure of the genus *Acinetobacter*. *FEMS Microbiol. Lett.* **124:**349–353.

Schroth, M. N., D. C. Hildebrand, and N. Panopoulos. 1992. Phytopathogenic pseudomonads and related plant-associated pseudomonas, p. 3104–3131. *In* A. Balows, H.-G. Trüper, M. Dworkin, W. Harder, and K.-H. Schleifer (ed.), *The Prokaryotes — A Handbook on the Biology of Bacteria: Ecophysiology, Isolation, Identification, Applications*. Springer, New York.

Segers, P., M. Vancanneyt, B. Pot, U. Torck, B. Hoste, D. Dewettinck, E. Falsen, K. Kersters, and P. De Vos. 1994. Classification of *Pseudomonas diminuta* Leifson and Hugh 1954 and *Pseudomonas vesicularis* Busing, Doll, and Freytag 1953 in *Brevundimonas* gen. nov. as *Brevundimonas diminuta* comb. nov. and *Brevundimonas vesicularis* comb. nov., respectively. *Int. J. Syst. Bacteriol.* **44:**499–510.

Stackebrandt, E., and B. Goebel. 1994. Taxonomic note: a place for DNA-DNA reassociation and 16S rRNA sequence analysis in the present species definition in bacteriology. *Int. J. Syst. Bacteriol.* **44:**846–849.

Stackebrandt, E., R. G. E. Murray, and H. G. Trüper. 1988. *Proteobacteria* classis nov., a name for the phylogenetic taxon that includes the "purple bacteria and their relatives." *Int. J. Syst. Bacteriol.* **38:**321–325.

Stanier, R. Y., N. J. Palleroni, and M. Doudoroff. 1966. The aerobic pseudomonads: a taxonomic study. *J. Gen. Microbiol.* **43:**159–271.

Tamaoka, J., D.-M. Ha, and K. Komagata. 1987. Reclassification *of Pseudomonas acidovorans* den Dooren de Jong 1926 and *Pseudomonas testosteroni* Marcus and Talalay 1956 as *Comamonas acidovorans* comb.

nov. and *Comamonas testosterioni* comb. nov., with an emended description of the genus *Comamonas*. *Int. J. Syst. Bacteriol.* **37:**52–59.

Urakami, T., H. Araki, H. Oyanagi, K. Suzuki, and K. Komagata. 1992. Transfer of *Pseudomonas aminovorans* (den Dooren de Jong 1926) to *Aminobacter* gen. nov. as *Aminobacter aminovorans* comb. nov. and description of *Aminobacter aganoensis* sp. nov. and *Aminobacter niigataensis* sp. nov. *Int. J. Syst. Bacteriol.* **42:**84–92.

Willems, A., J. Busse, M. Goor, B. Pot, E. Falsen, E. Jantzen, B. Hoste, M. Gillis, K. Kersters, G. Auling, and J. De Ley. 1989. *Hydrogenophaga*, a new genus of hydrogen-oxidizing bacteria that includes *Hydrogenophaga flava* comb. nov. (formerly *Pseudomonas flava*), *Hydrogenophaga palleronii* (formerly *Pseudomonas palleronii*), *Hydrogenophaga pseudoflava* (formerly *Pseudomonas pseudoflava* and "*Pseudomonas carboxydoflava*") and *Hydrogenophaga taeniospiralis* (formerly *Pseudomonas taeniospiralis*). *Int. J. Syst. Bacteriol.* **39:**384–398.

Willems, A., E. Falsen, B. Pot, E. Jantzen, B. Hoste, P. Vandamme, M. Gillis, K. Kersters, and J. De Ley. 1990. *Acidovorax*, a new genus for *Pseudomonas facilis*, *Pseudomonas delafieldii*, EF group 13, EF group 16, and several clinical isolates, with the species *Acidovorax facilis* comb. nov., *Acidovorax delafieldii* comb. nov., and *Acidovorax temperans* sp. nov. *Int. J. Syst. Bacteriol.* **40:**384–398.

Woese, C. R., W. G. Weisburg, C. M. Hahn, B. J. Paster, L. B. Zablen, B. J. Lewis, T. J. Macke, W. Ludwig, and E. Stackebrandt. 1985. The phylogeny of purple bacteria: the gamma subdivision. *Syst. Appl. Microbiol.* **6:**25–33.

Yabuuchi, E., Y. Kosako, H. Oyaizu, I. Yano, H. Hotta, Y. Hashimoto, T. Ezaki, and M. Arakawa. 1992. Proposal of *Burkholderia* gen. nov. and transfer of seven species of the genus *Pseudomonas* homology group II to the new genus, with the type species *Burkholderia cepacia* (Palleroni and Holmes 1981) comb. nov. *Microbiol. Immunol.* **36:**1251–1275.

Yabuuchi, E., I. Yano, H. Oyaizu, Y. Hashimoto, T. Ezaki, and H. Yamasato. 1990. Proposals of *Sphingomonas paucimobilis* gen. nov. and comb. nov., *Sphingomonas parapaucimobilis* sp. nov., *Sphingomonas yanoikuyae* sp. nov., *Sphingomonas adhaesiva* sp. nov., *Sphingomonas capsulata* comb. nov., and two genospecies of the genus *Sphingomonas*. *Microbiol. Immunol.* **34:**99–119.

Yamamoto, S., and S. Harayama. 1995. PCR amplification and direct sequencing of *gyrB* genes with universal primers and their application to the detection and taxonomic analysis of *Pseudomonas putida* strains. *Appl. Environ. Microbiol.* **61:**1104–1109.

Molecular Biology of Pseudomonads
Edited by T. Nakazawa et al.

Chapter 22

Chromosome Multiplicity in *Burkholderia cepacia*

William Hendrickson, Anette Hübner, and Andrew Kavanaugh-Black

Burkholderia (formerly *Pseudomonas*) *cepacia* is important in environmental microbiology and bioremediation of numerous toxic compounds (Lessie and Gaffney, 1986; Bhat et al., 1994; Shields and Reagin, 1992; Shields et al., 1995). It is also of increasing importance as a pathogen in cystic fibrosis cases and nosocomial infections (Steinbach et al., 1994; Sun et al., 1995; Smith et al., 1993). *B. cepacia* appears to possess a highly plastic genome with tremendous adaptive capacity. It is unclear how this capacity evolves and is maintained, but it has been proposed that genes are transferred laterally among *Burkholderia* and other genera and that new metabolic capabilities are produced by integration of genes as well as modification of existing pathways for degradation of toxic compounds (Holloway et al., 1990; Lessie et al., 1990).

B. cepacia AC1100 appears to have acquired, during prolonged selection in continuous culture, genes for the degradation and utilization of the herbicide 2,4,5-trichlorophenoxyacetic acid (2,4,5-T) (Kellogg et al., 1981; Kilbane et al., 1982). Thus, strain AC1100 is of particular interest because it can degrade a persistent environmental pollutant, and it provides an example of an organism that appears to have rapidly evolved and acquired genes originally present in a consortium. Genes at two loci specifying a portion of this pathway were cloned and sequenced, and the encoded enzymes were characterized (Danganan et al., 1994; Daubaras et al., 1995). The association of these genes with insertion sequence (IS) elements and their locations on the genome suggest that portions of the 2,4,5-T pathway may have evolved by separate translocation events stimulated by the IS elements. ISs seem to be a common general source for chromosomal instability in *B. cepacia. B. cepacia* isolate 17616 contains numerous copies of at least nine different IS elements that have been well characterized (Gaffney and Lessie, 1987; Ferrante and Lessie, 1991; Byrne and Lessie, 1994; Lessie et al., 1990). Many of these elements can activate transcription of adjacent genes in the chromosome, which is advantageous in the evolution of new metabolic pathways.

We are using physical mapping techniques to determine the overall structure of *B. cepacia* genomes and, in strain AC1100, the distribution and function of insertion

William Hendrickson, Anette Hübner, and Andrew Kavanaugh-Black • Department of Microbiology and Immunology, University of Illinois, Chicago, Illinois 60612.

elements and the location of the catabolic genes for 2,4,5-T. A detailed comparison of the genomes of different *B. cepacia* isolates and characterization of chromosomal rearrangements will provide a clearer understanding of the evolutionary dynamics of this species.

MULTIPLE CHROMOSOMES IN BACTERIA

"All bacteria possess a single, circular chromosome": such was the conventional wisdom for the past 3 decades. Recent advances in the technology for physically analyzing large DNA molecules have permitted investigators to map rapidly the genomes of an array of organisms. One conclusion from these data is that bacterial genomes are far more complex and plastic than previously appreciated. The greatest surprise was the observation of multiple large replicons with all the expected properties of true chromosomes.

Suwanto and Kaplan (1989) were the first to clearly establish the existence of bacterial chromosome multiplicity. The physical map of the genome of the photosynthetic bacterium *Rhodobacter sphaeroides* resolved into two replicons of 3.0×10^6 and 0.9×10^6 bp (3.0 and 0.9 Mb). The smaller replicon clearly is not a "megaplasmid" that would be dispensable for normal growth. Both replicons are present in equal stoichiometry, they are equally stable, and both carry tRNA and rRNA operons. Several genes for metabolic functions were genetically mapped to the smaller replicon, confirming its identity as a chromosome (Choudhary et al., 1994).

Subsequently, pulsed-field gel electrophoresis of whole replicons and physical mapping revealed the presence of multiple replicons in several additional species. The *Brucella melitensis* 16M genome consists of 2.1- and 1.1-Mb chromosomes (Michaux et al., 1993). Two sets of rRNA genes reside on the larger chromosome and one is on the smaller chromosome. Two chromosomal bands of similar sizes appeared in electrophoresis of the DNA of other *Brucella* species, suggesting that all have multiple chromosomes. *Agrobacterium tumefaciens* also has two chromosomes of 3.0 and 2.1 Mb. In this case, however, the larger chromosome has the usual circular structure, whereas the smaller one appears to be linear (Allardet-Servent et al., 1993). In *Leptospira interrogans,* the presence of an essential gene on a 530-kb replicon has led to the suggestion that it is a second chromosome (Zuerner et al., 1993). All of these organisms are members of the alpha subdivision of the family *Proteobacteriaceae,* but some members of this family contain single-chromosome genomes, so chromosome multiplicity is not a universal characteristic of this group.

B. CEPACIA REPLICONS

Cheng and Lessie (1994) demonstrated that chromosome multiplicity is not confined to the alpha subdivision of the *Proteobacteriaceae.* Mapping of large restriction nuclease fragments of DNA from *B. cepacia* 17616 (also called strain 249) defined three large circular replicons of 3.4, 2.5, and 0.9 Mb. Single- and multiple-enzyme digests of DNA with rare-cutting enzymes, along with Southern blot hybridization of junction fragments, were used to order the fragment map and clearly resolve the three separate linkage groups. rRNA genes were found on all three replicons, supporting the conclusion that all three are chromosomes. Transposon insertions into genes for the synthesis of several amino acids were mapped to the largest replicon, whereas the genes for phthalate, ribitol, and penicillin utilization and lysine synthesis were lost in a strain with a large deletion in the 2.5-Mb replicon.

The chromosomal map of an additional *B. cepacia* strain, 25416, confirmed the presence of three chromosomes (Rodley et al., 1995). Two-dimensional pulsed-field gel techniques were used to map replicons of 3.65, 3.17, and 1.07 Mb to an average resolution of about 100 kb. As found with strain 17616, all three replicons carry rRNA genes. However, there was no obvious conservation of restriction patterns, suggesting that substantial chromosomal rearrangement may occur in *B. cepacia*.

We have used pulsed-field gel electrophoresis to measure chromosome sizes of several *B. cepacia* isolates (A. Hübner, R. Edelstein, A. Black, and W. Hendrickson, manuscript in preparation). Gels were run in a contour-clamped homogeneous electric field (CHEF) apparatus for 22 h to obtain accurate size data for the small to medium replicons of 0.15 to 1.5 Mb (Table 1). Data for larger replicons were obtained with gels run for 170 h. Linear DNA up to 6 Mb can be resolved under the conditions used. Circular DNA does not run into these gels, so bands are only obtained for these molecules that have been linearized by a single random break. To increase the yield of DNA entering the gels from the agar plugs used for cell lysis, we introduced a freeze-thaw procedure during preparation of the DNA. This method increases the amount of DNA reproducibly entering the gels; however, it does not alter the band pattern or greatly increase the amount of highly fragmented DNA smeared in the gel lanes. From these gels we observed that the genome of strain AC1100 has five replicons of 4, 2.7, 0.53, 0.34, and 0.15 Mb (Table 1) (Hübner et al., in preparation). The total genome size is 7.7 Mb, which is intermediate in size compared with strains 17616 and 25416.

Restriction enzyme mapping demonstrates that the DNA replicons reported in Table 1 do not result from breaks in larger molecules, but are independent circular replicons. We are assembling a macrorestriction map of AC1100 using the rare-cutting restriction enzymes *Swa*I, *Pac*I, *Pme*I, *Ceu*I, and *Spe*I. Such a map will afford us a more detailed comparison of chromosome structure with the previously mapped strains 17616 and 25416. The map will be useful in analysis of chromosomal evolution and rearrangements. DNA

Table 1. Replicon sizes observed in *B. cepacia* strains

Strain	Replicon sizes[a] (Mb)	Total genome size (Mb)
AC1100	4.0, 2.7, 0.53, 0.34, 0.15	7.75
N2P5	5.3, 3.5, 0.5	9.3
PT88	4.1, 2.7, 0.56, 0.31, 0.15	7.85
17616 (249)	3.3, 2.5, 0.9, 0.17	6.9
249-2 (*lys*)	3.3, 1.76, 0.63	5.7
ATCC10661	3.7, 3.4, 1.6	8.7
B.c.1[b]	3.1, 2.4, 1.0	6.5
B.c.2[b]	4.9, 2.7, 0.2	7.8
B.c.3[b]	3.4, 3.0, 0.74	7.1

[a]Sizes of replicons greater than 1.0 Mb were determined in gels run for 170 h with a 500- to 3,400-s ramped pulse time at 50 V; sizes of replicons smaller than 1.0 Mb were determined in gels run for 22 h with a 50- to 90-s ramped pulse time at 200 V.
[b]Strains isolated from cystic fibrosis patients, provided by K. Williams and D. Allison.

from the undigested individual replicons and from restriction fragments was excised from pulsed-field gels, labeled, and used as probes for Southern blot hybridizations. *Swa*I- and *Ceu*I-digested DNA fragments were unambiguously assigned to separate replicons by using labeled whole replicon DNA fragments as probes. Then, fragment linkages within each replicon were determined. Physical maps for replicons 1 and 2 were constructed by this method and show that these replicons are independent, circular molecules. Restriction enzyme *Ceu*I cuts within the 23S rRNA sequences of many gram-negative organisms (Liu et al., 1992); therefore, the enzyme can be used to map the rRNA genes. A *Ceu*I digest of strain AC1100 produces three large DNA fragments and three small fragments of 500, 300, and 200 kb, all of which map to the two large replicons. This result suggests there are at least six rRNA genes that are not highly clustered. A 16S rRNA gene probe was produced by PCR using highly conserved primers and strain AC1100 DNA as template. With the 16S rRNA probe, the rRNA genes of strain AC1100 were found in the two largest replicons in positions consistent with the results of *Ceu*I digestions.

The replicon numbers and sizes vary considerably among the *B. cepacia* strains studied. On the basis of 16S rRNA homology, the phenanthrene-utilizing strain N2P5 is similar to strain AC1100 (R. Devereux, personal communication), but the replicon sizes are very different (Table 1). N2P5 has the largest total genome size found, 9.3 Mb, more than 20% larger than that of strain AC1100. It has the largest single replicon surveyed, 5.3 Mb, as well as 3.5- and 0.5-Mb molecules. Other isolates from the same collection of phenanthrene utilizers (provided by S. Lantz and R. Devereux) also had large genomes with variable chromosome sizes (not shown). The environmental isolate 10661 also has a large genome with three replicons of 1.6, 3.4, and 3.7 Mb. The two largest molecules run as a closely associated doublet on CHEF gels, but their presence is confirmed by genome size estimates from restriction fragment patterns. This was the only environmental isolate studied that did not appear to harbor small replicons of 1 Mb or less. Multiple chromosomes of *Burkholderia* were first demonstrated in *B. cepacia* 17616 (Cheng and Lessie, 1994). Our size estimates for the chromosomes of *B. cepacia* 17616 and the *lys* deletion derivative closely match the published values of Cheng and Lessie (1994), so the observed variations in size values among strains are likely to be real and not artifacts of the gel techniques. Overall, the sizes of individual replicons vary dramatically and the total genome size differs by over 3 Mb.

Analysis of clinical isolates (provided by K. Williams and D. G. Allison) from cystic fibrosis patients also revealed significant variation among strains (B.c.1 through B.c.3 in Table 1). Strain B.c.2 has the largest genome, 7.8 Mb, but it has only two chromosomes. It is not clear whether the smaller megabase replicon found in most strains is dispensable, or whether it can fuse with one of the other chromosomes. Additional clinical isolates are being analyzed to compare strains that were isolated from patients with very different clinical histories, and isolates obtained over time from the patient, to look for correlations of genome structure and disease state.

LOCATIONS OF *tft* GENES

B. cepacia AC1100 is capable of utilizing the defoliant 2,4,5-T as a sole source of carbon and energy. This capability is quickly lost in the absence of 2,4,5-T (Chatterjee et al., 1982). A metabolic pathway was suggested based on studies of intermediates produced by the parental and mutant strains (Sangodkar et al., 1988; Sangodkar et al., 1989). Two gene clusters involved in the catabolism of 2,4,5-T by strain AC1100 have been cloned and characterized. The *tftA* and *tftB* genes encode an oxygenase required for the first step, the conversion of 2,4,5-T to 2,4,5-trichlorophenol (TCP) (Fig. 1) (Haugland et al., 1991; Danganan et al., 1994). A second clone, containing genes designated *tftEFGH*, complements a transposon-induced mutant strain (PT88) unable to grow on 2,4,5-T (Sangodkar et al., 1988; Daubaras et al., 1995). The PT88 mutant accumulates 5-chloro-1,2,4-trihydroxybenzene (oxidized to 5-chlorohydroxyhydroquinone), which is thought to be an intermediate in the lower portion of the pathway. Based on amino acid homology, the enzyme activities of the *tftH* and *tftE* gene products have been suggested (Fig. 1) (Daubaras et al., 1995). The two sets of *tft* genes are flanked by insertion elements IS*931* and IS*932*, which may have been involved in the transfer of DNA into *B. cepacia*. We looked at the chromosomal location of the *tft* genes by Southern blot hybridization to whole replicons separated by pulsed-field gel electrophoresis. The *tftA* and *tftB* genes are located on the 0.34-Mb replicon, whereas the *tftEFGH* cluster is located on the 0.53-Mb replicon. The separate locations of genes for the upper and lower portions of the pathway and their association with IS elements are consistent with the possibility that the pathway was assembled in strain AC1100 by multiple insertional events. Alternatively, during the evolution of AC1100, a single gene cluster may have rearranged and split apart after a single initial genetic exchange. It will be interesting to determine the chromosomal locations of the remaining genes of the pathway.

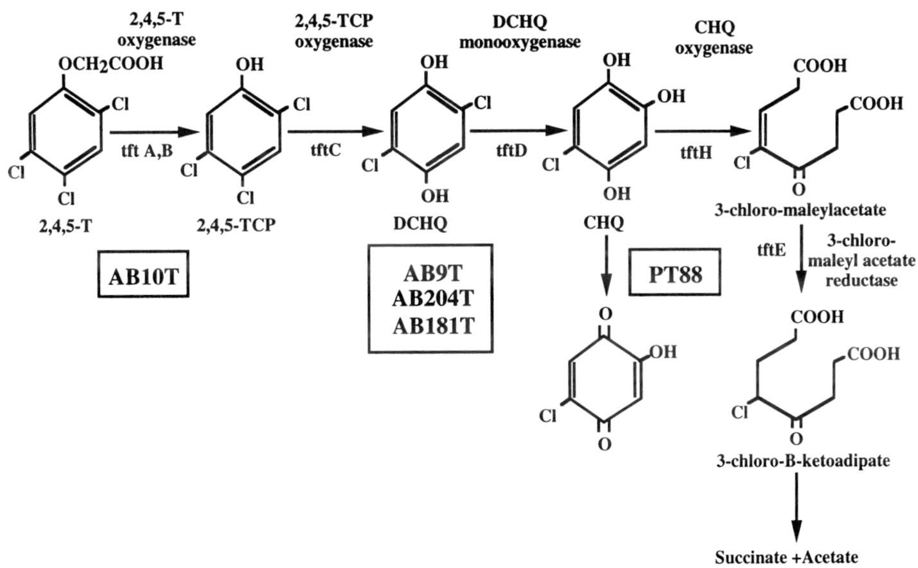

Figure 1. 2,4,5-T catabolic pathway. Gene names and proposed enzymatic activities are indicated. DCHQ, dichlorohydroquinone; CHQ, chlorohydroquinone. Names of mutant strains are boxed. PT88 is defective in chlorohydroquinone oxygenase, thus producing the oxidation product chlorohydroxyhydroquinone.

We are now mapping the locations of the IS elements and assessing whether specific portions of the genome (specific chromosomes?) are involved in deletion and insertion events. In at least one case this seems to be true. Strain PT88 was originally thought to result from a transposon insertion mutation of the *tftE* gene cluster (Haugland et al., 1991). We have shown, however, that PT88 has undergone considerable rearrangement, including deletion of the *tftE* gene cluster. Replicon 3 has increased in size by 30 kb, and 30 kb has been deleted from replicon 4 (Table 1; Fig. 2). DNA of the cloned *tftAB* and *tftEFGH* genes was used to probe Southern blots of PT88 replicons. Surprisingly, the *tftA* and *tftB* genes have translocated from replicon 4 to replicon 3. In the presence of 2,4,5-T, PT88 rapidly mutates to become *tftAB* deficient. These mutations are easily detected on plates by a failure to produce a pink-colored chlorohydroxyquinone intermediate that is excreted by PT88 cells. Colonies that failed to produce pink color on 2,4,5-T plates and in liquid media were isolated. In the *tftAB* mutants, a 300-kb deletion of

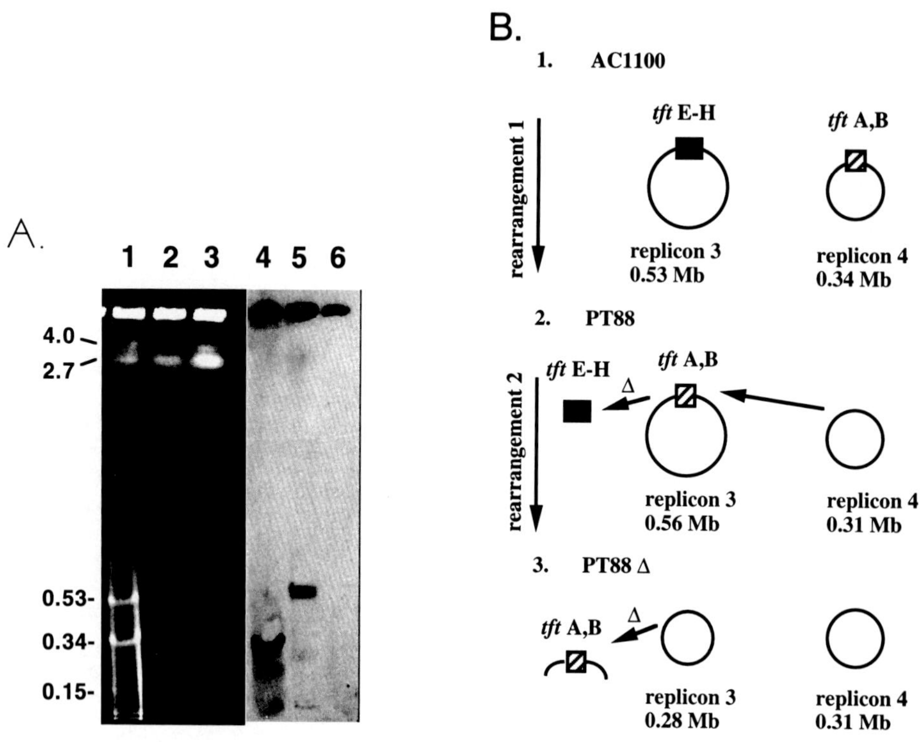

Figure 2. Chromosomal rearrangements in *B. cepacia* AC1100. (A) Southern blot analysis. Sizes in megabases of strain AC1100 chromosomes are indicated. Lanes 1 to 3, ethidium-stained CHEF gel; lanes 4 to 6, autoradiogram of Southern blot hybridization with probe carrying genes *tftA* and *tftB*. Lanes 1 and 4, AC1100 DNA; lanes 2 and 5, PT88 DNA; lanes 3 and 6, PT88 deletion. (B) Depiction of rearrangements observed in panel A. Solid box, genes *tftEFGH;* striped box, genes *tftA* and *tftB*. (1) Location of genes in strain AC1100; (2) deletion of *tftEFGH* in strain PT88 and translocation of *tftAB;* (3) deletion of *tftAB* in PT88Δ (data from W. Hendrickson, A. Hübner, and A. Kavanaugh-Black, manuscript in preparation).

replicon 3 had occurred in each of several candidates studied. The rearrangements are depicted in Fig. 2B. Thus, we could not find a small "cassette" capable of moving these catabolic genes, but the genome analysis allowed us to identify a larger rearrangement that occurs at high frequency. These events may be similar to the ones that established the genes in strain AC1100 initially, and they may be responsible for the rapid loss of 2,4,5-T catabolic potential when strain AC1100 is used in field studies (Chatterjee et al., 1982). Since the predominant rearrangements appear to be specifically directed toward certain chromosome locations, there may be elements such as ISs causing hyper-recombination.

TRANSPOSON MUTAGENESIS

Transposon mutants of strain AC1100 would be useful for obtaining genetic markers such as amino acid auxotrophs to create a combined genetic and physical map, as well as for identifying and cloning additional genes involved in 2,4,5-T metabolism. Strain AC1100 was mutagenized with a transposon, Tn*5*-751S, containing an *Swa*I site for physical mapping. Approximately 10,000 independent transposon mutants were obtained, and 10 different amino acid auxotrophs were identified. The corresponding complementing cosmid clones were isolated from an AC1100 cosmid library, and the clones are being used to construct a combined genetic and physical map.

A modification of the selection was used to isolate transposon mutants defective in metabolism of 2,4,5-T. Mutants that exhibited limited or no growth on 2,4,5-T as sole source of carbon, yet grew well on glucose or Casamino Acids, were screened for complementation with the two clones of 2,4,5-T degradation genes. These two loci, contained in the vectors pUS1010 (Sangodkar et al., 1988) and pRHC89 (Danganan et al., 1994), are required for growth on 2,4,5-T as sole carbon source. Six of the mutants were not complemented by the clones containing the previously identified *tft* genes. Two mutants produced a pale pink color, suggesting a block at the distal part of the pathway and accumulation of chlorohydroxyhydroquinone, but these mutants produced less color than strain PT88. Each candidate was tested for production of trichlorophenol, the product of the first step in the pathway, and for dechlorinase activity, the second and third steps. Mutant AB10T was not able to convert 2,4,5-T to 2,4,5-TCP; therefore, it is likely defective in the 2,4,5-T oxygenase (Fig. 1). Mutants AB9T and AB204T produced TCP but showed no dechlorinase activity, whereas AB181T had partial dechlorinase activity. These mutations are likely in the TCP or dichlorohydroquinone oxygenase genes or related regulatory functions (Fig. 1). Once the 2,4,5-T pathway was disrupted, all the mutants rapidly lost the *tftEFGH* genes, as observed in the PT88 mutant. Apparently, the genes of the lower portion of the pathway are highly unstable and could account for much of the loss of 2,4,5-T metabolic activity.

INSERTION ELEMENTS IN *B. CEPACIA* AC1100

Two insertion elements, IS*931* and IS*932*, were previously found associated with both of the cloned *tft* gene clusters (Haugland et al., 1990; Tomasek et al., 1989). Although IS*932* was not characterized, IS*931* was sequenced and shown to transpose and transcriptionally activate adjacent genes. A probe containing IS*931* was produced by

PCR and hybridized to the strain AC1100 replicons. IS*931* was found to be present in multiple copies in strain AC1100 on all four large replicons. It was absent from *B. cepacia* strains 17616, 25416, and N2P5 when analyzed by Southern blot hybridization under stringent conditions. A number of IS elements have been characterized in strain 17616 (Lessie et al., 1990; Wood et al., 1991), but hybridization with probes containing these elements indicated that they are not present in AC1100 or 25416. Thus, there is considerable segregation of IS elements among different *B. cepacia* strains.

We are using a "promoter trap" vector to observe IS activity and to look for additional IS elements with promoter activity. The vector has a promoterless streptomycin resistance gene that can be driven by promoters from elements inserted upstream of the translational start site (Bagdasarian et al., 1983). The vector, pKT240, was electroporated into strain AC1100, and cells were plated for high streptomycin resistance (800 μg/ml). PCR proved to be an easy and reliable method to screen plasmids for insertions. Primers were synthesized for the vector region between the *str* gene and a *kan* marker 1 kb upstream. An additional primer corresponding to the right end of IS*931* was also made. Colonies were picked and the cells were disrupted by microwave, followed directly by PCR. All the primers were used simultaneously so that any insertions were detected and the presence of IS*931* was also seen in the same sample. All candidates that contained IS elements but were negative for IS*931* were characterized by restriction nuclease analysis of the PCR products.

Of 211 candidates that were characterized, most appeared to carry IS*931* or IS*932* (Table 2) (A. Hübner and W. Hendrickson, manuscript in preparation). A new IS element was found, IS*1413*, and its DNA sequence was determined (data not shown). One insertion is a small fragment of 400 bp which retains the promoter activity of an IS element. It may have resulted from insertion of one IS element into another and then improper excision removing all but one end of the IS. This construct provides an interesting example of how a promoter could be "evolved" from an insertion element with little remaining evidence of the original insertion event. By measuring the size of the PCR product, an accurate measure of the distance of the IS element from the *str* gene start site was obtained. High-level transcriptional activity was observed with insertions up to 600 bp away. Another insertion trap vector, pUC800, contains the *sacB* gene, whose product is lethal in the presence of sucrose (Gay et al., 1985). Insertions inactivating *sacB* are selected because they impart sucrose tolerance. We found that IS*931* produced most of the insertion events in strain AC1100 with pUC800 even when promoter

Table 2. Transposition activity of strain AC1100 insertion elements

Characterization	No. of insertions found	Size of insert (bp)	Distance (bp) from promoter
No insertion in plasmid[a]	35	None	
IS*931* insertion	127	1,477	50 to 600
IS*932* insertion	46	3,400	ND[b]
IS*1413*	2	1,440	100 to 360
IS fragment	1	400	ND

[a]Streptomycin-resistant clones of strain AC1100 with no insertion upstream of the plasmid streptomycin gene.
[b]ND, not determined.

activity was not selected for. From these data we conclude that insertion elements continue to be highly active and that their transposition and recombination may drive much of the chromosomal instability of AC1100.

CONCLUSIONS AND PROSPECTS

B. cepacia genomes contain multiple chromosomes that vary in number and size. The total genome size varies by more than 3 Mb in the limited number of strains tested. At present there is no obvious conservation of restriction pattern among mapped strains, suggesting considerable chromosomal rearrangements. This is consistent with genetic studies using multilocus enzyme electrophoresis which revealed great genetic diversity among a freshwater population of *B. cepacia* (Wise et al., 1995). The existence of multiple chromosomes may play a role in the genetic plasticity of this organism and its adaptability. A comparison of more detailed physical and genetic maps is needed to determine whether the replicons or portions of the replicons can be grouped into more stable and variable domains. It is not clear whether chromosome number can change by chromosome fusions, or whether some replicons are dispensable under certain conditions.

The existence of chromosomal multiplicity raises new questions regarding our definition of chromosomes and plasmids. The presence of rRNA genes has been a prime criterion for a chromosome, but this is certainly not definitive. In several cases, extensive studies identifying essential genes involved in central metabolic functions have confirmed the designation of a chromosome. The replication and segregation of multiple chromosomes present problems not previously considered in bacteria. Are all the chromosomes controlled as independent replicons, or is there a single replication and segregation system?

Acknowledgments. We thank C. Danganan, D. Daubaras, A. Chakrabarty, and T. Lessie for invaluable help, materials, and discussions. We thank S. Lantz, R. Devereux, K. Williams, and D. Allison for strains. This work was supported by U.S. Environmental Protection Agency grant R822632.

REFERENCES

Allardet-Servent, A. S., S. Michaux-Characon, E. Jumas-Bilak, L. Karayan, and M. Ramuz. 1993. Presence of one linear and one circular chromosome in the *Agrobacterium tumefaciens* C58 genome. *J. Bacteriol.* **175:**7869–7874.

Bagdasarian, M. M., E. Amann, R. Lurz, B. Ruckert, and M. Bagdasarian. 1983. Activity of the hybrid *trp-lac(tac)* promoter of *Escherichia coli* in *Pseudomonas putida*. Construction of broad-host-range, controlled-expression vectors. *Gene* **26:**273–282.

Bhat, M. A., M. Tsuda, K. Horiike, M. Nozaki, C. S. Vaidyanathan, and T. Nakazawa. 1994. Identification and characterization of a new plasmid carrying genes for degradation of 2,4-dichlorophenoxyacetate from *Pseudomonas cepacia* CSV90. *Appl. Environ. Microbiol.* **60:**307–312.

Byrne, A. M., and T. G. Lessie. 1994. Characteristics of IS*401*, a new member of the IS*3* family implicated in plasmid rearrangements in *Pseudomonas cepacia*. *Plasmid* **31:**138–147.

Chatterjee, D. K., J. J. Kilbane, and A. M. Chakrabarty. 1982. Biodegradation of 2,4,5-trichlorophenoxyacetic acid in soil by pure culture of *Pseudomonas cepacia*. *Appl. Environ. Microbiol.* **44:**514–516.

Cheng, H.-P., and T. G. Lessie. 1994. Multiple replicons constituting the genome of *Pseudomonas cepacia* 17616. *J. Bacteriol.* **176:**4034–4042.

Choudhary, M., C. Mackenzie, K. S. Nereng, E. Sodergren, G. M. Weinstock, and S. Kaplan. 1994. Multiple chromosomes in bacteria: structure and function of chromosome II of *Rhodobacter sphaeroides* 2.4.1^{T}. *J. Bacteriol.* **176:**7694–7702.

Danganan, C. E., R. W. Ye, D. L. Daubaras, L. Xun, and A. M. Chakrabarty. 1994. Nucleotide sequence and functional analysis of the genes encoding 2,4,5-trichlorophenoxyacetic acid oxygenase in *Pseudomonas cepacia* AC1100. *Appl. Environ. Microbiol.* **60:**4100–4106.

Daubaras, D. L., C. D. Hershberger, K. Kitano, and A. M. Chakrabarty. 1995. Sequence analysis of a gene cluster involved in metabolism of 2,4,5-trichlorophenoxyacetic acid by *Burkholderia cepacia* AC1100. *Appl. Environ. Microbiol.* **61:**1279–1289.

Ferrante, A. A., and T. G. Lessie. 1991. Nucleotide sequence of IS*402* from *Pseudomonas cepacia. Gene* **102:**143–144.

Gaffney, T. D., and T. G. Lessie. 1987. Insertion-sequence-dependent rearrangements of *Pseudomonas cepacia* plasmid pTGL1. *J. Bacteriol.* **169:**224–230.

Gay, P., D. Le Coq, M. Steinmetz, T. Berkelman, and C. I. Kado. 1985. Positive selection procedure for entrapment of insertion sequence elements in gram-negative bacteria. *J. Bacteriol.* **164:**918–921.

Haugland, R. A., U. M. X. Sangodkar, and A. M. Chakrabarty. 1990. Repeated sequences including RS1100 from *Pseudomonas cepacia* AC1100 function as IS elements. *Mol. Gen. Genet.* **220:**222–228.

Haugland, R. A., U. M. X. Sangodkar, P. R. Sferra, and A. M. Chakrabarty. 1991. Cloning and characterization of a chromosomal DNA region required for growth on 2,4,5-T by *Pseudomonas cepacia* AC1100. *Gene* **100:**65–73.

Holloway, B. W., S. Dharmsthiti, C. Johnson, A. Kearney, V. Krishnapillai, A. F. Morgan, E. Ratnaninfsih, R. Saffery, M. Sinclair, D. Strom, and C. Zhang. 1990. Chromosome organization in *Pseudomonas aeruginosa* and *Pseudomonas putida*, p. 269–278. *In* S. Silver, A. M. Chakrabarty, B. Iglewski, and S. Kaplan (ed.), *Pseudomonas: Biotransformations, Pathogenesis, and Evolving Biotechnology.* American Society for Microbiology, Washington, D.C.

Kellogg, S. T., D. K. Chatterjee, and A. M. Chakrabarty. 1981. Plasmid-assisted molecular breeding: new technique for enhanced biodegradation of persistent toxic chemicals. *Science* **214:**1133–1135.

Kilbane, J. J., D. K. Chatterjee, J. S. Karns, S. T. Kellogg, and A. M. Chakrabarty. 1982. Biodegradation of 2,4,5-trichlorophenoxyacetic acid by a pure culture of *Pseudomonas cepacia. Appl. Environ. Microbiol.* **44:**72–78.

Lessie, T. G., and T. Gaffney. 1986. Catabolic potential of *Pseudomonas cepacia*, p. 439–481. *In* J. R. Sokatch and L. N. Ornston (ed.), *The Bacteria*, vol. 10: *The Biology of Pseudomonas.* Academic Press, Orlando, Fla.

Lessie, T. G., M. S. Wood, A. Byrne, and A. Ferrante. 1990. Transposable gene-activating elements in *Pseudomonas cepacia*, p. 279–291. *In* S. Silver, A. M. Chakrabarty, B. Iglewski, and S. Kaplan (ed.), *Pseudomonas: Biotransformations, Pathogenesis, and Evolving Biotechnology.* American Society for Microbiology, Washington, D.C.

Liu, S.-H., A. Hessel, and K. E. Sanderson. 1992. Genomic mapping with I-*Ceu*I, an intron-encoded endonuclease specific for genes for ribosomal RNA in *Salmonella* spp., *E. coli,* and other bacteria. *Proc. Natl. Acad. Sci USA* **90:**6874–6878.

Michaux, S., J. Paillisson, M.-J. Carles-Nurit, A. Bourg, A. Allardet-Servent, and M. Ramuz. 1993. Presence of two independent chromosomes in the *Brucella melitensis* 16M genome. *J. Bacteriol.* **175:**701–705.

Rodley, P., U. Römling, and B. Tümmler. 1995. A physical genome map of the *Burkholderia cepacia* type strain. *Mol. Microbiol.* **17:**57–67.

Sangodkar, U. M. X., T. L. Aldrich, R. A. Haugland, J. Johnson, R. K. Rothmel, P. J. Chapman, and A. M. Chakrabarty. 1989. Molecular basis of biodegradation of chloroaromatic compounds. *Acta Biotechnol.* **9:**301–316.

Sangodkar, U. M. X., P. J. Chapman, and A. M. Chakrabarty. 1988. Cloning, physical mapping and expression of chromosomal genes specifying degradation of the herbicide 2,4,5-T in *Pseudomonas cepacia* AC1100. *Gene* **71:**267–277.

Shields, M. S., and M. J. Reagin. 1992. Selection of a *Pseudomonas cepacia* strain constitutive for the degradation of trichloroethylene. *Appl. Environ. Microbiol.* **58:**3977–3983.

Shields, M. S., M. J. Reagin, R. R. Gerger, R. Campbell, and C. Somerville. 1995. TOM, a new aromatic degradative plasmid from *Burkholderia (Pseudomonas) cepacia* G4. *Appl. Environ. Microbiol.* **61:**1352–1356.

Smith, D. L., L. B. Gumery, E. G. Smith, D. E. Stableforth, M. E. Kaufmann, and T. L. Pitt. 1993. Epidemic of *Pseudomonas cepacia* in an adult cystic fibrosis unit: evidence of person-to-person transmission. *J. Clin. Microbiol.* **31:**3017–3022.

Steinbach, S., L. Sun, R. Z. Jiang, P. Flume, P. Gilligan, T. M. Egan, and R. Goldstein. 1994. Transmissibility of *Pseudomonas cepacia* infection in clinic patients and lung-transplant recipients with cystic fibrosis. *N. Engl. J. Med.* **331:**981–987.

Sun, L., R. Z. Jiang, S. Steinbach, A. Holmes, C. Campanelli, J. Forstner, U. Sajjan, Y. Tan, M. Riley, and R. Goldstein. 1995. The emergence of a highly transmissible lineage of *cbl*+ *Pseudomonas (Burkholderia) cepacia* causing CF centre epidemics in North America and Britain. *Nature Med.* **1:**661–666.

Suwanto, A., and S. Kaplan. 1989. Physical and genetic mapping of the *Rhodobacter sphaeroides* 2.4.1 genome: presence of two unique circular chromosomes. *J. Bacteriol.* **171:**5850–5859.

Tomasek, P. H., B. Frantz, U. M. X. Sangodkar, R. A. Haugland, and A. M. Chakrabarty. 1989. Characterization and nucleotide sequence determination of a repeat element isolated from a 2,4,5-T degrading strain of *Pseudomonas cepacia. Gene* **76:**227–238.

Wise, M. G., L. J. Shimkets, and J. V. McArthur. 1995. Genetic structure of a lotic population of *Burkolderia (Pseudomonas) cepacia. Appl. Environ. Microbiol.* **61:**1791–1798.

Wood, M. S., A. Byrne, and T. G. Lessie. 1991. IS*406* and IS*407*, two gene-activating insertion sequences for *Pseudomonas cepacia. Gene* **105:**101–105.

Zuerner, R. L., J. L. Herrmann, and I. Saint Girons. 1993. Comparison of genetic maps for two *Leptospira interrogans* serovars provides evidence for two chromosomes and intraspecies heterogeneity. *J. Bacteriol.* **175:**5445–5451.

Section V

ENVIRONMENTAL AND INDUSTRIAL MICROBIOLOGY

Molecular Biology of Pseudomonads
Edited by T. Nakazawa et al.

Chapter 23

Engineering Bacteria To Degrade Nylon Oligomers

Seiji Negoro, Irfan D. Prijambada, and Itaru Urabe

The production and distribution of synthetic compounds by the chemical industry lead to the problem of their safe disposal. Natural enzymes may have limited abilities to degrade such compounds. If novel metabolic abilities could evolve in microorganisms under laboratory conditions, these abilities would be interesting from the point of view of enzyme evolution and would also provide a means of studying the adaptation of microorganisms to xenobiotic compounds. We first overview the degradation of a xenobiotic compound, i.e., a by-product of the nylon-6 industry, and then describe the artificial expansion of the metabolic abilities of *Flavobacterium* and *Pseudomonas* spp. to degrade this compound through experimental evolution.

BIODEGRADATION OF NYLON BY-PRODUCTS

Nylon-6 is produced by ring cleavage polymerization of caprolactam and consists of monomeric units of 6-aminohexanoate (Ahx) (Fig.1). During the polymerization reaction, by-products such as the linear dimer (Ald) and the cyclic dimer (Acd) are produced. We previously isolated two microorganisms, *Flavobacterium* sp. strain K172 (Kinoshita et al., 1975) and *Pseudomonas* sp. strain NK87 (Kanagawa et al., 1989), that grow on Ald and Acd as the sole sources of carbon and nitrogen. The degradation of these xenobiotic compounds depends on specific enzymes, i.e., Acd hydrolase (EI) (Kinoshita et al., 1977; Tsuchiya et al., 1989), Ald hydrolase (EII) (Kinoshita et al., 1981; Kanagawa et al., 1993), and endo-type 6-aminohexanoate oligomer hydrolase (EIII) (Kakudo et al., 1993, 1995), and the responsible genes are encoded by a plasmid (Negoro et al., 1980; Negoro et al., 1983; Okada et al., 1983; Negoro et al., 1992). The degradative plasmid pOAD2 in *Flavobacterium* sp. strain KI72 comprises 45,519 bp and has a G+C content of 66.6% mol% (Kato et al., 1995). Four nylon oligomer (Nom) degradation genes (*nylA* [Acd hydrolase gene], *nylB* [Ald hydrolase gene], *nylB′* [a gene having 88% identity to *nylB* in amino acid sequences], and *nylC* [endo-type 6-aminohexanoate oligomer hydrolase gene]) are located on different parts of the plasmid (Fig. 2). A homology search of

Seiji Negoro, Irfan D. Prijambada, and Itaru Urabe • Department of Biotechnology, Faculty of Engineering, Osaka University, 2-1 Yamada-oka, Suita, Osaka 565, Japan.

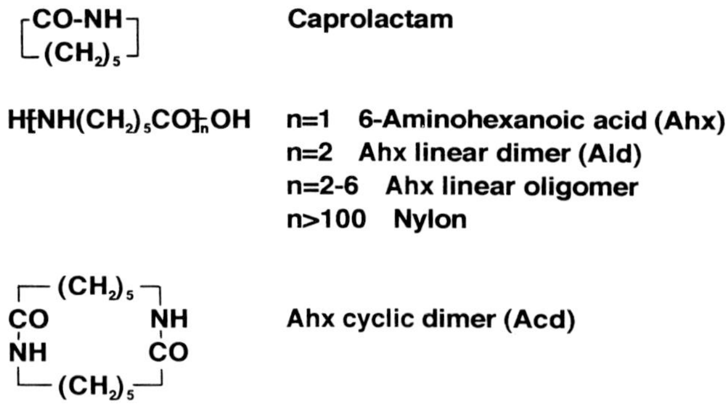

Figure 1. Chemical structures of Noms.

the DNA database revealed DNA regions homologous to the *opp* (oligopeptide uptake) gene clusters of *Salmonella* and *Bacillus* spp. (Hiles et al., 1987; Perego et al., 1991), *ftsX* (filamentation temperature sensitive) of *Escherichia coli* (Gill et al., 1986), *penDE* (isopenicillin *N*-acyltransferase) of *Penicillium* spp. (Tobin et al., 1990; Alvarez et al., 1993), and the *rep* (replication) genes of plasmid pTiB6S3 (Tabata et al., 1989), plasmid F (Mori et al., 1986), plasmid RK2 (Thomas and Smith, 1986), and bacteriophage P1 (Davis et al., 1992). In addition, the insertion sequence IS*6100* was found at five locations in this plasmid. Recombination between two insertion sequence elements resulted in the loss of 9 kb containing the entire *nylA* region (Negoro and Okada, 1982) (Fig. 2). This deletion plasmid, pOAD21, was used in the experiments described below.

EXPERIMENTAL EVOLUTION OF Nom DEGRADATIVE ENZYMES

Wild-type strain KI72 was readily cured of plasmid pOAD2 by mitomycin C treatment, with concomitant loss of the strain's ability to grow on Acd, Ald, and unfractionated Noms obtained from a nylon factory (Negoro and Okada, 1982; Negoro et al., 1992). Among the 1,000 Acd$^-$ clones obtained from KI72 with mitomycin C (0.5 μg/ml), one isolate (KI725) retained the ability to grow on Ald (Fig. 3). This strain harbors the 35-kb deletion plasmid pOAD21 lacking *nylA* (Fig. 2) (Kato et al., 1994). Since strain KI725 does not grow on Nom, we tested whether this strain could restore the ability to metabolize Nom. When KI725 cells were spread on Nom-minimal medium, colonies appeared spontaneously (Nom$^+$ phenotype, KI725R strains) at a frequency of 10^{-7} per cell after 14 days of incubation (Fig. 3). Plasmids from a Nom$^+$ revertant strain (KI725R1) were introduced into cured strain KI723 (pOAD2$^-$ Nom$^-$) by transformation, giving a Nom$^+$ phenotype; in one of the Nom$^+$ transformants (KI723T12), a 35-kb plasmid (pOAD21Nom$^+$) was detected in addition to the two cryptic plasmids (pOAD11 and pOAD3) already present in the recipient (Fig. 3). As a control experiment, an Ald$^+$ transformant (KI723T11) obtained with plasmids originating from strain KI725 showed no growth on Nom-minimal medium. These results suggest that one or several mutations occurred on pOAD21Nom$^+$. Since the 35-kb plasmids recovered from three independently isolated Nom$^+$ strains (KI725R1, KI7250R1, and KI7250R2) exhibited the same restriction pattern as the parental plasmid pOAD21 from two Nom$^-$ strains (KI725 and

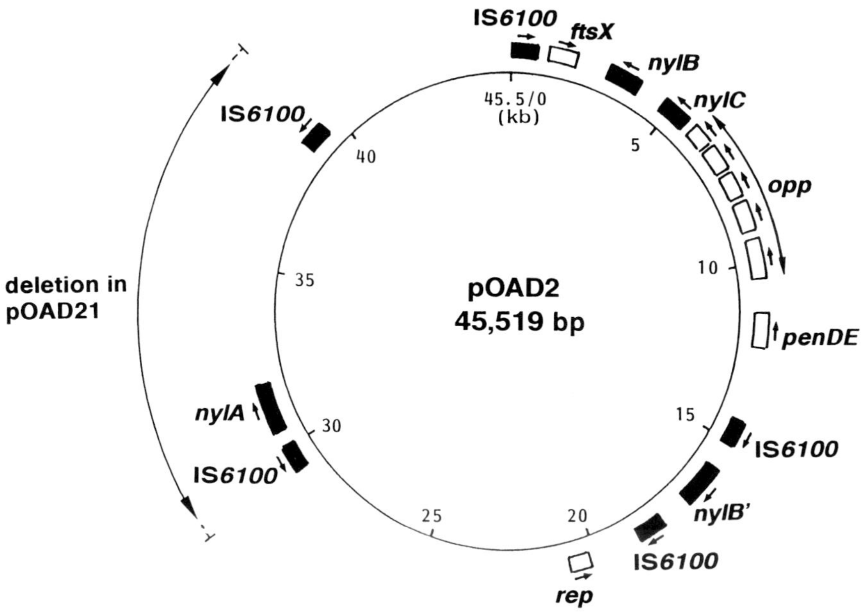

Figure 2. Functional map of plasmid pOAD2. ■, regions encoding the identified gene products, i.e., four Nom degradation genes (*nylA*, *nylB*, *nylB′*, and *nylC*) and IS*6100* sequences appearing five times on the plasmid (Kato et al., 1995); □, DNA regions with significant homology to sequences of the *opp* (oligopeptide permease), *ftsX*, *penDE*, and *rep* genes. Plasmid pOAD21 was obtained from pOAD2 by homologous recombination between the directly repeated IS*6100* sequences. The large arrow indicates the region deleted in pOAD21 (Kato et al., 1995).

KI7250), the pOAD21Nom$^+$ derivatives probably contain minor genetic alterations such as point mutations.

Cell extracts from two Nom$^-$ strains (KI725 and KI7250) had low levels of enzyme activity with Nom as a substrate (1 mU/mg of cellular protein, i.e., approximately 5% of the wild-type activity of KI72). However, this activity was two- to sixfold higher in the Nom$^+$ revertants KI725R1, KI7250R1, and KI7250R2. Several possibilities may explain the phenotypic differences between the KI725 and KI725R strains. Since Nom includes 6-aminohexanoate-cyclic oligomers as major components and since the activities for Nom increase in strain KI725R, it is conceivable that the enhanced level of *nylC* gene expression makes the cells Nom$^+$. However, the following possibilities cannot be ignored: (i) perhaps KI725R possesses an additional Nom degradation enzyme that is active toward a substrate included in Nom, but KI725 has no degradative ability toward the substrate; (ii) perhaps transport proteins of Noms are activated in KI725R; or (iii) perhaps the EIII proteins were altered by mutations in the coding region of the *nylC* gene, thereby changing the specific activities and/or substrate specificity of the enzyme. The last possibility should be negligible, because the nucleotide sequences of the *nylC* gene are identical in the KI72 and KI725R1 strains.

To see whether Nom degradation occurs in bacteria not related to *Flavobacterium* species, we also tested *Pseudomonas aeruginosa* PAO for its adaptation to nylon sub-

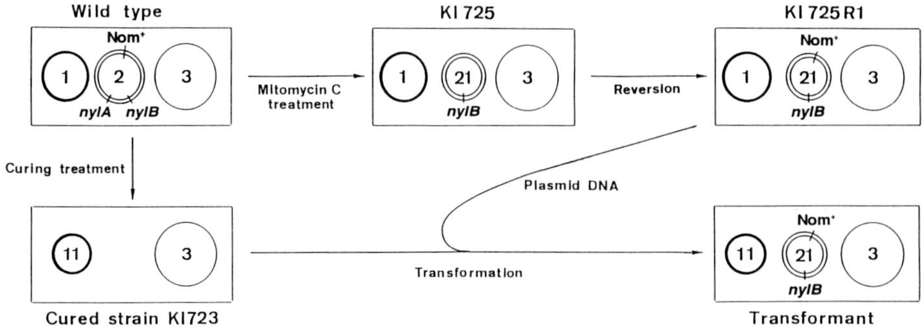

Figure 3. Genetic steps in the formation of cured and transformant strains. Strain KI725 possesses deletion plasmid pOAD21, derived from pOAD2 (see Fig. 2). 1, pOAD1; 2, pOAD2; 3, pOAD3; 21, pOAD21.

strates. Strain PAO, a clinical isolate from New Zealand, has been well studied biochemically and genetically (Holloway and Morgan, 1986). Ahx is poorly utilized, whereas neither Ald nor Acd is utilized by the wild-type PAO1. A mutant (named PAO5501) that grows fast on an Ahx-minimal plate was isolated from PAO1. Strain PAO5501 was then subjected to selective cultivation for 3 months, using Ald as a sole source of carbon and nitrogen, and one Ald^+ strain (designated PAO5502) was obtained. Strain PAO5502 grows to approximately 10^9 cells per ml in either Ald- or Acd-minimal medium within only 4 days (Prijambada et al., 1995).

In glucose-minimal medium, strains PAO1, PAO5501, and PAO5502 exhibit similar growth rates (0.29, 0.28, and 0.27 h^{-1}, respectively) in the exponential phase. In Acd-minimal medium, only strain PAO5502 grows up to 10^9 cells per ml within 3 to 4 days of cultivation, whereas strains PAO1 and PAO5501 show no detectable growth under the same conditions. These results suggest that strain PAO5502 has acquired a genetic alteration that accounts for the new metabolic activity.

Strains PAO1, PAO5501, and PAO5502 exhibit similar morphological and physiological characteristics. Moreover, two-dimensional gel electrophoresis (O'Farrell, 1975) of the total proteins from cell lysates of all three strains grown in glucose-minimal medium yields similar patterns, indicating that PAO5501 and PAO5502 are true derivatives of PAO1 (data not shown).

To check whether strain PAO5502 uses the pathway of Acd utilization found in *Flavobacterium* sp. strain KI72, the activities of Acd hydrolase EI and Ald hydrolase EII were analyzed by thin-layer chromatography. The enzymes in crude extracts were incubated with 10 mM Acd (EI assay) or 10 mM Ald (EII assay). After 20 h of incubation, the reaction mixtures were analyzed by thin-layer chromatography. The reaction products were detected by ninhydrin. A major spot corresponding to authentic Ahx was found in the reaction mixture containing Ald and extract from PAO5502. No Ahx was detected with an extract from PAO1 (Fig. 4). In the reaction mixture containing Acd and extract from PAO5502, a spot corresponding to Ahx was found after 20 h of reaction. In contrast, no spots for Ald or Ahx were found in the mixture containing the extract from PAO1. These results demonstrate that the ability of *P. aeruginosa* PAO5502 to utilize Acd is due to the existence of a newly evolved enzymatic system responsible for hydro-

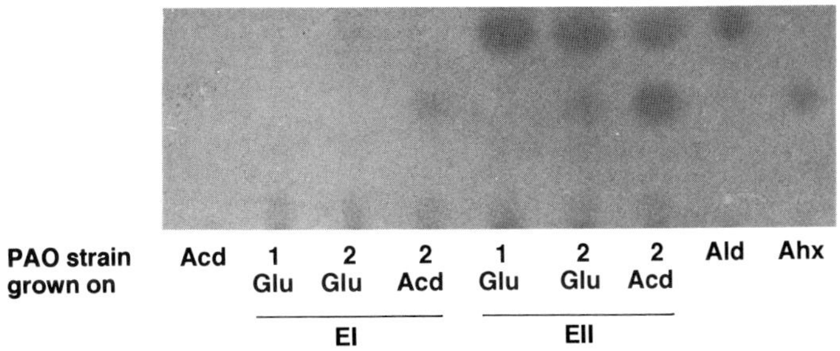

Figure 4. Thin-layer chromatography for the detection of degradation products from Acd and Ald. Cells (*P. aeruginosa* PAO1 and PAO5502) grown in glucose-minimal medium (Glu) or Acd-minimal medium (Acd) were lysed, and the lysates were incubated with 10 mM Acd (EI assay) or 10 mM Ald (EII assay). Acd lacking free amino groups gave no spots by ninhydrin (see text). 1, PAO1; 2, PAO5502.

lyzing Acd into Ald and further into Ahx. Since the enzyme activities in PAO5502 cells grown on Acd-minimal medium are higher than those in cells grown on glucose-minimal medium, the enzymes seem to be partially inducible.

MOLECULAR BASE FOR ADAPTATION TO A XENOBIOTIC COMPOUND

The adaptation of microorganisms to nonphysiological substrates has been extensively studied, and several molecular mechanisms are possible: (i) alteration of substrate specificity of an enzyme (Clarke and Slater, 1986), (ii) activation of a cryptic gene by mutation in the promoter region (Hall and Clarke, 1977), (iii) alteration of regulator specificity (Ramos et al., 1986), or (iv) alteration of uptake specificity. Although the molecular basis of Nom metabolism in strain PAO5502 is still unknown, environmental stress might favor this adaptation. DNA polymerase errors are known to give rise to some "adaptive" mutations that cause conversion from a Lac^- to a Lac^+ phenotype in *E. coli* (Foster and Trimarchi, 1994; Rosenberg et al., 1994), and furthermore, recombination appears to be involved in the phenomenon of "adaptive" mutation (Harris et al., 1994). Since the Nom has no detectable toxicity toward microorganisms, wild-type cells can be maintained in a starved condition for a long time. After the cells have undergone the required genetic alteration, they grow in the Nom medium.

We found that the EII enzyme and its probable antecedent, the EII′ protein encoded by pOAD2, have the same number of amino acid residues and are 88% identical in their amino acid sequences. However, the catalytic activity of the EII′ enzyme is only about 0.5% of that of the EII protein. Interestingly, two amino acid replacements, i.e., Gly-181 to Asp (EII type) and His-266 to Asn (EII type), in the EII′ protein suffice to increase the activity of EII′ to the level of the parental EII enzyme (Kato et al., 1991). In addition, the remaining 44 amino acid substitutions play no part in enzyme activity, although these 44 alterations included many nonsynonymous substitutions (Kato et al., 1991). Microorganisms may possess a cryptic gene such as the EII′ gene, and by increasing the activity of an enzyme degrading a xenobiotic compound, the microorganisms may be able to adapt to utilization of the compound.

Our experimental results show that the metabolic range of a bacterium can be expanded to include Nom degradation. This adaptation, which may be called "evolutionary engineering," took place under laboratory conditions and occurred at a higher frequency than was expected.

REFERENCES

Alvarez, E., B. Meesschaert, E. Montenegro, S. Gutierrez, B. Diez, J. L. Barredo, and J. F. Martin. 1993. The isopenicillin-N acyltransferase and isopenicillin-N amidohydrolase, 6-aminopenicillanic acid acyltransferase and penicillin amidase activities, all of which are encoded by the single *penDE* gene. *Eur. J. Biochem.* **215:**323–332.

Clarke, P. H., and J. H. Slater. 1986. Evolution of enzyme structure and function in *Pseudomonas*, p. 71–144. *In* J. R. Sokatch (ed.), *The Bacteria*, vol. 10. *The Biology of Pseudomonas*. Academic Press, Inc., Orlando, Fla.

Davis, M. A., K. A. Martin, and S. J. Austin. 1992. Biochemical activities of the *parA* partition protein of the P1 plasmid. *Mol. Microbiol.* **6:**1141–1147.

Foster, P. L., and J. M. Trimarchi. 1994. Adaptive reversion of a frameshift mutation in *Escherichia coli* by simple base deletions in homopolymeric runs. *Science* **265:**407–409.

Gill, D. R., G. F. Hartfull, and G. P. Salmond. 1986. A new cell division operon in *Escherichia coli*. *Mol. Gen. Genet.* **205:**134–145.

Hall, B. G., and N. D. Clarke. 1977. Regulation of newly evolved enzymes. III. Evolution of *ebg* repressor during selection for enhanced lactose activity. *Genetics* **85:**193–201.

Harris, R. S., S. Longerich, and S. M. Rosenberg. 1994. Recombination in adaptive mutation. *Science* **264:**258–260.

Hiles, I. D., M. P. Gallagher, D. J. Jamieson, and C. F. Higgins. 1987. Molecular characterization of the oligopeptide permease of *Salmonella typhimurium*. *J. Mol. Biol.* **195:**125–142.

Holloway, B. W., and A. F. Morgan. 1986. Genome organization in *Pseudomonas*. *Annu. Rev. Microbiol.* **40:**79–105.

Kakudo, S., S. Negoro, I. Urabe, and H. Okada. 1993. New nylon oligomer degradation gene, *nylC*, on plasmid pOAD2 from a *Flavobacterium* strain encodes endo-type 6-aminohexanoate-oligomer hydrolase: purification and characterization of the *nylC* gene product. *Appl. Environ. Microbiol.* **59:**3978–3980.

Kakudo, S., S. Negoro, I. Urabe, and H. Okada. 1995. Characterization of endo-type 6-aminohexanoate-oligomer hydrolase from *Flavobacterium* sp. *J. Ferment. Bioeng.* **80:**12–17.

Kanagawa, K., S. Negoro, N. Takada, and H. Okada. 1989. Plasmid dependence of *Pseudomonas* sp. strain NK87 enzymes that degrade 6-aminohexanoate-cyclic dimer. *J. Bacteriol.* **171:**3181–3186.

Kanagawa, K., M. Oishi, S. Negoro, I. Urabe, and H. Okada. 1993. Characterization of the 6-aminohexanoate-dimer hydrolase from *Pseudomonas* sp. NK87. *J. Gen. Microbiol.* **139:**787–795.

Kato, K., K. Fujiyama, H. S. Hatanaka, I. D. Prijambada, S. Negoro, I. Urabe, and H. Okada. 1991. Amino acid alterations essential for increasing the catalytic activity of the nylon-oligomer-degradation enzyme of *Flavobacterium* sp. *Eur. J. Biochem.* **200:**165–169.

Kato, K., K. Ohtsuki, Y. Koda, T. Maekawa, T. Yomo, S. Negoro, and I. Urabe. 1995. A plasmid encoding enzymes for nylon oligomer degradation: nucleotide sequence and analysis of pOAD2. *Microbiology* **141:**2585–2590.

Kato, K., K. Ohtsuki, H. Mitsuda, T. Yomo, S. Negoro, and I. Urabe. 1994. Insertion sequence IS*6100* on plasmid pOAD2, which degrades nylon oligomers. *J. Bacteriol.* **176:**1197–1200.

Kinoshita, S., S. Kageyama, K. Iba, Y. Yamada, and H. Okada. 1975. Utilization of a cyclic dimer and linear oligomers of ε-aminocaproic acid by *Achromobacter guttatus* KI72. *Agric. Biol. Chem.* **39:**1219–1223.

Kinoshita, S., S. Negoro, M. Muramatsu, V. S. Bisaria, S. Sawada, and H. Okada. 1977. 6-Aminohexanoic acid cyclic dimer hydrolase: a new cyclic amide hydrolase produced by *Achromobacter guttatus* KI72. *Eur. J. Biochem.* **80:**489–495.

Kinoshita, S., T. Terada, T. Taniguchi, Y. Takene, S. Masuda, N. Matsunaga, and H. Okada. 1981. Purification and characterization of 6-aminohexanoic acid oligomer hydrolase of *Flavobacterium* sp. KI72. *Eur. J. Biochem.* **116:**547–551.

Mori, H., A. Kondo, A Ohshima, T. Ogura, and S. Hiraga. 1986. Structure and function of the F plasmid genes essential for partitioning. *J. Mol. Biol.* **192:**1–15.

Negoro, S., S. Kakudo, I. Urabe, and H. Okada. 1992. A new nylon oligomer degradation gene (*nylC*) on plasmid pOAD2 of *Flavobacterium* sp. *J. Bacteriol.* **174:**7948–7953.

Negoro, S., and H. Okada. 1982. Physical map of nylon oligomer degradative plasmid pOAD2 harbored in *Flavobacterium* sp. KI72. *Agric. Biol. Chem.* **46:**745–750.

Negoro, S., H. Shinagawa, A. Nakata, S. Kinoshita, T. Hatozaki, and H. Okada. 1980. Plasmid control of 6-aminohexanoic acid cyclic dimer degradation enzymes of *Flavobacterium* sp. KI72. *J. Bacteriol.* **143:**238–245.

Negoro, S., T. Taniguchi, M. Kanaoka, H. Kimura, and H. Okada. 1983. Plasmid-determined enzymatic degradation of nylon oligomers. *J. Bacteriol.* **155:**22–31.

O'Farrell, P. H. 1975. High resolution two-dimensional electrophoresis of proteins. *J. Biol. Chem.* **250:**4007–4021.

Okada, H., S. Negoro, H. Kimura, and S. Nakamura. 1983. Evolutionary adaptation of plasmid-encoded enzymes for degrading nylon oligomers. *Nature* (London) **306:**203–206.

Perego, M., C. F. Higgins, S. R. Pearce, M. P. Gallagher, and J. A. Hoch. 1991. The oligopeptide transport system of *Bacillus subtilis* plays a role in the initiation of sporulation. *Mol. Microbiol.* **5:**173–185.

Prijambada, I. D., S. Negoro, T. Yomo, and I. Urabe. 1995. Emergence of nylon oligomer degradation enzymes in *Pseudomonas aeruginosa* PAO through experimental evolution. *Appl. Environ. Microbiol.* **61:**2020–2022.

Ramos, J. L., A. Stolz, W. Reineke, and K. N. Timmis. 1986. Altered effector specificities in regulators of gene expression: TOL plasmid *xylS* mutants and their use to engineer expansion of the range of aromatics degraded by bacteria. *Proc. Natl. Acad. Sci. USA* **83:**8467–8471.

Rosenberg, S. M., S. Longerich, P. Gee, and R. S. Harris. 1994. Adaptive mutation by deletions in small mononucleotide repeats. *Science* **265:**405–407.

Tabata, S., P. J. Hooykaas, and A. Oka. 1989. Sequence determination and characterization of the replicator region in the tumor-inducing plasmid pTiB6S3. *J. Bacteriol.* **171:**1665–1672.

Thomas, C. M., and C. A. Smith. 1986. The *trfB* region of broad host range plasmid RK2, the nucleotide sequence reveals *incC* and key regulatory gene *trfB/korA/korD* as overlapping genes. *Nucleic Acids Res.* **14:**4453–4469.

Tobin, M. B., M. D. Fleming, P. L. Skatrud, and J. R. Miller. 1990. Molecular characterization of the acyl-coenzymeA:isopenicillin-*N* acyltransferase gene (*penDE*) from *Penicillium chrysogenum* and *Aspergillus nidulans* and activity of recombinant enzyme in *Escherichia coli*. *J. Bacteriol.* **172:**5908–5914.

Tsuchiya, K., S. Fukuyama, N. Kanzaki, K. Kanagawa, S. Negoro, and H. Okada. 1989. High homology between 6-aminohexanoate-cyclic-dimer hydrolases of *Flavobacterium* and *Pseudomonas* strains. *J. Bacteriol.* **171:**3187–3191.

Molecular Biology of Pseudomonads
Edited by T. Nakazawa et al.

Chapter 24

Trichloroethylene Degradation Using Recombinant Bacteria Expressing Soluble Methane Monooxygenase from *Methylosinus trichosporium* OB3b

Deokjin Jahng, Adam K. Sun, Craig S. Kim, and Thomas K. Wood

Trichloroethylene (TCE) is manufactured in large quantities as a degreasing agent, dry cleaning fluid, fumigant, and cleanser (Ensley, 1991). Its widespread use and chemical stability have made it the most frequently detected groundwater contaminant on the National Priorities List of the U.S. Environmental Protection Agency (Little et al., 1988). Hence, the amount of TCE that must be remediated is enormous. For example, it is estimated that 4,840 metric tons of TCE contaminates the soil and groundwater at the Department of Energy Savannah River facility (Ensley and Kurisko, 1994). TCE is a confirmed carcinogen and is directly toxic (Ensley, 1991). It can cause central nervous system depression, anemia, kidney swelling, and liver changes (Mutti et al., 1992), and it is a U.S. Environmental Protection Agency priority pollutant (Wackett et al., 1989). Since the genes responsible for TCE degradation have been cloned and sequenced for many bacteria, molecular biology techniques can be used to create recombinant microorganisms that can readily degrade this pollutant (Jahng and Wood, 1994).

TCE DEGRADATION RATES

To select a suitable microorganism for TCE remediation, the maximum TCE degradation rate and the extent of TCE mineralization were determined in a similar manner for five prominent TCE-degrading strains. In the absence of copper ions, *Methylosinus trichosporium* OB3b expresses soluble methane monooxygenase (sMMO) for growth on methane (Tsien et al., 1989). With growth on phenol or toluene as a sole carbon source, *Burkholderia cepacia* G4 expresses toluene *ortho*-monooxygenase and mineralizes TCE to CO_2 (Nelson et al., 1987). *B. cepacia* G4 PR1, a transposon mutant of *B. cepacia* G4, constitutively expresses toluene *ortho*-monooxygenase (Shields and Reagin, 1992). *Pseudomonas putida* F1 degrades TCE by using toluene dioxygenase, with growth on

Deokjin Jahng, Adam K. Sun, Craig S. Kim, and Thomas K. Wood • Department of Chemical and Biochemical Engineering, University of California, Irvine, Irvine, California 92717-2575.

toluene supplied in the vapor phase as the sole carbon source (Wackett and Gibson, 1988). *Pseudomonas mendocina* KR1 expresses toluene *para*-monooxygenase, with growth on toluene or phenol as the sole carbon source, and can also degrade TCE completely (Ensley and Kurisko, 1994).

The V_{max} and K_m for TCE degradation by resting cells of these five strains (degradation in sealed vials that lack nutrients) are shown in Table 1. In addition, TCE mineralization by these same strains (compared uniformly at 25 μM TCE in the liquid phase) is shown in Fig. 1. It is clear that *M. trichosporium* OB3b induced with methane degrades TCE 25 times faster than other strains and completely mineralizes TCE better than the other TCE-degrading strains.

RECOMBINANT PSEUDOMONAD FOR TCE DEGRADATION

In addition to rapidly degrading and completely mineralizing TCE, sMMO from *M. trichosporium* OB3b can oxidize a wide range of compounds, including vinyl chloride, chloroform, dichloromethane, dichloroethanes, dichloroethylenes, styrene, benzene, toluene, carbon monoxide, naphthalene, ammonia, hydrochlorofluorocarbons, and hexane. Unfortunately, expression of sMMO is repressed by low concentrations of copper ion (0.25 μM) (Tsien et al., 1989), and concentrations of copper in excess of 0.25 μM have been found in polluted groundwater (Phelps et al., 1992). In addition, TCE degradation using sMMO is subject to competitive inhibition, since both TCE and methane compete for the active site (Oldenhuis et al., 1991), and *M. trichosporium* OB3b grows slowly (doubling time of >8.5 h). To overcome these intrinsic obstacles in the wild-type strain, the 5.3-kb *mmo* locus from *M. trichosporium* OB3b was cloned into *P. putida* F1 by using the broad-host-range plasmid pMMB277 (Morales et al., 1991) to form *P. putida* F1(pSMMO20) (Fig. 2), and active sMMO expression under control of the vector *ptac* promoter was observed after induction with isopropyl-β-D-thiogalactopyranoside (IPTG) (Jahng and Wood, 1994). In this recombinant system, copper repression, competitive inhibition, and slow growth of cells were eliminated.

For cloning sMMO, *Pseudomonas* species were chosen, since they are in general very robust, and their genetics are well known. Pseudomonads are also often used in bioremediation, because members of the genus are able to degrade and utilize a wide variety of common and exotic organic compounds. Furthermore, pseudomonads have relatively high growth rates, and those that degrade TCE have the ability to accommodate TCE and the intermediates of TCE oxidation (some of which, like chloral

Table 1. V_{max} and K_m for aerobic TCE degradation

Strain	V_{max} (nmol/min/mg of protein)	K_m (μM)	Reference(s)
M. trichosporium OB3b	456–600	145	Oldenhuis et al., 1991
B. cepacia G4	9	4	Sun and Wood, 1996;
	8	3	Folsom et al., 1990
B. cepacia G4 PR1	18	29	Sun and Wood, 1996
P. mendocina KR1	20	10	Sun and Wood, 1996
P. putida F1	8	5	Sun and Wood, 1996
P. putida F1(pSMMO20)	5	22	Jahng and Wood, 1994

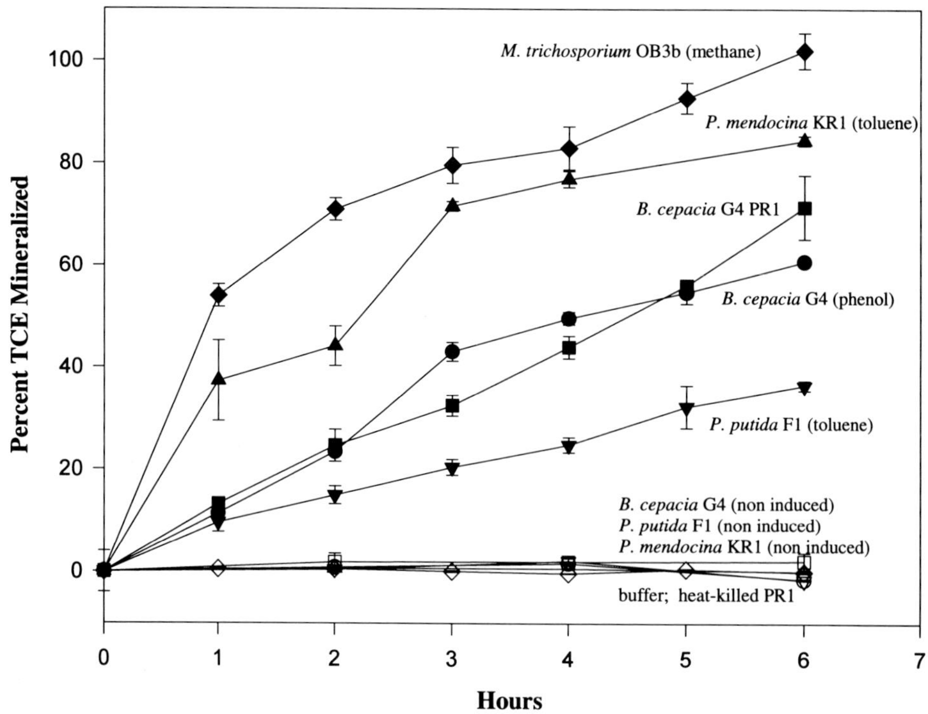

Figure 1. Extent of TCE (25 μM in phosphate buffer) mineralization by resting cells (25°C) as determined from chloride ion measurements. Data represent averages of duplicate or triplicate vials (standard deviation error bars are shown). For the noninduced negative controls, cultures were grown in M9–0.4% glucose.

hydrate, are potentially toxic to cells [Newman and Wackett, 1991]). In addition, the GC content of pseudomonads (especially *P. putida* [62%]) is similar to that of methanotrophs (62%).

Despite achieving whole sMMO activity for the first time in a recombinant host, sMMO activity in *P. putida* F1(pSMMO20) was low and inconsistent. The V_{max} and K_m for active cultures degrading TCE were 5 nmol/min/mg of protein and 22 μM, respectively. However, only 20% of the cultures degraded 35% of 20 μM TCE in 5 h, while 80% of the cultures degraded only 15% of the TCE in the same time (negative controls showed less than 6% decrease in 5 h) (Jahng and Wood, 1994). A single Luria broth culture gives rise to both efficient and nonefficient minimal-medium cultures, and both efficient and nonefficient phenotypes were not stable upon subcultivation. Attempts to isolate an efficient TCE-degrading colony failed. The plasmid appears to be maintained stably in the inefficient TCE-degrading cultures (pSMMO20 is clearly present in nonefficient cultures), and sMMO is synthesized in the inefficient TCE-degrading cultures, as shown by sodium dodecyl sulfate-polyacrylamide gel electrophoresis (SDS-PAGE) and Western immunoblotting. For efficient TCE-degrading cultures, about 15% of the sMMO appears to be active.

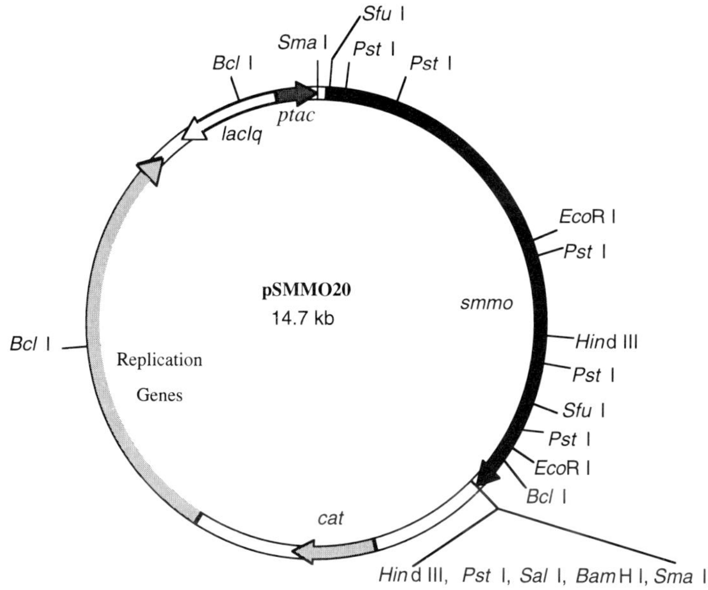

Figure 2. Restriction endonuclease site map of pSMMO20 (based on broad-host-range cloning vector pMMB277 [Morales et al., 1991]). Abbreviations: *cat*, gene encoding chloramphenicol acetyltransferase; *lacI*^{q}, gene encoding *Escherichia coli* lactose operon repressor (high-expression mutant); *ptac*, *trp-lac* hybrid promoter.

BIOCHEMISTRY OF TCE DEGRADATION

The best-studied TCE degradation system is the sMMO enzyme of *M. trichosporium* OB3b. In methanotrophs, sMMO (EC 1.14.13.25) converts methane to methanol. This is the first reaction in the oxidation of methane to CO_2, which yields both carbon and energy for these organisms (Fox et al., 1989):

$$CH_4 + NADH + H^+ + O_2 \xrightarrow{\text{sMMO}} CH_3OH + NAD^+ + H_2O$$

sMMO also fortuitously oxidizes TCE to produce (in vitro) primarily glyoxylate (5%), CO (53%), and formate (35%) (Fox et al., 1990). The overall, whole-cell reaction is (McFarland et al., 1992)

$$Cl_2C{=}CClH + NADH + H^+ + 2O_2 \xrightarrow{\text{sMMO}} 2CO_2 + NAD^+ + 3HCl$$

Pure cultures of both methanotrophs and pseudomonads completely mineralize TCE by converting it to CO_2. Furthermore, since the TCE degradation reaction depends on NADH supplied by the cell, another substrate must be present and used as an energy source to drive the degradation reaction; the reaction will not proceed in the presence of TCE alone.

The DNA sequence of the *mmo* locus of *M. trichosporium* OB3b was determined by Cardy et al. (1991). It is very similar to that of *Methylococcus capsulatus* (Bath). The 5.3-kb *mmo* locus is composed of six genes (*mmoXYBZC* and *orfY*), which code for the α, β, component B, γ, and reductase proteins, respectively (the product and function of *orfY* are not known, although the sequence appears to have conserved analogs in the phenol hydroxylase of *P. putida* CF600, the toluene 4-monooxygenase of *P. mendocina* KR1, and the toluene *ortho*-monooxygenase of *B. cepacia* G4). The hydroxylase, $(\alpha\beta\gamma)_2$, contains two oxygen-bridged, dinuclear iron clusters [Fe-OH-Fe], the reductase is a [2Fe-2S] flavoprotein, and component B mediates control of electron transfer (Fox et al., 1993; Rosenzwieg et al., 1995).

ENHANCING sMMO ACTIVITY

After inducing *P. putida*(pSMMO20) for 5 to 6 h with 1 mM IPTG, all five major sMMO proteins were visualized using SDS-PAGE and Western immunoblotting (Jahng and Wood, 1994). Expression of sMMO in the recombinant *P. putida*(pSMMO20) was high and comparable to that of wild-type *M. trichosporium* OB3b induced with methane in copper-free medium (~15% total-cell protein). Therefore, efforts were directed at producing active protein rather than increasing expression.

To obtain additional sMMO-expressing recombinant strains, the *mmo* locus was cloned into bacterial strains that are phylogenetically close to *M. trichosporium* OB3b (Jahng and Wood, in press). *M. trichosporium* OB3b is known to possess a 16S rRNA sequence that is highly homologous to the sequences of α-2 strains (Woese et al., 1984). Hence, other α-2 strains, including three facultative methylotrophs (bacteria that grow on single-carbon compounds; e.g., *Methylobacterium organophilum* XX), two methanotrophs (bacteria that grow on methane; e.g., *Methylocistus parvus* OBBP), *Agrobacterium tumefaciens* A114, and *Rhizobium meliloti* 102F34 were screened for sMMO activity (along with five pseudomonads and one non-α-2 methylotroph, for a total of 13 strains tried). For the methylotrophs, the *mmo* locus was placed under the control of the methanol dehydrogenase promoter of pHX200-47-m1 (Xu et al., 1993) to form pSMMO50, which was induced with methanol. Active sMMO was obtained in the *Agrobacterium* and *Rhizobium* strains with TCE degradation comparable to that of *P. putida* F1(pSMMO20).

To increase sMMO activity, a modified minimal medium was selected from various minimal and complex media on the basis of TCE degradation and growth rates and was improved by removing the sMMO-inhibiting metal ions [Cu(II), Ni(II), and Zn(II)] and chloramphenicol from the medium and supplementing the medium with 3.6 μM $Fe(NH_4)_2(SO_4)\cdot 6H_2O$ (Jahng and Wood, in press). A 4 to 12% increase in the extent of TCE degradation was observed when the inhibiting metals were removed, and the elimination of chloramphenicol from the culture medium increased TCE degradation by 25% for *P. putida* F1(pSMMO40). Ferrous ammonium sulfate was better for TCE degradation than other Fe(II) and Fe(III) compounds such as ferrous sulfate, ferric chloride, ferric ammonium citrate, or EDTA ferric-sodium salt.

To determine which component of sMMO is responsible for the low and inconsistent sMMO activity of *P. putida* F1(pSMMO20), sMMO activities of cell extracts were complemented with purified sMMO components of *M. trichosporium* OB3b (generously provided by J. D. Lipscomb, University of Minnesota) and examined by a propene oxidation assay (Jahng and Wood, in press). As shown in Table 2, addition of purified component B or reductase did not affect sMMO activity of the cell extracts, but addition of the purified hydroxylase to cell extracts of *P. putida* F1(pSMMO20) enhanced sMMO activity dramatically. Therefore, the low and inconsistent sMMO activity of *P. putida* F1(pSMMO20) is believed to be due to incomplete activity of the recombinant hydroxylase component.

Plasmid segregational instability was encountered when a large-scale batch culture (25 liters) of *P. putida* F1(pSMMO20) was attempted. To reduce the formation of plasmid-free cells, the post-segregational-killing locus from plasmid R1 (*hok-sok*; formerly *parB* [Pecota and Wood, 1996; Thisted et al., 1995]) was inserted into the *Bam*HI site downstream of the *mmo* locus of pSMMO20 to form pSMMO40 (Jahng and Wood, in press). This plasmid was electroporated into *P. putida* F1, *A. tumefaciens* A114, and *R. meliloti* 102F34. To measure the enhanced plasmid stability with the *hok-sok* locus, plasmid-containing cells from batch cultures were analyzed by a colony-lift hybridization using a 2.1-kb *Eco*RI fragment of the *mmo* locus. The complex medium did not contain antibiotics and was supplemented with 1 mM IPTG. Therefore, the *hok-sok* locus was the only plasmid selection pressure in the presence of a strong metabolic burden (recombinant protein expression enhances plasmid loss [Wu and Wood, 1994]). The *hok-sok* locus was most effective in *R. meliloti* 102F34 (e.g., after 17 h of cultivation with IPTG induction, 61% of the population contained *hok*$^+$ pSMMO40, whereas pSMMO20 [which lacks *hok*] was present in only 6% of the cells) but was not significantly effective in *A. tumefaciens* A114. This killing locus was also effective in *P. putida* F1 but was less effective there than in *R. meliloti* 102F34. In shake-flask experiments, TCE degradation in pSMMO40-containing cells (*hok-sok*$^+$) was only slightly higher than that in cells with pSMMO20 (which lacks *hok*) (Jahng and Wood, in press).

Table 2. Complementation of cell extracts of *P. putida* F1(pSMMO20) with purified sMMO components from *M. trichosporium* OB3b

sMMO source[a]	Relative activity[b]
H + B + R	1.0
Cell extract only	0[c]
Cell extract + H	0.09
Cell extract + B	0
Cell extract + R	0
Cell extract + H + B	0.13
Cell extract + H + R	0.14

[a] Amounts of purified sMMO components: 10 nmol of hydroxylase (H), 20 nmol of component B (B), and 10 nmol of reductase (R).

[b] Activity was measured after 18 min of incubation. Relative activity of 1 is 324 nmol of propene oxide per min per mg of hydroxylase.

[c] Propene oxide (oxidation product of propene by recombinant sMMO) was observed for longer incubation times (90 min).

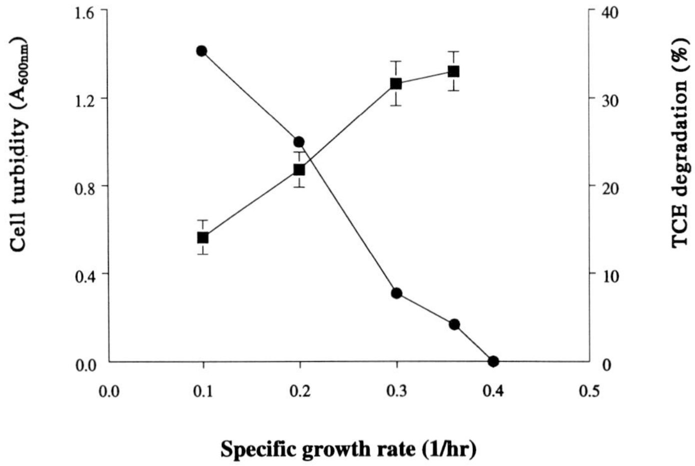

Figure 3. Effect of dilution rate on sMMO activity (assayed by extent of TCE degradation [n] and cell density [c]) for *P. putida* F1(pSMMO40). Data are averages of three samples at each dilution rate, and each error bar represents 1 standard deviation. Optimized minimal medium supplemented with 1 mM IPTG and 25 mg/ml kanamycin was used for chemostat growth (30°C). To determine the extent of TCE degradation (in 5 h at 25°C), cell broth was taken from the chemostat, adjusted to an absorbance at 600 nm (A_{600nm}) of 2, and placed in sealed vials containing TCE.

To further increase sMMO activity and discern the impact of cell metabolic state on sMMO activity, *P. putida* F1(pSMMO40) was cultivated in a chemostat fermentor containing the optimized minimal medium (no copper, nickel, or zinc) with 1 mM IPTG and 25 μg of kanamycin per ml (Jahng and Wood, submitted). As anticipated, cell density was higher at lower dilution rates (Fig. 3). More important, sMMO activity (assayed through extent of TCE degradation) was greater at higher dilution rates (Fig. 3). In addition, sMMO activity was consistent in that cells harvested at certain dilution rates always gave rise to the same amount of TCE degradation (unlike batch cultures). Therefore, chemostat culture is recommended for consistent recombinant sMMO activity. Plasmid stability was also examined in the chemostat, and pSMMO40 in *P. putida* F1 was 100% stable for at least 11 to 20 generations in the presence of kanamycin. These combined optimization efforts resulted in a twofold increase in the extent of TCE degradation and a more consistent sMMO activity.

Acknowledgments. This work was supported by the U.S. Army Research Office, the California Environmental Protection Agency, and the Fluor-Daniel Foundation.

REFERENCES

Cardy, D. L. N., V. Laidler, G. P. C. Salmond, and J. C. Murrell. 1991. The methane monooxygenase gene cluster of *Methylosinus trichosporium*: cloning and sequencing of the *mmoC* gene. *Arch. Microbiol.* **156:**477–483.

Ensley, B.D. 1991. Biochemical diversity of trichloroethylene metabolism. *Annu. Rev. Microbiol.* **45:**283–299.

Ensley, B. D., and P. R. Kurisko. 1994. A gas lift bioreactor for removal of contaminants from the vapor phase. *Appl. Environ. Microbiol.* **60:**285–290.

Folsom, B. R., P. J. Chapman, and P. H. Pritchard. 1990. Phenol and trichloroethylene degradation by *Pseudomonas cepacia* G4: kinetics and interactions between substrates. *Appl. Environ. Microbiol.* **56:**1279–1285.

Fox, B. G., J. G. Borneman, L. P. Wackett, and J. D. Lipscomb. 1990. Haloalkene oxidation by the soluble methane monooxygenase from *Methylosinus trichosporium* OB3b: mechanistic and environmental implications. *Biochemistry* **29:**6419–6427.

Fox, B. G., W. A. Froland, J. E. Dege, and J. D. Lipscomb. 1989. Methane monooxygenase from *Methylosinus trichosporium* OB3b. *J. Biol Chem.* **264:**10023–10033.

Fox, B. G., M. P. Hendrich, K. K Surerus, K. K. Anderson, W. A. Froland, J. D. Lipscomb, and E. Munck. 1993. Mössbauer, EPR, and ENDOR studies of the hydroxylase and reductase components of methane monooxygenase from *Methylosinus trichosporium* OB3b. *J. Am. Chem. Soc.* **115:**3688–3701.

Jahng, D., and T. K. Wood. 1994. Trichloroethylene and chloroform degradation by a recombinant pseudomonad expressing soluble methane monooxygenase from *Methylosinus trichosporium* OB3b. *Appl. Environ. Microbiol.* **60:**2473–2482.

Jahng, D., and T. K. Wood. Optimization of trichloroethylene degradation using soluble methane monooxygenase of *Methylosinus trichosporium* Ob3b expressed in recombinant bacteria. *Biotechnol. Bioeng.*, in press.

Little, C. D., A. V. Palumbo, S. E. Herbes, M. E. Lidstrom, R. L. Tyndall, and P. J. Gilmer. 1988. Trichloroethylene biodegradation by a methane-oxidizing bacterium. *Appl. Environ. Microbiol.* **54:**951–956.

McFarland, M. J., C. M. Vogel, and J. C. Spain. 1992. Methanotrophic cometabolism of trichloroethylene (TCE) in a two stage bioreactor system. *Water Res.* **26:**259–265.

Morales, V. M., A. Backman, and M. Bagdasarian. 1991. A series of wide-host-range low-copy-number vectors that allow direct screening for recombinants. *Gene* **97:**39–47.

Mutti, A., R. Alinovi, E. Bergamaschi, C. Biagini, S. Cavazzini, I. Franchini, R. R. Lauwerys, A. M. Bernard, H. Roles, E. Gelpi, J. Rossello, I. Ramis, R. G. Price, S. A. Taylor, M. DeBroe, G. D. Nuyts, H. Stolte, and L. M. Fels. 1992. Nephropathies and exposure to perchloroethylene in dry cleaners. *Lancet* **340:**189–193.

Nelson, M. J. K., S. O. Montgomery, W. R. Mahaffey, and P. H. Pritchard. 1987. Biodegradation of trichloroethylene and involvement of an aromatic biodegradative pathway. *Appl. Environ. Microbiol.* **53:**949–954.

Newman, L. M., and L. P. Wackett. 1991. Fate of 2,2,2-trichloroacetaldehyde (chloral hydrate) produced during trichloroethylene oxidation by methanotrophs. *Appl. Environ. Microbiol.* **57:**2399–2402.

Oldenhuis, R., J. Y. Oedzes, J. J. Van der Waarde, and D. B. Janssen. 1991. Kinetics of chlorinated hydrocarbon degradation by *Methylosinus trichosporium* OB3b and toxicity of trichloroethylene. *Appl. Environ. Microbiol.* **57:**7–14.

Pecota, D. C., and T. K. Wood. 1996. Exclusion of T4 phage by the *hok* or *sok* killer locus from plasmid R1. *J. Bacteriol.* **178:**2044–2050.

Phelps, P. A., S. K. Agarwal, G. E. Speitel, and G. Georgiou. 1992. *Methylosinus trichosporium* OB3b mutants having constitutive expression of soluble methane monooxygenase in the presence of high levels of copper. *Appl. Environ. Microbiol.* **58:**3701–3708.

Rosenzwieg, A. C., P. Nordlund, P. M. Takahara, C. A. Frederick, and S. J. Lippard. 1995. Geometry of the soluble methane monooxygenase catalytic diiron center in two oxidation states. *Chem. Biol.* **2:**409–418.

Shields, M. S., and M. J. Reagin. 1992. Selection of *Pseudomonas cepacia* strain constitutive for the degradation of trichloroethylene. *Appl. Environ. Microbiol.* **58:**3977–3983.

Sun, A. K., and T. K. Wood. 1996. Trichloroethylene degradation and mineralization by pseudomonads and *Methylosinus trichosporium* OB3b. *Appl. Microbiol. Biotechnol.* **45:**248–256.

Thisted, T., N. S. Sorensen, and K. Gerdes. 1995. Mechanism of post-segregational killing: secondary structure analysis of the entire hok mRNA from plasmid R1 suggests a fold-back structure that prevents translation and antisense RNA binding. *J. Mol. Biol.* **247:**859–873.

Tsien, H. C., G. A. Brusseau, R. S. Hanson, and L. P. Wackett. 1989. Biodegradation of trichloroethylene by *Methylosinus trichosporium* OB3b. *Appl. Environ. Microbiol.* **55:**3155–3161.

Wackett, L. P., G. A. Brusseau, S. R. Householder, and R. S. Hanson. 1989. Survey of microbial oxygenases: trichloroethylene degradation by propane-oxidizing bacteria. *Appl. Environ. Microbiol.* **55:**2960–2964.

Wackett, L. P., and D. T. Gibson. 1988. Degradation of trichloroethylene by toluene dioxygenase in whole-cell studies with *Pseudomonas putida* F1. *Appl. Environ. Microbiol.* **54:**1703–1708.

Woese, C. R., E. Stackebrandt, W. G. Weisburg, B. J. Paster, M. T. Madigan, V. J. Fowler, C. M. Hahn, P. Blanz, R. Gupta, K. H. Nealson, and G. E. Fox. 1984. The phylogeny of purple bacteria: the alpha subdivision. *Syst. Appl. Microbiol.* **5:**315–326.

Wu, K., and T. K. Wood. 1994. Evaluation of the *hok/sok* killer locus for enhanced plasmid stability. *Biotechnol. Bioeng.* **44:**912–921.

Xu, H. H., M. V. Viebahn, and R. S. Hanson. 1993. Identification of methanol-regulated promoter sequences from the facultative methylotrophic bacterium *Methylobacterium organophilum* XX. *J. Gen. Microbiol.* **139:**743–752.

Molecular Biology of Pseudomonads
Edited by T. Nakazawa et al.

Chapter 25

A New Mixotrophic Bacterium That Can Fix CO_2 and Assimilate Aliphatic and Aromatic Hydrocarbons Anaerobically

Tadayuki Imanaka and Masaaki Morikawa

It is generally accepted that many living organisms can degrade and assimilate chemically stable hydrocarbons by using oxygen as an electron acceptor. During the last decade, some bacteria have been reported to couple the anaerobic oxidation and utilization of heterocyclic aromatic hydrocarbons to the reduction of sulfate (Rabus et al., 1993; Beller et al., 1992; Szewzyk and Pfennig, 1987), nitrate (Evans et al., 1991; Dolfing et al., 1990; Payne, 1981), or Fe(III) (Lovley et al., 1989). Methanogenic mixed cultures also transform toluene and benzene to CO_2 and CH_4 (Grbić-Galić and Vogel, 1987). On the other hand, there are only a few reliable reports of the anaerobic degradation of aliphatic hydrocarbons, especially alkanes (Rueter et al., 1994; Aeckersberg et al., 1991), whose metabolic pathways have not been examined. The enzymatic oxidation of *n*-heptane to *n*-hept-1-ene without molecular oxygen was accomplished by using resting cells of the aerobe *Pseudomonas aeruginosa* (Chouteau et al., 1962). The partial purification of an NAD-dependent *n*-alkane dehydrogenase was performed by Parekh et al. (1977). Although the question of whether living organisms can degrade aliphatic hydrocarbons anaerobically remains in contention, these data suggested the possibility of finding new bacteria that could assimilate aliphatic hydrocarbons under anaerobic conditions.

SCREENING OF OIL-ASSIMILATING BACTERIA

Hydrocarbon-assimilating bacteria were isolated under anaerobic conditions as follows. Basal medium (BM) consisted of 0.5% (wt/vol) $(NH_4)_2SO_4$, 0.1% KH_2PO_4, and 0.05% $MgCl_2 \cdot 6H_2O$ in tap water. The pH was adjusted to 7.0 with NaOH. For plate culture, the medium was solidified with 1.5% (wt/vol) pure agarose. Agarose plates supplemented with light crude oil (Sagara Oil) on the surface were prepared in an anaerobic

Tadayuki Imanaka • Department of Biotechnology, Graduate School of Engineering, Osaka University, 2-1 Yamadaoka, Suita, Osaka 565, Japan. ***Masaaki Morikawa*** • Department of Material and Life Sciences, Graduate School of Engineering, Osaka University, 2-1 Yamadaoka, Suita, Osaka 565, Japan.

chamber and degassed three times (the final gas phase consisted of N_2-CO_2-H_2 at 90:5:5 mol%), and a Pd-Al catalyst removed residual oxygen continuously. Agarose plates were preincubated in the chamber overnight, soil samples from the area of an oil spill were streaked on them, and then the plates were incubated at 28 or 37°C for 2 weeks. Although many candidate bacteria appeared to grow on the plates, most of these bacteria were eliminated from further consideration because their cell growth was finally eliminated in the course of successive subculturing. Finally, three colonies were selected, and a pure culture was prepared from each colony. Since the characteristics of these three strains were similar, we finally selected one of them, HD-1, for further experimentation. This bacterium grew on CO_2 (carbon source) and H_2 (energy source) without oil in both plate and liquid cultures, but growth was clearly enhanced by the addition of oil. Cells attached to and grew on the surfaces of oil drops, as shown in Fig. 1. The optimum growth temperature was 37°C.

The enhancement of growth by oil was verified by liquid culture (200 ml) of the strain in BM with and without 1% tetradecane (*n*-TD). After the liquid medium had been autoclaved, a mixture of anaerobic gas was supplied overnight, and then 0.1% by volume of a preculture of strain HD-1 in BM was inoculated. The culture was kept free from oxygen contamination by continuously bubbling the anaerobic mixed gas through the culture. The gas was guaranteed oxygen free (<0.1 ppm). The cells were grown anaerobically, and the growth (estimated as final cell dry weight) was enhanced with the following pure saturated hydrocarbons: *n*-decane, *n*-dodecane, *n*-TD, *n*-hexadecane, and cyclohex-

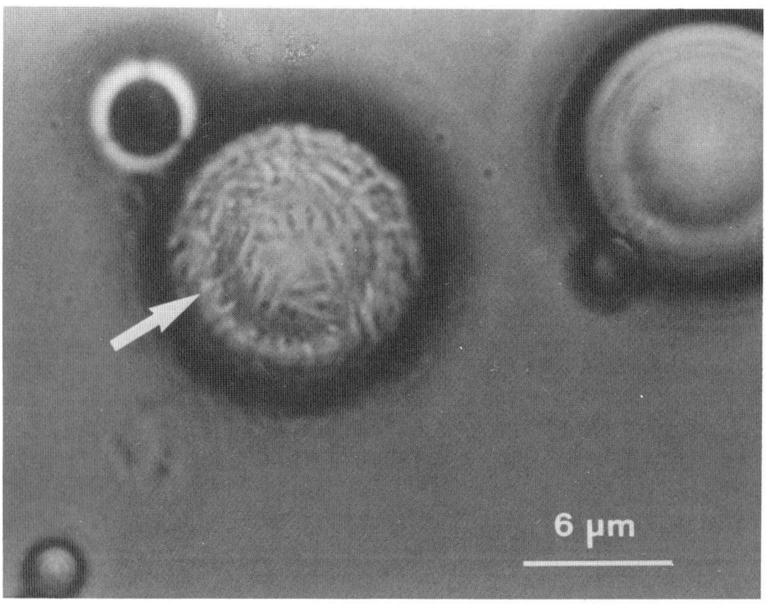

Figure 1. Micrographs of strain HD-1. Cells were grown anaerobically in BM supplemented with *n*-TD as a carbon source. Growth occurred mainly on the surface of *n*-TD, as indicated by an arrow.

ane. Toluene, a typical aromatic hydrocarbon, was also utilized by this strain. Since toluene is volatile, 0.1% (by volume) toluene was added anaerobically every 24 h.

ASSIMILATION OF *n*-TD AND TOLUENE

The increase in cell numbers on a droplet of *n*-TD could be observed microscopically (photograph not shown), but it was difficult to determine the total cell number in culture because of the culture's heterogeneity. Optical density methods were unsuitable, because emulsification occurred along with cell growth. Therefore, we confirmed anaerobic cell growth and its extent on *n*-TD or toluene by measuring the final dry cell weight with and without hydrocarbons.

After 15 days of cultivation, cells were centrifuged (10,000 × *g*, 20 min) and washed with water. In the case of the BM + *n*-TD culture, cells were washed with hexane after the water wash. The cell membrane was confirmed to be unbroken by hexane washing and microscopic observation. After lyophilization, dry cells were obtained (Table 1). The results indicated that cell growth was enhanced by the addition of *n*-TD or toluene. Anaerobic assimilation of *n*-TD and toluene should lead to an increase in both the lipophilic and the hydrophilic fractions compared with those in controls. Total weight of hydrophilic components derived from the cells in each culture was estimated to be 15 (*n*-TD), 10 (toluene), and 4.3 (control) mg/liter. The differences in hydrophilic fractions in cells grown with and without hydrocarbon (15 to 4.3 and 10 to 4.3 mg/liter) were the quantities of hydrophilic substances (e.g., protein, sugar, nucleic acid, etc.) due to the assimilation of each hydrocarbon.

When strain HD-1 was cultivated anaerobically in BM without CO_2 gas or H_2 gas, the cells eventually lysed (data not shown). This fact indicated that both CO_2 and H_2 were necessary as carbon and energy sources, respectively. In other words, HD-1 grown under that set of conditions was a chemoautotroph that could reduce and fix CO_2. The strain did not utilize light energy. When HD-1 was grown in L broth without *n*-TD, the lipophilic fraction content was 16 to 23%. This value was much higher than those reported for *Escherichia coli* (7%) and *Bacillus subtilis* (4%). *B. subtilis* and *E. coli* have one and two membranes, respectively. Assuming that about 3.5 to 4% of the lipophilic fraction corresponds to a cytoplasmic membrane, the newly isolated bacterium HD-1 was expected to have a thick membrane or several layers of membrane. This expectation was confirmed by electron microscopic observation of ultrathin sections of HD-1 cells (Fig. 2a). The cell surface was wavy and very thick (ca. 0.02 to 0.08 μm).

Table 1. Anaerobic assimilation of *n*-TD and toluene[a]

Medium	Dry cell wt (mg/liter)	LPF (mg/liter)	HPF (mg/liter)	LPF/dry cell wt
BM	7.5	3.2	4.3	0.42
BM + *n*-TD	30	15	15	0.50
BM + toluene	22	12	10	0.54

[a]HD-1 was cultivated in BM, BM + *n*-TD, or BM + toluene. Inoculated dry cell weight was 0.2 mg/liter. Data are average values from two independent experiments. LPF, lipophilic fraction (weight of chloroform/methanol-extractable components); HPF, hydrophilic fraction (difference between dry cell and LPF weights) (Kates, 1974).

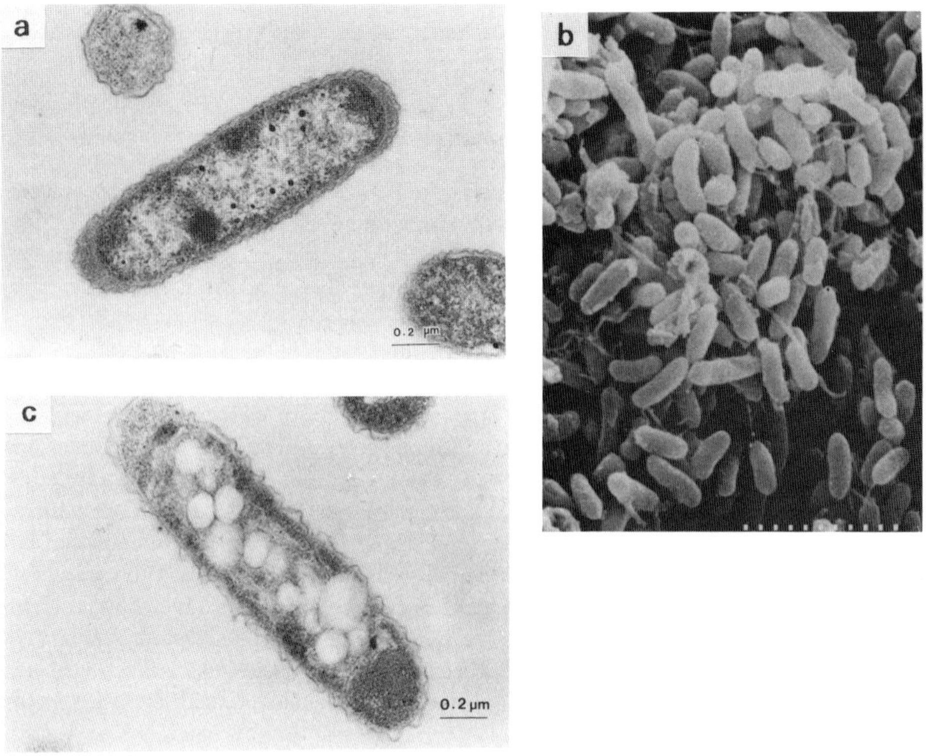

Figure 2. Electron micrographs of strain HD-1. (a) Ultrathin sections of cells grown aerobically in L broth. An electron microscope (type JEM1200Ex, JEOL, Tokyo) was used. (b) A scanning electron microscope (type S-570, Hitachi, Tokyo) was used. Cells were grown anaerobically in BM supplemented with *n*-TD. (c) Ultrathin sections of cells grown anaerobically in BM supplemented with *n*-TD.

After strain HD-1 was grown in BM + *n*-TD, the cells were analyzed by scanning electron microscopy (Fig. 2b). The cell was rod shaped (0.5×1.2 to 1.5 µm) and had a rough cell surface. The characteristics were the same as those of cells grown in L broth (photograph not shown). Ultrathin sections of cells were also analyzed by electron microscopy (Fig 2c). The cell surface was extraordinarily wavy. Many inclusions containing hydrophobic substances were found in the cytoplasmic space. de Andres et al. (1991) had shown similar electron microscopic data for the aerobic assimilation and accumulation of alkane or triglyceride by *P. aeruginosa* cells. Recently, strain HD-1 was found to produce poly-β-hydroxyalkanoate inside cells.

ANALYSIS OF *n*-TD METABOLIC PATHWAY

Strain HD-1 was grown anaerobically in BM supplemented with 1% (vol/vol) *n*-TD (Morikawa and Imanaka, 1993). Cells were cultivated for 14 days, centrifuged, washed with 50 mM sodium phosphate buffer (pH 7.0), and freeze-dried to prepare resting cells, which were used for accumulation and identification of early metabolites. *n*-TD degradation was examined as follows under anaerobic conditions. Screw-cap test tubes containing 50 mg of dried cells in 2.5 ml of sodium phosphate buffer and 40 µl of pure *n*-TD were degassed three times separately and then mixed (the final gas phase was completely changed to the anaerobic gas mixture). After the cap had been tightly closed, tubes were kept shaking at 37°C for 15, 30, and 60 min. Four milliliters of carbon tetrachloride was added to each tube to stop the reaction and extract the hydrocarbon-containing fraction. The extracts were analyzed with Fourier transform-infrared spectrometry (JIR-AQS2OM; JEOL, Tokyo, Japan). Characteristic absorption bands at 1,000 cm^{-1} (C-H deformation vibration) and 1,650 cm^{-1} (C=C stretching vibration) indicated the formation of substances that contained double bonds in the molecule and that reached their maximum amounts after 30 min of reaction. Since the modification of a double bond with a polar group is a useful technique for isolating and identifying the original structure of the alkene, the products from the 30-min reaction (R30) were modified by iodine chloride (ICl) according to the standard method of the Japan Oil Chemists' Society (1995). Gas chromatography (GC) (GC-14A equipped with a capillary column equivalent to OV-1; Shimadzu, Kyoto, Japan) and GC-mass spectrometry (MS)-EI (JMS-DX303; JEOL) analysis data for the 30-min sample modified by ICl (R30-ICl) are shown in Fig. 3. Several peaks eluting after *n*-TD in Fig. 3b are metabolites that originally contained double bonds in the molecule. No novel peaks appeared without a degradation reaction on *n*-TD by strain HD-1. Although the molecular ion peak could not be detected, a 2-mass-unit decrease of every fragment ion peak in the mass spectrum strongly suggested that P1 and P2 are alkenes. Unstable –I and –Cl must be eliminated during ionization to regenerate the double bond. ^{1}H-nuclear magnetic resonance analysis data of the ICl-modified 30-min sample indicated the existence of a terminal double bond in the alkene (figure not shown). The R30 sample was then oxidized with OsO_4 and modified with trimethyl chlorosilane according to the method of Capella and Zorzut (1968). When the resulting *O*-trimethylsilyl (OTMS) derivative was analyzed by GC-MS-EI, fragmentation occurred

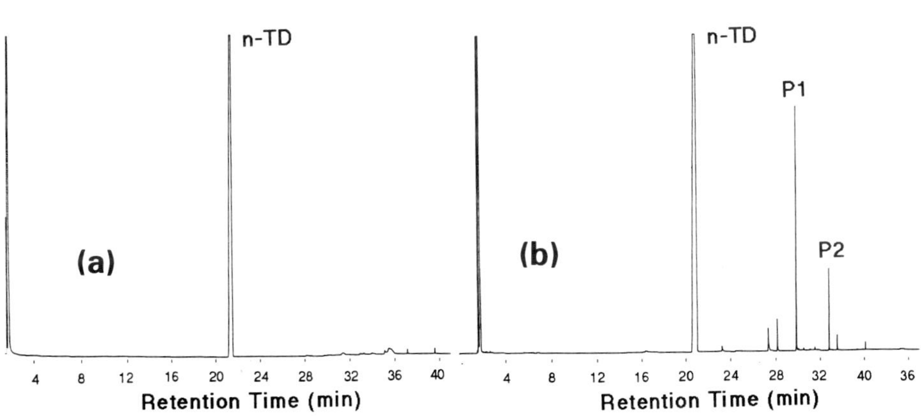

Figure 3. GC-flame ionization detection analysis of metabolites after ICl modification. (a) *n*-TD after treatment of ICl modification reaction. *n*-TD was not susceptible to the modification reaction, and peaks other than that for *n*-TD were absent. (b) *n*-TD degradation sample after 30 min (R30). P1 and P2 are major metabolites that originally contained double bonds in the molecule.

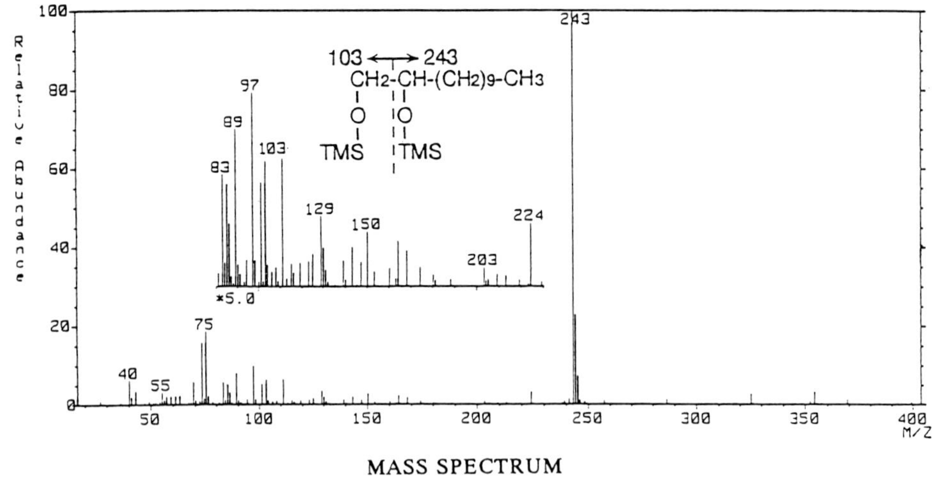

Figure 4. GC-MS-EI analysis of P1-OTMS. Assignments of OTMS-containing peaks and deduced structure are also shown. Standard 1-dodecene-OTMS derivative showed similar retention time and fragmentation pattern. TMS, trimethylsilyl.

specifically between two adjacent OTMS-bound carbons. The mass spectrum of R30-OTMS was analyzed, and fragment peaks were assigned as shown in Fig. 4. Finally, the major metabolite (P1) accumulating in the resting cells was identified as 1-dodecene. A standard 1-dodecene–ICl derivative gave exactly the same retention time in GC and a similar fragmentation pattern by GC-MS-EI (figure not shown). 1-Dodecene was not derived from de novo synthesis by the cell, because a control experiment omitting *n*-TD from the reaction mixture gave no 1-dodecene.

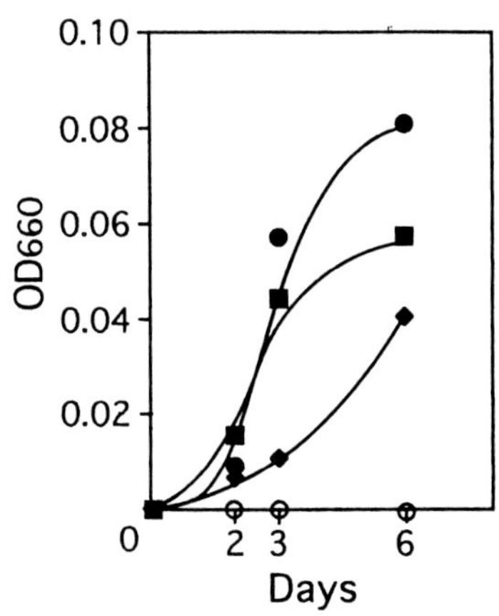

Figure 5. Growth curve of strain HD-1. Symbols, ●, BM + 1% *n*-TD/N_2+CO_2; ■, BM + 1% *n*-TD/N_2+H_2+CO_2; ♦, BM/N_2+H_2+CO_2; ○, BM/N_2+CO_2. Initial cell concentration corresponded to an optical density at 660 nm (OD660) of 0.000189. Culture was washed twice with equal volumes of ethanol-butanol-chloroform (10:10:1) to remove *n*-TD, and absorbance at 660 nm was measured.

n-TD was probably oxidized by alkane dehydrogenase under anaerobic condition, as was previously suggested for *Pseudomonas* sp. (Parekh et al., 1977). The strain could grow in mineral BM supplemented with n-TD and CO_2 in the absence of H_2 and light (Fig. 5). This result suggests that the cell utilizes hydrocarbon as an energy source rather than a carbon source.

ELECTRON ACCEPTORS

Sulfate, CO_2, or H_2O might be considered as a final electron acceptor in this system. During the growth of HD-1 in BM, sulfide production was tested by the method of Cline (1969): only 3 to 4 mM sulfide was detected. Since we adopted an anaerobic fermentation system, some portion of the sulfide formed might have been released into the air. Taking into consideration the high solubility of sulfide (258 ml/100 g of water at 20°C and 1 atm [1 atm = 101.29 kPa]), 4 mM is too small an amount to account for the total electron mass balance during HD-1 growth. We suppose the reason is that strain HD-1 can originally grow autotrophically in the absence of oxygen. CO_2 must be used as the main electron acceptor during hydrocarbon assimilation. For example, the reductive monocarboxylic acid cycle or reversible carbon monoxide dehydrogenase pathway may be utilized for dehydrogenation from hydrocarbons (Thauer et al., 1972, 1989). The electron transfer system needs to be clarified in the future.

IDENTIFICATION AND CHARACTERIZATION OF HD-1

The characteristics of this bacterium were tested according to methods given in *Bergey's Manual of Systematic Bacteriology* (Krieg and Holt, 1984) (Table 2). Strain HD-1 was placed in *Bergey's* section 4: gram-negative aerobic rods and cocci. The G+C content

Table 2. Characteristics of strain HD-1

Parameter	Description
Morphology	Rods
Size of cells	0.5 × 1.2–~1.5 μm
Oxygen demand	Facultative anaerobe
Gram staining	–
Motility	+
Spore formation	–
Methane production	–
Catalase	+
Oxidase	+
Tween 20 degradation	+
Tween 80 degradation	–
Tri-n-butyrin degradation (lipase)	+
Starch hydrolysis (amylase)	–
Na^+ requirement for growth	–
Growth temp	
30°C	+
37°C	+
48°C	–
Mol% G+C of DNA	67

and lack of carbohydrate-assimilating ability indicate that the strain is a pseudomonad. When HD-1 is grown in L broth, cells tend to become filamentous, i.e., up to five times longer than normal. Ethanol is the most effective carbon source. Lack of methane production and the anaerobic growth of the bacterium mean that this organism belongs to neither the methane-producing nor the hydrogen bacteria. It seems most unlikely that strain HD-1 could be classified as a sulfate-reducing bacterium, because it is a facultative anaerobe and can grow slightly even with $(NH_4)NO_3$ in place of $(NH_4)_2SO_4$. In the API 20NE system, the profile number of strain HD-1 was 0200044 (reduction of NO_3 [−]; indole production from tryptophan [−]; glucose utilization [−]; arginine dihydrase [−]; urease [+]; β-glucosidase [−]; protease [−]; β-galactosidase [−]; assimilation of glucose, arabinose, mannose, mannitol, *n*-acetylglucosamine, maltose, gluconate, caprate, adipate, citrate, or phenylacetate [−], but malate assimilation [+]; and cytochrome oxidase [+]). In addition, glycerol, sucrose, methanol, 1-pentanol, and 1-hexanol were not utilized. Ethanol, 1-propanol, 1-butanol, and oleic acid were assimilated aerobically. According to the API identification program and *Bergey's Manual of Systematic Bacteriology*, this strain is most likely one of the new species of *Pseudomonas* (Table 3), and it was tentatively designated *Pseudomonas anaerooleophila* HD-1.

Although strain HD-1 was identified as a possible *Pseudomonas* species, one characteristic disagrees with this result. Anaerobic growth of *Pseudomonas* spp. is reported only with nitrate reduction. According to the results of the API test, strain HD-1 is negative for nitrate reductase. Some sulfate-reducing bacteria, for example, *Desulfobacterium* sp., can also grow autotrophically (Brysch et al., 1987). However, strain HD-1 does not seem to be a *Desulfobacterium* species, because it grows under both anaerobic and aerobic conditions. Sequence analysis of 16S rRNA to identify its taxonomic position is now in progress.

PRODUCTION OF BIOSURFACTANT BY STRAIN HD-1

Researchers have known for many years that biosurfactants are isolated from oil fields (Kosaric and Gray, 1987). When microorganisms grow on hydrocarbons, the step of hydrocarbon uptake is strongly limited by the hydrophobic character of these compounds. Biosurfactants play an important role in the assimilation of hydrocarbons by microorganisms (Oberbremer et al., 1990). Biosurfactant producers are easily selected on an oil-agar plate by their propensity to form halos (Morikawa et al., 1992; Morikawa et al., 1993). In the plate culture of strain HD-1, oil-displaced halos formed around the colonies. This fact also supports the view that strain HD-1 takes up and assimilates hydrocarbons.

Table 3. Identification percentages of strain HD-1[a]

Candidates	ID%[b]
Pseudomonas mesophilica	76.3
Moraxella phenylpyruvica	9.3
Oligella ureolytica	8.5
CDC group C-2	2.2
Bordetella bronchiseptica	1.1

[a]The API identification program [API 20NE (V4.0)] was applied for the profile number of strain HD-1. *P. mesophilica* was judged to be the nearest strain. CDC, Centers for Disease Control and Prevention.
[b]ID%, identification percentage.

REFERENCES

Aeckersberg, F., F. Bak, and F. Widdel. 1991. Anaerobic oxidation of saturated hydrocarbons to CO_2 by a new type of sulfate-reducing bacterium. *Arch. Microbiol.* **156:**5–14.

Beller, H. R., M. Reinhard, and D. Grbić-Galić. 1992. Metabolic by-products of anaerobic toluene degradation by sulfate-reducing enrichment cultures. *Appl. Environ. Microbiol.* **58:**3192–3195.

Brysch, K., C. Schneider, G. Fuchs, and F. Widdel. 1987. Lithoautotrophic growth of sulfate-reducing bacteria, and description of *Desulfobacterium autotrophicum* gen. nov., sp. nov. *Arch. Microbiol.* **148:**264–274.

Capella, P., and C. M. Zorzut. 1968. Determination of double bond position in monounsaturated fatty acid esters by mass spectrometry of their trimethylsilyloxy derivatives. *Anal. Chem.* **40:**1458–1463.

Chouteau, J., E. Azoulay, and J. C. Senez. 1962. Anaerobic formation of hept-1-ene from n-heptane by resting cells of *Pseudomonas aeruginosa. Nature* (London) **194:**576–578.

Cline, J. D. 1969. Spectrophotometric determination of hydrogen sulfide in natural waters. *Limnol. Oceanogr.* **14:**454–458.

de Andres, C., M. J. Espuny, M. Robert, M. E. Mercade, A. Manresa, and J. Guinea. 1991. Cellular lipid accumulation by *Pseudomoas aeruginosa* 44T1. *Appl. Microbiol. Biothechnol.* **35:**813–816.

Dolfing, J., J. Zeyer, P. Binder-Eicher, and R. P. Schwarzenbach. 1990. Isolation and characterization of a bacterium that mineralizes toluene in the absence of molecular oxygen. *Arch. Microbiol.* **154:**336–341.

Evans, P. J., D. Mang, K. S. Kim, and L. Y. Young. 1991. Anaerobic degradation of toluene by a denitrifying bacterium. *Appl. Environ. Microbiol.* **57:**1139–1145.

Grbić-Galić, D., and T. M. Vogel. 1987. Transformation of toluene and benzene by mixed methanogenic cultures. *Appl. Environ. Microbiol.* **53:**254–260.

Kates, M. 1974. Lipid extraction procedures, p. 347–353. *In* T.S. Work and E. Work (ed.), *Techniques of Lipidology*. North-Holland, Amsterdam.

Kosaric, N., and N. C. C. Gray. 1987. *Biosurfactants and Biotechnology*. Marcel Dekker, New York.

Krieg, N. R., and J. G. Holt. 1984. *Bergey's Manual of Systematic Bacteriology*, vol. 1. The Williams & Wilkins Co., Baltimore.

Lovley, D. R., M. J. Baedecker, D. J. Lonergan, I. M. Cozzarelli, E. J. P. Phillips, and D. I. Siegel. 1989. Oxidation of aromatic contaminants coupled to microbial iron reduction. *Nature* (London) **339:**297–300.

Morikawa, M., H. Daido, T. Takao, S. Murata, T. Shimonishi, and T. Imanaka. 1993. A new lipopeptide biosurfactant produced by *Arthrobacter* sp. strain MIS38. *J. Bacteriol.* **175:**6459–6466.

Morikawa, M., and T. Imanaka. 1993. Isolation of a new mixotrophic bacterium which can fix CO_2 and assimilate aliphatic and aromatic hydrocarbons anaerobically. *J. Ferment. Bioeng.* **76:**280–283.

Morikawa, M., M. Ito, and T. Imanaka. 1992. Isolation of a new surfactin producer *Bacillus pumilus* A-1, and nucleotide sequence of the regulator gene, *psf-1. J. Ferment. Bioeng.* **74:**255–261.

Oberbremer, A., R. Muller-Hurtig, and F. Wagner. 1990. Effect of the addition of microbial surfactants on hydrocarbon degradation in a soil population in a stirred reactor. *Appl. Microbiol. Biotechnol.* **32:**485–489.

Parekh, V. R., R. W. Traxler, and J. M. Sobek. 1977. *n*-Alkane oxidation enzymes of a pseudomonad. *Appl. Environ. Microbiol.* **33:**881–884.

Payne, W. J. 1981. *Denitrification*. John Wiley & Sons, Inc., New York.

Phillips, E. J. P., and D. I. Siegel. 1989. Oxidation of aromatic contaminants coupled to microbial iron reduction. *Nature* (London) **339:**297–299.

Rabus, R., R. Nordhaus, W. Ludwig, and F. Widdel. 1993. Complete oxidation of toluene under strictly anoxic conditions by a new sulfate-reducing bacterium. *Appl. Environ. Microbiol.* **59:**1444–1451.

Rueter, P., R. Rabus, H. Wilkes, F. Aeckersberg, F. A. Rainey, H. W. Jannasch, and F. Widdel. 1994. Anaerobic oxidation of hydrocarbons in crude oil by new types of sulphate-reducing bacteria. *Nature* (London) **372:**455–458.

Szewzyk, R., and N. Pfennig. 1987. Complete oxidation of catechol by the strictly anaerobic sulfate-reducing *Desulfobacterium catecholicum* sp. nov. *Arch. Microbiol.* **147:**163–168.

Thauer, R. K., F. H. Kirchniawy, and K. A. Jungermann. 1972. Properties and function of the pyruvate-formate-lyase reaction in Clostridiae. *Eur. J. Biochem.* **27:**282–290.

Thauer, R. K., D. Möller-Zinkhan, and A. M. Spormann. 1989. Biochemistry of acetate catabolism in anaerobic chemotrophic bacteria. *Annu. Rev. Microbiol.* **43:**43–67.

The Japan Oil Chemists' Society. 1995. *Standard Method of the Japan Oil Chemists' Society*. 2.4.5.1-71. The Japan Oil Chemists' Society, Tokyo.

Molecular Biology of Pseudomonads
Edited by T. Nakazawa et al.

Chapter 26

Arrangement and Transcriptional Regulation of the Denitrification Genes in *Pseudomonas aeruginosa*

Hiroyuki Arai, Shinji Kawasaki, Yasuo Igarashi, and Tohru Kodama

The bacteria and fungi that are able to grow under anaerobic conditions by using nitrogen oxides as the respiratory substrate are distributed among various taxonomic groups, including pseudomonads (Jeter and Ingraham, 1991; Zumft, 1992). The anaerobic reduction of nitrate is divided into two categories based on the type of reduction mechanism: the assimilative reduction of nitrate yields ammonium (which is used as a nitrogen source), while the dissimilative reduction of nitrate usually yields gaseous products. Denitrification is commonly defined as the latter process. Complete denitrification consists of four sequential steps to reduce nitrate (NO_3^-) to dinitrogen gas (N_2) via nitrite (NO_2^-), nitric oxide (NO), and nitrous oxide (N_2O). This pathway is ecologically important because it is one of very few routes for generating atmospheric dinitrogen (Jeter and Ingraham, 1991). Each step of the pathway is catalyzed by individual metalloenzymes, i.e., nitrate reductase (NAR), nitrite reductase (NIR), nitric oxide reductase (NOR), and nitrous oxide reductase (N_2OR) (Zumft, 1992; Cuypers and Zumft, 1992). The reduction of nitrate to nitrite is a common step in both the assimilatory and the dissimilatory pathways, whereas the last three enzymes are specific for denitrification. Usually, denitrifying bacteria are facultative anaerobes that favor oxygen as a respiratory substrate, and the maxumum expression of the denitrification enzymes occurs in an environment of low oxygen concentration. In addition to anoxia, the presence of an N oxide such as nitrate or nitrite is required for the full expression of the denitrification enzymes. Work on the regulatory mechanisms of the denitrification system has primarily focused on three organisms: *Pseudomonas aeruginosa, Pseudomonas stutzeri,* and *Paracoccus denitrificans*. The structural genes corresponding to all three denitrification-specific enzymes and some of the regulatory genes have been identified in these organisms. In *P. stutzeri,* the genes for the three enzymes are clustered in a 30-kb region of chromosomal DNA (Braun and Zumft, 1992). In *P. aeruginosa* and *Paracoccus*

Hiroyuki Arai • Laboratory of Microbiology, The Institute of Physical and Chemical Research, 2-1 Hirosawa, Wako, Saitama 351-01, Japan. ***Shinji Kawasaki, Yasuo Igarashi, and Tohru Kodama*** • Department of Biotechnology, University of Tokyo, Yayoi 1-1-1, Bunkyo-ku, Tokyo 113, Japan.

denitrificans the genes for NIR and NOR are close to each other, but whether the genes for N_2OR lie in the same region is not known (Arai et al., 1995a; van Spanning et al., 1995). In this chapter, we describe the present state of knowledge concerning the arrangement and transcriptional regulation of the denitrification genes from *P. aeruginosa* (Fig. 1).

GENES FOR NITRITE RESPIRATION

Dissimilatory NIR is a key enzyme in denitrification because it separates the reducing pathway from the assimilatory route and produces the first gaseous product, nitric oxide. Two types of the enzyme, cytochrome cd_1 (EC 1.9.3.2) and a copper-containing protein (EC 1.7.2.1), have been identified (Coyne et al., 1989). NIR from *P. aeruginosa* was the first denitrification enzyme characterized (Yamanaka et al., 1960). It consists of two identical subunits, each containing a covalently attached heme *c* and a noncovalently bound heme d_1. The physiological electron donor for the enzyme is cytochrome c_{551}. A small blue copper protein, azurin, can also act as an electron donor in vitro (reviewed by Silvestrini et al., 1994). The structural gene for NIR (*nirS*, formerly *denA*) was first isolated and analyzed by Silvestrini et al. (1989). We found that the gene encoding cytochrome c_{551} (*nirM*, formerly *denB*) is located just downstream of *nirS* (Arai et al., 1990). The same observation was made independently by Nordling et al. (1990). The *nirM* gene is followed by a gene encoding another monoheme cytochrome *c* (*nirC*). The role of the *nirC* gene product has not been determined, but it must function as an indispensable factor for nitrite respiration, since similar genes have been found in the downstream regions of *nirS* genes of *P. stutzeri* (Jüngst et al., 1991) and *Paracoccus denitrificans* (de Boer et al., 1994). The *nirF* gene, which follows *nirC*, was also identified in *Paracoccus denitrificans*. No sequences homologous to those of the *nirF* gene product have been found in the protein databanks. Disruption of the gene causes the production in both bacteria of an inactive NIR protein that specifically lacks heme d_1, suggesting that the gene product takes part in the biosynthetic pathway of heme d_1 (Kawasaki et al., 1995; de Boer et al., 1994). Other genes with unknown functions might follow *nirF* in the same cluster.

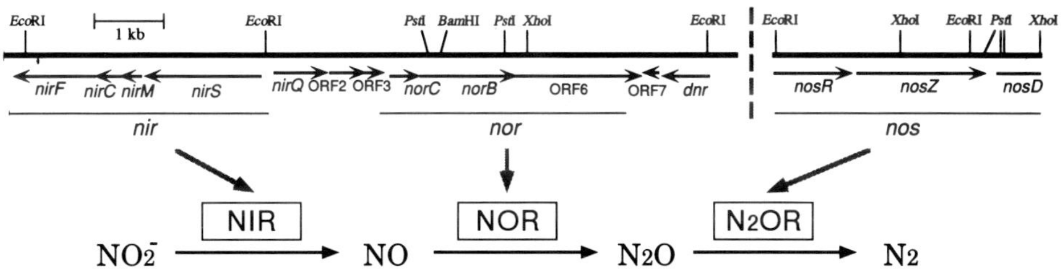

Figure 1. Physical map of the denitrification gene cluster from *P. aeruginosa*. Arrows show sizes and directions of transcription of denitrification genes. The genes for NO_2 reduction, NO reduction, and N_2O reduction are indicated by bars labeled *nir, nor,* and *nos*, respectively. Sources for sequence data: Silvestrini et al., 1989 (*nirS*); Arai et al., 1990, and Nordling et al., 1990 (*nirM*); Kawasaki et al., 1995 (*nirCF*); Arai et al., 1994 (*nirQ*, ORF2, and ORF3); Arai et al., 1995a (*norCB* and ORF6); Arai et al., 1995b (ORF7 and *dnr*); Zumft et al., 1992 (*nosRZD*).

GENES FOR NOR

NOR (EC 1.7.99.7) catalyzes the reduction of nitric oxide (NO) to nitrous oxide (N_2O). NO is highly toxic for cells, and the intracellular NO concentration must be kept very low. It has long been uncertain whether NO is an obligate intermediate, but recent studies have clarified that the production of NO from nitrite by NIR and the consumption of NO by NOR are concertedly regulated and that the concentration of free NO is kept at a minimum (Zumft, 1994; Ye et al., 1994). Bacterial NOR has been purified from *P. stutzeri* (Heiss et al., 1989), *Paracoccus denitrificans* (Dermastia et al., 1991), and *Achromobacter cycloclastes* (Jones and Hollocher, 1993). The enzymes of these three bacteria are classified as the same type, i.e., a membrane-bound cytochrome *bc* complex, even though the former two strains have a cytochrome cd_1-type NIR and the last one has a copper-containing NIR. NOR has also been found in the fungus *Fusarium oxysporum* (Nakahara et al., 1993), but there it is a cytochrome P-450 and different from the bacterial enzymes. In *P. aeruginosa,* the genes for NOR (*norCB*) are located about 2 kb upstream of *nirS* (Fig. 1) (Arai et al., 1995a), whereas in *P. stutzeri,* the *norCB* genes are located downstream of *nirS* (Braun and Zumft, 1992). Analyses of the nucleotide and deduced amino acid sequences of the genes for NOR gave detailed information on the structure of the enzyme (Zumft et al., 1994). The cytochrome *b* subunit (NorB) carries 12 hydrophobic transmembrane spans. The cytochrome *c* subunit (NorC) has an N-terminal hydrophobic portion that is expected to function either in anchoring the enzyme to the membrane or in interacting with NorB. The amino acid sequence of NorB is similar to that of FixN, a major subunit of a novel heme-copper oxidase in aerobic respiration (Saraste and Castresana, 1994; van der Oost et al., 1994). The FixN complex has an exceptionally high affinity for oxygen and is expressed under conditions of low oxygen concentration. FixN corresponds to subunit I of the cytochrome oxidases and carries the conserved six histidine residues that are known to be required for the binding of two hemes and of Cu_B. Though only two prosthetic groups, heme *c* and heme *b,* have been identified in the purified NOR, NorB from both *P. aeruginosa* and *P. stutzeri* has all six histidine ligands. The *norB* gene is followed by a gene, ORF6, encoding a hydrophilic protein. A similar gene is found in *P. stutzeri,* and a partial sequence has been reported (Zumft et al., 1994). ORF6 is thought to be indispensable for denitrification because a mutant of *P. aeruginosa* with a gene disruption could not grow on nitrate under anaerobic conditions (Arai, 1995).

THE *nirQ* OPERON

Three genes (*nirQ,* ORF2, and ORF3) are located between the structural genes of NIR and NOR (Fig. 1). These three genes are transcribed divergently from *nirS* under denitrifying conditions (Arai et al., 1994). The *nirQ* gene encodes a hydrophilic protein containing two nucleotide-binding motifs. Jüngst and Zumft (1992) investigated the role of the *nirQ* gene in *P. stutzeri* and found that a *nirQ* mutant of the bacterium simultaneously loses the activities of both NIR and NOR in vivo, although both reductase proteins are synthesized. When phenazine methosulfate was used as an electron donor, in vitro activity of NIR was detected, whereas that of NOR was not. These results indicate that the *nirQ* gene product mediates a functional coupling of NIR and NOR. Concerted expression of the two reductase activities is necessary in order to avoid accumulation of toxic NO. In fact, it has been reported that the loss of NIR enzyme activity causes a decrease in the NOR expression level and that the in vivo activity of NIR is severely reduced in the NOR^- mutant (Zumft et al., 1994). We believe that the *nirQ* gene product converts inactive NOR enzyme to an active form. The loss of in vivo NIR activity in the *nirQ* mutant may be due to the absence of the active NOR enzyme. The existence of such a posttranslational activation mechanism for the NOR enzyme in *P. stutzeri* has been suggested (Zumft et al., 1994). In this bacterium, the in vivo activity of NOR is much lower than that expected from the amount of the protein, indicating that much of the enzyme is catalytically inactive. Circumstantial evidence supporting the role of NirQ as a posttranslational activator of the enzyme was obtained by investigating the role of a NirQ homolog. We found a gene, *cbbQ*, highly similar to *nirQ*, in the downstream region of *cbbLS*, which are genes for the large and small subunits of ribulose-1,5-bisphosphate carboxylase/oxygenase (Rubisco) from the thermophilic hydrogen-utilizing bacterium *Pseudomonas hydrogenothermophila* (Yokoyama et al., 1995). The translated sequence of *cbbQ* shares 53% identity with the NirQ of *P. aeruginosa* and 49% identity with that of *P. stutzeri*. Although Rubisco activity was functionally expressed in *Escherichia coli* carrying the cloned *cbbLS* genes from *P. hydrogenothermophila*, the existence of *cbbQ* with *cbbLS* in *E. coli* apparently raised the activity without changing the concentration of the Rubisco protein (R. N. Hayashi, H. Arai, K.-S. Yoon, Y. Igarashi, and T. Kodama, unpublished data).

The hydropathy profiles of the translated sequences of ORF2 and ORF3 indicate that the gene products are membrane proteins carrying five and three hydrophobic spans, respectively. A homology search in the protein data banks showed that the translated sequence of ORF2 is similar to subunit III of the cytochrome oxidases. A *P. aeruginosa* mutant strain lacking the three genes *nirQ*, ORF2, and ORF3 could not grow under denitrifying conditions. Although ORF2 and ORF3 were transcribed with *nirQ* as one operon under denitrifying conditions, the growth of the mutant could be restored by introducing only the *nirQ* gene. Thus, ORF2 and ORF3 are not necessary for growth by denitrification. The role of these genes remains unexplained (Arai, 1995).

EVOLUTIONARY LINKS BETWEEN DENITRIFICATION AND AEROBIC RESPIRATION

Oxygen respiration may have developed from nitrate respiration (Egami, 1973). No obvious evidence supports nitrate respiration preceding aerobic respiration in the evolution of energy metabolism. However, the high degree of similarity between the cytochrome systems of denitrification and oxygen respiration indicates that the two energy-yielding mechanisms may have derived from the same evolutionary origin. Moreover, recent genetic studies on the structures of the denitrification enzymes reinforce the hypothesis of an evolutionary relationship between these two respiration pathways (Fig. 2).

Cytochrome oxidases, the terminal enzymes of the aerobic respiratory chain, such as cytochrome aa_3, consist of three major subunits (COI, COII, and COIII) and several minor subunits. The sites for electron transport and oxygen reduction are on COI and COII. Sequence similarity between the Cu_A domains of N_2OR and COII was shown by Zumft et al. (1992). The electron paramagnetic resonance spectra of the two enzymes are also similar (Lappalainen and Saraste, 1994). Sequence similarity supporting the evolu-

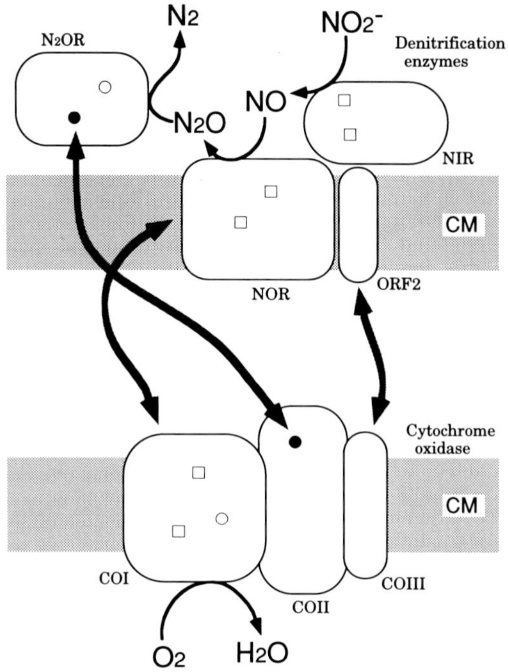

Figure 2. Evolutionary links (indicated by arrows) between denitrification enzymes (NIR, NOR, N_2OR) and subunits of cytochrome oxidase (COI, COII, COIII). Squares indicate heme groups, and circles indicate copper atoms. Closed circles are Cu_A. CM, cytoplasmic membrane. Comparison was based on similarities between the denitrification enzymes of *P. aeruginosa* or *P. stutzeri* and the subunits of mitochondrial or bacterial oxidases (cytochrome aa_3 and cytochrome *bo*). Sources for the evolutionary relationships: Saraste and Castresana, 1994, and van der Oost et al., 1994 (NOR-COI); Zumft et al., 1992 (N_2OR-COII); Arai et al., 1994 (ORF2-COIII).

tionary relationship between the denitrification enzymes and cytochrome oxidase has been found in the cytochrome *b* subunits (NorB) of NOR and COI (Saraste and Castresana, 1994; van der Oost et al., 1994). As mentioned previously, the primary structure of NorB is also similar to that of FixN, and the six histidine ligands for binding of two hemes and Cu_B are conserved in NorB, FixN, and COI. The FixN complex is an enzyme system that is highly adapted for respiration in a low-oxygen environment and is thought to be the oldest type of cytochrome *c* oxidase. From these observations, it could be proposed that the respiratory enzymes evolved from NOR to the ordinary cytochrome oxidases via the FixN complex as atmospheric oxygen accumulated (Saraste and Castresana, 1994). Another evolutionary link between these pathways is the similarity between the ORF2 gene product and COIII (Arai et al., 1994). COIII does not carry the redox center of the enzyme and is not necessarily required for enzyme activity. The role of the subunit has not been identified, but some data have indicated its participation either in proton translocation or in the assembly or maintenance of the cytochrome oxidase complex (Haltia et al., 1989). Although ORF2 is not essential for anaerobic growth of *P. aeruginosa* (Arai,1995), the role of the gene product may be similar to that of COIII.

TRANSCRIPTIONAL REGULATION OF THE *nir* AND *nor* GENES MEDIATED BY TWO CRP-FNR-RELATED REGULATORS

A CRP-FNR-related transcriptional regulator, ANR, is known to be required for denitrification, for the arginine deiminase pathway, and for hydrogen cyanide biosynthesis in *P. aeruginosa*. ANR is highly similar to FNR in *Escherichia coli*, with 51% of the amino acids being identical (Sawers, 1991; Zimmermann et al., 1991). FNR is an oxygen-sensing regulator that positively regulates the expression of the genes for anaerobic metabolism in *E. coli*. Four cysteine residues, which might be essential for chelation of Fe^{2+}, are necessary for the activity of FNR (Guest, 1992). All four cysteine residues are conserved in ANR, and the *anr* gene can functionally complement an *fnr* mutation in *E. coli*, suggesting that ANR regulates the anoxic induction of the genes involved in anaerobic metabolism in the same manner as FNR. The genes regulated by FNR carry a conserved binding motif (TTGATN_4ATCAA) in their promoter regions. The sequences that resemble the FNR-binding motif have also been found in anaerobically regulated promoters from *P. aeruginosa* (Table 1). A gene for an FNR homolog, *fnrA*, was isolated from *P. stutzeri* by using the *anr* gene of *P. aeruginosa* as a probe (Cuypers and Zumft, 1993). The amino acid sequence of FnrA is 81.6% identical to that of ANR. The denitrification genes from *P. stutzeri* carry the FNR-binding motif in their promoter regions, but expression of the denitrification enzymes is not affected by an *fnrA* mutation. A synthetic FNR-dependent promoter is still activated anaerobically in the *fnrA* mutant, suggesting the existence of another FNR homolog, tentatively designated FnrD, in *P. stutzeri* (Cuypers and Zumft, 1993).

In the region downstream of the *nor* genes of *P. aeruginosa*, we found a gene encoding a protein similar to the CRP-FNR family of transcriptional regulators (Fig. 3) (Arai et al., 1995b). Disruption of the gene results in the inability of the strain to grow on nitrate under anaerobic conditions, whereas aerobic growth is not affected by the mutation, suggesting that the gene product regulates the expression of denitrification genes in addition to ANR. This is the first finding that two CRP-FNR-related regulators are involved in denitrification in the same bacterium. We designated the gene *dnr* for dissimilatory nitrate respiration regulator or denitrification regulator. A similar gene has been

Table 1. Presumed ANR-binding sequences of genes for denitrification and the arginine deiminase pathway in *P. aeruginosa*

Putative recognition motif[a]	Gene(s)	Function	Reference
----TTGAT----ATCAA----	FNR consensus		Guest, 1992
aatcTTGATtccggTCAAgcaa[b]	*nirSMCF*	NIR	Arai et al., 1991a
ttgcTTGAccggaATCAAgatt[b]	*nirQ*-ORF2, ORF3	NIR-NOR activation	Arai et al., 1991a
aatcTTGATtgccATCAAgcgg	*norCB*-ORF6	NOR	Arai et al., 1995a
acaacTGATtcccgcCgtcgag	*nosZ*	N_2OR	Zumft et al., 1992
gagcTTGccgtgcgTCAAgatg	*dnr*	Transcriptional activator	Arai et al., 1995b
ccgcTTGATcgcggTCAAgcgc	ORF7	Unknown	Arai et al., 1995b
gggtTTGAcctgaATCAgtgga	*azu*	Azurin	Hoitink et al., 1990
gctaTTGAcgtggATCAgcatt	*arcDABC*	Anaerobic arginine catabolism	Galimand et al., 1991

[a]Nucleotides corresponding to the *E. coli* FNR consensus sequence are in capital letters.
[b]The motif for *nirQ* is a sequence that is complementary to that of the *nirS* promoter.

```
DNR      1:MEFQ-RVHQQLLQSHHLFEPLSPVQLQE-LLASSDLVNLDKGAYVFRQGEPAHAFYYLI-SG-CVKIYRL
CRP(E)   1:                M---------VLGKPQ---T--DPTLEWFLSHCHIHKYPSKSTLIHQGEKAETLYY
CRP(H)   1:                MSNELTEIDEVVTSSQEEATQRDPVLDWFLTHCHLHKYPAKSTLIHAGEDATTLYY
FNR      1:MIPEKRIIRRIQSGGCAIHCQDCSISQLCIPFTLNEHELDQLDNIIERKKPIQKGQTLFKAGDELKSLYA
ANR      1: MAE--TI-KVRALP-QAHCKDCSLAPLCLPLSLTVEDMDSLDEIVKRGRPLKKGEFLFRQGDPFGSVFA
NtcA     1:      MDQSLTQDRPLAAVFRRLG-SE-LMPPV-VETFDRSKTIFFPGDPAERVYFL-LKG-AVKLSRV
FixK     1:          MKPSVVMIEPNGHFCSDCAIRTSAVCSSLDAAELREFEHLGRRVHFSSGETVFSEEDITT
NNR      1:  MN-APLPEAVKKSVLLNGLTPEMRDK-LLKDAQRRSYREGETIFLQGDPARAVFIVL-NG-FIKLSRL

DNR     67:TPEG---QEKILEVTNE-RNTF----AE---AMMFMDTPNYVATAQAVVPSQLFRFSNKAYLRQLQDNTP
CRP(E)  43:IVKGSVAVLIKDEEGKEMILSYLNQGDFIGELGLFEEGQERSAWVRAKTACEVAEISYKKFRQLIQVNPD
CRP(H)  57:VIKGSVMVSSKDDEGKEMILTYLGAGQFFGEAGLFDEGSKRSAWVKTKTTCEIAEISYKKYRQLIQANPE
FNR     71:IRSGTIKSYTITEQGDEQITGF-HLAGDL-VGFDAIGSGHHPSFAQALETSMVCEIPFETLDDLSGKMPN
ANR     66:VRSGALKTFSITDAGEEQITGF-HLPSEL-VGLSGMDTETYPVSAQALETTSVCEIPFERLDELSEQLPQ
NtcA    60:YEAG---EEITVALLRE-NSVF----GVL-SLVTGQRSDRFYHAVAFTPVELLSAPIEQVEQAL-KEHPD
FixK    61:SFYNVLEGVMRLYKLLPDGRRQIVGFALPGDFLGMNLSGRHNFSADAIGAVTVCQFAKAPFGRFIEERPQ
NNR     65:TPNGS---EAVVAILGR-NRSF----AE---AMVLRGTP-YPVSAEAISDCTVLQIDGARLRQFLLENQE

                                                                    *********    *
DNR    126:LALALLAKLSTRLHQRIDEIETLSLKNATHRVVRYLLTLAAH-A-PG-ENCRVEIPVAKQLVAGHLSIQP
CRP(E) 113:ILMRLSAQMARRLQVTSEKVGNLAFLDVTGRIAQTLLNLAKQ-PDAMTHPDGMQIKITRQEIGQIVGCSR
CRP(H) 127:ILMFLTAQLARRLQNTSRQVTNLAFLDVAGRIAQTLMNLAKQ-PEAMTHPDGMQIKITRQEIGQMVGCSR
FNR    139:LRQQMMRLMSGEIKGDQDMILLLSKKNAEERLAAFIYNLSRRFAQRGFSPREFRLTMTRGDIGNYLGLTV
ANR    134:LRRQLMRLMSREIRDDQQMMLLLSKKTADERIATFLVNLSARFRARGFSAQQFRLAMSRNEIGNYLGLAV
NtcA   120:LSLLMLQGLSSRILQTEMMIETLAHRDMGSRLVSFLLILCRDFGVPAPDGIRIDLKLSHQAIAEAIGSTR
FixK   131:LLRRINELAIRELSQARDHMVLLGRRSADEKVAAFLLGWRERLLALKGASDTVPLPMSRQDIADYLGLTI
NNR    123:FAIGLLASTFVHLQGLVDQIERLKAHTGVQRVAQFLADLSDA-V-AGPA--EVRLPYNKRLIAGHLGMQP

           ************
DNR    193:ETFSRIMHRLGDEGIIHLDGREISILDRERLECFE          227
CRP(E) 182:ETVGRILKMLEDQNLISAHGKTIVVYGTR                210
CRP(H) 196:ETVGRIIKMLEDQNLIHAHGKTIVVYGAR                224
FNR    209:ETISRLLGRFQKSGMLAVKGKYITIENNDALAQLAGHTRNVA   250
ANR    204:ETVSRVFTRFQQNGLISAEGKEVHILDSIELCALAGGQLEG    244
NtcA   190:VTVTRLLGDLREGNMISITKKKITVHNPVALSQQFT         225
FixK   201:ETVSRTFTKLERHGAIAIIHGGISLLDPARVEALAAA        237
NNR    189:ESLSRAFARLRNDGVEIEADKAMIADIAELRMMAMD         224
```

Figure 3. Alignment of DNR with CRP of *E. coli* (E) and *Haemophilus influenzae* (H), FNR of *E. coli*, ANR of *P. aeruginosa*, NtcA of *Synechocystis* sp. strain PCC7120, FixK of *Bradyrhizobium japonicum*, and NNR of *Paracoccus denitrificans*. Identical residues are shaded, and gaps are indicated by hyphens. DNR showed the highest identity with NNR (33.3%). Cyclic AMP-binding residues of CRP and cysteine residues required for the activity of FNR and ANR are underlined. Asterisks indicate the helix-turn-helix motif (DNA binding domain).

found in *Paracoccus denitrificans* and designated *nnr*, for nitrite and nitric oxide reductases regulator (van Spanning et al., 1995). DNR carries neither the cysteine residues conserved in the FNR-type regulators nor the conserved cyclic AMP-binding residues of the CRP-type regulators. If an effector of DNR exists, it may be different from that of FNR or CRP. The regulatory function of DNR probably differs from the functions of the anaerobic or catabolite respression controls.

We examined the promoter activities of the *nirS, nirQ*, and *norCB* genes under various conditions, using either *xylE* or *lacZ* as a reporter gene (Arai, 1995; Arai et al., 1991a, 1991b, 1994). All of the promoters were expressed under anaerobic conditions in the presence of nitrite. Without nitrite, the activity was very low even under anaerobic conditions. These results suggest the existence of a nitrite-sensing mechanism in addition to an ANR-mediated oxygen-sensing mechanism. Significant induction of the promoter activity by nitrite was not detected under conditions of strong aeration when either of the two reporter genes was used. Although the maximum level of expression for denitrification activity is observed under anaerobic conditions, denitrification enzymes are expressed even under partially aerobic conditions in the presence of nitrate (Zennaro et al., 1993). This aerobic induction is thought to be due to a residual aerobic activity of ANR (Ye et al., 1995). Our promoter probing system consists of promoters carried by multicopy plasmids. Our failure to detect aerobic induction of the promoters may suggest a shortage of active ANR molecules under aerobic conditions. We confirmed the dependence of *nir* and *nor* gene expression on ANR by measuring promoter activity in an *anr* mutant of *P. aeruginosa* (Table 2) (Arai et al., 1995b). Transcription from all three promoters (*nirS, nirQ*, and *norCB*) is significantly reduced in the mutant strain PAO6261. Transcriptional activity of the genes is also very low in a *dnr* mutant, RM536 (Table 2). Whether the two CRP-FNR-related regulators, ANR and DNR, activate the transcription of the *nir* and *nor* genes directly is not known with certainty. Recently, the entire denitrification pathway of *P. aeruginosa* was shown to be under the control of ANR (Ye et al., 1995). NAR, however, does not seem to be under the control of DNR, since a significant amount of nitrite accumulated when the *dnr* mutant was grown under conditions of low aeration in the presence of nitrate (H. Arai, Y. Igarashi, and T. Kodama, unpublished data).

PERSPECTIVES

Expression of the denitrification enzymes is regulated by oxygen limitation and by N-oxide substrates. ANR, an analog of FNR, is involved in the anaerobic activation of the denitrification genes in *P. aeruginosa*. However, the direct interaction of ANR with denitrification promoters and the regulatory mechanism involved in sensing N oxides have not been demonstrated. In *E. coli*, expression of the genes for nitrate reduction is regulated by a two-component system consisting of dual-response regulators (NarL and NarP) and dual sensors (NarX and NarQ) (Rabin and Stewart, 1993). A similar system probably regulates the induction of NAR in denitrifying bacteria. Expression of NIR and NOR is controlled by *dnr* in *P. aeruginosa* (Arai et al., 1995b) and by *nnr* in *Paracoccus denitrificans* (van Spanning et al., 1995). An involvement of DNR and NNR in N-oxide regulation is not certain at present. NIR and NOR activity should be expressed coordinately to avoid accumulation of toxic NO; in *P. stutzeri*, the direct inducer of NOR is not nitrite but endogenous NO (Körner, 1993). The *nirQ* gene, which encodes a putative

Table 2. Both *dnr* and *anr* genes are required for transcription of *nir* and *nor* genes of *P. aeruginosa*[a]

Strain (genotype)	β-Galactosidase activity for promoters[b]		
	nirS	*nirQ*	*norCB*
PAO1 (wild type)	2.4	0.8	7.6
RM536 (*dnr*)	0.1	<0.05	<0.05
PAO6261 (*anr*)	0.1	<0.05	0.1

[a]From Arai et al., 1995b.

[b]Transcriptional activity was determined by using a *lacZ* promoter probe vector, pQF50 (Farinha and Kropinski, 1990), and measuring the activity of β-galactosidase, the gene product of *lacZ*. Specific activity of β-galactosidase is expressed in Miller kilounits. The data are mean values from three or four independent experiments. Cultivation was done under oxygen-limiting conditions in the presence of 5 mM sodium nitrite.

activator for NOR, also seems to be regulated by NO in *P. aeruginosa* (Arai, 1995). The divergent transcription of *nirQ* and *nirS* may facilitate the coordinate expression of NIR and NOR. NosR, a membrane-bound regulatory protein, is known to be essential for the expression of N_2OR (Cuypers et al., 1992). These observations indicate that each step of the denitrification pathway has an independent regulatory system responsive to its own substrate. A mechanism for the coordinate expression of the whole denitrification system should be present in order to accomplish the controlled reduction of nitrate to dinitrogen. Investigations of transcriptional control of the regulatory genes as well as the structural genes will be necessary in order to understand this complex regulatory network in denitrifying bacteria.

Acknowledgments. We thank M. Roberts for critical reading of the manuscript.

REFERENCES

Arai, H. 1995. Structure and regulation of the denitrification gene cluster from *Pseudomonas aeruginosa*. Ph.D. thesis. University of Tokyo, Tokyo.

Arai, H., Y. Igarashi, and T. Kodama. 1991a. Anaerobically induced expression of the nitrite reductase cytochrome *c*-551 operon from *Pseudomonas aeruginosa*. *FEBS Lett.* **280:**351–353.

Arai, H., Y. Igarashi, and T. Kodama. 1991b. Nitrite activates the transcription of the *Pseudomonas aeruginosa* nitrite reductase and cytochrome *c*-551 operon under the anaerobic conditions. *FEBS Lett.* **288:**227–228.

Arai, H., Y. Igarashi, and T. Kodama. 1994. Structure and ANR-dependent transcription of the *nir* genes for denitrification from *Pseudomonas aeruginosa*. *Biosci. Biotechnol. Biochem.* **58:**1286–1291.

Arai, H., Y. Igarashi, and T. Kodama. 1995a. The structural genes for nitric oxide reductase from *Pseudomonas aeruginosa*. *Biochim. Biphys. Acta* **1261:**279–284.

Arai, H., Y. Igarashi, and T. Kodama. 1995b. Expression of the *nir* and *nor* genes for denitrification of *Pseudomonas aeruginosa* requires a novel CRP/FNR related transcriptional regulator, DNR, in addition to ANR. *FEBS Lett.* **371:**73–76.

Arai, H., Y. Sanbongi, Y. Igarashi, and T. Kodama. 1990. Cloning and sequencing of the gene encoding cytochrome *c*-551 from *Pseudomonas aeruginosa*. *FEBS Lett.* **261:**196–198.

Braun, C., and W. G. Zumft. 1992. The structural genes of the nitric oxide reductase complex from *Pseudomonas stutzeri* are part of a 30-kilobase gene cluster for denitrification. *J. Bacteriol.* **174:**2394–2397.

Coyne, M. S., A. Arunakumari, B. A. Averill, and J. M. Tiedje. 1989. Immunological identification and distribution of dissimilatory heme cd_1 and nonheme copper nitrite reductases in denitrifying bacteria. *Appl. Environ. Microbiol.* **55:**2924–2931.

Cuypers, H., A. Viebrock-Sambale, and W. G. Zumft. 1992. NosR, a membrane-bound regulatory component necessary for expression of nitrous oxide reductase in denitrifying *Pseudomonas stutzeri*. *J. Bacteriol.* **174:**5332–5339.

Cuypers, H., and W. G. Zumft. 1992. Regulatory components of the denitrification gene cluster of *Pseudomonas stutzeri*, p. 188–197. *In* E. Galli, S. Silver, and B. Witholt (ed.), *Pseudomonas: Molecular Biology and Biotechnology*. American Society for Microbiology, Washington, D.C.

Cuypers H., and W. G. Zumft. 1993. Anaerobic control of denitrification in *Pseudomonas stutzeri* escapes mutagenesis of an *fnr*-like gene. *J. Bacteriol.* **175:**7236–7246.

de Boer, A. P. N., W. N. M. Reijnders, J. G. Kuenen, A. H. Stouthamer, and R. J. M. van Spanning. 1994. Isolation, sequencing and mutational analysis of a gene cluster involved in nitrite reduction in *Paracoccus denitrificans*. *Antonie van Leeuwenhoek* **66:**111–127.

Dermastia, M., T. Turk, and T. C. Hollocher. 1991. Nitric oxide reductase. Purification from *Paracoccus denitrificans* with use of a single column and some characteristics. *J. Biol. Chem.* **266:**10899–10905.

Egami, F. 1973. A comment to the concept on the role of nitrate fermentation and nitrate respiration in an evolutionary pathway of energy metabolism. *Z. Allg. Mikrobiol.* **13:**177–181.

Farinha, M. A., and A. M. Kropinski. 1990. Construction of broad-host-range plasmid vectors for easy visible selection and analysis of promoters. *J. Bacteriol.* **172:**3496–3499.

Galimand, M., M. Gamper, A. Zimmermann, and D. Haas. 1991. Positive FNR-like control of anaerobic arginine degradation and nitrate respiration in *Pseudomonas aeruginosa. J. Bacteriol.* **173:**1598–1606.

Guest, J. R. 1992. Oxygen-regulated gene expression in *Escherichia coli. J. Gen. Microbiol.* **138:**2253–2263.

Haltia, T., M. Finel, N. Harms, T. Nakari, M. Raitio, M. Wikström, and M. Saraste. 1989. Deletion of the gene for subunit III leads to defective assembly of bacterial cytochrome oxidase. *EMBO J.* **8:**3571–3579.

Heiss, B., K. Frunzke, and W. G. Zumft. 1989. Formation of the N-N bond from nitric oxide by a membrane-bound cytochrome *bc* complex of nitrate-respirating (denitrifying) *Pseudomonas stutzeri. J. Bacteriol.* **171:**3288–3297.

Hoitink, C. W. G., L. P. Woudt, J. C. M. Turenhout, M. van de Kamp, and G. W. Canters. 1990. Isolation and sequencing of the *Alcaligenes denitrificans* azurin-encoding gene: comparison with the gene encoding blue copper proteins from *Pseudomonas aeruginosa and Alcaligenes faecalis. Gene* **90:**15–20.

Jeter, R. M., and J. L. Ingraham. 1991. The denitrifying prokaryotes, p. 913–925. *In* M. P. Starr, H. Stolp, H. G. Trüper, A. Balows, and H. G. Schlegel (ed.), *The Prokaryotes. A Handbook on the Habitats, Isolation, and Identification of Bacteria.* Springer-Verlag KG., Berlin.

Jones, A. M., and T. C. Hollocher. 1993. Nitric oxide reductase of *Achromobacter cycloclastes. Biochim. Biophys. Acta* **1144:**359–366.

Jüngst, A., S. Wakabayashi, H. Matsubara, and W. G. Zumft. 1991. The *nirSTBM* region for cytochrome cd_1-dependent nitrite respiration of *Pseudomonas stutzeri* consists of a cluster of mono-, di, and tetraheme proteins. *FEBS Lett.* **279:**205–209.

Jüngst, A., and W. G. Zumft. 1992. Interdependence of respiratory NO reduction and nitrite reduction revealed by mutagenesis of *nirQ*, a novel gene in the denitrification gene cluster of *Pseudomonas stutzeri. FEBS Lett.* **314:**308–314.

Kawasaki, S., H. Arai, Y. Igarashi, and T. Kodama. 1995. Sequencing and characterization of the downstream region of the genes encoding nitrite reductase and cytochrome *c*-551 (*nirSM*) from *Pseudomonas aeruginosa:* identification of the gene necessary for biosynthesis of heme d_1. *Gene* **167:**87–91.

Körner, H. 1993. Anaerobic expression of nitric oxide reductase from denitrifying *Pseudomonas stutzeri. Arch. Microbiol.* **159:**410–416.

Lappalainen, P., and M. Saraste. 1994. The binuclear Cu_A centre of cytochrome oxidase. *Biochim. Biophys. Acta* **1187:**222–225.

Nakahara, K., T. Tanimoto, K. Hatano, K. Usuda, and H. Shoun. 1993. Cytochrome P-450 55AI (P-450dNIR) acts as nitric oxide reductase employing NADH as the direct electron donor. *J. Biol. Chem.* **268:**8350–8355.

Nordling, M., S. Young, B. G. Karlsson, and L. G. Lundberg. 1990. The structural gene for cytochrome c_{551} from *Pseudomonas aeruginosa.* The nucleotide sequence shows a location downstream of the nitrite reductase. *FEBS Lett.* **259:**230–232.

Rabin, R. S., and V. Stewart. 1993. Dual response regulators (NarL and NarP) interact with dual sensors (NarX and NarQ) to control nitrate- and nitrite-regulated gene expression in *Escherichia coli* K-12. *J. Bacteriol.* **175:**3259–3268.

Saraste, M., and J. Castresana. 1994. Cytochrome oxidase evolved by tinkering with denitrification enzymes. *FEBS Lett.* **341:**1–4.

Sawers, R. G. 1991. Identification and molecular characterization of a transcriptional regulator from *Pseudomonas aeruginosa* PAO1 exhibiting structural and functional similarity to the FNR protein of *Escherichia coli. Mol. Microbiol.* **5:**1469–1481.

Silvestrini, M. C., S. Falcinelli, I. Ciabatti, F. Cutruzzolà, and M. Brunori. 1994. *Pseudomonas aeruginosa* nitrite reductase (or cytochrome oxidase): an overview. *Biochimie* **76:**641–654.

Silvestrini, M. C., C. L. Galeotti, M. Gervais, E. Schininà, D. Barra, F. Bossa, and M. Brunori. 1989. Nitrite reductase from *Pseudomonas aeruginosa:* sequence of the gene and the protein. *FEBS Lett.* **254:**33–38.

van der Oost, J., A. P. N. de Boer, J.-W. L. de Gier, W. G. Zumft, A. H. Stouthamer, and R. J. M. van Spanning. 1994. The heme-copper oxidase family consists of three distinct types of terminal oxidases and is related to nitric oxide reductase. *FEMS Microbiol. Lett.* **121:**1–10.

van Spanning, R. J. M., A. P. N. de Boer, W. N. M. Reijnders, S. Spiro, H. V. Westerhoff, A. H. Stouthamer, and J. Van der Oost. 1995. Nitrite and nitric oxide reduction in *Paracoccus denitrificans* is under the control of NNR, a regulatory protein that belongs to the FNR family of transcriptional activators. *FEBS Lett.* **360:**151–154.

Yamanaka, T., A. Ota, and K. Okunuki. 1960. Nitrite reductase activity of *Pseudomonas* cytochrome oxidase. *Biochim. Biophys. Acta* **44:**397–398.

Ye, R. W., B. A. Averill, and J. M. Tiedje. 1994. Denitrification: production and consumption of nitric oxide. *Appl. Environ. Microbiol.* **60:**1053–1058.

Ye, R. W., D. Haas, J.-O. Ka, V. Krishnapillai, A. Zimmermann, C. Baird, and J. M. Tiedje. 1995. Anaerobic activation of the entire denitrification pathway in *Pseudomonas aeruginosa* requires Anr, an analog of Fnr. *J. Bacteriol.* **177:**3606–3609.

Yokoyama, K., N. R. Hayashi, H. Arai, S.-Y. Chung, Y. Igarashi, and T. Kodama. 1995. Genes encoding RubisCO in *Pseudomonas hydrogenothermophila* are followed by a novel *cbbQ* gene similar to *nirQ* of the denitrification gene cluster from *Pseudomonas* species. *Gene* **153:**75–79.

Zennaro, E., I. Ciabatti, F. Cutruzzola, R. D'Alessandro, and M. C. Silvestrini. 1993. The nitrite reductase gene of *Pseudomonas aeruginosa:* effect of growth conditions on the expression and construction of a mutant by gene disruption. *FEMS Microbiol. Lett.* **109:**243–250.

Zimmermann, A., C. Reimmann, M. Galimand, and D. Haas. 1991. Anaerobic growth and cyanide synthesis of *Pseudomonas aeruginosa* depend on *anr*, a regulatory gene homologous with *fnr* of *Escherichia coli. Mol. Microbiol.* **5:**1483–1490.

Zumft, W. G. 1992. The denitrifying prokaryotes, p. 554–582. *In* A. Balows, H. G. Trüper, M. Dworkin, W. Harder, and K.-H. Schleifer (ed.), *The Prokaryotes. A Handbook on the Biology of Bacteria: Ecophysiology, Isolation, Identification, Applications*, 2nd ed. Springer-Verlag, New York.

Zumft, W. G. 1994. The biological role of nitric oxide in bacteria. *Arch. Microbiol.* **160:**253–264.

Zumft, W. G., C. Braun, and H. Cuypers. 1994. Nitric oxide reductase from *Pseudomonas stutzeri.* Primary structure and gene organization of a novel bacterial cytochrome *bc* complex. *Eur. J. Biochem.* **219:**481–490.

Zumft, W. G., A. Dreusch, S. Löchelt, H. Cuypers, B. Friedrich, and B. Schneider. 1992. Derived amino acid sequence of the *nosZ* gene (respiratory N_2O reductase) from *Alcaligenes eutrophus, Pseudomonas aeruginosa* and *Pseudomonas stutzeri* reveal potential copper-binding residues. Implications for the Cu_A site of N_2O reductase and cytochrome-*c* oxidase. *Eur. J. Biochem.* **208:**31–40.

Section VI

PROTEIN STRUCTURE AND ENGINEERING

Molecular Biology of Pseudomonads
Edited by T. Nakazawa et al.

Chapter 27

Three-Dimensional Structure of the 2,3-Dihydroxybiphenyl Dioxygenase (BphC Enzyme) from the Polychlorinated Biphenyl-Degrading Organism *Pseudomonas* sp. Strain KKS102

Toshiya Senda and Yukio Mitsui

Polychlorinated biphenyls (PCBs) are widely distributed environmental pollutants because of their toxicity and carcinogenicity. PCBs are strongly resistant to biodegradation because of their chemical stability. The total amount of PCBs that has been released into the biosphere is ca. 750,000 tons (1 ton = 0.907 metric tons). Some of this amount has accumulated and concentrated in the bodies of fishes, birds, and even humans. Toxic symptoms caused by PCBs include headache, pain in joints, and hypertension. Since 1973, a number of microorganisms that can degrade PCBs have been isolated and characterized (Ahmed and Focht, 1973; Furukawa and Matsumura, 1976; Furukawa and Chakrabarty, 1982; Furukawa, 1982; Bedard et al., 1986; Furukawa and Miyazaki, 1986; Bedard et al., 1987a; Bedard et al., 1987b; Kimbara et al., 1989; Fukuda, 1993).

The BphC enzyme (2,3-dihyroxybiphenyl dioxygenase), one of the key enzymes in the biodegradation pathway of PCBs, catalyzes the extradiol ring cleavage of 2,3-dihydroxybiphenyl. To date, a number of extradiol ring cleavage enzymes have been characterized in the metabolic pathways for a variety of aromatic compounds. There are several lines of evidence indicating that each of these extradiol-type dioxygenases has a ferrous [Fe(II)] iron in its active site (reviewed by Howard and Rees [1991]). The details of the catalytic mechanism of the extradiol-type dioxygenases, however, are not well understood because of a total lack of three-dimensional structural information for this type of enzyme. Several spectroscopic studies have been published (Arciero and Lipscomb, 1986; Mabrouk et al., 1991; Bertini et al., 1994; Shu et al., 1995). The crystal structure of the BphC enzyme from *Pseudomonas* sp. strain KKS102 (hereafter referred to as the KKS102 BphC enzyme or simply the BphC enzyme) has been solved by our group in close cooperation with another group at Nagaoka University of Technology led by M. Fukuda, K. Kimbara, and the late K. Yano. The structure preliminarily reported by

Toshiya Senda and Yukio Mitsui • Department of BioEngineering, Nagaoka University of Technology, Nagaoka, Niigata 940-21, Japan.

Sugiyama et al. (1995) is the first three-dimensional structure for the extradiol-type dioxygenases. This structure gave new insights into the structure-activity relationship and the catalytic mechanism of the extradiol dioxygenases.

OVERALL STRUCTURE OF THE BphC ENZYME

The KKS102 BphC enzyme is an octameric enzyme in which the eight subunits are related to each other by a 442-point group symmetry (Sugiyama et al., 1995). The enzyme as a whole is a thick-walled cylinder with a diameter of ca. 110 Å (1 Å = 0.1 nm) and a height (fourfold axis direction) of ca. 93 Å. A barrel-shaped central cavity penetrates the molecule. The inner diameter of the central cavity is ca. 25 Å at the top (and bottom) of the cylinder and ca. 25 Å at the middle of the cylinder. The octamer can be regarded as a stack of two planar rings, each composed of four subunits arranged by a fourfold rotational symmetry. A more complete description of the BphC structure has recently appeared (Senda et al., 1996).

SUBUNIT STRUCTURE

The polypeptide chain folding in the subunit of the BphC enzyme is shown in Fig. 1. The three-dimensional structure of the subunit may be described as belonging to one of the $\alpha + \beta$ folding categories as classified by Orengo and Thornton (1993). Each subunit of the BphC enzyme consists of two domains, domain 1 (N-terminal part; residues 1 to 135) and domain 2 (C-terminal part; residues 136 to 292). Each domain contains two repetitions of a unique folding motif, each consisting of ca. 55 amino acid residues (in domain 2, an additional β-strand is attached to each motif, providing an outermost β-strand). The unique folding motif may be classified as an α-sandwich structure (Orengo and Thornton, 1993) having a βαβββ motif. The βαβββ motif has so far been identified only in the struture of the bleomycin resistance protein (Dumas et al., 1994). In each domain, the first β-strand in one of such motifs and the corresponding β-strand in the

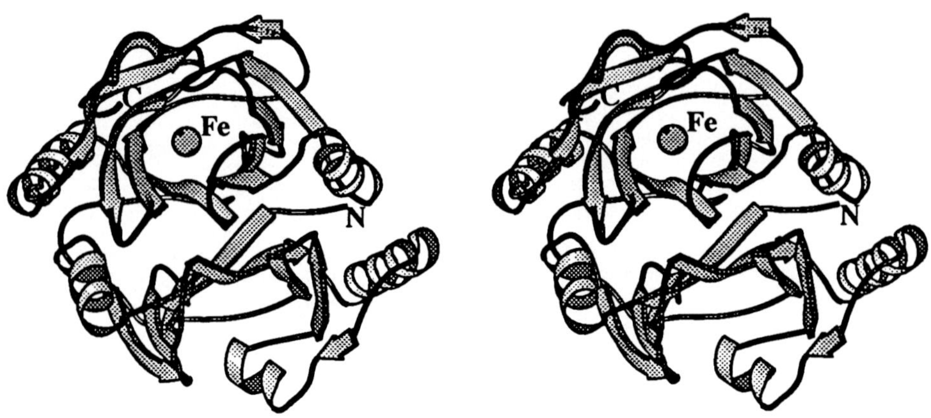

Figure 1. Schematic ribbon drawing (stereo pair) of the subunit of the BphC enzyme (Sugiyama et al., 1995). The Fe ion and the N and C termini are marked. This figure was prepared by using the program MOLSCRIPT (Kraulis, 1991).

other motif provide an intermotif interaction by forming an antiparallel β-sheet. As a result of this intermotif interaction, each domain has a β-barrel-like structure which is composed of 8 (domain 1) or 10 (domain 2) β-strands.

Least-squares fitting of the four independent βαβββ motifs in one subunit shows that these motifs are well fit except for the second β-strand and the loop region between the second and third β-strands. Amino acid sequence alignments of motifs A through D based on the three-dimensional structures of these motifs show only a weak (especially in the C-terminal part) sequence homology (7 to 21%) between any pair of the four motifs. Thus, it appears that the two-step duplication of the basic gene (corresponding to one βαβββ motif), which must have ensured similar chain folds, was a relatively old event allowing enough subsequent sequence variation.

LOCATION OF THE ACTIVE SITE

The active site of the BphC enzyme is located deep inside the barrel structure of domain 2 (the upper part of the molecule shown in Fig. 1), where the Fe ion coordinates the side chains of His-145, His-209, and Glu-260. Thus, none of the catalytic residues can be exposed to the surface of the molecule. The amino acid residues which bind the Fe ion are completely conserved among the related enzymes. In addition to these amino acid residues, two water molecules are bound to the Fe ion in the crystals of the BphC enzyme prepared without adding the substrates. For the enzymatic reaction to occur, the substrates must penetrate the barrel structure of domain 2 through some entranceway. Examining the present crystal structure, we have found a candidate for the entranceway, which is surrounded by the side chains of Ile-174, Phe-201, His-208, Tyr-249, and Thr-280. The essentially hydrophobic character of the entranceway may be important for the initial recognition of substrates which are highly hydrophobic.

THE Fe ION COORDINATION SYSTEM

For crystals of the BphC enzyme prepared by adding the substrate 2,3-dihydroxybiphenyl (2,3-DHBP) or 3-methylcatechol (3-MCT), we observed the substrate bound to the Fe ion in the active site. This happened apparently because the BphC enzyme in the crystal specimens used was in the inactive form, having a ferric (rather than ferrous, as would be expected for the active state) iron in the active site. Now that we have three-dimensional structures of the BphC enzyme complexed with its substrate (2,3-DHBP or 3-MCT), we should be able to discuss the structural origin of the substrate specificity and the reaction mechanism for the BphC and related enzymes.

The shape of the coordination polyhedron of the BphC enzyme complexed with its substrate, 2,3-DHBP, as shown in Fig. 2, may be described as a distorted trigonal bipyramid. Since the oxidation state of the Fe ion in this crystal specimen is different from that in the normal active state of the enzyme, the details of the coordination geometry may deviate slightly from the present crystal structure. However, several lines of evidence from studies on the mutated enzymes indicate that the presently observed geometry must be at least topologically valid for the active state. To determine the precise geometry of the coordination sphere of the BphC enzyme in the active state, structure determination for crystals having ferrous irons must be performed, preferably at a higher resolution.

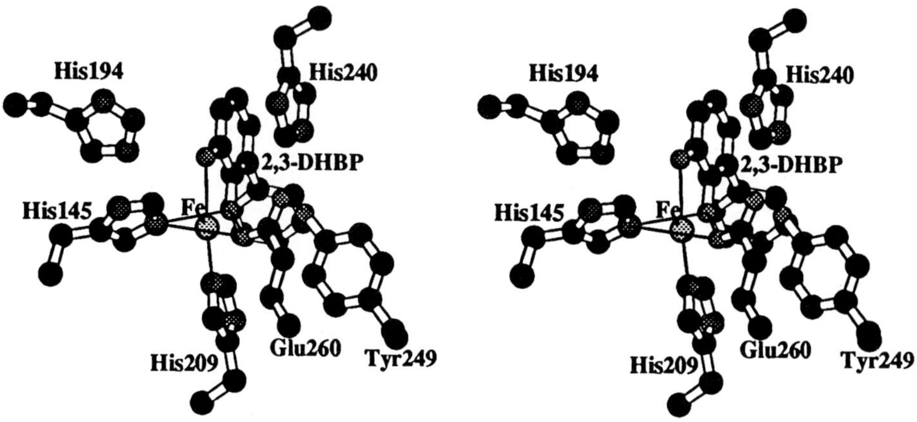

Figure 2. Schematic drawing (stereo pair) of the Fe coordination sphere found in the BphC enzyme complexed with 2,3-DHBP. This figure was prepared by using the program MOLSCRIPT (Kraulis, 1991).

ENZYME-SUBSTRATE INTERACTION

The amnio acid residues, His-194, His-240, and Tyr-249, interacting with the catechol ring of the substrate (2,3-DHBP or 3-MCT) are well conserved. Since the catechol ring moiety is always the target for the extradiol-type dioxygenases, including the BphC enzyme, these conserved residues must be important for enzymatic activities, and the catalytic mechanisms must be common to the related enzymes. The benzene ring moiety of 2,3-DHBP, on the other hand, interacts with less well conserved residues such as Ile-174, Phe-201, and Thr-280. These and other varied residues must be responsible for varied substrate specificities among the related enzymes.

OXYGEN BINDING SITE AND THE REACTION MECHANISM

Previous spectroscopic studies (Arciero et al., 1985; Arciero and Lipscomb, 1986; Mabrouk et al., 1991) suggest that in the initial stage of the reaction, first the hydroxyl groups of the substrate and then an O_2 molecule bind to the ferrous iron, resulting in the enzyme-substrate-O_2 ternary complex. On the basis of the present three-dimensional structures obtained for the crystals prepared in both the presence and the absence of the substrates, we propose a three-dimensional model for the ternary complex composed of the BphC enzyme, a substrate molecule, and an O_2 molecule as shown in Fig. 3. Considering the van de Waals radii of the atom around the Fe ion, we concluded that the oxygen-binding cavity must be located around Ala-197 and Val-147 (see the legend to Fig. 3).

On the basis of spectroscopic studies and analyses with model compounds, some reaction mechanisms for the extradiol-type dioxygenases have been proposed (Howard and Rees, 1991; Harayama et al., 1992). Initially the two hydroxyl groups of the substrate and then an O_2 molecule bind to the ferrous iron, resulting in the activation of the O_2 molecule, which, in turn, attacks the C-1 position of the catechol ring in the substrate (Fig. 3). This reaction scheme appears to be consistent with the present crystal structure

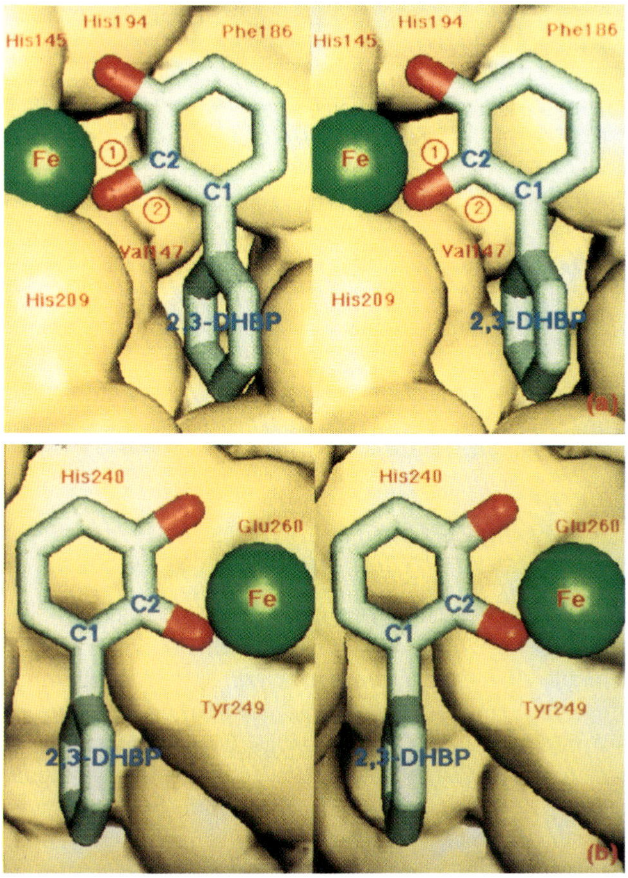

Figure 3. The van der Waals inner surface of the cavity enclosing the bound substrate, 2,3-DHBP (shown as a skeleton), is shown as a pair of half-cut nutshells (stereo pair). Panel a shows the surface behind the substrate. Proposed binding sites for the two oxygen atoms of the attacking O_2 molecule (sites 1 and 2 [circled]) are indicated. These sites are located in the oxygen-binding cavity. Note that the line connecting the two oxygen atoms is approximately parallel to the C-1 and C-2 bond of the 2,3-DHBP molecule. The surface in front of (in the sense of the view in panel a) the substrate is shown in panel b as a view 180° rotated around the in-plane vertical diad. Attack of the C-1 carbon by an oxygen atom would best be carried out from site 2, indicated in panel a. Then the benzene ring moiety of the substrate would be tilted towards the front (back in the view in panel b) surface as a result of the imposed tetrahedral configuration at the C-1 site. From the view shown in panel b, it is judged that such a benzene ring moiety would easily be accommodated in the cavity seen in the lower left. This cavity is what we named the entranceway (see text).

of the BphC enzyme complexed with its substrate in the following way. (i) The proposed orientation of the O_2 ligand (circled number in Fig. 3), which is approximately parallel to the C-1–C-2 bond of the catechol ring, is consistent with the geometries required for the reaction mechanisms proposed so far. (ii) Model-building studies show that the benzene ring, which in the intermediate step would be connected to the catechol ring through a tetrahedral carbon in position 1, can be accommodated in the enzyme active site without a large conformation change (see legend to Fig. 3). This statement assumes that the attack of the C-1 by an oxygen atom at site 2 occurs from "behind" the substrate (Fig. 3a). If, for some reason, this attack occurred from the "front" side of the substrate, statement ii would not hold.

Besides the amino acid residues that directly bind to the Fe ion (His-145, His-209, Glu-260), His-194 and Tyr-249 are also completely conserved among the related enzymes. Upon substrate binding, the imidazole ring of His-194, which may play some role in the enzymatic reaction of the extradiol-type dioxygenases, moves toward the hydroxyl group of the catechol ring. The phenol ring of Tyr-249, on the other hand, is located opposite the imidazole ring of His-194 with respect to the catechol ring of the substrate (Fig. 2). The hydroxyl group of Tyr-249 is located close to the active center (the Oη atom being ca. 4 Å from the Fe ion). This fact might show that the hydroxyl group of Tyr-249 also plays some role in the enzymatic reaction.

DIFFERENCE BETWEEN THE STRUCTURES OF THE INTRA- AND EXTRADIOL DIOXYGENASES

Two types of dioxygenases, intradiol and extradiol, have been known to be engaged in aromatic ring cleavage reactions. However, the amino acid sequences of the two types of enzymes are completely different from each other. Moreover, certain multigene modifications exist among the extradiol-type dioxygenases. The crystal structure of an intradiol-type dioxygenase (protocatechuate 3,4-dioxygenase from *Pseudomonas aeruginosa*, hereafter referred to as the 3,4-PCD enzyme) has been determined (Ohlendorf et al., 1988; Ohlendorf et al., 1994). Comparing this structure with the present structure, we find that they are completely unrelated to each other not only with respect to amino acid sequence but also with respect to subunit composition and the polypeptide chain folding found in each subunit. Thus, the 3,4-PCD enzyme (an intradiol-type dioxygenase) contains 12 subunits composed of six α- and six β-subunits with similar but distinct patterns of chain folding, while the BphC enzyme (an extradiol-type dioxygenase) is composed of eight identical subunits. The pattern of the polypeptide chain folding found in the subunit of the BphC enzyme is completely different from either that found in the α-subunit or that found in the β-subunit of the 3,4-PCD enzyme. It has been known that the intradiol-type dioxygenases (e.g., the 3,4-PCD enzyme) require a ferric iron for enzymatic activity, while the extradiol-type dioxygenases (e.g., the BphC enzyme) require a ferrous iron for activity (reviewed by Howard and Rees [1991]). Despite these differences, the coordination system around the Fe ion found in the BphC enzyme and that found in the 3,4-PCD enzyme exhibit considerable geometric and electrostatic similarity.

In the crystal structure of the 3,4-PCD enzyme, two His residues (His-460 and His-462), two Tyr residues (Tyr-408 and Tyr-447), and one water molecule were found to bind to the ferric iron (Ohlendorf et al., 1994). The shape of the coordination polyhedron is approximately that of a trigonal bipyramid (Ohlendorf et al., 1994), similar to that found in the BphC-substrate complexes. Surprisingly, the two trigonal bipyramids found in the 3,4-PCD and BphC enzymes can be superimposed with the root-mean-square deviation of only 0.39 Å. It is surprising that they perform quite different types of ring cleavage reactions despite such similarity in coordination geometry.

Ohlendorf et al. (1994) suggested that in the course of the reaction catalyzed by the 3,4-PCD enzyme, the two Fe ligands, one a hydroxyl group (probably from Tyr-447) and the other a water molecule, might be replaced by the two hydroxyl groups of the substrate molecule. If this is the case, the Fe coordination geometry in the substrate-bound 3,4-PCD enzyme may be similar to that found in the present structure of the substrate-bound BphC enzyme. Despite the overall similarity in Fe coordination geometry, there do exist two important differences, which must be responsible for the difference in the types of enzymatic reactions catalyzed by the two enzymes. First, the oxidation states of the Fe ions are different: a ferric iron must be present in the 3,4-PCD enzyme, while a ferrous iron must be present in the BphC enzyme. Second, in the trigonal bipyramidal Fe coordination sphere, four ligands (two imidazole nitrogens and two hydroxyl groups of the substrates) are common to the two types of enzymes, while the remaining ligand is different (a carboxylate group [Glu-260] in the BphC enzyme and a hydroxyl group [Tyr-408] in the 3/4-PCD enzyme).

In the present crystals of the BphC enzyme prepared by adding the substrates, the substrates were found intact in the active site presumably because the Fe ion was in a ferric form, as indicated by electron spin resonance studies (M. Sato, unpublished data). This means that the extradiol-type dioxygenases, despite being quite similar in overall coordination geometry, cannot have intradiol-type ring-cleaving activity even if the Fe ion is oxidized to the ferric state. As mentioned above, the only conspicuous difference in the Fe coordination sphere between the oxidized BphC and 3,4-PCD enzymes is the difference in one amino acid ligand bound to the ferric iron. Therefore the difference in pK_a values between the side chains of Tyr-408 in the 3,4-PCD enzyme and Glu-260 in the BphC enzyme might be mainly responsible for the fact that the oxidized BphC enzyme does not have an intradiol-type ring-cleaving activity. It has been proposed that the intradiol-type dioxygenases activate the bound substrate, while the extradiol-type dioxygenases activate the dioxygen bound to the ferrous iron (Howard and Rees, 1991). The higher pK_a value of the hydroxyl group of Tyr as an Fe ligand might be favorable for the activation of the substrate in the intradiol-type dioxygenase. On the other hand, the lower pK_a value of the carboxyl group of Glu-260 as an Fe ligand might be favorable for the activation of the dioxygen which is required to attack the C-1 position of the catechol ring of the substrate. It should be noticed that the amino acid residue corresponding to Glu-260 of the BphC enzyme is completely conserved among the related extradiol-type dioxygenases.

Acknowledgments. We thank T. Nonaka of our group for discussions related to crystallography. We also thank K. Kobayashi, of Nagaoka University of Technology, for stimulating discussions on the reaction mechanism of the BphC enzyme.

REFERENCES

Ahmed, M., and D. D. Focht. 1973. Degradation of polychlorinated biphenyls by two species of *Achromobacter*. *Can. J. Microbiol.* **19:**47–52.

Arciero, D. M., and J. D. Lipscomb. 1986. Binding of ^{17}O-labeled substrate and inhibitors to protocatechuate 4,5-dioxygenase-nitrosyl complex. *J. Biol. Chem.* **261:**2170–2178.

Arciero, D. M., A. M. Orville, and J. D. Lipscomb. 1985. [^{17}O]water and nitric oxide binding by protocatechuate 4,5-dioxygenase and catechol 2,3-dioxygenase. *J. Biol. Chem.* **260:**14035–14044.

Bedard, D. L., M. L. Haberl, R. J. May, and M. J. Brennan. 1987a. Evidence for novel mechanisms of polychlorinated biphenyl metabolism in *Alcaligenes eutrophus* H850. *Appl. Environ. Microbiol.* **53:**1103–1112.

Bedard, D. L., R. Unterman, L. H. Bopp, M. J. Brennan, M. L. Haberl, and C. Johnson. 1986. Rapid assay for screening and characterizing microorganisms for the ability to degrade polychlorinated biphenyls. *Appl. Environ. Microbiol.* **51:**761–768.

Bedard, D. L., R. E. Wagner, M. J. Brennan, M. L. Haberl, and J. F. Brown, Jr. 1987b. Extensive degradation of Aroclors and environmentally transformed polychlorinated biphenyls by *Alcaligenes eutrophus* H850. *Appl. Environ. Microbiol.* **53:**1094–1102.

Bertini, I., F. Briganti, S. Mangani, H. F. Nolting, and A. Scozzafava. 1994. X-ray absorption studies on catechol 2,3-dioxygenase from *Pseudomonas putida* mt-2. *Biochemistry* **33:**10777–10784.

Dumas, P., M. Bergdoll, C. Cagnon, and M.-M. Masson. 1994. Crystal structure and site-directed mutagenesis of a bleomycin resistance protein and their significance for drug sequestering. *EMBO J.* **13:**2483–2492.

Fukuda, M. 1993. Diversity of chloroaromatic oxygenases. *Curr. Opin. Biotechnol.* **4:**339–343.

Furukawa, K. 1982. Microbial degradation of polychlorinated biphenyls, p. 33–57. *In* A. M. Chakrabarty (ed.), *Biodegradation and Detoxification of Environmental Pollutants.* CRC Press, Inc., Boca Raton, Fla.

Furukawa, K., and A. M. Chakrabarty. 1982. Involvement of plasmids in total degradation of chlorinated biphenyls. *Appl. Environ. Microbiol.* **44:**619–626.

Furukawa, K., and F. Matsumura. 1976. Microbial metabolism of polychlorinated biphenyls. Studies on the relative degradability of polychlorinated biphenyl components by *Alcaligenes* sp. *J. Agric. Food Chem.* **42:**543–548.

Furukawa, K., and T. Miyazaki. 1986. Cloning of a gene cluster encoding biphenyl and chlorobiphenyl degradation in *Pseudomonas pseudoalcaligenes. J. Bacteriol.* **166:**392–398.

Harayama, S., M. Kok, and E. L. Neidle. 1992. Functional and evolutionary relationships among diverse oxygenases. *Annu. Rev. Microbiol.* **46:**565–601.

Howard, J. B., and D. C. Rees. 1991. Perspectives on non-heme iron protein chemistry. *Adv. Protein Chem.* **42:**199–280.

Kimbara, K., T. Hashimoto, M. Fukuda, T. Koana, M. Takagi, M. Oishi, and K. Yano. 1989. Cloning and sequencing of two tandem genes involved in degradation of 2,3-dihydroxybiphenyl to benzoic acid in the polychlorinated biphenyl-degrading soil bacterium *Pseudomonas* sp. strain KKS102. *J. Bacteriol.* **171:**2740–2747.

Kraulis, P. J. 1991. MOLSCRIPT: a program to produce both detailed and schematic plots of protein structures. *J. Appl. Crystallogr.* **24:**946–950.

Mabrouk, P. A., A. M. Orville, J. D. Lipscomb, and E. I. Solomon. 1991. Variable-temperature variable-field magnetic circular dichroism studies of the Fe(II) active site in metapyrocatechuase: implications for the molecular mechanism of extradiol dioxygenase. *J. Am. Chem. Soc.* **113:**4053–4061.

Ohlendorf, D. H., A. M. Orville, and J. D. Lipscomb. 1994. Structure of protocatechuate 3,4-dioxygenase from *Pseudomonas aeruginosa* at 2.15 Å resolution. *J. Mol. Biol.* **244:**586–608.

Ohlendorf, D. H., A. M. Orville, and P. C. Weber. 1988. Structure and assembly of protocatechuate 3,4-dioxygenase. *Nature* (London) **336:**403–405.

Orengo, C. A., and J. M. Thornton. 1993. Alpha plus beta folds revisited: some favoured motifs. *Structure* **1:**105–120.

Senda, T., K. Sugiyama, H. Narita, T. Yamamoto, K. Kimbara, M. Fukuda, M. Sato, K. Yano, and Y. Mitsui. 1996. Three-dimensional structures of free form and two substrate complexes of an extradiol ring-cleavage type dioxygenase, the BphC enzyme from *Pseudomonas* sp. strain KKS102. *J. Mol. Biol.* **255:**735–752.

Shu, L., Y.-M. Chiou, A. M. Orville, M. A. Miller, J. D. Lipscomb, and L. Que, Jr. 1995. X-ray absorption spectroscopic studies of the Fe(II) active site of catechol 2,3-dioxygenase. Implications for the extradiol cleavage mechanism. *Biochemistry* **34:**6649–6659.

Sugiyama, K., T. Senda, H. Narita, T. Yamamoto, K. Kimbara, M. Fukuda, K. Yano, and Y. Mitsui. 1995. Three-dimensional structure of 2,3-dihydroxybiphenyl dioxygenase (BphC enzyme) from *Pseudomonas* sp. strain KKS102 having polychlorinated biphenyl (PCB)-degrading activity. *Proc. Jpn. Acad.* **71B:**32–35.

Molecular Biology of Pseudomonads
Edited by T. Nakazawa et al.

Chapter 28

Lipase of *Pseudomonas aeruginosa*: Molecular Biology and Biotechnological Application

Karl-Erich Jaeger, Bernd Schneidinger, Klaus Liebeton, Dieter Haas, Manfred T. Reetz, Statis Philippou, Gijs Gerritse, Stéphane Ransac, and Bauke W. Dijkstra

Pseudomonas aeruginosa is thought to be the most numerous organism on earth (Costerton and Anwar, 1994), and one of its intriguing properties is the potential to synthesize and secrete a variety of extracellular products. Among them are at least 10 different enzymes, 3 of which are lipolytic: a hemolytic and a nonhemolytic phospholipase C and a lipase (EC 3.1.1.3). The phospholipases C have been studied in great detail both biochemically and with respect to their regulation (Vasil et al., 1990; Vasil et al., 1994). Present knowledge about *P. aeruginosa* lipase has been described in recent review articles (Gilbert, 1993; Jaeger et al., 1994). Here, we summarize mainly the results of our own work, which started with purification and biochemical characterization of the lipase from *P. aeruginosa* PAC1R (Stuer et al., 1986). In parallel, the lipase gene from *P. aeruginosa* PAO1 was cloned, sequenced (Wohlfarth et al., 1992), and overexpressed (Jaeger et al., 1993b). In the meantime, we have shown by comparison of biochemical properties and Western blotting (immunoblotting) that the lipases of *P. aeruginosa* PAC1R and PAO1 are probably identical. We built a three-dimensional (3D) structural model, which now serves as a basis for identifying functionally important amino acids. Recently, we have begun to understand the regulation of lipase gene expression. An applied aspect of our work concerns the biotechnological potential of *P. aeruginosa* lipase to catalyze a variety of important reactions in organic chemistry.

Karl-Erich Jaeger, Bernd Schneidinger, and Klaus Liebeton • Lehrstuhl Biologie der Mikroorganismen, Ruhr-Universtität, D-44780 Bochum, Germany. ***Dieter Haas*** • Laboratoire de Biologie Microbienne, Université de Lausanne, CH-1015 Lausanne, Switzerland. ***Manfred T. Reetz*** • Max-Planck Institut für Kohlenforschung, D-45470 Mülheim, Germany. ***Statis Philippou*** • Institut für Pathologie, Ruhr-Universität, D-44780 Bochum, Germany. ***Gijs Gerritse*** • Genencor, NL-2600 MA Delft, The Netherlands. ***Stéphane Ransac and Bauke W. Dijkstra*** • Laboratory of Biophysical Chemistry, NL-9747 AG Groningen, The Netherlands.

BIOCHEMISTRY

P. aeruginosa lipase is an M_r-29,000 protein which has been purified from culture supernatants by analytical isoelectric focusing (Stuer et al., 1986). Table 1 shows some relevant biochemical properties, including the comparably high specific activity against both monoacylester (*para*-nitrophenylpalmitate) and triglygeride (trioleoylglycerol) substrates. A remarkable feature of this enzyme is its close association with lipopolysaccharide (LPS), which gives rise to large aggregates of M_r 0.1×10^6 to 1×10^6 (Jaeger et al., 1991a). Recently, we have developed a preparative purification protocol allowing us to prepare about 80 mg of purified lipase, which is now used for crystallization (Misset et al., 1994).

P. aeruginosa lipase, like most bacterial lipases, has a broad substrate specificity accepting triglyceride substrates with fatty acyl chain lengths varying for C_6 to C_{18}. However, this particular lipase proved to be 100% stereoselective for position *sn*-1 of the substrate trioctanoin (Rogalska et al., 1993). This result was recently confirmed by measurement of the hydrolysis of both the racemic and the chiral triglyceride substrates 1-butyroyl-2-stearoyl-3-palmitoyl-*sn*-glycerol, which clearly indicated the stereospecific hydrolysis of the *sn*-1 position of the triglyceride (Fig. 1) by *P. aeruginosa* lipase (Villeneuve et al., 1995).

MOLECULAR BIOLOGY AND SECRETION

Two genes, *lipA* and *lif* (formerly named *lipH*), are needed to obtain enzymatically active lipase. They presumably form a bicistronic operon. The structural gene *lipA* encodes the lipase (285 amino acids; M_r, 30,139). The two-component T7 expression system (Brunschwig and Darzins, 1992) was used to clone the lipase operon into plasmid

Table 1. Biochemical properties of *P. aeruginosa* lipase

Property	Value or description	Reference
No. of subunits	1	Stuer et al., 1986
No. of amino acids	285	Wohlfarth et al., 1992
Mol wt		
Sodium dodecyl sulfate-polyacrylamide gel electrophoresis	29,000	Stuer et al., 1986
DNA sequence	30,139	Wohlfarth et al., 1992
Isoelectric point	5.9	Stuer et al., 1986
pH optimum	8.0	Stuer et al., 1986
Disulfide bridge	1	Jaeger et al., 1993a
Sp act (U/mg)[a]		
p-Nitrophenylpalmitate	45,600	Misset et al., 1994
Triolein	22,800	Misset et al., 1994
Fatty acid chain length specificity[b]	Unspecific	Jaeger et al., 1991b
Stereoselectivity[c]	*sn*-1 in triglycerides	Rogalska et al., 1993 Villeneuve et al., 1995

[a]One unit corresponds to 1 μmol of fatty acid released from substrate per min.

[b]Determined with *p*-nitrophenyl esters of various-chain-length fatty acids as substrates.

[c]Determined with substrates trioctanoin and 1-butyroyl-2-stearoyl-3-palmitoyl *sn*-glycerol.

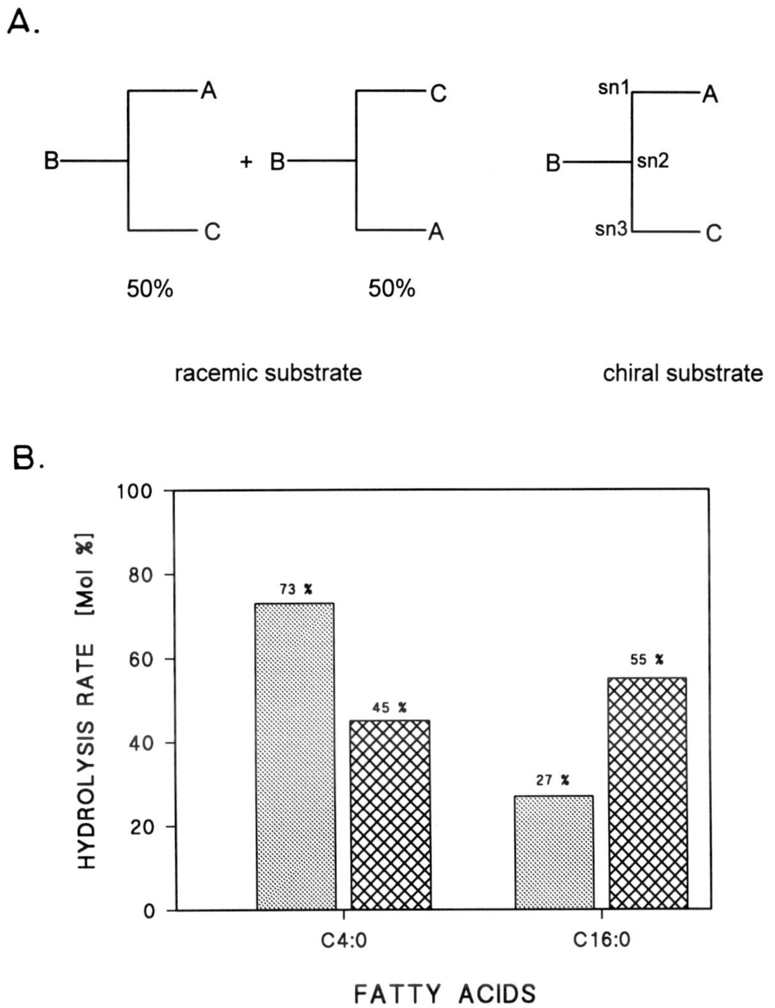

Figure 1. Stereospecificity of *P. aeruginosa* lipase (Villeneuve et al., 1995). (A) The substrates were a racemic mixture of 1-*A* 2-*B* 3-*C* and 1-*C* 2-*B* 3-*A* *sn*-glycerol and chiral substrate 1-*A* 2-*B* 3-*C* *sn*-glycerol with the substituents butyric acid (A), stearic acid (B), and palmitic acid (C) (BSP). (B) The amount of fatty acids released from the substrate after 30 s of incubation with *P. aeruginosa* lipase was determined with gas chromatography coupled to mass spectrometry. Shaded bars, chiral BSP; cross-hatched bars, racemic BSP.

pEB12 and overexpress it in *P. aeruginosa* ADD1976. Extracellular lipase was produced by strain ADD1976 at 0.02 µg/ml and by the overexpressing strain at 200 µg/ml (Jaeger et al., 1993b).

A unique feature of *Pseudomonas* lipases belonging to homology groups I and II is the requirement for a lipase-specific foldase protein, Lif. In *P. aeruginosa*, the *lif* gene product has 340 amino acids (M_r, 37,500), and the gene is located 49 nucleotides downstream of the lipase structural gene (for a review of different *lipA-lif* systems in *Pseudomonas* spp., see Jaeger et al., 1994). It appears that Lif is anchored to the cytoplasmic membrane via its hydrophobic N-terminal part. Recently, Lif proteins from *Burkholderia cepacia* (formerly, *Pseudomonas cepacia*) (Amand et al., 1994), *P. aeruginosa* (Schneidinger and Jaeger, 1994), and *Pseudomonas* sp. strain 109 (Ihara et al., 1995) were cloned in separate expression vectors and expressed independently in *Escherichia coli*, and their interactions with lipase were studied. In the case of *B. cepacia*, a 1:1 complex between prelipase and Lif protein was needed to ensure correct processing, folding, and secretion of lipase into the periplasm. A Lip/Lif ratio of 1:4 was found to be optimal for renaturation of urea-denatured lipase in *Pseudomonas* sp. strain 109. These results and those obtained with *P. aeruginosa* Lif further demonstrated that a truncated form of the Lif protein lacking its hydrophobic N-terminal part was still able to support in vitro renaturation of denatured lipase protein, although the recovered enzyme activity was less than 10% of the original activity (Amand et al., 1994).

P. aeruginosa lipase is secreted into the medium via an *xcp*-mediated secretion system which is composed of at least 12 different gene products (Tommassen et al., 1992; Lazdunski et al., this volume). Experimental evidence supporting an involvement of this so-called general secretion pathway in lipase export is as follows: (i) the presence of a 26-amino-acid signal sequence in prelipase, (ii) the occurrence of periplasmic intermediates during secretion, and (iii) the complete absence of any extracellular lipase in a *P. aeruginosa pilD* (=*xcpA*) mutant (K.-E. Jaeger and S. Lory, unpublished data). A simplified schematic presentation of the secretion mechanism for *P. aeruginosa* lipase is shown in Fig. 2A. After being translocated through the cytoplasmic membrane by means of the *sec* system, lipase makes contact with the Lif protein. The next step is the Lif-assisted folding in the periplasm, including the correct formation of the disulfide bond which is present in *Pseudomonas* group I and II lipases containing two cysteine residues. At present, there is no direct experimental evidence for an involvement of disulfide oxidoreductases analogous to DsbA, DsbB, and DsbC of *E. coli* (Bardwell, 1994). A *P. aeruginosa* strain presumed to be mutated in a *dsbB*-analogous gene (Hoang and Schweizer, 1995) showed no alteration in lipase activity compared with the wild-type strain *P. aeruginosa* PAO1 (K.-E. Jaeger and H. P. Schweizer, unpublished data). However, in the case of *Acinetobacter calcoaceticus* lipase, a periplasmic disulfide oxidoreductase termed PdoA is required to obtain enzymatically active lipase (Kok et al., 1995). The last step of the secretion process is the translocation of lipase through the outer membrane, which may be mediated by the XcpQ protein. It is interesting that at least part of the lipase always remains bound to the bacterial cell (Fig. 2B), presumably entrapped in a matrix composed mainly of LPS. The ratio of cell-bound to extracellular lipase varies: if *P aeruginosa* is grown at 30°C in nutrient broth medium in an Erlenmeyer flask with shaking, a ratio of 10% bound to 90% free lipase is observed, whereas growth in a fermentor in a minimal salts medium supplied with a triglyceride may give the inverse ratio of 90% bound to 10% free lipase.

The folding and secretion of *P. aeruginosa* lipase is a complex and possibly highly regulated process which requires the presence of at least 20 different functionally active gene products (Sec, Xcp, signal peptidase, foldase, and probably disulfide oxidoreductase). This fact provides an explanation for the difficulties encountered by many investigators in obtaining enzymatically active lipase protein by overexpression of the *lipA* and *lif* genes in heterologous hosts.

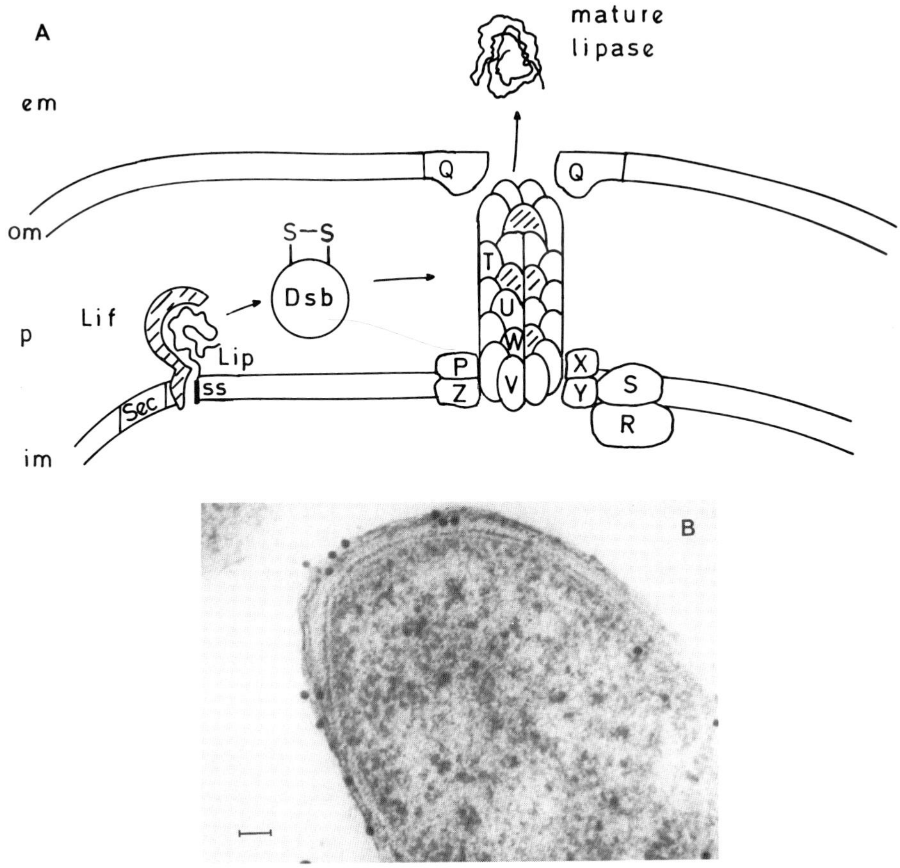

Figure 2. (A) Model for the *P. aeruginosa* lipase secretion pathway. Lipase (Lip) is secreted as prelipase through the bacterial inner membrane (im) by a *sec*-dependent mechanism which removes the signal sequence (ss). Interaction with the lipase-specific foldase (Lif) assists folding in the periplasm (p). A hypothetical disulfide oxidoreductase (Dsb) catalyzes the correct formation of the disulfide bond. Lipase is finally secreted through the outer membrane (om) to reach the extracellular medium (em). Components of the secretion machinery (XcpQ-T-U-V-W-P-X-Y, and -Z and Sec) are drawn as described elsewhere (Mattick and Alm, 1995; Lazdunski et al., this volume); the location and function of the Lif protein are as proposed for *B. glumae* LipB (Frenken et al., 1993). (B) Localization of *P. aeruginosa* lipase by immunoelectron microscopy. Stationary-phase cells were fixed with glutaraldehyde and embedded with LR white. Ultrathin sections were treated with antilipase antiserum and a colloidal gold-labeled second antibody (particle diameter; 10 nm) and examined with a Zeiss IM 900 transmission electron microscope (magnification, ×115,000; bar, 40 nm).

REGULATION

A variety of conditions stimulate or repress the synthesis and secretion of *P. aeruginosa* lipase. Triglycerides and detergents act as inducers, whereas long-chain fatty acids repress lipase production (Gilbert et al., 1991). In our laboratory, *P. aeruginosa* was grown in a 1-liter dialysis fermentor; extracellular lipase production was determined, and temperature, pH, conductivity, redox potential, and the concentrations of O_2, K^+, Mg^{2+}, and Ca^{2+} were continuously recorded. We observed that the release of extracellular lipase began when the redox potential decreased from +80 mV to −25mV, the O_2 concentration decreased from 8 to 4 mg/ml, and, interestingly, the concentration of Mg^{2+} ions sharply decreased from 1.3 μg/ml to zero (Koch, 1990). This Mg^{2+} effect, which was also observed in shake cultures grown in Erlenmeyer flasks, may be explained by the need of Mg^{2+} ions to stabilize lipase-LPS complexes as soon as they appear in the bacterial outer membrane.

The concentration of iron (Fe^{3+}) is known to influence the yield of different extracellular enzymes in *P. aeruginosa* (Bjorn et al., 1979). Extracellular lipase production was repressed in the presence of 50 μmol of Fe^{3+}, whereas depletion in the growth medium of Fe^{3+} [e.g., by addition of the iron chelator ethylenediamine-di(*o*-hydroxyphenylacetic acid)] resulted in a 10-fold increase in extracellular lipase activity. Gel shift assays using the iron-regulated Fur protein of *P. aeruginosa* (Prince et al., 1993) demonstrated that Fur did not bind to the DNA region upstream of the lipase structural gene, indicating that the lipase gene is not directly regulated by Fur (U. A. Ochsner, M. L. Vasil, and K.-E. Jaeger, unpublished data).

A search for regulatory sequences preceding the translational start site of the lipase structural gene revealed the presence of an RpoN consensus sequence at nucleotide positions −108 to −92 with respect to the translational start site (Fig. 3), with the invariant GG and GC dinucleotides separated by 10 nucleotides (Merrick, 1993). *P. aeruginosa* PAK-N1 carrying a tetracycline cassette inside the *rpoN* structural gene (Totten et al., 1990) did not produce any extracellular lipase, and a translational *lipA-lacZ* fusion showed no β-galactosidase activity when harbored by this *rpoN* mutant strain (Schneidinger et al., in preparation). We conclude that transcription of the *P. aeruginosa* lipase gene requires an RNA polymerase holoenzyme containing the alternative sigma factor RpoN (σ^{54}).

```
PpuxylS    T G G C G T T A T T T T T G C T
           | | | |                 | | | |
PpuxylCAB  T G G C A T G G C G G T T G C T
           | | |   |               | | | |
Ppucss     T G G A A C A G A T T T T G C T
           | | |   |               | | | |
Pspcpg2    T G G C A C T C G A A T T G C T
           | | | | |               | | | |
PaepilA    T G G C A T G G T A A G T G C T
           | | | | |               | | |
PaelipA    T G G C A C G G T T C C T G C G

                     C
Consensus  T G G C A   N g N N N t T G C T
                     T
```

Figure 3. Consensus DNA sequence recognized by the alternative sigma factor RpoN. Promoter sequences of RpoN-regulated genes *xylS, xylCAB*, and *css* from *Pseudomonas putida* (PpuxylS, PpuxylCAB, and Ppucss) (Deretic et al., 1989; Kim et al., 1995), *cpg*-2 of *Pseudomonas* sp. (Pspcpg2) (Minton and Clarke, 1985), and *pilA* of *P. aeruginosa* (PaepilA) (Nunn et al., 1990) were aligned with the sequence upstream of the *lipA* gene of *P. aeruginosa* (PaelipA).

Cell-to-cell communication by low-molecular-weight *N*-acyl-homoserine lactones termed autoinducers is a mechanism known to regulate the expression of extracellular protease genes in *P. aeruginosa* (Passador et al., 1993). The transcriptional activator LasR and the LasI protein directing the synthesis of *N*-oxododecanoyl-homoserine lactone are involved in the production of elastase and alkaline protease. At present, at least two additional autoinducer molecules and a second regulator/inducer (R/I)-type system (VsmR/I equivalent to RhlR/I) have been identified in *P. aeruginosa* (Pearson et al., 1994; Pearson et al., 1995; Salmond et al., 1995; Latifi et al., 1995; Williams et al., this volume). In a wide variety of bacterial species, similar regulatory circuits involving different R/I-type proteins and autoinducer molecules regulate a number of discrete metabolic processes in a cell density-dependent manner (for a review, see Salmond et al., 1995). We examined *P. aeruginosa* strains carrying mutations in the transcriptional activators LasR1 (Passador et al., 1993) and RhlR (Ochsner et al., 1994) and a strain impaired in autoinducer synthesis (Latifi et al., 1995) and observed that the activity of extracellular lipase was either significantly lower than in the wild-type strains or absent. To determine lipase gene expression, we measured β-galactosidase activities of a translational *lipA-lacZ* fusion in these mutants (Schneidinger et al., in preparation). In the *P. aeruginosa* mutant PANO67, the expression level of the *lipA-lacZ* fusion was low. Strain PANO67 is defective in the synthesis of two autoinducers, *N*-butanoyl-homoserine lactone and *N*-hexanoyl-homoserine lactone, and can be complemented partially by the cloned *vsmR/I* genes. However, the mutational defect of this strain is unknown (Latifi et al., 1995; Williams et al., this volume). Figure 4 shows a model for the regulation of the lipase operon in *P. aeruginosa*. The iron-Fur and autoinducer VsmR complexes might exert their regulatory effects by regulating the expression of a hypothetical regulator protein termed LipR, which, presumably in concert with RpoN, might then bind to a regulatory region upstream of the lipase operon.

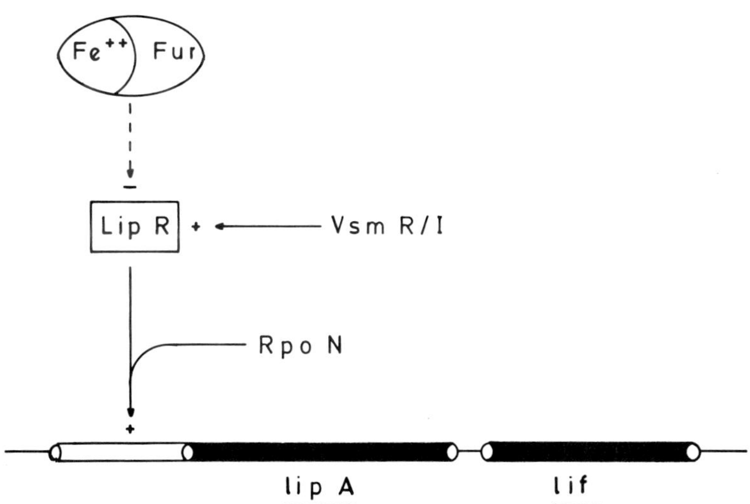

Figure 4. Putative regulating network controlling expression of the lipase gene *lipA* in *P. aeruginosa* (see text for details).

3D STRUCTURAL MODEL

A 3D structural model for *P. aeruginosa* lipase was constructed on the basis of the alignment of 50-amino-acid sequences of lipases and other hydrolases and coordinates of experimentally determined X-ray structures of different lipases (Jaeger et al., 1993a). During this work, the first X-ray structure of a bacterial lipase, that of *B. glumae* (formerly *Pseudomonas glumae*), was reported (Noble et al., 1993). We have used the coordinates of this structure to refine our model (Misset et al., 1994), which is shown in Fig. 5A. The characteristic features include a core structure of seven central β-strands, one of them antiparallel, and a catalytic triad consisting of amino acid residues S-82, D-229, and H-251. Close to the active site is bound a Ca^{2+} ion, which is stabilized by cooperative binding to residues D-209 and D-253 and to main chain oxygens O-257 and O-261. One disulfide bridge is formed between residues C-183 and C-235. An α-helix extending from S-132 to L-145 which could serve as a possible lid covering the active site is marked in yellow (top of Fig. 5A). Previously, without any structural information, we had predicted the presence of both a hydrophobic and a hydrophilic part on the surface of *P. aeruginosa* lipase to account for the interaction with amphipathic LPS molecules (Jaeger et al., 1991b; Jaeger et al., 1992). The 3D structural model reveals the existence of two

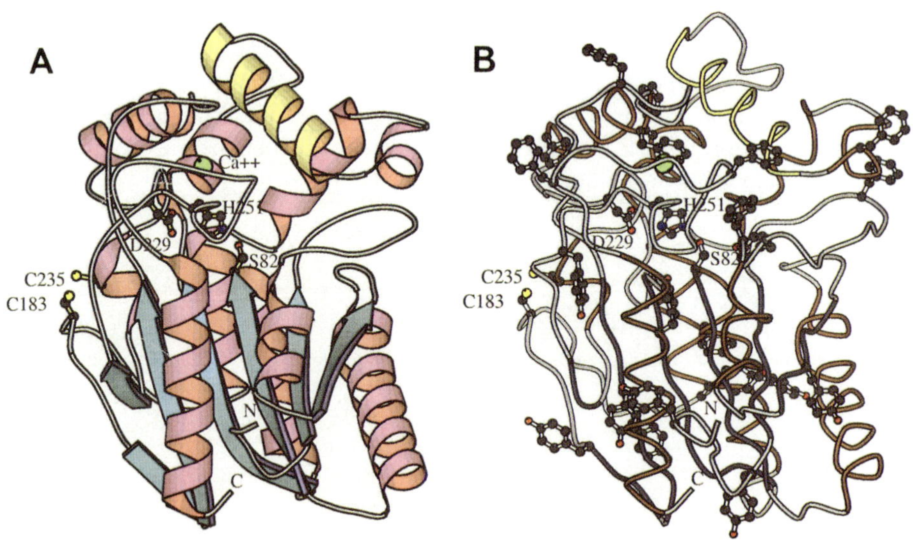

Figure 5. Structural model of *P. aeruginosa* lipase. (A) Ribbon plot drawn with MOLSCRIPT (Kraulis, 1991). The catalytic triad residues S-82, D-229, and H-251 and residues C-183 and C-235 forming a disulfide bond are numbered and drawn in a ball-and-stick presentation. The Ca^{2+} ion is shown as a green ball, and the α-helix presumed to represent a lid covering the active site is shown in yellow. Amino (N) and carboxy (C) termini of the lipase are indicated. (B) C_α backbone with the catalytic triad, C residues, and lid numbered and labeled as in panel A. Nine F residues representing the hydrophobic upper domain and 11 Y-residues forming the hydrophilic lower domain of the lipase are shown in a ball-and-stick presentation, with the red balls indicating the hydroxyl-oxygen atoms of tyrosines.

clearly distinguishable domains: a hydrophilic one characterized by 11 surface-exposed tyrosine residues (Fig. 5B, bottom) and a hydrophobic domain with 9 surface-exposed phenylalanine residues (Fig. 5B, top).

BIOTECHNOLOGICAL APPLICATION

Lipases represent a biotechnologically important class of enzymes. Their broad substrate specificity and high enantioselectivity enable chemists to produce enantiomerically pure compounds to be used as starting materials for the synthesis of a variety of pharmaceuticals and agrochemicals (Vulfson, 1994). *P. aeruginosa* lipase has proved to be stereospecific for position *sn*-1 in triglyceride substrates (see Biochemistry, above), suggesting that it could be useful for enantioselective hydrolysis reactions.

Immobilization in hydrophobic sol-gel-derived silica matrices stabilizes lipases (Reetz et al., 1995). In a matrix consisting of propyltrimethoxysilane and tetramethoxysilane in a ratio of 5:1, *P. aeruginosa* lipase retained its ability to catalyze the esterification of lauric acid with 1-octanol in *iso*-octane. The immobilized enzyme preparation (as well as free enzyme) was used for enantioselective acetylation of chiral amines with acetic acid ethyl ester as the acylating agent (Fig. 6A), and the kinetic resolutions resulted in an 87 to 95% enantiomeric excess of the acyl amide (Fig. 6B). At present, we are optimizing the reaction conditions for kinetic resolution of amines and testing the potential of the lipase to selectively acetylate *meso*-dialcohols (Jaeger et al., in preparation).

A.

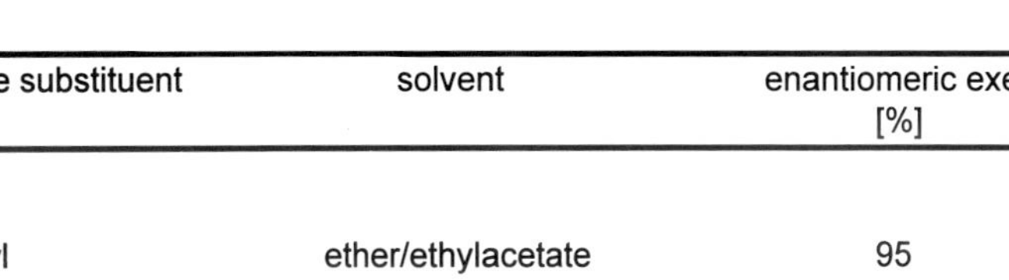

B.

amine substituent [R]	solvent	enantiomeric exess [%]
pentyl	ether/ethylacetate	95
pentyl	ethylacetate	90
phenylethyl	ethylacetate	87

Figure 6. Kinetic resolution of racemic amines with *P. aeruginosa* lipase. (A) Reaction scheme. (B) Enantiomeric excess of different primary amines. AcOEt, acetic acid ethyl ester; Et_2O, diethyl ether.

CONCLUSION

The present state of knowledge of molecular biology, regulation of gene expression, and structure of *P. aeruginosa* lipase allows (i) overexpression and large-scale purification of the enzyme, (ii) use of the enzyme for biotechnological applications, and (iii) the rational modification of its primary structure with respect to desired biochemical properties. However, there are still many questions to be answered, and the simplest one is probably the most important: What is the physiological role of lipase for *P. aeruginosa* cells? Continuing studies will be needed to understand why the bacterial cells use such a remarkable regulatory network to control the expression of a simple enzyme protein.

Acknowledgments. This work was supported by the European Commission under contract BIOT-CT91-272 as part of the BRIDGE T project on lipases. K.-E.J. expresses his gratitude to Robert Verger and to Stephen Lory for their continuous support and encouragement. We thank Barbara Iglewski, Andrée Lazdunski, Urs Ochsner, and Paul Williams for generously supplying strains and plasmids; Pierre Villeneuve for permission to prepare Fig. 1; and Dietmar Lang for help in preparing Fig. 5.

REFERENCES

Amand, J. L., A. H. Hobson, C. M. Buckley, S. T. Jørgensen, B. Diderichsen, and D. J. McConnell. 1994. Chaperone-mediated activation in vivo of a *Pseudomonas cepacia* lipase. *Mol. Gen. Genet.* **245:**556–564.

Bardwell, J. C. A. 1994. Building bridges: disulphide bond formation in the cell. *Mol. Microbiol.* **14:**199–205.

Bjorn, M. J., P. A. Sokol, and B. H. Iglewski. 1979. Influence of iron on yields of extracellular products in *Pseudomonas aeruginosa* cultures. *J. Bacteriol.* **138:**193–200.

Brunschwig, E., and A. Darzins. 1992. A two-component T7 system for the overexpression of genes in *Pseudomonas aeruginosa*. *Gene* **111:**35–41.

Costerton, J. W., and H. Anwar. 1994. *Pseudomonas aeruginosa*: the microbe and the pathogen, p. 1–20. *In* A. L. Baltch and R. P. Smith (ed.), *Pseudomonas aeruginosa Infections and Treatment*. Marcel Dekker, Inc., New York.

Deretic, V., W. M. Konyecsni, D. C. Mohr, D. W. Martin, and N. S. Hibler. 1989. Common denominators of promoter control in *Pseudomonas* and other bacteria. *Bio/Technology* **7:**1249–1254.

Frenken, L. G. J., A. de Groot, J. Tommassen, and C. T. Verrips. 1993. Role of *lipB* gene product in the folding of the secreted lipase of *Pseudomonas glumae*. *Mol. Microbiol.* **9:**591–599.

Gilbert, E. J. 1993. *Pseudomonas* lipases: biochemical properties and molecular cloning. *Enzyme Microb. Technol.* **15:**634–645.

Gilbert, E. J., A. Cornish, and C.W. Jones. 1991. Purification and properties of extracellular lipase from *Pseudomonas aeruginosa* EF2. *J. Gen. Microbiol.* **137:**2223–2229.

Hoang, T. T., and H. P. Schweizer. 1995. Genetic analysis of a *Pseudomonas aeruginosa dsbB* homologue, abstr. D-95, p. 185. *In Abstracts of the 95th General Meeting of the American Society for Microbiology, 1995*. American Society for Microbiology, Washington, D. C.

Ihara, F., I. Okamoto, K. Akao, T. Nihira, and Y. Yamada. 1995. Lipase modulator protein (LimL) of *Pseudomonas* sp. strain 109. *J. Bacteriol.* **177:**1254–1258.

Jaeger, K.-E., F.-J. Adrian, H. E. Meyer, R. E. W. Hancock, and U. K. Winkler. 1992. Extracellular lipase from *Pseudomonas aeruginosa* is an amphiphilic protein. *Biochim. Biophys. Acta* **1120:**315–321.

Jaeger, K.-E., A. Kharazmi, and N. Høiby. 1991a. Extracellular lipase of *Pseudomonas aeruginosa*: biochemical characterization and effect on human neutrophil and monocyte function *in vitro*. *Microb. Pathog.* **10:**173–182.

Jaeger, K.-E., K. Liebeton, A. Zonta, K. Schimossek, and M. T. Reetz. Biotechnological application of *Pseudomonas aeruginosa* lipase: efficient kinetic resolution of amines and alcohols. *Appl. Microbiol. Biotechnol.*, in press.

Jaeger, K.-E., S. Ransac, B. W. Dijkstra, C. Colson, M. van Heuvel, and O. Misset. 1994. Bacterial lipases. *FEMS Microbiol. Rev.* **15:**29–63.

Jaeger, K.-E., S. Ransac, H. B. Koch, F. Ferrato, and B. W. Dijkstra. 1993a. Topological characterization and modeling of the 3D structure of lipase from *Pseudomonas aeruginosa*. *FEBS Lett.* **332:**143–149.

Jaeger, K.-E., B. Schneidinger, R. Faschian, and U. K. Winkler. 1993b. Extracellular lipase of *Pseudomonas aeruginosa*: molecular cloning, overexpression, and regulation, abstr. Pl.5. *In Abstracts of the International Workshop: Characterization of Lipases for Industrial Applications: 3D-Structure and Catalytic Mechanism.* The Commisson of the European Communities, Elsinore, Denmark.

Jaeger, K.-E., S. Wohlfarth, and U. K. Winkler. 1991b. Extracellular lipase of *Pseudomonas aeruginosa*, p. 381–384. *In* L. Alberghina, R. D. Schmid, and R. Verger (ed.), *Lipases: Structure, Mechanism and Genetic Engineering*. GBF Monographs, vol. 16. Verlag Chemie, Weinheim, Germany.

Kim, Y., L. S. Watrud, and A. Matin. 1995. A carbon starvation survival gene of *Pseudomonas putida* is regulated by σ^{54}. *J. Bacteriol.* **177:**1850–1859.

Koch, H. B. 1990. Isolation and characterization of polyclonal antibodies against extracellular lipase of *Pseudomonas aeruginosa*. Diploma thesis. Ruhr University, Bochum, Germany.

Kok, R., G., J. J. van Thor, I. M. Nugteren-Roodzant, B. Vosman, and K. J. Hellingwerf. 1995. Characterization of lipase-deficient mutants of *Acinetobacter calcoaceticus* BD413: identification of a periplasmic lipase chaperone essential for production of extracellular lipase. *J. Bacteriol.* **177:**3295–3307.

Kraulis, P. J. 1991. MOLSCRIPT: a program to produce both detailed and schematic plots of proteins. *J. Appl. Crystallogr.* **24:**946–950.

Latifi, A., M. K. Winson, M. Foglino, B. W. Bycroft, G. S. A. B. Stewart, A. Lazdunski, and P. Williams. 1995. Multiple homologues of LuxR and LuxL control expression of virulence determinants and secondary metabolites through quorum sensing in *Pseudomonas aeruginosa* PAO1. *Mol. Microbiol.* **17:**333–343.

Mattick, J. S., and R. A. Alm. 1995. A common architecture of type 4 fimbriae and complexes involved in macromolecular traffic. *Trends Microbiol.* **3:**411–413.

Merrick, M. J. 1993. In a class of its own—the RNA polymerase sigma factor σ^{54} (σ^{N}). *Mol. Microbiol.* **10:**903–909.

Minton, N. P., and L. E. Clark. 1985. Identification of the promoter of the *Pseudomonas* gene coding for carboxypeptidase G2. *J. Mol. Appl. Genet.* **3:**26–35.

Misset, O., G. Gerritse, K.-E. Jaeger, U. Winkler, C. Colson, K. Schanck, E. Lesuisse, V. Dartois, M. Blaauw, S. Ransac, and B. W. Dijkstra. 1994. The structure-function relationship of the lipases from *Pseudomonas aeruginosa* and *Bacillus subtilis*. *Protein Eng.* **7:**523–529.

Noble, M. E. M., A. Cleasby, L. N. Johnson, M. R. Egmond, and L. G. J. Frenken. 1993. The crystal structure of triacylglycerol lipase from *Pseudomonas glumae* reveals a partially redundant catalytic aspartate. *FEBS Lett.* **331:**123–128.

Nunn, D., S. Bergman, and S. Lory. 1990. Products of three accessory genes, *pilB*, *pilC*, and *pilD*, are required for biogenesis of *Pseudomonas aeruginosa* pili. *J. Bacteriol.* **172:**2911–2919.

Ochsner, U. A., A. K. Koch, A. Fiechter, and J. Reiser. 1994. Isolation and characterization of a regulatory gene affecting rhamnolipid biosurfactant synthesis in *Pseudomonas aeruginosa*. *J. Bacteriol.* **176:**2044–2054.

Passador, L., J. M. Cook, M. J. Gambello, L. Rust, and B. H. Iglewski. 1993. Expression of *Pseudomonas aeruginosa* virulence genes requires cell-to-cell communication. *Science* **260:**1127–1130.

Pearson, J. P., K. M. Gray, L. Passador, K. D. Tucker, A. Eberhard, B. H. Iglewski, and E. P. Greenberg. 1994. Structure of the autoinducer required for expression of *Pseudomonas aeruginosa* virulence genes. *Proc. Natl. Acad. Sci. USA* **91:**197–201.

Pearson, J. P., L. Passador, B. H. Iglewski, and E. P. Greenberg. 1995. A second N-acylhomoserine lactone signal produced by *Pseudomonas aeruginosa*. *Proc. Natl. Acad. Sci. USA* **92:**1490–1494.

Prince, R. W., C. D. Cox, and M. L. Vasil. 1993. Coordinate regulation of siderophore and exotoxin A production: molecular cloning and sequencing of the *Pseudomonas aeruginosa fur* gene. *J. Bacteriol.* **175:**2589–2598.

Reetz, M. T., A. Zonta, and J. Simpelkamp. 1995. Efficient heterogenous biocatalysts by immobilization of lipases in hydrophobic sol-gel materials. *Angew. Chem.* **107:**373–376.

Rogalska, E., C. Cudrey, F. Ferrato, and R. Verger. 1993. Stereoselective hydrolysis of triglycerides by animal and microbial lipases. *Chirality* **5:**24–30.

Salmond, G. P. C., B. W. Bycroft, G. S. A. B. Stewart, and P. Williams. 1995. The bacterial 'enigma'; cracking the code of cell-cell communication. *Mol. Microbiol.* **16:**615–624.

Schneidinger, B., D. Haas, and K.-E. Jaeger. Manuscript in preparation.

Schneidinger, B., and K.-E. Jaeger. 1994. Overexpression and purification of Lif protein from *Pseudomonas aeruginosa*, p. 96. *In Abstracts of the International Workshop: Characterization of Lipases for Industrial*

Applications: 3D-Structure and Catalytic Mechanism. The Commission of the European Communities, Bandol, France.

Stuer, W., K.-E. Jaeger, and U. K. Winkler. 1986. Purification of extracellular lipase from *Pseudomonas aeruginosa. J. Bacteriol.* **168:**1070–1074.

Tommassen, J., A. Filloux, M. Bally, M. Murgier, and A. Lazdunski. 1992. Protein secretion in *Pseudomonas aeruginosa. FEMS Microbiol. Rev.* **103:**73–90.

Totten, P. A., J. C. Lara, and S. Lory. 1990. The *rpoN* gene product of *Pseudomonas aeruginosa* is required for expression of diverse genes, including the flagellin gene. *J. Bacteriol.* **172:**389–396.

Vasil, M. L., A. E. Pritchard, and R. M. Ostroff. 1990. Molecular biology of exotoxin A and phospholipase C of *Pseudomonas aeruginosa*, p. 3–14. *In* S. Silver, A. M. Chakrabarty, B. Iglewski, and S. Kaplan (ed.), *Pseudomonas: Biotransformations, Pathogenesis, and Evolving Biotechnology.* American Society for Microbiology, Washington, D.C.

Vasil, M. L., A. I. Vasil, and V. D. Shortridge. 1994. Phosphate and osmoprotectants in the pathogenesis of *Pseudomonas aeruginosa*, p. 126–132. *In* A. Torriani-Gorini, E. Yagil, and S. Silver (ed.), *Phosphate in Microorganisms: Cellular and Molecular Biology.* American Society for Microbiology, Washington, D.C.

Villeneuve, P., M. Pina, D. Montet, and J. Graille. 1995. Determination of lipase specificities through the use of chiral triglycerides and their racemics. *Chem. Phys. Lipids* **76:**109–113.

Vulfson, E. N. 1994. Industrial applications of lipases, p. 271–288. *In* P. Wooley and S. B. Petersen (ed.), *Lipases—Their Structure, Biochemistry and Application.* Cambridge University Press, Cambridge.

Wohlfarth, S., C. Hoesche, C. Strunk, and U. K. Winkler. 1992. Molecular genetics of the extracellular lipase of *Pseudomonas aeruginosa* PAO1. *J. Gen. Microbiol.* **138:**1325–1335.

Molecular Biology of Pseudomonads
Edited by T. Nakazawa et al.

Chapter 29

Structure, Regulation, and Functions of the Amidase Operon of *Pseudomonas aeruginosa*

Robert Drew, Bernard O'Hara, and Rachel Williams

Pseudomonas aeruginosa PAC1 is able to grow on a narrow range of short-chain-length aliphatic amides by virtue of a chromosomally located amidase (EC 3.5.1.4) (Kelly and Clarke, 1962). Amidase activity is inducible by some of these amides, but the inducer and substrate specificities of the system are distinct (Table 1) (Brammar and Clarke, 1964). Thus, whereas acetamide and propionamide are both good inducers of amidase expression and good substrates for the enzyme, butyramide is a very poor substrate and is active as an analog corepressor of amidase expression. Other amides such as lactamide and *N*-acetylacetamide are good inducers of enzyme activity but poor enzyme substrates (Table 1). The amidase system is of interest first because of the way the system has been selectively evolved to allow cell growth on an extended range of amide substrates (Clarke and Drew, 1988) and second because of the novel system regulating operon expression (Drew and Wilson, 1992).

Studies with the wild-type strain PAC1 and constitutive mutants have shown that in addition to the amide-dependent regulation of amidase synthesis, expression is also subject to catabolite repression (Smyth and Clarke, 1975) but not apparently to the general nitrogen regulation control system, although nitrogen regulation of amidase expression is seen in strain PAO1 (Janssen et al., 1982). A variety of mutants of the amidase system have been isolated and classified into two major groups. Regulatory mutants of several types include amidase negative, high or low constitutive, formamide or butyramide inducible, resistant to butyramide repression, and temperature sensitive. A second group of mutants consists of those involving the amidase structural gene (*amiE*), which include amidase-negative and substrate specificity mutants allowing growth on butyramide, valeramide, or phenylacetamide (Clarke and Drew, 1988). Catabolite repression-resistant mutants have also been isolated, but all of these appear to be unlinked to the locus.

Characterization of regulator temperature-sensitive mutations showed initially that amidase expression was primarily regulated via a positive control system by *amiR* (Farin and Clarke, 1978). Subsequently, a second negative controlling regulatory gene (*amiC*)

Robert Drew, Bernard O'Hara, and Rachel Williams • Department of Biochemistry and Molecular Biology, University College London, Gower Street, London WC1E 6BT, United Kingdom.

Table 1. Amides as substrates, inducers, and analog corepressors of the amidase system of *P. aeruginosa* PAC1 and amide binding to purified AmiC

Amide	Relative activity[a]			
	Substrate	Inducer	Corepressor	K_d (μM)[b]
Formamide	+	+	+	ND
Acetamide	++	++	0	3.7
Propionamide	++	++	0	3.1
Butyramide	Tr	0	+	0.03
Lactamide	+	++	0	0.03
N-Acetylacetamide	Tr	++	0	ND

[a]Tr, trace. Data are from Clarke and Drew (1988).
[b]Binding of amides to AmiC (Wilson et al., 1993). ND, not done.

was identified, mutations in which led to an amidase constitutive phenotype (Wilson and Drew, 1991). The amidase genes have been isolated on a 5.3-kb *Hin*dIII-*Sal*I DNA fragment from a high-expressing constitutive mutant, PAC433 (Drew et al., 1980), and the wild-type strain, PAC1 (Wilson and Drew, 1991). The *amiE* gene was initially found to lie at one end of the DNA fragment (Fig. 1), and subsequently the amidase nucleotide and amino acid sequences were determined (Clarke et al., 1981; Brammar et al., 1987; Ambler et al., 1987). The two regulatory genes which lie downstream of *amiE* were then identified and sequenced (Cousens et al., 1987; Lowe et al., 1989; Wilson and Drew, 1991). *amiR* was first identified as a positive regulator of amidase expression and thereafter shown to encode a transcription antitermination factor which, under inducing conditions, mediates the extension of an otherwise short, constitutively produced leader transcript through a rho-independent transcription terminator and into the amidase operon (Drew and Lowe, 1989; Wilson and Drew, 1995). *amiC*, encoding the negative regulator, has been overexpressed, the protein has been isolated and crystallized, and the structure has been solved (Wilson and Drew, 1991; Wilson et al., 1991; Pearl et al., 1994). The operon contains two other substantial open reading frames (ORFs), *aimB* and *amiS*, studies of which are described below.

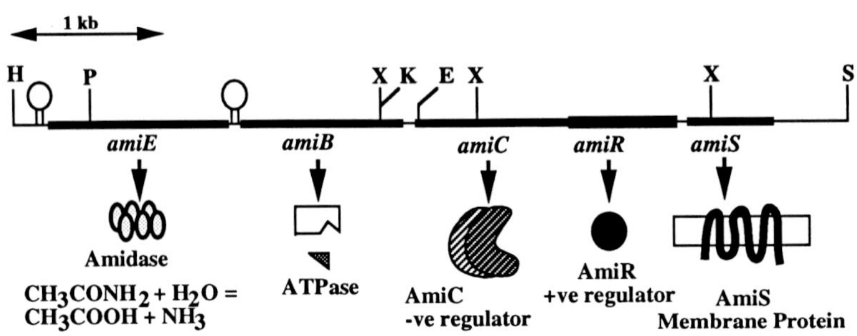

Figure 1. Structure-function map of the amidase operon of *P. aeruginosa*. Restriction sites: H, *Hin*dIII; P, *Pst*I; X, *Xho*I; K, *Kpn*I; E, *Eco*RV; S, *Sal*I. Rho-independent transcription terminator sequences are shown. –ve, negative; +ve, positive.

TRANSCRIPTION ANALYSIS AND ANTITERMINATION

The DNA sequence of the *amiE* upstream region shows an *Escherichia coli*-like σ^{70} promoter sequence some distance upstream of the gene itself, a short ORF of 35 amino acids of unknown function containing a rho-independent transcription terminator sequence, followed by the *amiE* Shine-Dalgarno sequence and gene (Fig. 2). The identification of the antitermination mechanism came from the analysis of a constructed terminator deletion which led to amide-independent, AmiR-independent constitutive amidase expression (Drew and Lowe, 1989). The model has now been confirmed by mapping the transcription start point to the promoter region and showing constitutive production of the leader mRNA (Wilson and Drew, 1995). Northern (RNA) blot analysis and S1 mapping have shown, in addition, that *amiE* transcripts are 50% terminated at a newly identified terminator site located between *amiE* and *amiB* (Fig. 1), and the remaining transcripts are of a length indicating that termination occurs downstream of *amiS*. Under these circumstances, it is difficult to envisage a simple model explaining how operon expression is turned on, since there must be a requirement for *amiC* and *amiR* expression. One way to ensure induction would be by the presence of a separate *amiCRS* transcription unit, and DNA sequence analysis has shown the presence of two potential RpoN-dependent promoter sequences upstream of *amiC*. However, we have been unable to map any transcripts originating from these postulated promoters, although in assays using an amidase promoter probe vector in vivo, the 650-bp *Xho*I fragment containing this region (Fig. 1) shows low constitutive promoter activity. Thus, although poorly defined at present, the *amiCRS* transcription unit may exist (Wilson and Drew, 1995).

Folding the leader region mRNA sequence (residues 1 to 100) shows the presence of two large stem-loop structures with a relatively unstructured central region (Fig. 3). The leader ORF starts with an AUG in the up-stem of stem-loop 1 and terminates downstream of the sequence shown. Stem-loop 2 is the previously determined transcription termination sequence. We have used in vitro mutagenesis to make changes in the leader region to investigate the role of both the leader region ORF and the RNA sequences in the antitermination reaction. Analysis of the changes in vivo, in both the presence and the absence of *amiR*, has shown that the ORF plays no apparent role in the antitermination reaction (R. Drew, unpublished observations). In contrast, sequences at the left end of the unstructured central region (residues 35 to 40) and the small stem-loop region (residues 53 to 62) are critical. Multiple changes in either of these regions can lead to the

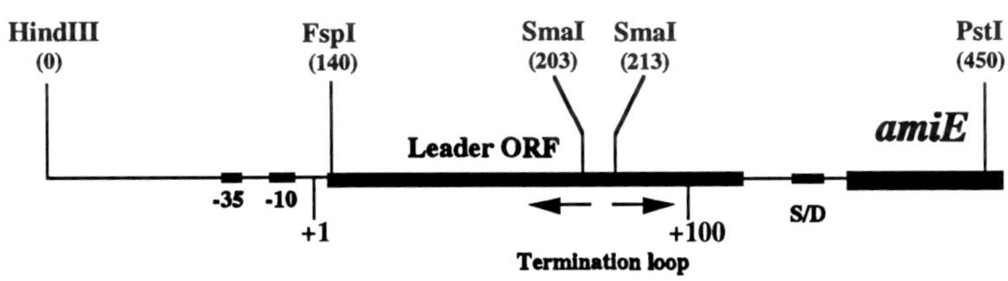

Figure 2. Structural map of the amidase operon leader region. Locations of the σ^{70} promoter sequences, the leader ORF, the rho-independent transcription terminator, the *amiE* gene Shine-Dalgarno sequence (S/D), the start of the *amiE* gene, and some of the restriction enzyme target sites are shown (Wilson and Drew, 1995).

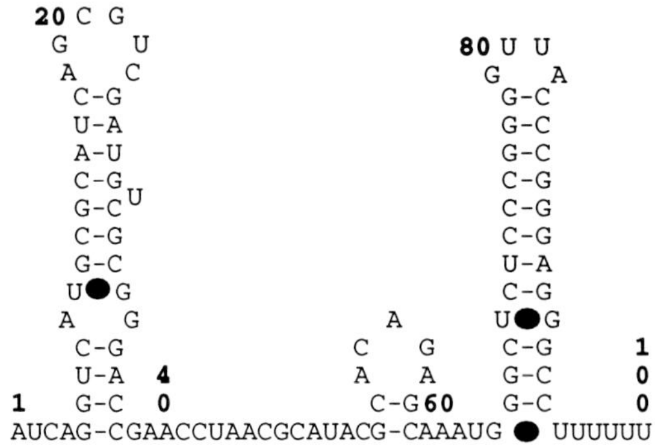

Figure 3. RNA fold of the leader region transcript. Residues 1 to 100 are shown. Complementary residues are shown by lines, and G-U interactions are indicated by filled circles. Drawn from folds predicted by Mufold (Zuker, 1989; Jaeger et al., 1989a, 1989b).

abolition of antitermination in vivo (Drew, unpublished observations). Experiments to isolate the antiterminator protein AmiR for use in in vitro studies have so far been unsuccessful. The *amiR* gene has been overexpressed in a variety of systems, but the protein appears to be very insoluble and is always found in an aggregated form. However, some preliminary successful in vitro investigations of the AmiC-AmiR interaction have been carried out with purified AmiC and crude cell extracts containing AmiR. These studies have shown that the two proteins appear to be closely associated in the presence of both inducing and repressing amides (Drew, unpublished observations).

THE CRYSTAL STRUCTURE OF AmiC

The finding of an amidase constitutive phenotype in a constructed *amiC* mutant was the initial evidence that the gene encoded a negative regulator (Wilson and Drew, 1991). Complementation studies have shown that the AmiR antitermination reaction is independent of inducing and/or repressing amides (Cousens et al., 1987; Wilson and Drew, 1991), and it has been established that AmiC binds amides (Wilson et al., 1993). Additional complementation studies of PAC1 with broad-host-range *amiC* and *amiR* expression vectors have shown that there is an apparent stoichiometry between the two proteins regulating operon expression. Thus, PAC1(pSW41) (*amiC*$^+$) shows a noninducible amidase phenotype, and PAC1(pSW40) (*amiR*$^+$) shows a semiconstitutive but further inducible phenotype (Wilson and Drew, 1991). These results indicate that AmiC and AmiR could form a regulatory pair, with signal transduction occurring by a noncovalent protein-protein interaction. Thus, inducing and/or repressing amides interact with AmiC, and it is the change in AmiC conformation that may regulate the antitermination activity of AmiR and subsequent operon expression.

amiC has been overexpressed, the protein has been isolated and crystallized in the presence of acetamide (Wilson et al., 1991), and the structure has been solved at 2.0 Å (0.2 nm) (Pearl et al., 1994). The butyramide crystal form has also been obtained and solved under different conditions (B. O'Hara, unpublished observations). AmiC consists of a single polypeptide chain of 385 residues folded into two domains, each with an alternating β-α-β topology. There are five parallel β-strands forming a slightly twisted β-sheet in each domain, surrounded on both faces by α-helices and separated by a central cleft. The two domains are closed down with a trapped acetamide molecule in the cleft (Fig. 4).

The AmiC fold is very similar in topology to members of the periplasmic binding protein family, particularly LivJ, the leucine/isoleucine/valine-binding protein from *E. coli*, even though there is less than 20% sequence identity (Wilson et al., 1993). The acetamide-bound AmiC structure is in an almost completely closed conformation (Pearl et al., 1994). There is a structural equivalence between AmiC and LivJ with respect to the N and C domains except that LivJ is in a more open conformation, the difference between the acetamide-bound AmiC form and the ligand-free LivJ being a 35° rigid body movement (Pearl et al., 1994).

Periplasmic binding proteins have been shown to close down upon binding to their target molecules (Newcomer et al., 1981; Vermersch et al., 1991; Jacobsen et al., 1991), and AmiC in the presence of the inducing molecule acetamide is found in a similar configuration. The binding of acetamide to AmiC is very favorable, with a binding constant (K_d) of 3.66 μM (Table 1) (Wilson et al., 1993). In structural terms, the ligand geometry of acetamide binding to AmiC is exquisitely precise. The key interactions that test for the geometric fidelity of the fit are exerted through hydrogen bonding and van der Waals interactions. There are four key interactions (Fig. 5): (i) the acetamide carbonyl is hydrogen bonded to Tyr-150 and Ser-85; (ii) the acetamide amine group makes four hydrogen bonds, to Ser-85, Pro-170, Tyr-104, and Tyr-83; (iii) the plane of the acetamide molecule packs against the plane of Tyr-152 to position the molecule; (iv) finally, the amide alkyl chain simultaneously permits the van der Waals interactions between the side chain of Thr-233 and the side chain of Tyr-152.

The result is that the acetamide substituents and the AmiC ligand binding sites are energetically satisfied. These four interactions allow the C domain and the N domain to form the closed-down conformation. This form of AmiC with acetamide represents the molecular state for induction of amidase operon expression, i.e., the switched-on state.

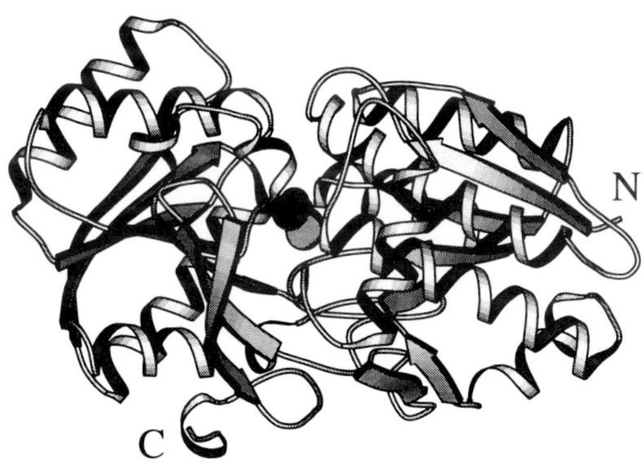

Figure 4. A secondary structure cartoon of the AmiC molecule with acetamide bound. The N and C domains each consist of a twisted β-sheet flanked on both sides by α-helices. The bound acetamide molecule sits in a cleft between the two domains. The figure was generated by using MOLSCRIPT (Kraulis, 1991).

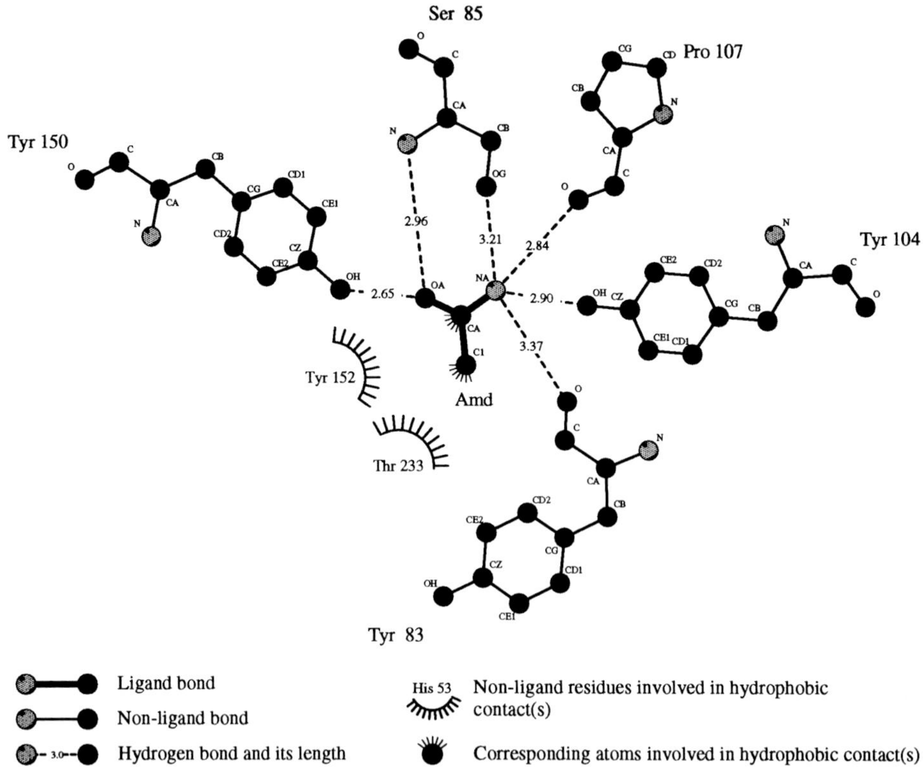

Figure 5. The AmiC ligand binding site with acetamide bound. Hydrogen bonding and van der Waals interactions with acetamide are shown. The figure was generated by using the program LIGPLOT (Wallace et al., 1993).

The structure of AmiC with butyramide, which has a lower binding constant (K_d = 0.03 μM; Table 1) (Wilson et al., 1993), has also been solved (O'Hara, unpublished observations). The molecule shows a more open conformation, with the two domains showing a slight interdomain movement, although not as large as that found in LivJ. The hydrogen bond network is satisfied for the butyramide amino and carbonyl substituents: however, the van der Waals interactions fail to be satisfied in the following way. The larger alkyl group of butyramide severely obstructs the packing of the side chain of Thr-233 (the residue that senses the alkyl group size) and Tyr-152, thus breaking up the van der Waals interaction network and destabilizing the closed-down conformation. The AmiC-butyramide complex is thus more open and represents the repressing form of AmiC, the switched-off state.

The analogy that one could use is the Cinderella story. The ugly sister, the one with large butyramide feet, can fit into the AmiC molecular shoe only by pushing the two domains slightly further apart, whereas the Cinderella molecule acetamide, with smaller feet, fits neatly into the molecular cleft of AmiC.

These two molecular states of AmiC suggest a model for the signal transduction pathway. AmiC in the open (noninducing) conformation could bind AmiR to prevent its interaction with the nascent mRNA, and hence transcription termination occurs, inhibiting operon expression. The binding of acetamide switches AmiC into the closed conformation, which would be unable to bind to AmiR. The released AmiR would then be able to function in the antitermination reaction, resulting in consequent operon expression. The structure of AmiC with the two forms described suggests a molecular mechanism for the first step in the process of induction and repression of the amidase operon.

STUDIES WITH AmiB AND AmiS

DNA sequencing has identified two additional genes within the operon, *amiB* and *amiS,* which are located downstream of *amiE* and *amiC,* respectively (Wilson et al., 1995). The intergenic regions upstream of both *amiB* and *amiS* include ribosome binding sites but no known promoter sequences, indicating that these two genes are expressed coordinately with the rest of the operon from the promoter, pE, situated upstream of *amiE* (Fig. 1).

The *amiB* gene encodes a substantially hydrophilic 371-amino-acid (42-kDa) protein which contains parts A and B of the Walker consensus nucleotide-binding motif (Walker et al., 1982). The amino acid sequence of AmiB shows extensive homology with an uncharacterized ORF adjacent to the amidase gene from the gram-positive bacterium *Rhodococcus erythropolis* (Soubrier et al., 1992) (39% identity, 60% similarity) and with the C-terminal ATP-binding domain of the subfamilies of the Clp regulatory proteins (Squires and Squires, 1992), including the heat shock response protein from *Saccharomyces cerevisiae* (Parsell et al., 1994). Threading analysis (Jones et al., 1992) has indicated that the tertiary structure of AmiB would adopt a three-dimensional structure similar to that of the ATP-binding protein adenylate kinase (Wilson et al., 1995).

In an attempt to ascertain a role for AmiB, a 400-bp internal deletion was made within the *amiB* gene. Comparison studies between *P. aeruginosa* PAC452 (which has a chromosomal deletion of the amidase locus), containing either pSW101 (which carries the whole amidase operon from PAC1) or the *amiB* deletion derivative pMW22, indicate that AmiB neither is a regulator protein involved in the induction of amidase expression (Wilson et al., 1995) nor is involved in protecting the amidase protein against heat shock (R. Williams, unpublished observations).

The nucleotide binding motif (Walker et al., 1982) within AmiB and the proposed structural homology with adenylate kinase suggest that AmiB may be capable of ATP hydrolysis. The AmiB protein has been overexpressed in *P. aeruginosa*, but sodium dodecyl sulfate-polyacrylamide gel electrophoresis analysis shows the presence of an additional band with a calculated molecular mass of 40 kDa only in the insoluble fraction (Wilson et al., 1995). Thus, in *P. aeruginosa*, AmiB appears to aggregate when overexpressed. To overcome the problems of protein refolding and isolation, enzymatic analysis of AmiB has been carried out with purified maltose-binding protein (MBP)-AmiB fusion protein. The MBP-AmiB fusion protein has been shown to have intrinsic ATPase activity with calculated K_m and V_{max} values of 174 ± 15 μM and 2.4 ± 0.1 μmol/min/mg, respectively. The fusion protein also exhibits slight GTPase activity but is unable to hydrolyze CTP. The ATPase activity of MBP-AmiB is dependent on the presence of magnesium ions, and whereas manganese ions can partially substitute for magnesium, the fusion cannot hydrolyze ATP with Ca-ATP or Zn-ATP complexes as substrates.

Finally, both ADP and ammonium vanadate were shown to be strong inhibitors of the ATPase activity of MBP-AmiB, most likely by competing with ATP for the substrate binding site. This intrinsic ATPase activity is similar to that shown by MalK, the ATP-binding component of the maltose ABC-type transporter *in Salmonella typhimurium* (K_m = 70 μM; V_{max} = 1.3 μmol/min/mg) (Morbach et al., 1993). Additionally, the MalK and MBP-AmiB ATPase activities share characteristic features such as substrate specificities, dependence on Mg^{2+} ions, and sensitivity to ADP; however, the MalK activity is resistant to inhibition by ammonium vanadate (Morbach et al., 1993).

The *amiS* gene encodes a protein of 171 amino acids with a calculated molecular mass of 18 kDa. Searches of the SwissProt and EMBL databases have identified two homologs of unknown function. The first is an uncharacterized ORF (40% identity, 68% similarity) adjacent to the amidase gene in the gram-positive organism *Mycobacterium smegmatis* (Mahenthiralingam et al., 1993), and the second is the *ureI* gene product (37% identity, 63% similarity) from the urease operon of the gram-negative organism *Helicobacter pylori* (Cussac et al., 1992). Analysis of AmiS and its two homologs reveals that (i) all three proteins contain hydrophobic regions of 18 to 20 amino acids, characteristic of transmembrane helices, with variable-length hydrophilic loop regions, suggesting that the three proteins are integral membrane proteins; (ii) AmiS and the *ureI* gene product appear to contain six transmembrane helices, and the larger *M. smegmatis* gene product contains seven transmembrane helices; and (iii) MEMSAT analysis (Jones et al., 1994) of AmiS and its homologs predicts the transmembrane regions and determines that the N terminus would be external for each protein. Multiple sequence alignment (Fig. 6) indicates significant homology among all three proteins, although in the UreI sequence insertions are present in predicted nonmembrane loop regions.

From the foregoing analyses and the high level of homology between these proteins, it has been proposed that they represent a novel family of integral membrane proteins (Wilson et al., 1995). Within the amidase operon of *P. aeruginosa*, two new genes have now been identified, one encoding an ATPase and the other encoding an integral membrane protein, both of which are specifically expressed in response to inducing amides in the growth medium. Further, the AmiB and AmiS homologs identified are located within operons involved in the utilization of amides from both gram-positive and gram-negative organisms.

An obvious role for AmiB and AmiS would be as an ABC-type transport system located within the plasma membrane and involved in the uptake of amides. ABC-type transporters, which are involved in both import and export processes, have been identified in both prokaryotes and eukaryotes, and they all have a basic anatomy in common (Higgins, 1992). In outline, these transporters consist of two domains: an integral membrane domain with six to eight transmembrane helices and a cytoplasmic domain with an ATP-binding motif and, in some cases, measured ATPase activity. The domains are found either as a single polypeptide chain or as two or more distinct polypeptides. Together, these proteins form a tetrameric complex which includes two copies of the cytoplasmic ATP-binding protein. Therefore, AmiS could represent the integral membrane domain and AmiB could represent the cytoplasmic ATP-binding component of an ABC-type transporter. In this case, we would expect the presence of an *amiB* homolog in the *M. smegmatis* amidase operon and the *H. pylori* urease operon. At present, the sequencing of the *M. smegmatis* operon is incomplete, and although there is no *amiB* homolog

```
            OUT         I            IN           II
           1                                               50
     amiS  MLGLVLLYVGAVLFLNAVWLLGKISGREVAVINFLVGVLSACVAFYLIFS
  M.s ORF  MGGVGLFYVGAVLIIDGLMLLGRISPRGATPLNFFVGGLQVVTPTVLILQ
     ureI  MLGLVLLYVGIVLISNGICGLTKVDPKSTAVMNFFVGGLSIICNVVVITY
           *:*::*:***:**: :*  :*::::::  :::**:**:*:     ::*

                   OUT                   III             IN
          51                                              100
     amiS  AAAGQ.................GSLKAGALTLLFAFTYLWVAANQFLEVD
  M.s ORF  SGGDA.................AVIFAASGLYLFGFTYLWVAINNVTDWD
     ureI  SALNPTAPVEGAEDIAQVSHHLTNFYGPATGLLFGFTYLYAAINHTFGLD
           ::                        : :  :**:****::*:*     *

                    IV                 OUT
         101                                              150
     amiS  GKGLGWFCLFVSLTACTVAIESF.AGA.......SGPFGLWNAVNWTVWA
  M.s ORF  GEGLGWFSLFVAIAALGYSWHAFTAEA...........DPAFGVIWLLWA
     ureI  WRPYSWYSLFVAINTIPAAILSHYSDMLDDHKVLGITEGDWWAIIWLAWG
           : :::*::***:: :   :: :: : :             :* ::*:

                V        IN            VI            OUT
         151                                              200
     amiS  LLWFCFFLLLGLSR.GIQKPVAYLTLASAIFTAWLPGLLLLGQVLKA*..
  M.s ORF  VLWFMLFLLLGLGHDALGPAVGFVAVAEGVITAAVPAFLIVSGNWETGPL
     ureI  VLWLTAFIENIL.KIPLGKFTPWLAIIEGILTAWIPAWLLFIQHWV*...
           :**:  *::::*    *:: :  :: :::: **: *: *:    :

                  VII                IN
         201                                      242
     amiS  ..........................................
  M.s ORF  PAAVIAVIGFAAVVLAYPIGRRLAAPSVTNPPPAALAATTR*
     ureI  ..........................................
```

Figure 6. Alignment of the AmiS sequence and homologs. Conserved residues in all three sequences are indicated by asterisks, and residues conserved in two sequences are indicated by colons. The transmembrane regions predicted by MEMSAT (Jones et al., 1994) are indicated by the shaded regions, and each potential transmembrane helix is numbered. The proposed orientation (IN, internal; OUT, external) of the nonmembrane loops, predicted by MEMSAT, is shown above the sequence. *M.s* ORF, an ORF in the *M. smegmatis* amidase operon (Mahenthiralingam et al., 1993); *ureI*, the *ureI* gene from *H. pylori* (Cussac et al., 1992).

within the *H. pylori* urease operon the *ureG* gene product possesses an ATP-binding motif (Cussac et al., 1992). Additionally, an *amiS* homolog has been identified in the *R. erythropolis* amidase operon, within which an a*miB* homolog has been previously found (H. Choubrier, personal communication).

In addition to the above-specified components, bacterial ABC-type transporters involved in the import of substrates usually have a periplasmic binding protein which binds and delivers the ligand to the integral membrane complex. There does not appear to be a periplasmic binding protein encoded by the amidase operon of *P. aeruginosa*. However, as described above, the negative regulator protein, AmiC, is structurally homologous to the leucine/isoleucine/valine periplasmic binding protein (LivJ) of *E. coli* (Wilson et al., 1993). It is therefore possible that AmiC has changed roles during evolution from being a periplasmic amide receptor in a transport system to forming the cytoplasmically located sensory component of a sensor-regulator pair involved in the regulation of amidase expression. At present, no putative periplasmic binding protein has been identified in any of the operons containing *amiB* and/or *amiS* homologs. It is therefore possible that these examples represent a novel subfamily of ABC-type transporters without the requirement for a periplasmic binding protein, present in both gram-positive and gram-negative organisms.

Acknowledgments. The transcription analysis and antitermination studies were supported by funds from the Wellcome Trust (to R.D. and Laurence Pearl); structural studies of the amidase regulator proteins are supported by the Science and Engineering Research Council (B.O'H; to Laurence Pearl and R.D.), and R.W. is the recipient of a Medical Research Council research studentship.

REFERENCES

Ambler, R. P., A. D. Auffret, and P. H. Clarke. 1987. The amino acid sequence of the aliphatic amidase from *Pseudomonas aeruginosa. FEBS Lett.* **215:**285–290.

Brammar, W. J., I. G. Charles, M. Matfield, L. Cheng-Pin, R. E. Drew, and P. H. Clarke. 1987. The nucleotide sequence of the *amiE* gene of *Pseudomonas aeruginosa. FEBS Lett.* **215:**291–294.

Brammar, W. J., and P. H. Clarke. 1964. Induction and repression of *Pseudomonas aeruginosa* amidase. *J. Gen. Microbiol.* **37:**307–319.

Clarke, P. H., and R. E. Drew. 1988. An experiment in enzyme evolution. Studies with *Pseudomonas aeruginosa* amidase. *Biosci. Rep.* **8:**103–120.

Clarke, P. H., R. E. Drew, C. Turberville, W. J. Brammar, R. P. Ambler, and A. D. Auffret. 1981. Alignment of the cloned *amiE* gene of *Pseudomonas aeruginosa* with the N-terminal sequence of amidase. *Biosci. Rep.* **1:**299–307.

Cousens, D. J., P. H. Clarke, and R. E. Drew. 1987. The amidase regulatory gene (*amiR*) of *Pseudomonas aeruginosa. J. Gen. Microbiol.* **133:**2041–2052.

Cussac, V., R. Ferrero, and A. F. Labigne. 1992. Expression of *Helicobacter pylori* urease genes in *Escherichia coli* grown under nitrogen-limiting conditions. *J. Bacteriol.* **175:**2466–2473.

Drew, R. E., P. H. Clarke, and W. J. Bammar. 1980. The construction *in vitro* of derivatives of bacteriophage lambda carrying the amidase genes *of Pseudomonas aeruginosa. Mol. Gen. Genet.* **177:**311–320.

Drew, R. E., and N. Lowe. 1989. Positive control of *Pseudomonas aeruginosa* amidase synthesis is mediated by a transcription anti-termination mechanism. *J. Gen. Microbiol.* **135:**817–823.

Drew, R. E., and S. A. Wilson. 1992. Regulation of amidase expression *in Pseudomonas aeruginosa*, p. 207–213. *In* E. Galli, S. Silver, and B. Witholt (ed.), *Pseudomonas: Molecular Biology and Biotechnology.* American Society for Microbiology, Washington, D.C.

Farin, F., and P. H. Clarke. 1978. Positive regulation of amidase synthesis in *Pseudomonas aeruginosa. J. Bacteriol.* **135:**379–392.

Higgins, C. F. 1992. ABC transporters: from microorganisms to man. *Annu. Rev. Cell Biol.* **8:**67–113.

Jacobsen, B. L., J. J. He, P. S. Vermersch, D. D. Lemon, and F. A. Quiocho. 1991. Engineered interdomain disulphide in the periplasmic receptor for sulphate transport reduces flexibility. *J. Biol. Chem.* **266:**522–525.

Jaeger, J. A., D. H. Turner, and M. Zuker. 1989a. Improved predictions of secondary structures for RNA. *Proc. Natl. Acad. Sci. USA* **86:**7706–7710.

Jaeger, J. A., D. H. Turner, and M. Zuker. 1989b. Predicting optimal and suboptimal secondary structure for RNA. *Methods Enzymol.* **183:**281–306.

Janssen, D. B., P. M. Herst, H. M. L. J. Joostein, and C. van der Drift. 1982. Regulation of amidase formation in mutants from *Pseudomonas aeruginosa* PAO lacking glutamine synthetase activity. *Arch. Microbiol.* **131:**344–346.

Jones, D. T., W. R. Taylor, and J. M. Thornton. 1992. A new approach to protein fold recognition. *Nature* (London) **358:**86–89.

Jones, D. T., W. R. Taylor, and J. M. Thornton. 1994. A model recognition approach to the prediction of all-helical membrane protein structure and topology. *Biochemistry* **33:**3038–3049.

Kelly, M., and P. H. Clarke. 1962. An inducible amidase produced by a strain of *Pseudomonas aeruginosa. J. Gen. Microbiol.* **27:**305–316.

Kraulis, P. J. 1991. MOLSCRIPT—a program to produce both detailed and schematic plots of protein structures. *J. Appl. Crystallogr.* **24:**946–950.

Lowe, N., P. M. Rice, and R. E. Drew. 1989. Nucleotide sequence of the aliphatic amidase regulator gene (*amiR*) of *Pseudomonas aeruginosa*. *FEBS Lett.* **246:**39–43.

Mahenthiralingam, E., P. Draper, E. O. Davis, and M. J. Colston. 1993. Cloning and sequencing of the gene which encodes the highly inducible acetamidase of *Mycobacterium smegmatis*. *J. Gen. Microbiol.* **139:**575–583.

Morbach, S., S. Tebbe, and E. Schneider. 1993. The ATP-binding cassette (ABC) transporter for maltose/maltodextrins of *Salmonella typhimurium*. *J. Biol. Chem.* **268:**18617–18621.

Newcomer, M. E., B. A. Lewis, and F. A. Quiocho. 1981. The radius of gyration of L-arabinose-binding protein decreases upon binding of ligand. *J. Biol. Chem.* **256:**13218–13222.

Parsell, D. A., A. S. Kowal, M. A. Singer, and S. Lindquist. 1994. Protein desegregation mediated by heat-shock protein Hsp104. *Nature* (London) **372:**475–478.

Pearl, L., B. O'Hara, R. Drew, and S. Wilson. 1994. Crystal structure of AmiC: the controller of transcription antitermination in the amidase operon of *Pseudomonas aeruginosa*. *EMBO J.* **13:**5810–5817.

Smyth, P. F., and P. H. Clarke. 1975. Catabolite repression of *Pseudomonas aeruginosa* amidase: the effect of carbon source on amidase synthesis. *J. Gen. Microbiol.* **90:**81–90.

Soubrier, F., S. Levy-Schil, J.-F. Mayaux, D. Petre, A. Arnaud, and J. Crouzet. 1992. Cloning and primary structure of the wide-spectrum amidase from *Brevibacterium* sp. R312: high homology to the *amiE* product from *Pseudomonas aeruginosa*. *Gene* **116:**99–104.

Squires, C., and C. L. Squires. 1992. The Clp proteins: proteolysis or molecular chaperones? *J. Bacteriol.* **174:**1081–1085.

Vermersch, P. S., J. J. G. Tesemer, D. D. Lemon, and F. A. Quiocho. 1991. A pro to gly mutation in the hinge of the arabinose-binding protein enhances binding and alters specificity. *J. Biol. Chem.* **265:**16592–16603.

Walker, J. E., M. Saraste, M. J. Runswick, and N J. Gay. 1982. Distantly related sequences in the α- and β-subunits of ATP synthase, myosin, kinases and other ATP requiring enzymes and a common nucleotide-binding fold. *EMBO J.* **1:**945–951.

Wallace, A. C., R. A. Laskowski, and J. M. Thornton. 1993. LIGPLOT: a program to generate schematic diagrams of protein-ligand interactions. *Protein Eng.* **8:**283–290.

Wilson, S. A., N. E. Chayen, A. M. Hemmings, R. E. Drew, and L. H. Pearl. 1991. Crystallization of and preliminary X-ray data for the negative regulator (AmiC) of the amidase operon of *Pseudomonas aeruginosa*. *J. Mol. Biol.* **222:**869–871.

Wilson, S. A., and R. E. Drew. 1991. Cloning and DNA sequence of *amiC*, a new gene regulating expression of the *Pseudomonas aeruginosa* aliphatic amidase, and purification of the *amiC* product. *J. Bacteriol.* **173:**4914–4921.

Wilson, S. A., and R. E. Drew. 1995. Transcriptional analysis of the amidase operon from *Pseudomonas aeruginosa*. *J. Bacteriol.* **177:**3052–3057.

Wilson, S. A., S. J. Wachira, R. E. Drew, D. Jones, and L. H. Pearl. 1993. Antitermination of amidase expression in *Pseudomonas aeruginosa* is controlled by a novel cytoplasmic amide-binding protein. *EMBO J.* **12:**3637–3642.

Wilson, S. A., R. J. Williams, L. H. Pearl, and R. E. Drew. 1995. Identification of two new genes in the *Pseudomonas aeruginosa* amidase operon, encoding an ATPase (AmiB) and a putative integral membrane protein (AmiS). *J. Biol. Chem.* **270:**18818–18824.

Zuker, M. 1989. On finding all suboptimal foldings of an RNA molecule. *Science* **244:**48–52.

Molecular Biology of Pseudomonads
Edited by T. Nakazawa et al.

Chapter 30

Pseudomonas Cytochrome P-450 Oxygenases: Progress toward De Novo Design for Bioremediation

Stephen G. Sligar, Ernest J. Mueller, and Paul J. Loida

The use of *Pseudomonas* species for bioremediation has undergone an explosion in interest over the years. Recent investigations have been focused on the ability of these bacteria to degrade polyaromatic hydrocarbons (Davison et al., 1994; Providenti et al., 1995), nitrites and cyano compounds (Dubey and Holmes, 1995; Chapatwala et al., 1995), aliphatics and petroleum-based mixtures (Alhadhrami et al., 1995; Banat 1995), aromatic nitro compounds (Gorontzy et al., 1994), and both halogenated aromatic (Brazil et al., 1995; Demnerova et al., 1994; Nishino et al., 1994; Middaugh et al., 1994) and halogenated aliphatic (Feidieker et al., 1994; Picardal et al., 1995) species. *Pseudomonas* species appear to be especially well adapted to biodegradation of organics, as they have the unusual ability to modify the fatty acid content of the outer membrane, which reduces permeability enough to allow the bacteria to survive in contaminated environments (Heipieper et al., 1994). This resistance, and the ability to degrade a large number of compounds, makes the genus an attractive host for future efforts in designed biotransformations.

Often, however, microbial degradations have the limitation that the enzymes carrying out the desired chemistry have less than optimal specificities, and they may degrade only some compounds of a mixture (Feidieker et al., 1994; Su and Kafkewitz, 1994). In addition, laboratory-constructed microbes with enzyme processes may not be able to compete effectively with the indigenous microbial population (Winkler et al., 1995). Thus, the effective realization of a microbially based catalyst requires optimization on all three sides of the triangle: the enzyme, the target substrate, and the indigenous environment. The enzyme must have an activity toward the target compound yet must also be carried by a host cell which can effectively survive in the remediation environment. The substrate also must have transport properties consistent with the environment and microbial host.

One approach to optimization of enzymatic processes for remediation of recalcitrant compounds is to utilize the power of genetic engineering to alter existing specificities

Stephen G. Sligar • Beckman Institute for Advanced Science and Technology, University of Illinois, Urbana, Illinois 61801. ***Ernest J. Mueller*** • Sigma Chemical Company, 3500 DeKalb Street, St. Louis, Missouri 63178. ***Paul J. Loida*** • Abbott Laboratories, Abbott Park, Illinois 60064.

and stabilities to more desired parameters. In this chapter, we explore the substrate-enzyme interaction process in an attempt to understand the basic principles of anaerobic and aerobic dehalogenation chemistry as carried out by the cytochrome P-450 class of oxygenases. The natural reductive dehalogenation of haloalkanes catalyzed by the cytochromes P-450 provides an attractive system with which to begin engineering enzymes for bioremediation. Haloalkanes represent an almost ubiquitous groundwater environmental pollutant because of the historical widespread use of these compounds in cleaning agents and industrial solvents (Abelson, 1985; Paulsen and Ornstein, 1994). The P-450 enzymes, which are responsible for xenobiotic metabolism and hormone biosynthesis (Guengerich, 1990), can degrade halohydrocarbons by a variety of mechanisms and have received considerable attention over the past two decades (Wolf et al., 1980; Castro et al., 1988).

The mechanisms of dehalogenation have many poorly understood features (Wackett et al., 1994; Nastainczyk et al., 1981). Both carbene and carbanion intermediates have been implicated, depending on the substrate and P-450 isozyme (Artaud et al., 1990; Castro et al., 1985; Hildebrandt et al., 1988; Mansuy et al., 1974; Mansuy et al., 1977; Ruf et al., 1984). The reactions of cytochromes P-450 with halogenated ethanes are illustrative of the general reaction. Dehalogenation reaction products are derived from either direct substitution of halide with a proton or β-elimination in which a second halide separates from the adjacent carbon to give the corresponding olefin (Fig. 1). The elimination reaction pathway is generally preferred over substitution, but partitioning can be modulated by the lability of the leaving group (Castro et al., 1988; Li and Wackett, 1993). For example, the fully chlorinated substrate hexachloroethane reacts with the *Pseudomonas* P-450cam system under anaerobic conditions to give only tetrachloroethylene, while the partially fluorinated analog 1,1,1-trichloro-2,2,2-trifluoroethane undergoes both the β-elimination and substitution reactions. Electronic effects have also been implicated in the metabolism of halogenated methanes, as the brominated compounds undergo more facile reduction than the corresponding chlorinated and fluorinated species (Castro et al., 1985; Li and Wackett, 1993). Such is the case of bromodichloromethane, which is a substrate for P-450 turnover, while chloroform is not metabolized.

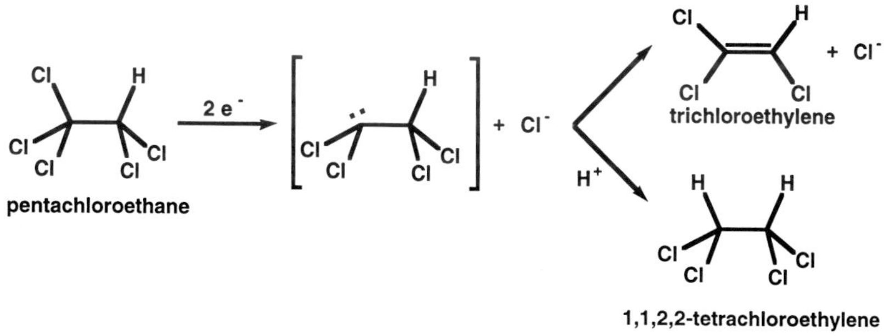

Figure 1. Reaction pathway for reductive dehalogenation. The more common elimination branch on the top results in a net loss of two halides and the production of the corresponding olefin.

A wide variety of halogenated small molecules are substrates for the *Pseudomonas* cytochrome P-450cam (Ruf et al., 1984). Chlorinated methanes and ethanes make up a representative set of substrates with large differences in the free energy of binding and reactivity. The equilibrium spin conversion, which is induced by the dissociation of the water ligand to the heme iron as a result of steric complementarity of substrate and binding pocket, and the dissociation constants for the series chloroform through hexachloroethane correlate with the number of chlorines on the carbon skeleton; more heavily chlorinated compounds show a higher affinity and larger spin state change upon binding. Of all the haloethanes, hexachloroethane binds most like the native substrate of P-450cam, D-camphor, in that it displays a micromolar dissociation constant and nearly complete conversion to the high-spin form. With respect to reactivity, it is interesting that 1,1,1,2-tetrachloroethane is a poor substrate of P-450cam (Table 1) and 1,1,2,2-tetrachloroethane is not. The steric and electronic characteristics of the P-450cam active site responsible for discriminating between these two isomers, and different halocarbons in general, presumably limit access of the substrate to a reactive conformation. Understanding the origins of these differential activities could facilitate the process engineering a novel cytochrome P-450 with a broader substrate specificity and higher catalytic efficiency for application in bioremediation.

The alteration of an enzyme active site to a predefined substrate has been a popular goal since the advent of recombinant DNA technology. Obviously, complementarity between protein and substrate dictates the specificity of the overall reaction. Equally important in the case of the cytochromes P-450, however, is the coupling of reducing equivalents into the enzyme system for the ultimate production of product. The absence of substrate-protein complementarity can lead to a variety of uncoupling reactions in which the reducing equivalents derived from pyridine nucleotide are released to superoxide, peroxide, or additional water molecules rather than to the normal oxygenase stoichiometry (Atkins and Sligar, 1987; Loida and Sligar, 1993a, 1993b) (Fig. 2). Earlier mutagenesis efforts in our laboratory have yielded a qualitative understanding of the

Table 1. Equilibrium binding constants and maximal spin conversion for P-450cam mutants with chlorinated alkanes

Substrate[a]	K_d (μM), maximum spin conversion (%) (mean ± SD)				
	Wild type	T101M	V247M	T185F	T101M-V247M-T185F
Carbon tetrachloride	160 ± 4, 49 ± 2	700 ± 140, 24 ± 1	ND[b]	ND	480 ± 180, 28 ± 2
1,1,1-Trichloroethane	300 ± 37, 46 ± 3	630 ± 68 20 ± 1	ND	ND	330 ± 56, 21 ± 2
1,1,1,2-Tetrachloroethane	150 ± 10,[c] 50	360 ± 15, 14 ± 1	155 ± 10, 45 ± 1	50 ± 3, 22 ± 2.5	240 ± 50, 20 ± 4
Pentachloroethane	10 ± 5, 68 ± 2	45 ± 12, 21 ± 4	18 ± 1, 53 ± 1	14 ± 3, 21 ± 1	61 ± 5, 29 ± 1
Camphor	1.4 ± 0.3,[d] 100	52 ± 4, 63 ± 1	3.3 ± 1,[d] 74	13 ± 2,[d] 24	74 ± 7,[d] 49 ± 1

[a]For structures, see Fig. 1.
[b]ND, not determined.
[c]From Li and Wackett (1993).
[d]From Loida and Sligar (1993a).

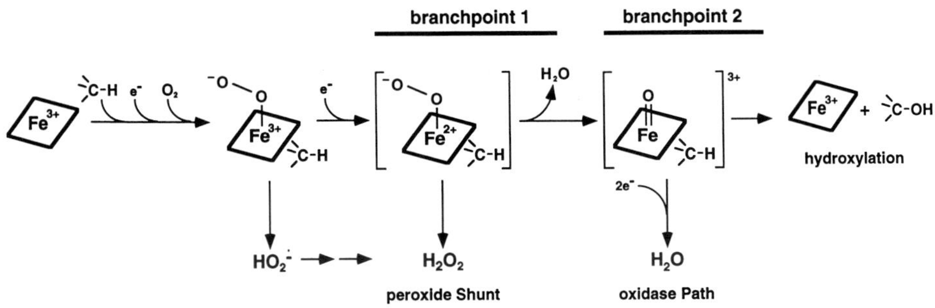

Figure 2. Branch points in the reaction cycle of the cytochromes P-450 leading to reduced oxygen products.

factors responsible for controlling the various branch points that lead to uncoupling. In the case of ethylbenzene metabolism by P-450cam, these effects can be described by reference to the enzyme active-site structure and grouping those residues which contact the substrate into tiers (Fig. 3). In this scheme, mutations in residues nearest the heme plane, tier 1, which add steric bulk, tend to lower the efficiency of product formation and increase the production of a second water molecule, essentially an oxidase activity. Conceptually, this effect could be due to an effective movement of the substrate away from

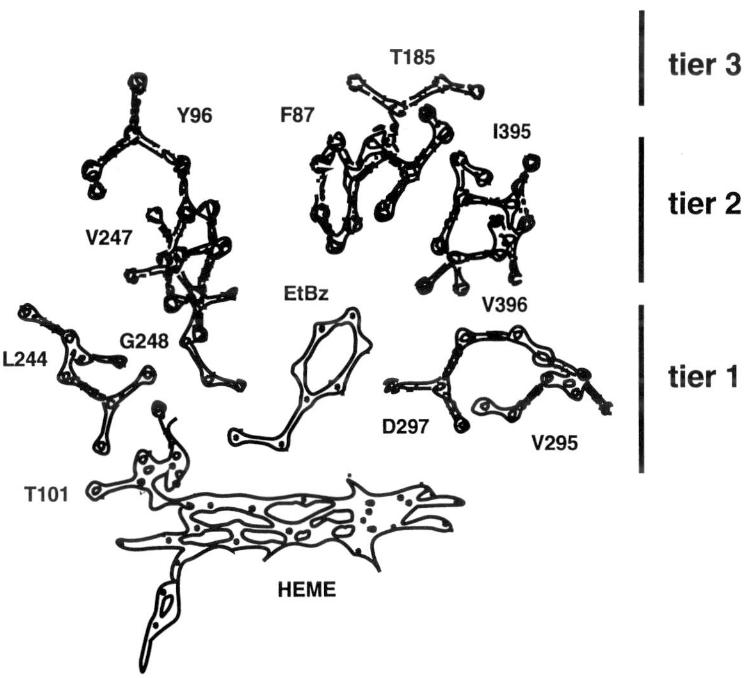

Figure 3. The active-site pocket of P-450cam as determined by the crystal structure (Poulos et al., 1985). Ethylbenzene (EtBz) is illustrated as the substrate in an energy-minimized conformation (Loida and Sligar, 1993b). The amino acid side chains lining the pocket are classified in tiers by their distances from the heme pocket (Loida and Sligar, 1993a).

the putative high-valence metal-oxo complex responsible for initiating substrate oxidation. The high-valence iron-oxo species could then decompose to water with the addition of two additional redox equivalents from the pyridine nucleotide-coupled electron transport chain. Tier 1 residues in cytochrome P-450cam include Thr-101, Leu-244, Asp-297, and Val-295. In contrast, tier 2 residues, Val-247, Val-396, Val-1395, and Phe-87, when mutated to bulkier amino acids, tend to favor product formation and decrease the loss of electrons resulting from uncoupling at the oxidase branch point (Loida et al., 1995). Residue T-185, which lies directly above the natural substrate along the Fe-camphor C5 axis (Poulos et al., 1985), constitutes tier 3; when altered to increase steric size, it decreases water production as well (Loida and Sligar, 1993a, 1993b).

Thus, the reengineering of a cytochrome P-450 for new specificity must also take into consideration the effect of active-site alteration on the total coupling of reducing equivalents to the desired product pathway. Such concerns may be even more critical in a reductive dehalogenation mode. We were interested in knowing whether the qualitative picture of tiers that rationalized the observations for oxidative ethylbenzene metabolism by P-450cam was also applicable to the reductive dehalogenation chemistry of this enzyme. Therefore, the rates of reductive dehalogenations for a series of chlorinated methanes and ethanes were determined for a set of active-site mutations of P-450cam. An obvious goal is to rationally select active-site mutations in a cytochrome P-450 which enhance catalytic efficiency of reductive dechlorinations.

For these experiments, between 20 and 40 μl of P-450cam (typically 1 mM) was exchanged into a buffer (10 mM Tris-HCl [pH 7.4], 5 mM β-mercaptoethanol) by using an equilibrated sizing column. The apparent equilibrium binding constant was determined by adding successive amounts of substrate into a septum-covered enzyme solution. Optical spectra allowed calculation of the fraction of high-spin heme induced by the addition of substrate to saturation as well as the dissociation constant for the reaction (Sligar, 1976). The rate of reductive dehalogenation of chlorinated methanes and ethanes was measured by headspace analysis of the substrate and product as a function of reaction time (Thompson et al., 1985). Typical reactions were reconstituted under anaerobic conditions in a sealed serum vial containing 50 mM Tris-HCl (pH 7.4), 0.5 mM substrate, 150 mM KCl, 1 μM putidaredoxin reductase, 5 μM putidaredoxin, and 3 μM P-450cam to a final volume of 1 ml. The reaction was initiated with NADH, and product was assayed every 2 to 6 min by headspace extraction and gas chromatography-mass spectrometry.

The apparent equilibrium binding constants of wild-type P-450cam and several mutants were determined for carbon tetrachloride, 1,1,1-trichloroethane, 1,1,1,2-tetrachloroethane, and pentachloroethane. Saturation curves were reproducible for most of the haloalkanes tested. A mutation in tier 1 (T101M) increased the dissociation constant for several haloalkanes, a mutation in tier 2 (V247M) had minor effects, and a mutation in tier 3 (T185F) decreased the dissociation constants relative to the wild type (Table 1). This trend generally follows that observed in the reaction of P-450cam with ethylbenzene (Loida and Sligar, 1993a, 1993b). Converting dissociation constants to differential binding free energies to each of these mutant classes reveals that the sum of the energy effects for each of the individual mutants is nearly equal to that of a triple mutant, T101M-V247M-T185F, suggesting that the mutations create independent perturbations of the substrate binding site. Substrate turnover by wild-type and mutant

P-450cam (Li and Wackett, 1993) was linear for all substrates and products over the relevant concentration range.

In the cytochrome P-450cam mutants described above, large hydrophobic side chains such as leucine, isoleucine, methionine, and phenylalanine have been substituted for the small nonpolar residue valine or small polar residue threonine (Loida and Sligar, 1993a, 1993b). The mutations are distributed over the surface of the active site, with two, T-101 and V-295, located near the plane of the heme and two, V-247 and T-185, positioned a longer distance from the heme group in the upper region of the binding pocket (Fig. 3). As judged from the volume of the amino acid side chains and the molecular volume of camphor, the single substitutions decrease the open volume of the P-450cam active site by 10 to 25%, with the triple mutant closing the binding pocket to nearly one-half of its original size (Raag and Poulos, 1991; Ponder and Richards, 1987).

These active-site mutants of P-450cam are effective in changing the efficiency of reductive dehalogenation, with the reaction rate correlated with the position of the mutation in the active site (Table 2). With 1,1,1,2-tetrachloroethane, amino acid substitutions in tier 2 and tier 3 result in a 150% increase in the rate of 1,1-dichloroethylene production. Mutations introducing larger bulk in tier 1 reduce the rate by fourfold. Similar but less dramatic changes are seen for these mutants in the dehalogenation reactions of pentachloroethane. These observations are also consistent with the effects seen in the hydroxylation of ethylbenzene (Loida and Sligar, 1993a, 1993b). Mutations adding bulk to the top of the pocket appear to "push" the substrate toward the heme iron and increase the probability of catalysis. Steric bulk added near the heme tends to block the access of the substrate to the iron, resulting in a slowed reaction rate. These data clearly show that the relationship between the steric constraints of the pocket and the catalytic rate of the enzyme is not confined to one substrate or reaction chemistry. We would thus predict that the efficiency of cytochrome P-450cam in both the oxidative and the reductive mode would be altered in a similar manner by changing the orientation of the substrate in the active site. While the detailed steps of P-450 catalysis are, by the nature of the reaction, very different in the absence of oxygen, these results serve to point out the similarities in the mechanisms of substrate recognition for anaerobic dehalogenation and oxidative hydroxylation. Perhaps the simplest interpretation of the data is that the site for electron transfer from the P-450cam heme to the substrate during anaerobic reductive dehalogenation is through the top face accessible to the substrate access channel.

Table 2. Dehalogenation efficiencies of P-450 mutants with chloroalkanes

Substrate[a]	k_{cat}/k_d (μM^{-1})[b]				
	Wild type	T101M	V247M	T185F	T101M-V247M-T185F
Carbon tetrachloride	0.063	0.012	ND	ND	0.020
1,1,1-Trichloroethane	NR	NR	NR	NR	NR
1,1,1,2-Tetrachloroethane	0.025	0.0027	0.042	0.12	0.046
Pentachloroethane	0.61	0.017	0.23	0.26	0.10
Camphor	860	15	ND	ND	ND

[a]For structures, see Fig. 1.
[b]ND, not determined; NR, no reaction.

Future work in the redesign of enzyme substrate specificity should be aided by a variety of computational models which have already been used to predict the interaction of P-450cam with a number of substrates (Loida et al., 1995; Harris and Loew, 1995; Fruetel et al., 1994; Chang et al., 1993; Paulsen et al., 1993). Theoretical calculations for the binding of 1,1,1-trichloroethane with this P-450 isozyme predict a nonproductive binding, with the chlorinated methyl group away from the heme iron (Paulsen and Ornstein, 1994). This may explain why none of the mutants tested in this study were able to react with this substrate. Predictions of the effects of mutation on P-450cam are beginning to emerge in the literature, and these results will be invaluable toward the goal of rational enzyme design.

Acknowledgments. We thank Aretta Weber for editorial assistance. This work was supported by grants GM 33775 and GM 31756 from the National Institutes of Health.

REFERENCES

Abelson, P. H. 1985. Chemicals from waste dumps. *Science* **229:**335.

Alhadhrami, M. N., H. M. Lappinscott, and P. J. Fisher. 1995. Bacterial survival and N-alkane degradation within omani crude oil and a mousse. *Mar. Pollut. Bull.* **30:**403–408.

Artaud, I., N. Gregoire, P. Leduc, and D. Mansuy. 1990. Formation and fate of iron-carbene complexes in reactions between a diazoalkane and iron-porphyrins: relevance to the mechanism of formation of N-substituted hemes in cytochrome P-450 dependent oxidation of sydnones. *J. Am. Chem. Soc.* **112:**6899–6905.

Atkins, W., and S. Sligar. 1987. Metabolic switching in cytochrome P-450cam: deuterium isotope effects on regiospecificity and the monoxygenase/oxidase ratio. *J. Am. Chem. Soc.* **109:**3754–3760.

Banat, I. M. 1995. Biosurfactants production and possible uses in microbial enhanced oil recovery and oil pollution remediation—a review. *Bioresource Technol.* **51:**1–12.

Brazil, G. M., L. Kenefick, M. Callanan, A. Haro, V. DeLorenzo, D. N. Dowling, and F. Ogara. 1995. Construction of a rhizosphere pseudomonad with potential to degrade polychlorinated biphenyls and detection of *bph* gene expression in the rhizosphere. *Appl. Environ. Microbiol.* **61:**1946–1952.

Castro, C. E., R. S. Wade, and N. O. Belser. 1985. Biodehalogenation: reactions of cytochrome P-450 with polyhalomethanes. *Biochemistry* **24:**204–210.

Castro, C. E., R. S. Wade, and N. O. Belser. 1988. Dehalogenation: reductive reactivities of microbial and mammalian cytochromes P-450 compared with heme and whole-cell models. *J. Agric. Food Chem.* **36:**915–919.

Chang, Y. T., G. H. Loew, A. E. Rettie, T. A. Baillie, P. R. Sheffel, and P. R. Ortiz de Montellano. 1993. Binding of flexible ligands to proteins: valproic acid and its interaction with cytochrome P450cam. *Int. J. Quantum Chem.* **20:**161–180.

Chapatwala, K. D., G. R. V. Babu, E. R. Armstead, E. M. White, and J. H. Wolfram. 1995. Bioremediation of sodium cyanide and acetonitrile by free and immobilized cells of *Pseudomonas putida. Appl. Biochem. Biotechnol.* **51:**717–726.

Davison, A. D., H. Csellner, P. Karuso, and D. A. Veal. 1994. Synergistic growth of two members from a mixed microbial consortium growing on biphenyl. *FEMS Microbiol. Ecol.* **14:**133–146.

Demnerova, K., B. Kralova, and D. L. McBeth. 1994. Introduction of biodegradative plasmids to indigenous bacteria from polluted sites in the Czech Republic. *Int. Biodeterior. Biodegrad.* **33:**311–318.

Dubey, S. K., and D. S. Holmes. 1995. Biological cyanide destruction mediated by microorganisms. *World J. Microbiol. Biotechnol.* **11:**257–265.

Feidieker, D., P. Kampfer, and W. Dott. 1994. Microbiological and chemical evaluation of a site contaminated with chlorinated aromatic compounds and hexachlorocyclohexanes. *FEMS Microbiol. Ecol.* **15:**265–278.

Fruetel, J., Y. T. Chang, J. Collins, G. Loew, and P. R. Oritiz de Montellano. 1994. Thioanisol sulfoxidation by cytochrome P450(cam) (CYP101): experimental and calculated absolute stereochemistries. *J. Am. Chem. Soc.* **116:**11643–11648.

Gorontzy, T., O. Drzyzga, M. W. Kahl, D. Brunsnagel, J. Breitung. E. Von Loew, and K. H. Blotevogel. 1994. Microbial degradation of explosives and related compounds. *Crit. Rev. Microbiol.* **20:**265–284.

Guengerich, F. P. 1990. Enzymatic oxidation of xenobiotic chemicals. *Crit. Rev. Biochem.* **25:**97–153.

Harris, D., and G. Loew. 1995. Prediction of regiospecific hydroxylation of camphor analogs by cytochrome P450(cam). *J. Am. Chem. Soc.* **117:**2738–2746.

Heipieper, H. J., F. J. Weber, J. Sikkema, H. Keweloh, and J. A. M. Debont. 1994. Mechanisms of resistance of whole cells to toxic organic solvents. *Trends Biotechnol.* **12:**409–415.

Hildebrandt, P., H. Garda, A. Stier, M. Stockburger, and R. A. Van Dyke. 1988. Resonance raman study of the cytochrome P-450_{LM} 2-halothane intermediate complex. *FEBS Lett.* **237:**15–20.

Li, S., and L. P. Wackett. 1993. Reductive dehalogenation by cytochrome P450cam: substrate binding and catalysis. *Biochemistry* **32:**9355–9361.

Loida, P. J., and S. G. Sligar. 1993a. Molecular recognition in cytochrome P-450: mechanism for the control of uncoupling reactions. *Biochemistry* **32:**11530–11538.

Loida, P. J., and S. G. Sligar. 1993b. Engineering cytochrome P-450cam to increase the stereospecificity and coupling of aliphatic hydroxylation. *Protein Eng.* **2:**207–212.

Loida, P. J., S. G. Sligar, M. D. Paulsen, G. E. Arnold, and R. L. Ornstein. 1995. Stereoselective hydroxylation of norcamphor by cytochrome P450(cam): experimental verification of molecular dynamics simulations. *J. Biol. Chem.* **270:**5326–5330.

Mansuy, D., M. Lange, J. Chottard, and P. Guerin. 1977. Reaction of carbon tetrachloride with 5,10,15,20-tetraphenylporphinatoiron (II): evidence for the formation of the carbene complex [(TPP)Fe(II)(CCl_2)]. *J. Chem. Soc. Chem. Commun.* **459:**648–649.

Mansuy, D., W. Nastainczyk, and V. Ullrich. 1974. The mechanism of halothane binding to microsomal P-450. *Arch. Pharmacol.* **285:**315–324.

Middaugh, D. P., S. E. Lantz, C. S. Heard, and J. G. Mueller. 1994. Field-scale testing of a 2-stage bioreactor for removal of creosote and pentachlorophenol from ground water—chemical and biological assessment. *Arch. Environ. Contam. Toxicol.* **26:**320–328.

Nastainczyk, W., H. R. Ahr, and V. Ullrich. 1981. The reductive metabolism of halogenated alkanes by liver microsomal cytochrome P-450. *Biochem. Pharmacol.* **31:**391–396.

Nishino, S. F., J. C. Spain, and C. A. Pettigrew. 1994. Biodegradation of chlorobenzene by indigenous bacteria. *Environ. Toxicol. Chem.* **13:**871–887.

Paulsen, M. D., D. Filipovic, S. G. Sligar, and R. L. Ornstein. 1993. Controlling the regiospecificity and coupling of cytochrome P450cam: T185F mutant increases coupling and abolishes 3-hydroxynorcamphor production. *Protein Sci.* **2:**357–365.

Paulsen, M. D., and R. L. Ornstein. 1994. Active-site mobility inhibits reductive dehalogenation of 1,1,1-trichloroethane by cytochrome P-450cam. *J. Comput. Aided Mol. Des.* **8:**389–404.

Picardal, F., R. G. Arnold, and B. B. Huey. 1995. Effects of electron donor and acceptor conditions on reductive dehalogenation of tetrachloromethane by *Shewanella putrefaciens* 200. *Appl. Environ. Microbiol.* **61:**8–12.

Ponder, J. W., and F. M. Richards. 1987. Tertiary templates for proteins. *J. Mol. Biol.* **193:**775–791.

Poulos, T. L., B. C. Finzel, I. C. Gunsalus, G. C. Wagner, and J. Kraut. 1985. The 2.6-Å crystal structure of *Pseudomonas putida* cytochrome P-450. *J. Biol. Chem.* **260:**16122–16130.

Providenti, M. A., C. W. Greer, H. Lee, and J. T. Trevors. 1995. Phenanthrene mineralization by *Pseudomonas* sp. UG14. *World J. Microbiol. Biotechnol.* **11:**271–279.

Raag, R., and T. L. Poulos. 1991. Crystal structures of cytochrome P-450cam complexed with camphane, thiocamphor, and adamantane: factors controlling P-450 substrate hydroxylation. *Biochemistry* **30:**2674–2684.

Ruf, H. H., H. Ahr, W. Nastainczyk. V. Ullrich, D. Mansuy, J. P. Battioni, R. Monteil-Montoya, and A. Trautwein. 1984. Formation of a ferric carbanion complex from halothane and cytochrome P-450: electron spin resonance, electronic spectra and model complexes. *Biochemistry* **25:**5300–5306.

Sligar, S. G. 1976. Coupling of spin, substrate, and redox equilibria in cytochrome P-450. *Biochemistry* **15:**5399–5406.

Su, J. J., and D. Kafkewitz. 1994. Utilization of toluene and xylenes by a nitrate-reducing strain of *Pseudomonas maltophilia* under low oxygen and anoxic conditions. *FEMS Microbiol. Ecol.* **15:**249–257.

Thompson, J. A., B. Ho, and S. L. Mastovich. 1985. Dynamic headspace analysis of volatile metabolites from the reductive dehalogenation of trichloro- and tetrachloroethanes by hepatic microsomes. *Anal. Biochem.* **145:**376–384.

Wackett, L. P., M. J. Sadowsky, L. M. Newman, H. Hur, and L. Shuying. 1994. Metabolism of polyhalogenated compounds by a genetically engineered bacterium. *Nature* (London) **368:**627–629.

Winkler, J., K. N. Timmis, and R. A. Snyder. 1995. Tracking the response of *Burkholderia cepacia* GA 5223-PR1 in aquifer microcosms. *Appl. Environ. Microbiol.* **61:**448–455.

Wolf, C. R., W. G. Harrelson, W. M. Nastainczyk, R. M. Philpot, B. Kalyanraman, and R. P. Mason. 1980. Metabolism of carbon tetrachloride in hepatic microsomes and reconstituted monooxygenase systems and its relationship to lipid peroxygenation. *Mol. Pharmacol.* **18:**553–558.

Section VII

CELL ENVELOPE, TRANSPORT, AND RESISTANCES

Molecular Biology of Pseudomonads
Edited by T. Nakazawa et al.

Chapter 31

Multidrug Efflux Pumps Make a Major Contribution to Drug Resistance in Pseudomonads

Hiroshi Nikaido, Haruko Okusu, Dzwokai Ma, and Xian-Zhi Li

Pseudomonads, especially fluorescent pseudomonads, are known to show high levels of intrinsic resistance to a wide variety of antibiotics and chemotherapeutic agents. The *Pseudomonas aeruginosa* outer membrane displays very low permeability coefficients toward hydrophilic solutes (about two orders of magnitude lower than those of the *Escherichia coli* outer membrane) (Angus et al., 1982; Yoshimura and Nikaido, 1982). In spite of low permeability, however, solutes equilibrate across the outer membrane relatively rapidly, in part because of the large surface-to-volume ratio in small bacterial cells. Thus the periplasmic concentrations of the more permeable cephalosporins are expected to reach 50% of the external concentration in 10 to 20 s in *P. aeruginosa* (Nikaido, 1989). Low permeability of the outer membrane, therefore, is not a complete explanation for the high intrinsic levels of resistance in *P. aeruginosa*. Clearly, additional mechanisms must exist (Nikaido, 1989). The chromosomally encoded periplasmic β-lactamases function as an additional mechanism for those β-lactam compounds that induce these enzymes and are readily hydrolyzed by them. In fact, with *E. coli,* the synergistic interaction of the outer membrane barrier and β-lactamase can quantitatively explain the levels of resistance achieved (Nikaido and Normark, 1987). However, this quantitative model does not work with at least some strains of *P. aeruginosa* (Livermore and Davy, 1991). Furthermore, no such additional contributing mechanism was known for agents other than β-lactams in most wild-type strains of *P. aeruginosa* (Nikaido, 1989). This article describes the discovery of one major mechanism, multidrug efflux pumps (Nikaido, 1994), in *P. aeruginosa,* with some reference to studies performed in other gram-negative bacteria.

Hiroshi Nikaido and Haruko Okusu • Department of Molecular and Cell Biology, University of California, Berkeley, California 94720. ***Dzwokai Ma*** • Department of Physiology, University of California, San Francisco, California 94143. ***Xian-Zhi Li*** • Department of Microbiology, University of Saskatchewan, Saskatoon, Saskatchewan, Canada S7N 0W0.

E. COLI AcrAB SYSTEM AS A MULTIDRUG EFFLUX PUMP

It has been known for several decades that the *acrA* mutation makes *E. coli* cells hypersusceptible to various dyes (e.g., acridines) and lipophilic antibiotics. Since the only mechanism that was known to alter resistance or susceptibility to a wide range of agents was the outer membrane barrier, the outer membrane of *acrA* mutants was studied in many laboratories, but no reproducible correlations were discovered. When the *acrA* gene was cloned and sequenced in a collaborative work between two laboratories (Ma et al., 1993), we found an operon consisting of *acrA* together with a downstream gene, *acrB*. AcrB belongs to a transporter family called the resistance-nodulation-division, or RND family (Saier et al., 1994). Members of this family are proteins with 12 transmembrane helices and use the proton motive force to catalyze the efflux of cations, drugs, and presumably nodulation signals. This suggested that AcrAB made *E. coli* more resistant to dyes and antibiotics by catalyzing their active efflux, rather than by decreasing passive influx through the outer membrane barrier. Similar observations were reported independently (Xu et al., 1993). Ma et al. (1993) further showed that the steady-state accumulation levels of acriflavine in *acrA*$^+$ *E. coli* cells were much lower than in the *acrA* mutant cells. This result can best be explained by assuming the presence of an active efflux process. Finally, the difference in accumulation levels completely disappeared when the presumptive pump was inhibited by the addition of a proton conductor, carbonyl cyanide *p*-chlorophenylhydrazone (CCCP) (Ma et al., 1993), a result consistent with the hypothesis that the two strains differed in the levels of efflux activity (see Fig. 1). (In retrospect, Nakamura [1966], who isolated the first *acrA* mutant, found early that the mutant had a higher steady-state accumulation level of acriflavine and that the accumulation level in the wild-type cells could be increased by starvation, by the addition of metabolic poisons, or by lowering the temperature to 0°C, but it was impossible to interpret these data at that time.) The AcrAB system appears to pump out an extremely wide range of compounds including antibiotics (such as tetracycline, chloramphenicol, penicillin, erythromycin, fluoroquinolones, fusidic acid, mitomycin C, and novobiocin), dyes (such as acriflavine, ethidium bromide, and crystal violet), and surfactants (such as sodium dodecyl sulfate, fatty acids, and bile salts) (Ma et al., 1993; Ma et al., 1995; H. Nikaido, unpublished data).

AcrA protein is a periplasmic protein anchored to the cytoplasmic membrane through its N-terminal lipid moiety (Ma et al., 1993). Its function is suggested by its sequence homology to *E. coli* HlyD, which is thought to function by bridging between the inner membrane transporter and an outer membrane channel, TolC, so that a large protein, hemolysin, can be exported directly into the medium (Wandersman and Delepelaire, 1990). Sequence comparison of AcrA and other homologs led to the establishment of the membrane fusion protein (MFP) family. Members of this family are thought to bring together an inner membrane transporter and an outer membrane channel so that transport processes can bypass the porin channels in the outer membrane. The sequence homology between the MFP family and a paramyxovirus membrane fusion protein strengthens the hypothesis that these proteins function by locally fusing two membranes together (outer and inner membranes, in the case of the MFP family proteins) (Dinh et al., 1994).

MexAB-OprM MULTIDRUG EFFLUX PUMP OF *P. AERUGINOSA*

We, as well as D. M. Livermore in London, were interested in the mechanism of resistance of carbenicillin-resistant clinical isolates of *P. aeruginosa*. Isolates from the United Kingdom did not produce plasmid-coded β-lactamase and yet were resistant to most β-lactam compounds as well as to tetracycline, chloramphenicol, novobiocin, and floroquinolones (Williams et al., 1984). Livermore and Davy (1991) showed convincingly that the outer membrane permeability of these resistant isolates is not decreased in comparison with the more susceptible isolates.

Single-step mutants exhibiting resistance to all of the drugs mentioned above were selected as spontaneous mutants (Li et al., 1994a). The drug resistance phenotype of these single-step mutants was reminiscent of that of the *nalB* mutants (Rella and Haas, 1982). When the kinetics of accumulation of antibiotics such as tetracycline, chloramphenicol, and norfloxacin was followed in clinical isolates as well as in the laboratory-isolated *nalB*-type mutant, the steady-state accumulation level was significantly lower in the strains with elevated levels of resistance (Li et al., 1994a). This observation cannot be explained by an increased exclusion by the outer membrane alone, because that would only slow down the process of accumulation and would not affect the steady-state accumulation level (Fig. 1). Moreover, when CCCP was added to deenergize the active pumping process in the cytoplasmic membrane, the low steady-state accumulation levels in the resistant strains increased to the higher levels seen in the most susceptible strains. Since CCCP did not increase the permeability of the outer membrane (Li et al., 1994a), these results can only be explained by the active efflux.

Active efflux was shown to be essential not only for the elevated resistance of the *nalB*-type mutants, but also for the intrinsic resistance of wild-type *P. aeruginosa* strains. Reminiscent of the findings with *E. coli acrA* mutants, the drug hypersusceptibility of a multistep mutant strain, *P. aeruginosa* Z61 (Zimmermann, 1980), was initially believed to be a result of elevated outer membrane permeability, but the drug accumulation assay showed that it is primarily caused by lack of active efflux processes (Li et al., 1994a).

Elevated resistance in *nalB*-type mutants could result from overproduction (or activation) of a single efflux system with a wide substrate specificity, or of many efflux systems each of which has narrow specificity. Analysis of overproduced membrane proteins showed that such mutants expressed elevated levels of MexA-MexB-OprM, products of the *mexAB-oprM* operon, characterized independently by Poole et al. (1993) as a multidrug efflux pump during study of pyoverdine-dependent iron transport. (The outer membrane protein gene, originally thought to be *oprK*, was later found to be *oprM* [Gotoh et al., 1995]). MexB is a homolog of AcrB, and thus MexB is likely to be an efflux pump driven by the proton motive force. MexA is a homolog of AcrA and thus presumably links the pump to an outer membrane channel. Most importantly, the operon contains a gene for the presumed outer membrane channel protein, OprM. This suggested that the three proteins coded for by the operon might produce a multisubunit complex traversing both the outer and the inner membranes (Fig. 2), so that the system could extrude the drug directly into the medium without its accumulation in the periplasm. In contrast, the *acrAB* operon does not contain a gene for an outer membrane channel, but such a channel coded by an unlinked gene may be shared by various efflux systems. TolC is already known to be used by more than one protein export system (Fath and Kolter, 1993) and is

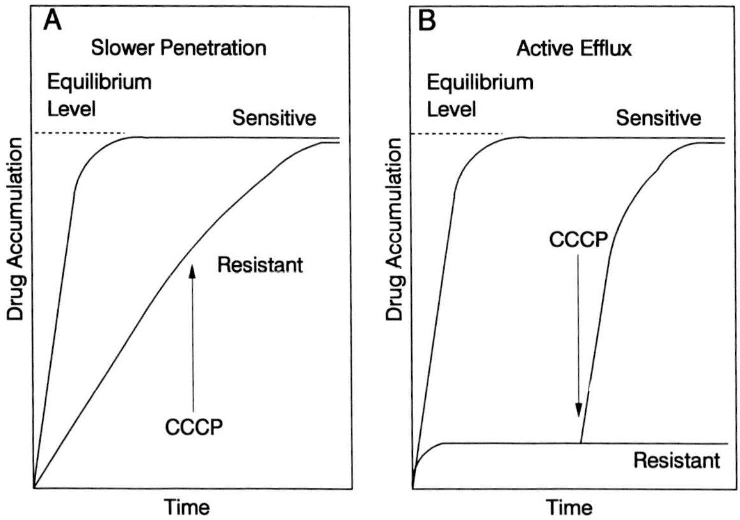

Figure 1. Expected time course of accumulation of drugs in an otherwise isogenic sensitive/resistant pair of bacterial strains. (A) Resistance is assumed to be due to increased barrier properties of the cell envelope or outer membrane. In both strains the intracellular level of the drug reaches equilibrium with the external concentration (broken line), although the attainment of equilibrium is delayed in the resistant strain. CCCP, an uncoupler of proton motive force, has no effect on the accumulation process. (B) Resistance is assumed to be due to an increased active efflux of the drug. The resistant strain will reach a steady-state concentration that is lower than in the sensitive strain. The addition of CCCP will inhibit the active efflux process, and the accumulation level in the resistant strain will reach the equilibrium level. Accumulation of chloramphenicol, tetracycline, norfloxacin, and benzylpenicillin in *P. aeruginosa* strains behaved more or less as shown in panel B (Li et al., 1994a; Li et al., 1994b).

a candidate for use by the AcrAB system. Indeed, the inactivation of *tolC* makes cells hypersusceptible to detergents, dyes, and antibiotics (Nagel de Zwaig and Luria, 1967; Davies and Reeves, 1982), most of which probably are substrates of the AcrB pump.

The involvement of the MexAB-OprM system in drug resistance was confirmed by the observation that inactivation of any of the three genes increased the steady-state accumulation levels of various drugs and converted *P. aeruginosa* into an organism more susceptible to most antibiotics than the average *E. coli* strain (Li et al., 1995). Conversely, overproduction of the MexAB-OprM system in *nalB*-type mutants elevated resistance levels to a wide variety of antibiotics, as described above (Li et al., 1994a; Li et al., 1994b; Li et al., 1995).

One surprising feature of these *nalB*-type, carbenicillin-resistant strains was their elevated resistance to β-lactams, since these agents act outside the cytoplasmic membrane and many are thought (and indeed shown experimentally [Li et al., 1994b]) not to traverse the cytoplasmic membrane. It seems likely that these agents are "grabbed" by the efflux pump before they enter the cytoplasm, possibly while they are partly inserted into the outer leaflet of the plasma membrane bilayer (Fig. 2). This mechanism is not so strange as it sounds and in fact is related to the mechanism by which the multidrug resistance

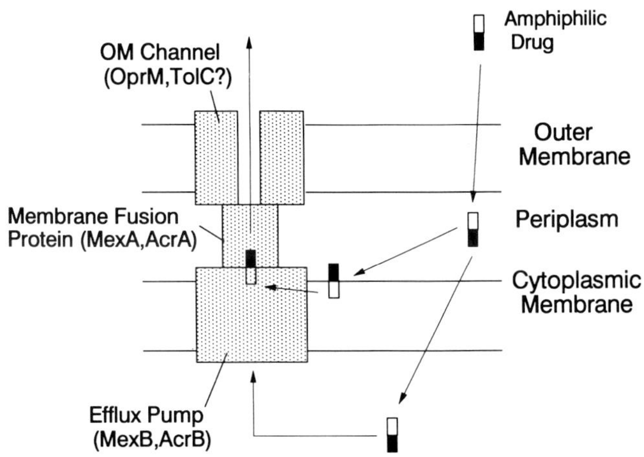

Figure 2. Model for the multidrug efflux complex in gram-negative bacteria. The RND-type chemiosmotic efflux pumps (such as AcrB or MexB) are connected to outer membrane channels (such as TolC [presumably] or OprM) by proteins that belong to the MFP family (such as AcrA or MexA). Drugs can be exported from the cytoplasm directly into the external medium. In addition, amphiphilic drugs (with the lipophilic portion shown as an empty rectangle) can be captured by the pump assembly while they are partially inserted into the outer surface of the cytoplasmic membrane; this is proposed to be the predominant pathway for the elimination of most β-lactams. Modified after Li et al. (1994a).

human P-glycoprotein captures its substrates while they are partially inserted into the bilayer, that is, before they enter the cytoplasm (Fojo et al., 1985; Homolya et al., 1993). The active efflux of β-lactams explains the resistance, which could become very highly elevated in MexAB-OprM overproducing mutants, of *P. aeruginosa* to those agents that are either poor substrates (e.g., carbenicillin or cefsulodin) or poor inducers (e.g., ceftriaxone or azlocillin) of the chromosomally encoded β-lactamase of this organism (Livermore and Yang, 1987).

SYNERGISM BETWEEN OUTER MEMBRANE BARRIER AND EFFLUX PUMPS

We have described two examples of drug hypersensitivity phenotypes, *acrA* mutants of *E. coli* and the Z61 mutant of *P. aeruginosa,* which were originally thought to be caused by the increased permeability of the outer membrane but are now thought to be caused primarily by defects in efflux pumps. This does not mean that the outer membrane barrier is not important. Because the AcrAB-(plus TolC?) and MexAB-OprM efflux machineries pump drugs directly into the medium, they become more effective if the influx is slowed by the presence of an effective outer membrane barrier. Mathematical modeling showed that, to produce identical resistance levels for tetracycline in *E. coli,* these direct-extrusion-type pumps composed of three proteins need only about 1% of the activity of a Tet-type pump, which is a single protein that is located in the inner membrane and exports the drug into the periplasm (Thanassi et al., 1995). With the less permeable outer membrane of *P. aeruginosa,* the direct-extrusion-type pumps are even more effective in producing resistance (Ma et al., 1993).

OTHER EFFLUX PUMPS

MexA-MexB-OprM is not the only multidrug efflux pump produced by *P. aeruginosa*. Masuda et al. (1995) characterized the phenotypes of single-step, multidrug-resistant mutants of *P. aeruginosa* (see Table 1). The first system shows resistance to various cephalosporins, fluoroquinolones, chloramphenicol, and tetracycline, a phenotype characteristic of the *nalB* regulatory mutants located at about 20 min on the *P. aeruginosa* chromosome (Rella and Haas, 1982). These strains overproduce OprM, and the phenotype is that shown by the MexAB-OprM overproduction mutant PAO4098E (Li et al., 1995). The second system shows a phenotype characteristic of the *nfxB* mutants that map at 4 to 8 min on the chromosome (Hirai et al., 1987), characterized by resistance to fluoroquinolones but not to conventional cephalosporins. Some *nfxB* strains are hypersusceptible to cephalosporins and some aminoglycosides. Interestingly, they appear to be more resistant to some newly introduced cephalosporins, such as cefpirome and cefozopran (Masuda et al., 1995). The resistant mutant K385 (Poole et al., 1993) shows a similar phenotype and moreover overproduces a 54-kDa outer membrane protein that was called OprK (Poole et al., 1993) or OprJ (Masuda et al., 1995). The third system shows resistance to fluoroquinolones and also to carbapenems, but not to the conventional cephalosporins, a phenotype corresponding to that of the *nfxC* mutation shown to map at 46 min on the chromosome (Fukuda et al., 1990).

The *nfxB* type strains are known, from the analysis of strain K385 (Poole et al., 1993; Li et al., 1994a), to overproduce proteins similar in size to MexA, MexB, and OprM. The outer membrane protein overproduced (OprJ) appears to share much amino acid sequence homology with OprM (Poole et al., 1993). Thus the *nfxB* mutants overproduce an efflux machinery that is probably homologous to MexAB-OprM. We provisionally call it MexCD-OprJ. Possibly the *nfxC* mutants overproduce another set of homologs that catalyze the multidrug efflux process.

Another example of the multidrug efflux pump of the RND type was found in *Neisseria gonorrhoeae*. Pan and Spratt (1994) found a gene complex, *mtr*, consisting of *mtrC* and

Table 1. Multidrug resistance in *P. aeruginosa* presumably caused by multidrug efflux process[a]

Presumed regulator	Efflux pump	Resistance[b] to: Penams/ cephems	4th-generation cephems[c]	Carba- penems	Fluoro- quinolones	Tetra- cycline	Chloram- phenicol	Gentamicin
NalB	MexA-MexB-OprM	R	U	U	R	R	R	U
NfxB	MexC-MexD-OprJ	U/S	R	U	R	R/U	R/U	U/S
NfxC	?-?-OprN	U	U	R	R	U	U	U

[a]Based on data compiled by Li et al. (1994a) and more recently by Masuda et al. (1995).

[b]R, more resistant (than in the wild type); S, more susceptible; U, unchanged.

[c]"Fourth-generation cephems" include cefpirome, cefepime, cefclidin, and cefozopran. These are the most recently developed compounds that have low affinity to chromosomally coded β-lactamases of gram-negative bacteria. This property is usually achieved by adding a bulky, positively charged group at the C-3 position of the cephem nucleus.

mtrD, which are homologs of *acrA*/*mexA* and *acrB*/*mexB*, respectively. Overexpression of these genes made the strain more resistant to several antibiotics, dyes, and surfactants (such as free fatty acids).

Many drug efflux proteins have been identified in *E. coli* (Ma et al., 1994). First, there are several homologs of AcrAB, belonging to the RND family. Second, there are transporters belonging to the major facilitator (MF) family, such as EmrB and EmrD. The *emrB* gene occurs together with a gene coding for a member of the MFP family, *emrA* (Lewis, 1994). EmrAB, when overproduced, makes *E. coli* cells more resistant to various uncouplers, some dyes, and an antibiotic, thiolactomycin (Lewis, 1994), but the disruption of these genes does not have detectable effects on the susceptibility of *E. coli* to most of the clinically significant antibiotics (Nikaido, unpublished). Finally, there is an unusually small transporter protein, EmrE (MvrC), which is predicted to span the membrane only four times. The disruption of the *emrE* gene makes *E. coli* hypersusceptible to tetraphenylphosphonium and to dyes such as methylviologen and ethidium bromide (reviewed by Lewis [1994]). The overproduction of the EmrE protein makes the strain marginally more resistant to tetracycline, erythromycin, and sulfadiazine (Yerushalmi et al., 1995). It appears, from this brief summary, that in *E. coli, P. aeruginosa,* and *N. gonorrhoeae* clinically important antibiotics are removed from cellular compartments predominantly by pumps of the RND family, although there are pumps of other families that are important in the removal of uncouplers and dyes.

EXPRESSION OF RND-FAMILY EFFLUX TRANSPORTERS

Several global regulatory systems in *E. coli,* including *marRAB* and *soxRS,* are known to affect the antibiotic resistance of the organism. MarRAB is thought to be the regulatory mechanism by which *E. coli* increases the expression of genes involved in intrinsic resistance when antibiotics are present in the environment (Cohen et al., 1993). Increase in the level of the positive activator MarA decreases the expression of the larger channel porin OmpF, thereby decreasing the drug influx, and at the same time presumably increases the expression of the drug efflux pump(s). In this context, it is interesting that *acrAB* transcription was increased by high levels of MarA (Ma et al., 1995). Furthermore, we recently found that increases in the level of MarA, caused by the inactivation of the repressor MarR, had no effect on the antibiotic resistance of a Δ*acrAB* mutant, although they increased the resistance of the *acrAB*$^+$ strain (Okusu et al., 1996). Thus the efflux through the RND-type pump AcrAB explains most of the drug resistance phenotype of *mar* mutants and Mar-mediated elevation of resistance in *E. coli.*

The transcription level of *acrAB* appears increased by other "global" regulatory signals, such as perturbation by entry into stationary phase or addition of 0.5 M NaCl or 4% ethanol to the medium (Ma et al., 1995). It also is increased by the presence of inhibitors that exist in the natural environment of *E. coli,* such as free fatty acids. These responses are mediated by regulatory proteins that remain to be identified.

In *P. aeruginosa,* mutations such as *nalB, nfxB,* and *nfxC* increase levels of resistance to multiple drugs presumably by elevating the level of transcription of genes coding for pumps. The increased expression of pump, linker, and outer membrane channel proteins is such that they can be easily detected by sodium dodecyl sulfate-polyacrylamide gel electrophoresis (Poole et al., 1993; Li et al., 1994a; Masuda et al., 1995). Alteration in the promoter region of the efflux pump genes themselves can cause such an overexpression, as shown for a multidrug-resistant Mtr strain of *N. gonorrhoeae* (Hagman and Shafer, 1995). However, in most other cases the mutations responsible for pump overexpression appear to occur in regulatory genes that are separate from the structural genes for the pumps. The sequence of the *nfxB* gene has been determined (Okazaki and Hirai, 1992). NfxB resembles the MarA/SoxS/MerR family in its small size and the position of the helix-turn-helix motif.

CONCLUSION

Active efflux has been known as a major mechanism of plasmid-coded tetracycline resistance, and the process is known to be present even in plasmid-free *E. coli* strains (Levy, 1992). However, the realization (i) that many additional pumps are multidrug efflux machineries of unexpectedly wide specificity (including even β-lactams among the substrates), (ii) that they are usually organized as multisubunit complexes spanning both the inner and the outer membranes and pump out drugs directly into the external medium, and (iii) that their expression is controlled by global regulatory mechanisms in response to general stress conditions as well as to the presence of antibiotics (through the Mar system) and of oxidants (through the Sox system) provides a novel perspective on their importance in the interaction of gram-negative bacteria with the environment (Nikaido, 1994). Mathematical modeling shows that the outer membrane barrier alone cannot produce the intrinsic resistance level found even in the wild-type strains of *P. aeruginosa,* and thus the multidrug efflux systems are essential. It seems likely that similar multidrug efflux pumps are present in practically all gram-negative bacteria and play important roles in baseline-level resistance as well as in the elevated levels of antibiotic resistance found in clinical isolates. Homologs of *acrA* and *acrB* have been found in the first complete sequence of the genome of a gram-negative bacterium, *Haemophilus influenzae* (Fleischmann et al., 1995).

Acknowledgments. We are grateful to K. Poole and D. M. Livermore for sharing results and concepts and to J. E. Hearst for enthusiastic collaboration. The experimental study in the laboratory of H.N. has been supported by a grant from the U.S. Public Health Service (AI-09644).

REFERENCES

Angus, B. L., A. M. Carey, D. A. Caron, A. M. B. Kropinski, and R. E. W. Hancock. 1982. Outer membrane permeability in *Pseudomonas aeruginosa:* comparison of a wild-type with an antibiotic-supersusceptible mutant. *Antimicrob. Agents Chemother.* **21:**299–309.

Cohen, S. P., H. Hächler, and S. B. Levy. 1993. Genetic and functional analysis of the multiple antibiotic resistance (*mar*) locus in *Escherichia coli*. *J. Bacteriol.* **176:**1484–1492.

Davies, J. K., and P. Reeves. 1992. Genetics of resistance to colicins in *Escherichia coli* K-12: cross-resistance among colicins of group A. *J. Bacteriol.* **123:**102–117.

Dinh, T., I. T. Paulsen, and M. H. Saier, Jr. 1994. A family of extracytoplasmic proteins that allow transport of large molecules across the outer membranes of gram-negative bacteria. *J. Bacteriol.* **176:**3825–3831.

Fath, M. J., and R. Kolter. 1993. ABC transporters: bacterial exporters. *Microbiol. Rev.* **57:**995–1017.

**Fleischmann, R. D., M. D. Adams, O. White, R. A. Clayton, E. F. Kirkness, A. R. Kerlavage, C. J. Bult, J. F. Tomb, B. A. Dougherty, J. M. Merrick, K. McKenney, G. Sutton, W. FitzHugh, C. Fields, J. D. Gocayne, J. Scott, R. Shirley, L.-I. Liu, A. Glodek, J. M. Kelley, J. F. Weidman, C. A. Phillips, T. Spriggs, E. Hedblom, M. D. Cotton, T. R. Utterback, M. C. Hanna, D. T. Nguyen, D. M. Saudek, R. C. Brandon, L.

D. Fine, J. L. Fritchman, J. L. Fuhrman, N. S. M. Geohagen, C. L. Gnehm, L. A. McDonald, K. V. Small, C. M. Fraser, H. O. Smith, and J. C. Venter. 1995. Whole-genome random sequencing and assembly of *Haemophilus influenzae* Rd. *Science* **269:**496–512.

Fojo, A., S. Akiyama, M. M. Gottesman, and I. Pastan. 1985. Reduced drug accumulation in multiply drug-resistant human KB carcinoma cell lines. *Cancer Res.* **45:**3002–3007.

Fukuda, H., M. Hosaka, K. Hirai, and S. Iyobe. 1990. New norfloxacin resistance gene in *Pseudomonas aeruginosa* PAO. *Antimicrob. Agents Chemother.* **34:**1757–1761.

Gotoh, N., H. Tsujimoto, K. Poole, J.-I. Yamagishi, and T. Nishino. 1995. The outer membrane protein OprM of *Pseudomonas aeruginosa* is encoded by *oprK* of the *mexA-mexB-oprK* multidrug resistance operon. *Antimicrob. Agents Chemother.* **39:**2567–2569.

Hagman, K. E., and W. M. Shafer. 1995. Transcriptional control of the *mtr* efflux system of *Neisseria gonorrhoeae*. *J. Bacteriol.* **177:**4162–4165.

Hirai, K., S. Suzue, T. Irikura, S. Iyobe, and S. Mitsuhashi. 1987. Mutations producing resistance to norfloxacin in *Pseudomonas aeruginosa*. *Antimicrob. Agents Chemother.* **31:**582–586.

Homolya, L., Z. Hollo, U. A. Germann, I. Pastan, M. M. Gottesman, and B. Sarkadi. 1993. Fluorescent cellular indicators are extruded by the multidrug resistance protein. *J. Biol. Chem.* **268:**21493–21496.

Levy, S. B. 1992. Active efflux mechanisms for antimicrobial resistance. *Antimicrob. Agents Chemother.* **36:**695–703.

Lewis, K. 1994. Multidrug resistance pumps in bacteria: variations on a theme. *Trends Biochem. Sci.* **19:**119–123.

Li, X.-Z., D. M. Livermore, and H. Nikaido. 1994a. Role of efflux pump(s) in intrinsic resistance of *Pseudomonas aeruginosa:* resistance to tetracycline, chloramphenicol, and norfloxacin. *Antimicrob. Agents Chemother.* **38:**1732–1741.

Li, X.-Z., D. Ma, D. M. Livermore, and H. Nikaido. 1994b. Role of efflux pump(s) in intrinsic resistance of *Pseudomonas aeruginosa:* active efflux as a contributing factor to β-lactam resistance. *Antimicrob. Agents Chemother.* **38:**1742–1752.

Li, X.-Z., H. Nikaido, and K. Poole. 1995. The role of MexA-MexB-OprM in antibiotic efflux in *Pseudomonas aeruginosa*. *Antimicrob. Agents Chemother.* **39:**1948–1953.

Livermore, D. M., and K. W. M. Davy. 1991. Invalidity for *Pseudomonas aeruginosa* of an accepted model of bacterial permeability to β-lactam antibiotics. *Antimicrob. Agents Chemother.* **35:**916–921.

Livermore, D. M., and Y.-J. Yang. 1987. β-Lactamase lability and inducer power of newer β-lactam antibiotics in relation to their activity against β-lactamase-inducibility mutants of *Pseudomonas aeruginosa*. *J. Infect. Dis.* **155:**775–782.

Ma, D., D. N. Cook, M. Alberti, N. G. Pon, H. Nikaido, and J. E. Hearst. 1993. Molecular cloning and characterization of *acrA* and *acrE* genes of *Escherichia coli*. *J. Bacteriol.* **175:**6299–6313.

Ma, D., D. N. Cook, M. Alberti, N. G. Pon, H. Nikaido, and J. E. Hearst. 1995. Genes *acrA* and *acrB* encode a stress-induced efflux system of *Escherichia coli*. *Mol. Microbiol.* **16:**45–55.

Ma, D., D. N. Cook, J. E. Hearst, and H. Nikaido. 1994. Efflux pumps and drug resistance in Gram-negative bacteria. *Trends Microbiol.* **2:**489–493.

Masuda, N., E. Sakagawa, and S. Ohya. 1995. Outer membrane proteins responsible for multiple drug resistance in *Pseudomonas aeruginosa*. *Antimicrob. Agents Chemother.* **39:**645–649.

Nagel de Zwaig, R., and S. E. Luria. 1967. Genetics and physiology of colicin-tolerant mutants of *Escherichia coli*. *J. Bacteriol.* **94:**1112–1123.

Nakamura, H. 1966. Acriflavine-binding capacity of *Escherichia coli* in relation to acriflavine sensitivity and metabolic activity. *J. Bacteriol.* **92:**1447–1452.

Nikaido, H. 1989. Outer membrane barrier as a mechanism of antimicrobial resistance. *Antimicrob. Agents Chemother.* **33:**1831–1836.

Nikaido, H. 1994. Prevention of drug access to bacterial targets: role of permeability barriers and active efflux. *Science* **264:**382–388.

Nikaido, H., and S. Normark. 1987. Sensitivity of *Escherichia coli* to various β-lactams is determined by the interplay of outer membrane permeability and degradation by periplasmic β-lactamases: a quantitative predictive treatment. *Mol. Microbiol.* **1:**29–36.

Okazaki, T., and K. Hirai. 1992. Cloning and nucleotide sequence of the *Pseudomonas aeruginosa nfxB* gene, conferring resistance to new quinolones. *FEMS Microbiol. Lett.* **97:**197–202.

Okusu, H., D. Ma, and H. Nikaido. 1996. AcrAB efflux pump plays a major role in the antibiotic resistance phenotype of *Escherichia coli* Mar mutants. *J. Bacteriol.* **178:**306–308.

Pan, W., and B. G. Spratt. 1994. Regulation of the permeability of the gonococcal cell envelope by the mtr system. *Mol. Microbiol.* **11:**769–775.

Poole, K., K. Krebes, C. McNally, and S. Neshat. 1993. Multiple antibiotic resistance in *Pseudomonas aeruginosa:* evidence for involvement of an efflux operon. *J. Bacteriol.* **175:**7363–7372.

Rella, M., and D. Haas. 1982. Resistance of *Pseudomonas aeruginosa* PAO to nalidixic acid and low levels of β-lactam antibiotics: mapping of chromosomal genes. *Antimicrob. Agents Chemother.* **22:**242–249.

Saier, M. H., Jr., R. Tam, A. Reizer, and J. Reizer. 1994. Two novel families of bacterial membrane proteins concerned with nodulation, cell division and transport. *Mol. Microbiol.* **11:**841–847.

Thanassi, D. G., G. S. B. Suh, and H. Nikaido. 1995. Role of outer membrane barrier in efflux-mediated tetracycline resistance of *Escherichia coli. J. Bacteriol.* **177:**998–1007.

Wandersman, C., and P. Delepelaire. 1990. TolC, an *Escherichia coli* outer membrane protein required for hemolysin secretion. *Proc. Natl. Acad. Sci USA* **87:**4776–4780.

Williams, R. J., D. M. Livermore, M. A. Lindridge, A. A. Said, and J. D. Williams. 1984. Mechanism of beta-lactam resistance in British isolates of *Pseudomonas aeruginosa. J. Med. Microbiol.* **17:**283–293.

Xu, J., M. L. Nilles, and K. P. Bertrand. 1993. The *Escherichia coli acrAB* and *acrEF* genes: a new family of multidrug efflux pumps. Abstr. K-169, p. 290. *Abstr. Gen. Meet. Am. Soc. Microbiol. 1993.*

Yerushalmi, H., M. Lebendiker, and S. Schuldiner. 1995. EmrE, an *Escherichia coli* 12-kDa multidrug transporter, exchanges toxic cations and H^+ and is soluble in organic solvents. *J. Biol. Chem.* **270:**6856–6863.

Yosimura, F., and H. Nikaido. 1982. Permeability of *Pseudomonas aeruginosa* outer membrane to hydrophilic solutes. *J. Bacteriol.* **152:**636–642.

Zimmermann, W. 1980. Penetration of β-lactam antibiotics into their target enzymes in *Pseudomonas aeruginosa:* comparison of a highly sensitive mutant with its parent strain. *Antimicrob. Agents Chemother.* **18:**94–100.

Molecular Biology of Pseudomonads
Edited by T. Nakazawa et al.

Chapter 32

Protein D2, a Multifunctional Channel-Forming Outer Membrane Protein of *Pseudomonas aeruginosa*

Taiji Nakae, Eisaku Yoshihara, Hiroshi Yoneyama, and Junko Ishii

High and broad antibiotic resistance of *Pseudomonas aeruginosa* is a major problem in hospitals. The cause of this antibiotic resistance is attributed largely to low outer membrane permeability, production of antibiotic-modifying enzymes, and more recently active drug efflux. An antibiotic-modifying enzyme, such as β-lactamase, confers resistance against only antibiotics with structural similarities. Antibiotic resistance due to low outer membrane permeability or high efflux appears to be broad and exhibits low stereochemical discrimination of antibiotics. Low outer membrane permeability is most likely attributable to lack of porins with a large pore (Caulcott et al., 1984; Yoneyama et al., 1986; Yoneyama and Nakae, 1986). In other words, the *P. aeruginosa* porins predominantly form small pores that exclude most bulky antibiotics. Alternatively, it was reported that the outer membrane of *P. aeruginosa* contains a large pore-forming porin, but diffusion through this porin is very inefficient (Bellido et al., 1992; Nikaido et al., 1991; Benz and Hancock, 1981; Hancock and Nikaido, 1978). Among these, involvement in antibiotic diffusion has been demonstrated only for the *P. aeruginosa* porin, protein D2. This short review focuses on the structure and functions of protein D2.

GENERAL PROPERTIES OF PROTEIN D2

Protein D2 is an outer membrane protein that was found to have apparent M_rs of 36,000 and 46,000 in a sodium dodecyl sulfate (SDS)-polyacrylamide gel electrophoretogram when the protein was solubilized at 25 and 95°C, respectively (Yoshihara et al., 1991). This result suggests that the protein retains a native conformation at 25°C in SDS. Protein D2 appeared to exist as trimeric aggregates in the native outer membrane, in the reconstituted liposome membranes, and in a solution containing a nonionic surfactant, as demonstrated by chemical cross-linking and light scattering experiments (Yoshihara et

Taiji Nakae, Eisaku Yoshihara, Hiroshi Yoneyama, and Junko Ishii • The Department of Molecular Life Science, Tokai University School of Medicine, Isehara 259-11, Japan.

al., 1991). Native protein D2 showed a β-strand-rich conformation as generally observed in many other porins (E. Yoshihara and T. Nakae, unpublished data). The protein disaggregates into monomers in SDS solution at concentrations above 0.1%, and the trimers readily reassemble upon dilution of SDS to concentrations below 0.1% with a solution containing a nonionic surfactant or upon reconstitution into liposome membranes. Reassembled protein D2 forms a channel that is indistinguishable in solute diffusion from that of native protein D2 trimers.

When protein D2 was subjected to mild trypsin treatment, native 46,000-molecular-weight (46K) protein was cleaved into two domains with apparent M_rs of 27,000 and 19,000 (Yoshihara and Nakae, 1992). The 27K domain was responsible for channel formation. Protein D2 exhibited two single-channel conductances in planar lipid bilayers; these were 30 and 400 pS in 1 M NaCl when membranes were reconstituted from only phosphatidylcholine and phosphatidylcholine plus lipopolysaccharide (LPS), respectively (Ishii and Nakae, 1993). The protein seems to have calcium binding sites, and binding of calcium may affect the efficiency of the channel (Yoshihara and Nakae, 1993). A protein D2 structure was predicted to have 16 β-strands in analyses using multiple alignments, structural prediction, and amphipathic calculations (Huang et al., 1995). The proposed model has seven short loops at the periplasmic side and eight longer loops at the cell surface. Deletion mutations were inserted into proposed loop 1 (L1), L2, L5, and L7, and the strains were tested for imipenem susceptibility. Only a mutant having a deletion at L2 was found to be partially imipenem resistant in an *oprD*::Ω background. Data suggested a possible involvement of L2 in imipenem recognition. This L2 coincided with a trypsin-susceptible site.

The gene encoding protein D2, *oprD,* was cloned and sequenced (Yoneyama and Nakae, 1991; Yoneyama et al., 1992; Huang et al., 1992). An open reading frame contained a 1,332-bp sequence encoding 443 amino acid residues. Mature protein D2 consisted of 420 amino acid residues corresponding to an M_r of 46,016. The amino acid sequence showed low overall homology to the *Escherichia coli* porin OmpF or OmpC but high homology to another *P. aeruginosa* porin, OprE1. The protein D2-defective mutant was 8 to 32 times more resistant to imipenem than the protein D2-positive counterpart (Büscher et al., 1987; Lynch et al., 1987; Quinn et al., 1986; Satake et al., 1991), and the imipenem susceptibility was fully restored by transformation of the plasmid-borne *oprD* into the protein D2-deficient strain (Yoneyama and Nakae, 1991).

THE ROLE OF PORINS IN ANTIBIOTIC DIFFUSION

Among the outer membrane proteins of *P. aeruginosa,* proteins C, D2, and E1 are porins that form small diffusion pores (Yoshihara and Nakae, 1989). Protein F was reported to be the porin forming a large but inefficient pore (Bellido et al., 1992; Nikaido et al., 1991; Benz and Hancock, 1981; Hancock and Nikaido, 1978). The role of these porins in antibiotic susceptibility was tested by introducing genetically defined deletion mutations into the wild-type strain PAO1 chromosomal porin genes by means of a gene replacement technique or by selecting for imipenem resistance and determining the MICs of antibiotics (Yoneyama et al., 1995). Mutants having a deletion in either one of these porin genes or mutants having multiple deletion mutations in all possible combinations of these genes exhibited MICs of fluoroquinolones, chloramphenicol, tetracycline, and most β-lactam antibiotics (except for carbapenem susceptibility in the protein D2 deletion mutants) that were fully comparable with those of the wild-type strain (Table 1). MICs of all antibiotics so far tested in the protein F deletion strains were identical to those for their parents (Gotoh et al., 1989). These results indicate that all of the porins identified so far play a small role, if any, in the diffusion of antibiotics across the outer membrane of *P. aeruginosa,* except for the permeation of carbapenems through the protein D2 channel.

Protein D2 was lacking in a clinically isolated strain of *P. aeruginosa* obtained from patients for whom imipenem therapy was unsuccessful (Büscher et al., 1987; Lynch et al., 1987; Quinn et al., 1986; Satake et al., 1991). In vitro selection of imipenem-resistant mutants from several strains resulted in the deletion of protein D2 (Huang and Hancock, 1993; Satake et al., 1991; Trias et al., 1989). These imipenem-resistant mutants showed unaltered susceptibility toward most other antibiotics. Some fluoroquinolone-resistant mutants lacked protein D2 and became cross-resistant to imipenem (Fukuda et al., 1990; Michéa-Hamzehpour et al., 1987; Rådberg et al., 1990). Accordingly, it was assumed that protein D2 specifically facilitates the diffusion of carbapenem. However, a newly synthesized carbapenem, BMS-181139, seems to diffuse through the outer membrane mainly via a non-protein D2 pathway (Fung-Tomc et al., 1995). To test the solute selectivity of protein D2, purified protein D2 was reconstituted into liposome membranes and the diffusion of various solutes was tested. It was found in the liposome swelling assay that the diffusion rate of carbapenem was the highest among the antibiotics tested (Satake et al., 1990; Studemeister and Quinn, 1988; Trias and Nikaido, 1990a).

SOLUTE SELECTIVITY OF PROTEIN D2

Because of the cationic nature of imipenem at neutral pH and the high probability that the drug has structural resemblance to basic amino acids, interference with imipenem permeability by various amino acids was determined in intact cells. It was found that basic amino acids, such as lysine and arginine, competed with imipenem permeability with K_i values of about 0.6 mM (Trias and Nikaido, 1990b). Interestingly, basic amino acids with the D-configuration exhibited lower K_i values than those with the L-configuration. The K_d values of L-lysine and L-arginine for highly purified protein D2 appeared to be 0.23 and 0.06 mM, respectively, as determined by the equilibrium dialysis method (Table 2) (Yoshihara and Nakae, unpublished data).

The MIC of imipenem determined in Mueller-Hinton agar appeared to be 0.78 μg/ml, while that determined in minimal salt medium was 0.2 μg/ml (Fukuoka et al., 1991; Fukoka et al., 1993). This result was interpreted as meaning that the basic amino acids in Mueller-Hinton agar inhibited imipenem diffusion. In fact, when 50 mM L-lysine was added to minimum salt medium, the MIC of imipenem increased to a level eightfold higher than that in Mueller-Hinton agar (Fukuoka et al., 1991). Thus, it was concluded that imipenem and basic amino acids compete for diffusion through the protein D2 channel. Involvement of L2 in imipenem recognition was proposed by Huang et al. (1995).

To address the question of why the imipenem-resistant strains efficiently eliminate protein D2, the following experiments were performed. A plasmid with cloned *oprD* was transformed into the *P. aeruginosa* host TNP031, which produces an undetectable level of chromosomally encoded protein D2. Next, the imipenem-resistant mutants were se-

Table 1. Antibiotic susceptibilities of porin gene deletion mutants of *P. aeruginosa*[a]

Strain	Phenotype	MIC (μg/ml)									
		CAZ	CFS	LMOX	IPM	MPM	CBPC	OFLX	TFLX	CP	GM
PAO1	Wild type	0.78	1.56	12.5	0.78	0.39	25	0.78	0.2	25	1.56
TNP064	$OprC^-$	1.56	1.56	12.5	0.78	0.39	50	0.78	0.2	50	0.78
TNP004	$OprD^-$	1.56	1.56	12.5	12.5	3.13	50	0.78	0.2	50	3.13
YY100	$OprE^-$	1.56	1.56	12.5	0.78	0.39	25	0.78	0.2	25	1.56
TNP065	$OprC^-$ $OprD^-$	1.56	1.56	12.5	12.5	1.56	25	0.78	0.2	50	0.78
TNP066	$OprC^-$ $OprE^-$	1.56	3.13	12.5	0.78	0.39	50	0.78	0.2	25	1.56
YY200	$OprD^-$ $OprE^-$	1.56	1.56	12.5	12.5	3.13	50	0.78	0.2	25	1.56
TNP067	$OprC^-$ $OprD^-$ $OprE^-$	1.56	1.56	12.5	12.5	3.13	50	0.78	0.2	25	1.56
PAO2354[b]	$OprF^+$	0.78	0.78	12.5	0.78		6.25	0.78		100	0.78
KG1079[b]	$OprF^-$	0.39	0.78	6.25	0.78		6.25	0.39		50	0.39

[a]From Yoneyama et al., 1995, except as noted otherwise. Abbreviations: CAZ, ceftazidime; CFS, cefsulodin; LMOX, latamoxef; IPM, imipenem; MPM, meropenem; CBPC, carbenicillin; OFLX, ofloxacin; TFLX, tosfloxacin; CP, chloramphenicol; GM, gentamicin.

[b]From Gotoh et al., 1989.

Table 2. Interaction of protein D2 with ligands

Ligand	Equilibrium dialysis (K_d) (μM)	Membrane bilayer (K_d) (μM)[a]	Competition with imipenem (K_i) (μM)[b]	MIC (M)
D-Lysine	90		300	
L-Lysine	230		600	
L-Arginine	60	32,000		
Imipenem		630		2.6
DX8739		350		1.4
Ofloxacin		770		2.2

[a]From Ishii and Nakae, 1996.
[b]From Trias and Nikaido, 1990b.

lected from the partial diploid cells (Yoneyama and Nakae, 1993). All of the mutants selected were devoid of protein D2 despite the fact that they harbored the plasmid, suggesting that the plasmid-borne *oprD* had acquired a mutation. Nucleotide sequencing of these plasmids revealed that all of the *oprD* genes had deletion mutations (Yoneyama and Nakae, 1993); one type was a 12-bp deletion in the coding region generating a frameshift and a nonsense codon, and another type had a large deletion including the region upstream of *oprD*, the *oprD* promoter, and the coding region. Neither type of mutant produced detectable protein D2.

GATING ACTIVITY OF THE PROTEIN D2 CHANNEL

When trypsin-digested protein D2 was subjected to the permeability assay, its permeability was found to be roughly 10 times higher than that of native protein D2, without any effect on its apparent pore size (Yoshihara and Nakae, 1992). The 27K domain was identified as responsible for the channel formation. This result was interpreted to mean that protein D2 is equipped with the channel and gate and that they are located in separate domains.

When highly purified intact protein D2 was incorporated into a planar lipid bilayer of phosphatidylcholine, stepwise conductance increments of 30 pS in 1 M NaCl were recorded (Ishii and Nakae, 1993). This channel size barely allows the passage even of pentoses. When the protein was incorporated into a lipid bilayer consisting of phosphatidylcholine and deep rough LPS, the conductance level increased to 400 pS in 1 M NaCl (Ishii and Nakae, 1993). These results were interpreted to indicate that conductances of 30 and 400 pS represented the closed and open states, respectively, of the protein D2 channel. The channels opened more frequently as a negative potential was applied at the *cis* chamber to which the probe was immersed and closed when a positive potential was applied (Ishii and Nakae, 1993).

EFFECTS OF ANTIBIOTICS ON THE SINGLE-CHANNEL CONDUCTANCE OF PROTEIN D2

The effects of carbapenems and fluoroquinolones on the channel activity of protein D2 were investigated by adding the ligands into the subphases of the bathing solution of planar lipid bilayers with reconstituted protein D2. Carbapenems at concentrations in the range of 0.7 to 0.8 mM began to lower the probability of channel opening and the level of channel conductance, and a carbapenem concentration of 3 mM caused total closure of all open channels (Table 2) (Ishii and Nakae, 1996). Fluoroquinolones such as ofloxacin, levofloxacin, and ciprofloxacin exhibited a similar effect in the concentration range of 1 to 3 mM (Table 2) (Ishii and Nakae, 1996). The latter observation answers the question of why some of the fluoroquinolone-resistant strains lacked protein D2 but does not answer the question of why imipenem-selected protein D2-defective strains remain fluoroquinolone susceptible. Since protein D2-independent permeation of a carbapenem was reported (Fung-Tomc et al., 1995), it is likely that this carbapenem mainly diffuses through the same pathway as do fluoroquinolones. Other antibiotics, including ampicillin, piperacillin, latamoxef, and tetracycline, showed no detectable effect on channel activity. When similar experiments were conducted in the presence of lysine or arginine, the concentrations of these amino acids required to shut down the protein D2 channel completely appeared to be 50 mM. Net neutral or acidic amino acids exerted no detectable effect on the channel activity at concentrations of 50 mM or less.

ENZYMATIC ACTIVITY OF PROTEIN D2

The notion emerged that protein D2 may have a serine protease-like property, since it seems to have an affinity toward basic amino acids. When highly purified protein D2 was incubated with synthetic protease substrates, the hydrolysis of substrates was observed (Table 3) (Yoshihara et al., submitted for publication). Protein D2 hydrolyzed peptides containing arginine or lysine residues, and the K_m of protein D2 for BOC-Gln-Ala-Arg-MCA (*tert*-butoxycarbonyl–Gln–Ala–Arg–7-amino-4-methylcoumarin) appeared to be 9×10^{-6} M. However, the K_{cat} value was very low, 8×10^{-6} s^{-1}. A specific serine protease inhibitor, diisopropyl fluorophosphate (DFP), at the concentration of 1 mM at 37°C for 60 min completely inactivated the enzyme activity, and [^{3}H]DFP specifically

Table 3. Proteolytic activities of protein D2 toward various synthetic substrates[a]

Substrate[b]	Relative rate
Bz-Arg-MCA	57
Bz-Arg-Arg-MCA	7
BOC-Gln-Ala-Arg-MCA	100[c]
BOC-Gln-Arg-Arg-MCA	11
BOC-Glu(OBzl)-Ala-Arg-MCA	60
BOC-Gln-Gly-Arg-MCA	97
Z-Phe-Arg-MCA	42
BOC-Val-Leu-Lys-MCA	24
Suc-Ala-Ala-Pro-Phe-MCA	0
Suc-Ala-Pro-Ala-MCA	3
Suc-Ala-Ala-Pro-Val-MCA	0

[a]From Yoshihara and Nakae, submitted for publication.

[b]Bz, benzoyl; OBzl, γ-benzyl; Z, carbobenzoxy.

[c]The proteolytic activity toward BOC-Gln-Ala-Arg-MCA was 1.1×10^{-5} μmol/min/mg of protein at 37°C in 5 mM $C_{12}E_8$ (octaethyleneglycol dodecylether)–10 mM *N*-2-hydroxyethylpiperazine-*N*-2-ethanesulfonic acid (HEPES; pH 7.5).

and covalently modified protein D2, as analyzed by fluorography of the SDS-polyacrylamide gel electrophoretogram of protein D2 incubated with [^{3}H]DFP. Furthermore, monoclonal antibodies raised against protein D2 inhibited the protease activity. Although the protease activity of protein D2 was firmly established, the specific role of protease remains to be elucidated.

As has been described throughout this chapter, protein D2 of *P. aeruginosa* is multifunctional. The most prominent property is the channel function, which exhibited frequent opening and closing. The channel-forming domain could be separated from the gate-forming domain by simple trypsin treatment, resulting in elevated channel activity. Protein D2 facilitates the diffusion of carbapenem antibiotics and possibly that of peptides containing basic amino acids. Protein D2 exhibited protease activity, suggesting that it may cleave off peptides containing basic amino acids. Thus, it is likely that the specificity of protein D2 toward basic amino acids is derived from its protease function.

REFERENCES

Bellido, F., N. L. Martin, R. J. Siehnel, and R. E. W. Hancock. 1992. Reevaluation, using intact cells, of the exclusion limit and role of porin OprF in *Pseudomonas aeruginosa* outer membrane permeability. *J. Bacteriol.* **174:**5196–5203.

Benz, R., and R. E. W. Hancock. 1981. Properties of the large ion-permeable pores formed from protein F of *Pseudomonas aeruginosa* in lipid bilayer membranes. *Biochim. Biophys. Acta* **646:**298–308.

Büscher, K.-H., W. Cullmann, W. Dick, and W. Opferkuch. 1987. Imipenem resistance in *Pseudomonas aeruginosa* resulting from diminished expression of an outer membrane protein. *Antimicrob. Agents Chemother.* **31:**703–708.

Caulcott, C. A., M. R. W. Brown, and I. Gonda. 1984. Evidence for small pores in the outer membrane of *Pseudomonas aeruginosa. FEMS Microbiol. Lett.* **21:**119–123.

Fukuda, H., M. Hosaka, K. Hirai, and S. Iyobe. 1990. New norfloxacin resistance gene in *Pseudomonas aeruginosa* PAO. *Antimicrob. Agents Chemother.* **34:**1757–1761.

Fukuoka, T., N. Masuda, T. Takenouchi, N. Sekine, M. Iijima, and S. Ohya. 1991. Increase in susceptibility of *Pseudomonas aeruginosa* to carbapenem antibiotics in low-amino-acid media. *Antimicrob. Agents Chemother.* **35:**529–532.

Fukuoka, T., S. Ohya, T. Narita, M. Katsuta, M. Iijima, N. Masuda, H. Yasuda, J. Trias, and H. Nikaido. 1993. Activity of the carbapenem panipenem and role of the OprD (D2) protein in its diffusion through the *Pseudomonas aeruginosa* outer membrane. *Antimicrob. Agents Chemother.* **37:**322–327.

Fung-Tomc, J. C., E. Gradelski, B. Kolek, B. Minassian, M. Pucci, R. E. Kessler, and D. P. Bonner. 1995. Activity of carbapenem BMS-181139 against *Pseudomonas aeruginosa* is not dependent on porin protein D2. *Antimicrob. Agents Chemother.* **39:**386–393.

Gotoh, N., H. Wakebe, E. Yoshihara, T. Nakae, and T. Nishino. 1989. Role of protein F in maintaining structural integrity of the *Pseudomonas aeruginosa* outer membrane. *J. Bacteriol.* **171:**983–990.

Hancock, R. E. W., and H. Nikaido. 1978. Outer membranes of gram-negative bacteria. XIX. Isolation from *Pseudomonas aeruginosa* PAO1 and use in reconstitution and definition of the permeability barrier. *J. Bacteriol.* **136:**381–390.

Huang, H., and R. E. W. Hancock. 1993. Genetic definition of the substrate selectivity of outer membrane porin protein OprD of *Pseudomonas aeruginosa. J. Bacteriol.* **175:**7793–7800.

Huang, H., D. Jeanteur, F. Pattus, and R. E. W. Hancock. 1995. Membrane topology and site-specific mutagenesis of *Pseudomonas aeruginosa* porin OprD. *Mol. Microbiol.* **16:**931–941.

Huang, H., R. J. Siehnel, F. Bellido, E. Rawling, and R. E. W. Hancock. 1992. Analysis of two gene regions involved in the expression of the imipenem-specific, outer membrane porin protein OprD of *Pseudomonas aeruginosa. FEMS Microb. Lett.* **97:**267–274.

Ishii, J., and T. Nakae. 1993. Lipopolysaccharide promoted opening of the porin channel. *FEBS Lett.* **320:**251–255.

Ishii, J., and T. Nakae. 1996. Specific interaction of the protein-D2 porin of *Pseudomonas aeruginosa* with antibiotics. *FEMS Microbiol. Lett.* **136:**85–90.

Lynch, M. J., G. L. Drusano, and H. L. T. Mobley. 1987. Emergence of resistance to imipenem in *Pseudomonas aeruginosa. Antimicrob. Agents Chemother.* **31:**1892–1896.

Michéa-Hamzehpour, M., P. Auckenthaler, P. Regamey, and J.-C. Pechère. 1987. Resistance occurring after fluoroquinolone therapy of experimental *Pseudomonas aeruginosa* peritonitis. *Antimicrob. Agents Chemother.* **31:**1803–1808.

Nikaido, H., K. Nikaido, and S. Harayama. 1991. Identification and characterization of porins in *Pseudomonas aeruginosa. J. Biol. Chem.* **266:**770–779.

Quinn, J. P., E. J. Dudek, C. A. DiVincenzo, D. A. Lucks, and S. A. Lerner. 1986. Emergence of resistance to imipenem during therapy for *Pseudomonas aeruginosa* infections. *J. Infect. Dis.* **154:**289–294.

Rådberg, G., L. E. Nilsson, and S. Svensson. 1990. Development of quinolone-imipenem cross resistance in *Pseudomonas aeruginosa* during exposure to ciprofloxacin. *Antimicrob. Agents Chemother.* **34:**2142–2147.

Satake, S., H. Yoneyama, and T. Nakae. 1991. Role of OmpD2 and chromosomal β-lactamase in carbapenem resistance in clinical isolates of *Pseudomonas aeruginosa. J. Antimicrob. Chemother.* **28:**199–207.

Satake, S., E. Yoshihara, and T. Nakae. 1990. Diffusion of β-lactam antibiotics through liposome membranes reconstituted from purified porins of the outer membrane of *Pseudomonas aeruginosa. Antimicrob. Agents Chemother.* **34:**685–690.

Studemeister, A. E., and J. P. Quinn. 1988. Selective imipenem resistance in *Pseudomonas aeruginosa* associated with diminished outer membrane permeability. *Antimicrob. Agents Chemother.* **32:**1267–1268.

Trias, J., J. Dufresne, R. C. Levesque, and H. Nikaido. 1989. Decreased outer membrane permeability in imipenem-resistant mutants of *Pseudomonas aeruginosa. Antimicrob. Agents Chemother.* **33:**1201–1206.

Trias, J., and H. Nikaido. 1990a. Outer membrane protein D2 catalyzes facilitated diffusion of carbapenems and penems through the outer membrane of *Pseudomonas aeruginosa. Antimicrob. Agents Chemother.* **34:**52–57.

Trias, J., and H. Nikaido. 1990b. Protein D2 channel of the *Pseudomonas aeruginosa* outer membrane has a binding site for basic amino acids and peptides. *J. Biol. Chem.* **265:**15680–15684.

Yoneyama, H., A. Akatsuka, and T. Nakae. 1986. The outer membrane of *Pseudomonas aeruginosa* is a barrier against the penetration of disaccharides. *Biochem. Biophys. Res. Commun.* **134:**106–112.

Yoneyama, H., and T. Nakae. 1986. A small diffusion pore in the outer membrane of *Pseudomonas aeruginosa. Eur. J. Biochem.* **157:**33–38.

Yoneyama, H., and T. Nakae. 1991. Cloning of the protein D2 gene of *Pseudomonas aeruginosa* and its functional expression in the imipenem-resistant host. *FEBS Lett.* **283:**177–179.

Yoneyama, H., and T. Nakae. 1993. Mechanism of efficient elimination of protein D2 in outer membrane of imipenem-resistant *Pseudomonas aeruginosa. Antimicrob. Agents Chemother.* **37:**2385–2390.

Yoneyama, H., Y. Yamano, and T. Nakae. 1995. Role of porins in the antibiotic susceptibility of *Pseudomonas aeruginosa:* construction of the mutants having deletions in the multiple porin genes. *Biochem. Biophys. Res. Commun.,* **210:**356–362.

Yoneyama, H., E. Yoshihara, and T. Nakae. 1992. Nucleotide sequence of the protein D2 gene of *Pseudomonas aeruginosa. Antimicrob. Agents Chemother.* **36:**1791–1793.

Yoshihara, E., N. Gotoh, T. Nishino, and T. Nakae. Protease activity in bacterial porin. Submitted for publication.

Yoshihara, E., and T. Nakae. 1989. Identification of porins in the outer membrane of *Pseudomonas aeruginosa* that form small diffusion pores. *J. Biol. Chem.* **264:**6297–6301.

Yoshihara, E., and T. Nakae. 1992. Separation of gate- and channel-forming domains in the pore-forming protein of the outer membrane of *Pseudomonas aeruginosa. FEBS Lett.* **306:**5–8.

Yoshihara, E., and T. Nakae. 1993. Calcium ion-mediated opening of the channel gate in the *Pseudomonas aeruginosa* porin. *Biochem. Biophys. Res. Commun.* **194:**1460–1465.

Yoshihara, E., H. Yoneyama, and T. Nakae. 1991. *In vitro* assembly of the functional porin trimer from dissociated monomers in *Pseudomonas aeruginosa. J. Biol. Chem.* **266:**952–957.

Molecular Biology of Pseudomonads
Edited by T. Nakazawa et al.

Chapter 33

Siderophore-Mediated Iron Transport in *Pseudomonas aeruginosa*

Keith Poole, Charles Dean, David Heinrichs, Shadi Neshat, Kathleen Krebes, Lisa Young, and Laurie Kilburn

IRON AND BACTERIAL GROWTH

All bacteria except the lactobacilli require iron for growth. This need for iron is complicated by the very low solubility of iron under aerobic conditions at neutral pH. It has been estimated that the concentration of soluble, bioavailable Fe^{3+} under these conditions is 10^{-18} M, several magnitudes less than what is generally needed to support growth (Neilands et al., 1987). Although bacteria employ a variety of mechanisms to acquire iron, a common mechanism involves the synthesis of high-affinity iron chelators called siderophores (Neilands, 1981b). Released extracellularly, these molecules chelate available iron and deliver it back to the bacterial cell, facilitating iron acquisition under the most dilute of conditions. In gram-negative organisms, outer membrane receptors specific for the iron-siderophore complex function in the initial recognition and internalization of the complex, which is subsequently transported to the cell cytoplasm by periplasmic and cytoplasmic membrane-associated transport components (Neilands, 1982; Braun et al., 1987; Silver and Walderhaug, 1992). The iron is ultimately released from the siderophore by reductive or degradative mechanisms (e.g., Brickman and McIntosh, 1992; Halle and Meyer, 1992), and the siderophore may be recycled (Braun et al., 1984). Production of siderophores and their cognate transport components is typically regulated by environmental iron concentrations, increasing with iron starvation (Neilands, 1981a; Neilands, 1981b; Venturi et al., 1995b). In some instances, the siderophores themselves regulate expression of the corresponding transport components (Zimmermann et al., 1984; Poole et al., 1990; Gensberg et al., 1992; Koster et al., 1993).

IRON ACQUISITION BY *PSEUDOMONAS AERUGINOSA*

P. aeruginosa is a ubiquitous soil and water organism also associated with debilitating infections of humans (Fick, 1993). The search for essential iron is complicated, in

Keith Poole, Charles Dean, David Heinrichs, Shadi Neshat, Kathleen Krebes, Lisa Young, and Laurie Kilburn • Department of Microbiology and Immunology, Queen's University, Kingston, Ontario K7L 3N6, Canada.

nature, by competition from other microorganisms and, in animal hosts, by the presence of iron-binding proteins (lactoferrin and transferrin) and the intracellular sequestration of iron (Sawatzki, 1987). The ability to utilize transferrin-bound iron (Ankenbauer et al., 1985; Sriyosachati and Cox, 1986; Wolz et al., 1994) as well as intracellular iron sources such as heme and hemoglobin (Bullen et al., 1974; K. Poole and S. Neshat, unpublished data) undoubtedly contributes to *P. aeruginosa*'s in vivo growth capability. Still, a major source of iron for the organism growing in nature or the animal host is that captured by siderophores. *P. aeruginosa* is known to produce two siderophores, pyochelin (Cox, 1980) and pyoverdine (Cox and Adams, 1985) (Fig. 1), and is able to utilize a number of heterologous siderophores of bacterial and fungal origin (Meyer, 1992), including enterobactin (Poole et al., 1990).

The receptors for ferric pyoverdine, ferric pyochelin, and ferric enterobactin are well studied (see below). In addition to their characteristic negative regulation by iron, mediated by the Fur repressor (Prince et al., 1993), expression of all three receptors is positively regulated by the corresponding siderophore (Dean and Poole, 1993b; Gensberg et al., 1992; Heinrichs et al., 1991). The siderophore-dependent expression of the ferric enterobactin receptor makes sense, since enterobactin is not produced by *P. aeruginosa* and the receptor would be useful only if and when the organism encountered enterobactin in the environment. Siderophore-dependent expression of receptors for the endogenous

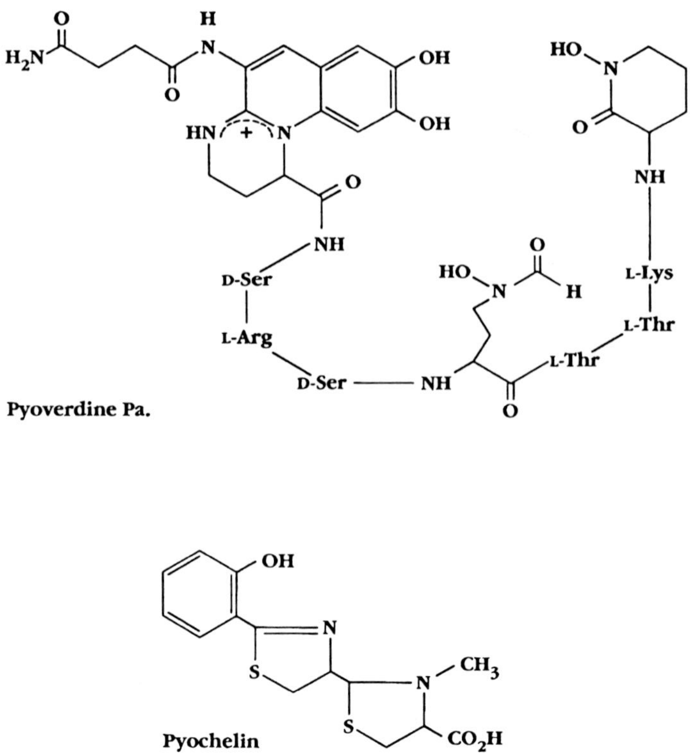

Figure 1. Structures of the *P. aeruginosa* siderophores pyochelin and pyoverdine.

siderophores pyoverdine and pyochelin, on the other hand, is best understood in the context of an organism being capable of producing two distinct iron chelators but needing only one at any particular moment to fulfill its iron requirements. Perhaps *P. aeruginosa* selects the appropriate uptake system on the basis of whichever siderophore is successful in acquiring iron in a given environment, specifically upregulating the corresponding transport system.

PYOVERDINE

Mixed hydroxamate-catecholate siderophores produced by the so-called fluorescent group of pseudomonads, pyoverdines (also called pseudobactins [Teintze et al., 1981]) are characterized by a conserved hydroxyquinoline moiety (the chromophore) and an amino acid tail of variable length and composition (Fig. 1) (Budzikiewicz, 1993). It is differences in the side chain which differentiate the various pyoverdines and are likely responsible for the observed specificity of pyoverdine utilization by individual strains of *P. aeruginosa* (Hohnadel and Meyer, 1988). The siderophore is highly water soluble, binds iron in a 1:1 stoichiometry with high affinity (stability constant of 10^{24} at pH 7) (Meyer and Abdallah, 1978), and is able to remove transferrin-bound iron in vitro (Sriyosachati and Cox, 1986). This ability may contribute to the observed ability of *P. aeruginosa* to grow in the presence of human serum (Ankenbauer et al., 1985). Recent in vivo studies demonstrated that pyoverdine production correlates with enhanced virulence in the burned mouse model of infection (Meyer et al., 1996), emphasizing the importance of iron acquisition to in vivo growth and, ultimately, pathogenesis. In studies using the rat lung model of infection, colonization of rat lungs was also shown to be dependent on the production of pyoverdine (Table 1). Thus, pyoverdine is important for iron acquisition and growth in the lung environment and thus likely contributes to the pathogenesis of chronic pulmonary *P. aeruginosa* infections seen in patients with cystic fibrosis (McCubbin and Fick, 1993).

Synthesis of the pyoverdine chromophore is hypothesized to involve a condensation of D-tyrosine and L-2,4-diaminobutyric acid (Budzikiewicz, 1993), while synthesis of the peptide moiety apparently involves a nonribosomal mechanism (Merriman et al., 1995). Studies of mutants have identified two loci involved in pyoverdine biosynthesis (Ankenbauer et al., 1986; Hohnadel et al., 1986), at 23 and 47 min on the recalibrated *P. aeruginosa* PAO map (O'Hoy and Krishnapillai, 1987). More recently, genes involved

Table 1. Pyoverdine-dependent growth of *P. aeruginosa* in rat lung[a]

Strain[b]	Phenotype	Pyoverdine[c]	No. of rats colonized
PAO25	*argF10 leu-10*	+	8
IA130	PAO25 *pvd-5*	–	0
PAO1	Prototroph	+	9
IAJ40M1	PAO1 *pvd-10*	–	0

[a]Cells of *P. aeruginosa* (10^4 CFU) were incorporated into agar beads and introduced into the lungs of Sprague-Dawley rats (10 rats per strain of *P. aeruginosa*) as described previously (Cash et al., 1979). After 7 days, the lungs of individual animals were examined for *P. aeruginosa* as evidence of colonization. *pvd,* inability to synthesize pyoverdine.

[b]Strains are from Ankenbauer et al. (1986).

[c]+, produces pyoverdine, –, pyoverdine deficient.

in pyoverdine biosynthesis have been cloned and mapped to the 65- to 70-min region of the chromosome (Stintzi et al., in press). A 103-kb fragment of chromosomal DNA from the 47-min region, dubbed the *pvd* region, has been cloned and shown to carry several genes involved in pyoverdine biosynthesis (Tsuda et al., 1995), including *pvdA*, encoding an L-ornithine N^5-oxygenase (Visca et al., 1994), *pvdD*, encoding a putative peptide synthetase (Merriman et al., 1995), and *pvdE*, whose product remains to be characterized (I. L. Lamont, personal communication). This region was first cloned by Rombel and Lamond (1992), who demonstrated that the pyoverdine biosynthetic genes exhibited homology with the corresponding biosynthetic genes of *Pseudomonas syringae* (Loper et al., 1984), *Pseudomonas putida* (Marugg et al., 1985), and *Pseudomonas* sp. strain B10 (Moores et al., 1984). These genes, as well as the pseudobactin biosynthetic genes from *Pseudomonas* sp. strain M114 (O'Sullivan et al., 1990), have been cloned as large gene clusters, in keeping with the expected complexity of pyoverdine biosynthesis.

The *P. aeruginosa* outer membrane receptor for ferric pyoverdine is a 86-kDa protein encoded by the *fpvA* gene (Poole et al., 1991; Poole et al., 1993). Additional ferric pyoverdine receptors have been found in this organism (Meyer et al., 1990; Gensberg et al., 1992), and although these are likely homologs of FpvA, *P. aeruginosa*, like *P. putida* (Koster et al., 1995), is able to utilize multiple pyoverdines (Hohnadel and Meyer, 1988) and so may synthesize multiple ferric pyoverdine receptors. The FpvA product shows homology to the ferric pseudobactin receptors PupA and PupB of *P. putida* and the coprogen/rhodotorulic acid receptor FhuE of *Escherichia coli* (Poole et al., 1993). As with previously described ferric siderophore receptors (Bäumler and Hantke, 1992), this homology is repeated in a somewhat regular pattern along the FpvA sequence, in regions predicted to exist in β-sheet, particularly amphipathic β-sheet. As such, these regions likely represent transmembranous domains of the protein (Bäumler and Hantke, 1992; Jeanteur et al., 1991). On the basis of these predictions of transmembranous regions and information supporting a disposition of the N and C termini at the periplasmic side of the outer membrane (Bäumler and Hantke, 1992, and references therein), a model for FpvA folding in the membrane has been developed (Fig. 2). As with previous models of ferric siderophore receptors (Murphy et al., 1990; Bäumler and Hantke, 1992; Koebnik and Braun, 1993), the periplasmic loops are minimal in size whereas the extracellular loops are quite extensive. Insertion of protease cleavage sites throughout the FpvA sequence has permitted identification of a region in the vicinity of the alanine residue at position 404 (Fig. 2) which is apparently surface exposed and is essential for ferric pyoverdine uptake (Kilburn et al., manuscript in preparation).

Expression of the *fpvA* gene is inducible under conditions of iron limitation, although the gene lacks a consensus Fur binding sequence and therefore is probably not directly regulated by the *P. aeruginosa* Fur repressor (Poole et al., 1993). Pyoverdine positively regulates expression of the ferric pyoverdine receptor: pyoverdine-deficient strains demonstrate a decrease in receptor levels which is reversible upon pyoverdine supplementation (Gensberg et al., 1992). The positive regulatory gene *pvdS*, required for pyoverdine production (Cunliffe et al., 1995; Miyazaki et al., 1995), is not sufficient for expression of an *fpvA-lacZ* fusion (Poole and Neshat, unpublished results), suggesting that some other gene(s) may be responsible for pyoverdine-dependent activation of *fpvA* gene expression. PvdS homologs have been reported for *P. putida* (PfrI [Venturi et al., 1995a]) and *Pseudomonas* sp. strain M114 (PbrA [Sexton et al., 1995]), in which they are re-

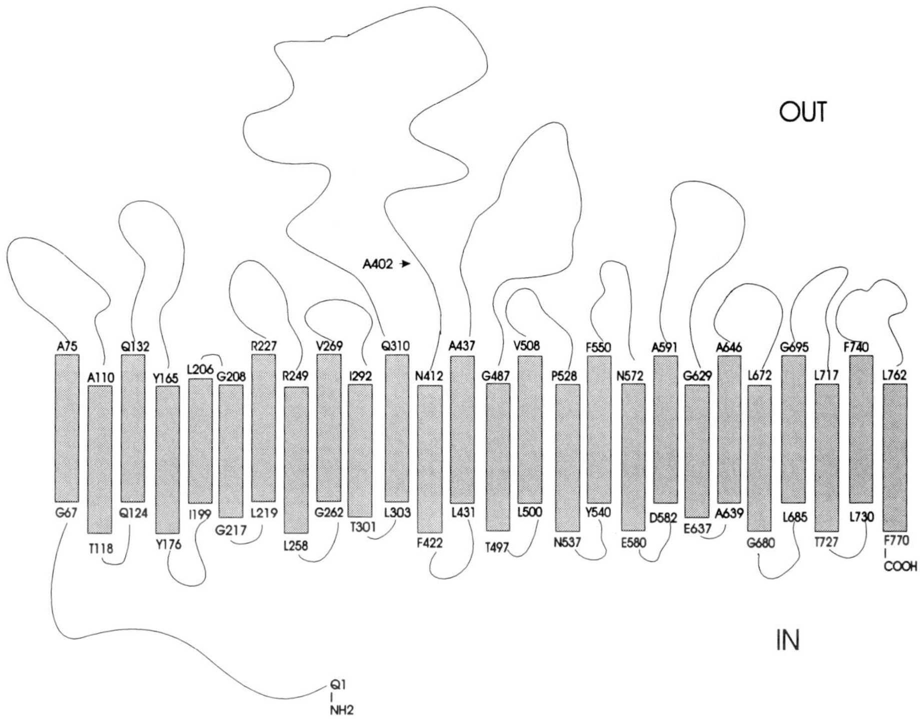

Figure 2. Model of the topology of FpvA in the outer membrane. Amino acid residues bordering the respective transmembranous β-sheet domains (shaded bars) are indicated. The N- and C-terminal residues are highlighted, as is a residue, alanine at residue 402 (A402), in a region confirmed as being surface exposed and important for ferric pyoverdine uptake.

quired for pseudobactin production. The role of PfrI in receptor gene expression has not been addressed, although PbrA was shown to activate expression of *pbuA*, the ferric pseudobactin receptor gene in strain M114 (Sexton et al., 1995).

FpvA exhibits sequence homology to the family of TonB-dependent receptors, which includes a variety of ferric siderophore receptors in *E. coli* and other gram-negative bacteria, such as members of the fluorescent pseudomonads (Bitter et al., 1991; Morris et al., 1994), and the *E. coli* vitamin B_{12} receptor BtuB, all of which share conserved regions of homology designated I to IV (Lundrigan and Kadner, 1986). It was predicted, therefore, that siderophore receptor function in *P. aeruginosa* utilizes a TonB-dependent energy transduction mechanism as has been elucidated for *E. coli* (reviewed in Postle, 1993) and, more recently, *P. putida* (Bitter et al., 1993). Indeed, a *P. aeruginosa tonB* homolog has been cloned and characterized (Poole et al., in press). Interestingly, FpvA lacks homology region I, the so-called TonB box implicated in binding to the TonB protein in *E. coli* (Schramm et al., 1987; Heller et al., 1988). It is possible, however, that secondary structure in this region is more important than primary sequence conservation or that FpvA interacts with a *P. aeruginosa* TonB protein in a manner different from that seen in *E. coli*. FpvA is predicted, for example, to possess an atypical N-terminal periplasmic extension (Q-1 to G-67; Fig. 2) as has been reported for the ferric pseudobactin receptors PupA (Bitter et al., 1991) and PupB (Koster et al., 1993) of *P. putida* WCS358. This region of PupB is critical for the observed PupB-dependent activation of *pupB* gene expression, mediated by the products of the *pupIR* operon. A proposed model predicts that TonB-dependent transport of ferric pseudobactin via PupB produces a conformational change in the receptor, facilitating the interaction of this N-terminal domain with PupR, a predicted cytoplasmic membrane protein. The latter then activates PupI, in an unknown but phosphorylation-independent manner, which functions as a transcriptional activator of *pupB* gene expression (Koster et al., 1994). Although PupI and PupR homologs have not been identified in *P. aeruginosa,* FpvA knockout mutants fail to express an *fpvA-lacZ* fusion (K. Poole, unpublished data), indicating that *fpvA* expression, like *pupB* expression, is receptor dependent. Whether control of *fpvA* expression involves a PupB-like mechanism remains to be seen.

PYOCHELIN

Pyochelin is a poorly water soluble, phenolate (related to the catecholates) siderophore of low molecular mass (325 Da) (Fig. 1) which binds iron in a 2:1 stoichiometry (Cox and Graham, 1979; Cox et al., 1981). Unlike pyoverdine, it exhibits a low affinity for iron in vitro (association constant of 2×10^5). Still, pyochelin production has been correlated with increased virulence and in vivo growth (Cox, 1982). Although it may be important for iron acquisition in vivo, the recent demonstration that pyochelin promotes free-radical formation and damage of endothelial cells (Britigan et al., 1992) suggests that its contribution to virulence may be unrelated to iron acquisition. Little is known about the biosynthesis of pyochelin, although salicylic acid has been implicated as an intermediate (Ankenbauer and Cox, 1988), and no genes have been cloned.

Early work implicated a 14-kDa outer membrane protein as the receptor for ferric pyochelin in *P. aeruginosa* (Sokol and Woods, 1983), but the contribution of this protein to ferric pyochelin uptake is likely to be marginal at best. Recent evidence implicates a 75-kDa iron-regulated outer membrane protein, encoded by the *fptA* gene (Ankenbauer, 1992; Ankenbauer and Quan, 1994), as the major receptor for ferric pyochelin. Mutants lacking this receptor are defective in ferric pyochelin uptake, and trypsin protection assays have demonstrated a specific interaction with ferric pyochelin (Heinrichs et al., 1991). Moreover, pyochelin is actually growth inhibitory for mutants lacking the 75-kDa receptor, a result which suggests that this protein is the sole receptor for ferric pyochelin in *P. aeruginosa* (Heinrichs and Poole, 1996).

The FptA protein shows homology to the TonB-dependent family of receptor proteins (Ankenbauer, 1992; Ankenbauer and Quan, 1994) although it, too, lacks the TonB box, again suggesting that this region is not important for interactions with TonB or that TonB-receptor interactions in *P. aeruginosa* differ from those in *E. coli.* Surprisingly, FptA shows the highest homology to the FpvA, PupA, PupB, and FhuE receptors (which bind hydroxamate-containing siderophores) and not to other catecholate receptors such as FepA or FatA (Ankenbauer and Quan, 1994), the latter having as its substrate anguibactin, a siderophore which shows some resemblance to pyochelin (Jalal et al., 1989). Sequence homology among receptor proteins is thus a poor predictor of siderophore or siderophore class specificity. A Fur consensus binding sequence is present upstream of the *fptA* coding region, and, as expected, *fptA* transcription is negatively regulated by iron (Ankenbauer and Quan, 1994; Heinrichs and Poole, 1996).

Characterization of a mutant deficient in FptA revealed that the positive regulatory gene *pchR* was required for maximal expression of FptA (Heinrichs and Poole, 1993), mediating the observed pyochelin-dependent expression of the receptor (Gensberg et al., 1992). *pchR* knockout mutants lack observable FptA protein (Heinrichs and Poole, 1993) and exhibit low levels of *fptA* expression (as measured by using a *fptA-lacZ* fusion) (Heinrichs and Poole, 1996). The *pchR* product is an apparently soluble protein of 31 kDa which exhibits homology to the AraC family of regulatory proteins (Heinrichs and Poole, 1993). Members of this family share a conserved C terminus characterized by a helix-turn-helix motif implicated in DNA binding. In addition to its role as an activator of *fptA* expression, which is apparent only in strains proficient in pyochelin production, PchR can also function as a repressor. Strains devoid of pyochelin, for example, fail to express detectable *fptA,* while mutational loss of *pchR* in these strains actually increases *fptA* expression (Heinrichs and Poole, 1996).

The *pchR* gene is iron regulated, consistent with the presence of a Fur binding site (confirmed by DNase I footprinting with *P. aeruginosa* Fur [M. L. Vasil and U. A. Ochsner, unpublished data]) upstream of this gene. *pchR* knockout mutants show increased expression of a *pchR-lacZ* fusion in pyochelin-producing and pyochelin-deficient strains, indicating that PchR negatively regulates its own expression (Heinrichs and Poole, 1996). PchR-mediated repression and activation of gene expression are, however, dependent on the FptA receptor protein (Heinrichs and Poole, 1996), suggesting that PchR may not respond directly to pyochelin but rather that FptA senses pyochelin and influences PchR activity (or expression) accordingly.

ENTEROBACTIN

P. aeruginosa is able to utilize a variety of siderophores produced by other microorganisms (Meyer, 1992). The best-characterized heterologous siderophore uptake system is that of ferric enterobactin. The uptake system is inducible by growth in the presence of enterobactin (Poole et al., 1990), which undoubtedly explains apparently conflicting observations of enterobactin-promoted growth in artificially iron-limited growth medium but a lack of enterobactin-mediated iron transport into this organism (Meyer, 1992) (since the latter experiments were performed on cells grown without enterobactin). The ferric enterobactin receptor is a 80-kDa iron-regulated, enterobactin-inducible outer membrane protein (Poole et al., 1990) encoded by the *pfeA* gene (Dean and Poole, 1993b). Highly homologous to the FepA receptor of *E. coli* (60% identity), PfeA is able to functionally replace FepA in *fepA* mutant strains of *E. coli* (Dean and Poole, 1993b). In contrast to FpvA and FptA, PfeA shares all four homology regions with the TonB-dependent family of receptors, including the so-called TonB box. It is not known whether conservation of the TonB box is significant for the observed activity of PfeA in *E. coli,* although it is expected that such activity would require that PfeA interact with *E. coli* TonB. Again, the *pfeA* gene is preceded by a consensus Fur binding sequence, which likely explains its regulation by iron.

The enterobactin-dependent expression of PfeA requires the products of an operon, *pfeRS,* which show homology to the superfamily of phosphorylation-dependent two-component regulatory protein pairs (Dean and Poole, 1993a). The cloned *pfeRS* genes are sufficient to drive expression of high levels of cloned PfeA in *E. coli*, and a *pfeR* mutant of *P. aeruginosa* fails to express detectable PfeA. A Fur box occurs upstream of *pfeRS*, overlapping the start site of the *pfeR* coding region, suggesting that this operon is iron regulated. Recent data indicate that *P. aeruginosa* Fur binds to the *pfeRS* promoter region (Vasil and Ochsner, unpublished data). PfeS, a predicted cytoplasmic membrane-associated histidine-kinase sensor, is expected to activate (via phosphorylation of a conserved aspartate residue) the regulator component, PfeR, in response to an environmental (periplasmic) stimulus, presumably ferric enterobactin. PfeR, in turn, apparently activates expression of *fptA* by binding upstream of this gene. Gel shift assays have confirmed this binding ability of PfeR (Dean et al., submitted for publication). Although ferric enterobactin must cross the outer membrane to reach PfeS in ultimately stimulating *pfeA* expression, PfeA knockout mutants still exhibit enterobactin-dependent expression of a *pfeA-lacZ* fusion, suggesting the existence of another route by which ferric enterobactin can cross the outer membrane (Dean et al., submitted). Consistent with this finding, PfeA mutants are still able to acquire ferric enterobactin (Dean et al., submitted). A model detailing the regulation of *pfeA* expression is shown in Fig. 3.

IDENTIFICATION OF A FatA HOMOLOG IN *P. AERUGINOSA*

During attempts at cloning the ferric pyoverdine receptor, K. Krebes and K. Poole (unpublished data) cloned a gene whose product showed substantial homology (36% identity, 15% conserved changes) to the FatA ferric anguibactin receptor of *Vibrio anguillarum* (Koester et al., 1991). As expected, this 83-kDa protein exhibits the con-

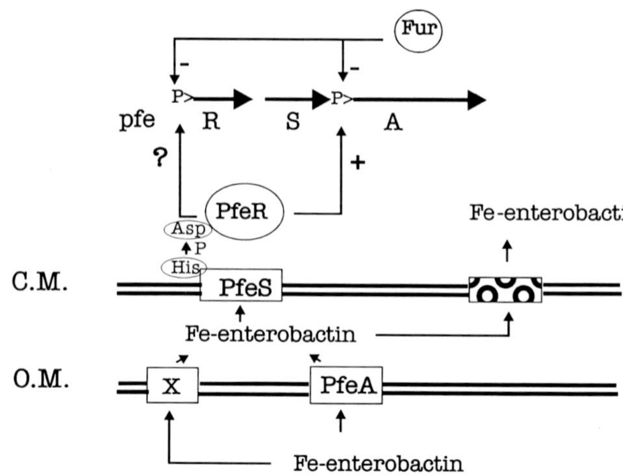

Figure 3. Model depicting the regulation of *pfeRSA* expression by Fur and PfeR. O.M., outer membrane; C.M., cytoplasmic membrane; P>, promoter; X, an unidentified protein able to transport ferric enterobactin across the outer membrane. The histidine (His) and aspartate (Asp) residues of PfeS and PfeR which are the sites of autophosphorylation and phosphotransfer (↑P) in this family of regulators are highlighted.

```
UfrA                                  AEAPAASSARSYDIAPG  17

UfrA  PLGRTLSAFASDNGVSLAFDPALTEGRRSAALRGRYAPVEALHRLLLGSG  67

UfrA  LELQQRSDGSYTLVRAATDGALELQSSLITAQAAGAETLPAE--------  109
FatA                                  LPISITHAEEQADESITVYGQA  22

UfrA  ---YAGGQVARGARLGMLGNADVMDAPFSITSYTARTIEQQQARSVADLL  156
FatA  NEAYAAGKISKASSIGMLGDKDFLDTPFNAIGYTDKHIQDQHAQDISDVI  72

UfrA  QANDPSVRVVGGRGDLVDSYTIRGFSVQNADVAFNGLYGLLPFWRVPIEF  206
FatA  SASDPSVFTSGETGLNKESFKIRGFSSDIGDVMFNGLYGIAPYYRSSPEM  122

UfrA  AERVEVLKGPNALLGGISPGGSVGGTINLVPKRADDQPLTRVSVDWTQRG  256
FatA  YQRIDVLKGPASLLNGMPPNGSVGGSINLVTKRAQEAPITSFTGTYMSDS  172

UfrA  QLGTHLDIGRRFGENNAFGVRFNGVYRNGDTAVDHQSREFPMLSLGLDFR  306
FatA  QFGGHIDIGRRFGENEQFGVRFNGVFRDGDASVDGQSRKAQLASLSLDWR  222

UfrA  GERLRLSSDLLYQKESLEGVVRPLLTGPGTTHIPHAPDSKTRFGLRDSYL  356
FatA  NDIALIEADLYFSTERVDGPNRGLSIASGVDV-PSPPSSDTLLSPSWAYN  271

UfrA  DQEDYSMVNRGEYDLADNLTAFASIGG-RQSNYETIAANSILVGNQGDIV  405
FatA  DSEDKGMMIRAELDLSNSVTAYGAVGASRTDFDSNVPQRVKIIDDSGTLE  321

UfrA  NSLARQRGDRRTYSAEVGLRGNFDTGPLRHDWTLSANRLHERLGMVYAFT  455
FatA  VSLGSVKLESKRTSGEVGIRSSFDTGPIEHYLVLNSTYFREDKNDSPTGN  371

UfrA  GMQSGNLYQTSPHTPLPDFSSLDGSIPKTNETDLGGVALADRLSFLEDRV  505
FatA  NNPGSWNPNIYNPVWGPEDSTYDNYYELPVDSTQISFGVADTLSLANGKY  421

UfrA  QVTLGVRRQQI--ESRNYDQTSGARTSHDKRHVWTPMASVLVKPLQDLSL  553
FatA  QVTLGLRHQSIDYESGVTWNGNAFPTTKLKESTYTPAIVALYKVSDSVSL  471

UfrA  YANYIQGLSQGEAAPMTAANAGQVLAPYKAEQYEIGAKYDLGGFTTTLAL  603
FatA  YGNYTEGLTNGKTAGSGAANVGEAFEPQKTKQTEAGLKLDMNDFAHTFSL  521

UfrA  FEIRKPNAYTDAS-NVFRADGEQRNRGVELSLYGEPLDGVRVMAGATYIK  652
FatA  FEIKKPNGYQDPDTNIYSFGGEQRNRGIEWGFYGTVLEDYTLTGGIAYTD  571

UfrA  PEQNKTGDPASEGKDAPGVARRQANLGVSWDTPFVDGLTLDSRWIYTGSA  702
FatA  AEITKATDVTTEGKQATKLPDLQAKLALEWNLPVMRQLTLIGQANYMSEQ  621

UfrA  YVDSANALAVPHWNRVDLGAAYAFQVAGKPLVARANLENALGKDYWTAAN  752
FatA  YIDAQNTQSLSAQTIFDLGARYNSTIANQSVIWRLAVNNVTDEAYWTTTH  671

UfrA  GY-LSISSPRTLSLSLTADF  771
FatA  YASLALGAPRTVMLSATADF  691
```

Figure 4. Alignment of the amino acid sequences of an unidentified ferric siderophore receptor (UfrA) from *P. aeruginosa* and the ferric anguibactin receptor FatA of *V. anguillarum*. The UfrA sequence was translated from a cloned and sequenced open reading frame of unknown function (GenBank accession number U33150). Exact matches (|) and conserved changes (·) are highlighted.

served regions typical of TonB-dependent receptors and is likely a ferric siderophore receptor. Alignment of FatA and this novel ferric siderophore receptor (here referred to as UfrA [unknown ferric siderophore receptor]) reveals that the homology exists throughout the length of the proteins, although UfrA possesses additional sequences at the N terminus which are absent in FatA (Fig. 4). It is interesting to speculate that this N-terminal extension, reminiscent of similar extensions in FpvA, PupA, and PupB, may be involved in a signal transduction cascade necessary for *ufrA* expression. Although anguibactin shows some structural similarities to pyochelin, no evidence was obtained for a role for UfrA in ferric pyochelin uptake. Indeed, *ufrA* knockout mutants exhibited no defects in growth, iron acquisition, or expression of any previously identified iron-regulated outer membrane proteins (K. Poole and E. Blouin, unpublished data). It is likely, therefore, that *ufrA* encodes an inducible receptor for a yet to be identified heterologous siderophore.

Acknowledgments. We thank Don Woods (Department of Microbiology and Infectious Disease, University of Calgary, Calgary, Alberta, Canada) for carrying out the rat lung colonization studies presented in Table 1 and Charles Cox (Department of Microbiology, University of Iowa, Iowa City) for providing the strains used in this study. The structure of pyoverdine shown in Fig. 1 was kindly provided by Mohammed Abdallah (Laboratoire de Chimie Microbienne, associé au CNRS, Institut de Chimie, Université Louis Pasteur). The continuing support of the Medical Research Council of Canada and the Canadian Cystic Fibrosis Foundation is also gratefully acknowledged.

REFERENCES

Ankenbauer, R. G. 1992. Cloning of the outer membrane high-affinity Fe(III)-pyochelin receptor of *Pseudomonas aeruginosa. J. Bacteriol.* **174:**4401–4409.

Ankenbauer, R. G., and C. Cox. 1988. Isolation and characterization of *Pseudomonas aeruginosa* mutants requiring salicylic acid for pyochelin biosynthesis. *J. Bacteriol.* **170:**5364–5367.

Ankenbauer, R., L. F. Hanne, and C. D. Cox. 1986. Mapping of mutations in *Pseudomonas aeruginosa* defective in pyoverdin production. *J. Bacteriol.* **167:**7–11.

Ankenbauer, R. G., and H. N. Quan. 1994. FptA, the Fe(III)-pyochelin receptor of *Pseudomonas aeruginosa:* a phenolate siderophore receptor homologous to hydroxamate siderophore receptors. *J. Bacteriol.* **176:**307–319.

Ankenbauer, R., S. Sriyosachati, and C. D. Cox. 1985. Effects of siderophores on the growth of *Pseudomonas aeruginosa* in human serum and transferrin. *Infect. Immun.* **49:**132–140.

Bäumler, A. J., and K. Hantke. 1992. Ferrioxamine uptake in *Yersinia enterocolitica:* characterization of the receptor protein FoxA. *Mol. Microbiol.* **6:**1309–1321.

Bitter, W., J. D. Marugg, L. A. de Weger, J. Tommassen, and P. J. Weisbeek. 1991. The ferric-pseudobactin receptor PupA of *Pseudomonas putida:* homology to TonB-dependent *Escherichia coli* receptors and specificity of the protein. *Mol. Microbiol.* **5:**647–655.

Bitter, W., J. Tommassen, and P. J. Weisbeek. 1993. Identification and characterization of the *exbB, exbD* and *tonB* genes of *Pseudomonas putida* WCS358: their involvement in ferric-pseudobactin transport. *Mol. Microbiol.* **7:**117–130.

Braun, V., C. Brazel-Faisst, and R. Schneider. 1984. Growth stimulation of *Escherichia coli* in serum by iron(III) aerobactin:recycling of aerobactin. *FEMS Microbiol. Lett.* **21:**99–103.

Braun, V., K. Hantke, K. Eick-Helmerich, W. Köster, U. Pressler, M. Sauer, S. Schäffer, H. Schöffler, H. Staudenmaier, and L. Zimmerman. 1987. Iron transport systems in *Escherichia coli,* p. 35–51. *In* G. W. Winkelmann, D. van der Helm, and J. B. Neilands (ed.), *Iron Transport in Microbes, Plants and Animals.* VCH Verlagsgesellschaft, Weinheim, Germany.

Brickman, T. J., and M. A. McIntosh. 1992. Overexpression and purification of ferric enterobactin esterase from *Escherichia coli. J. Biol. Chem.* **267:**12350–12355.

Britigan, D. E., T. L. Roeder, G. T. Rasmussen, D. M. Shasby, M. L. McCormick, and C. D. Cox. 1992. Interaction of the *Pseudomonas aeruginosa* secretory products pyocyanin and pyochelin generates hydroxyl radical and causes synergistic damage to endothelial cells. *J. Clin. Invest.* **90:**2187–2196.

Budzikiewicz, H. 1993. Secondary metabolites from fluorescent pseudomonads. *FEMS Microbiol. Rev.* **104:**209–228.

Bullen, J. J., C. G. Ward, and S. N. Wallis. 1974. Virulence and the role of iron in *Pseudomonas aeruginosa* infection. *Infect. Immun.* **10:**443–450.

Cash, H. A., D. E. Woods, B. McCullough, W. G. Johanson, Jr., and J. A. Bass. 1979. A rat model of chronic respiratory infection with *Pseudomonas aeruginosa. Am. Rev. Respir. Dis.* **119:**453–459.

Cox, C. D. 1980. Iron uptake with ferripyochelin and ferric citrate by *Pseudomonas aeruginosa. J. Bacteriol.* **142:**581–587.

Cox, C. D. 1982. Effect of pyochelin on the virulence of *Pseudomonas aeruginosa. Infect. Immun.* **36:**17–23.

Cox, C. D., and P. Adams. 1985. Siderophore activity of pyoverdin for *Pseudomonas aeruginosa. Infect. Immun.* **48:**130–138.

Cox, C. D., and R. Graham. 1979. Isolation of an iron-binding compound from *Pseudomonas aeruginosa. J. Bacteriol.* **137:**357–364.

Cox, C. D., K. L. Rinehart, Jr., M. L. Moore, and J.-C. Cooke, Jr. 1981. Pyochelin: novel structure of an iron-chelating growth promoter for *Pseudomonas aeruginosa. Proc. Natl. Acad. Sci. USA* **78:**4256–4260.

Cunliffe, H. E., T. R. Merriman, and I. L. Lamont. 1995. Cloning and characterization of *pvdS*, a gene required for pyoverdine synthesis in *Pseudomonas aeruginosa:* PvdS is probably an alternate sigma factor. *J. Bacteriol.* **177:**2744–2750.

Dean, C. R., and K. Poole. 1993a. Expression of the ferric enterobactin receptor (PfeA) of *Pseudomonas aeruginosa:* involvement of a two-component regulatory system. *Mol. Microbiol.* **8:**1095–1103.

Dean, C. R., and K. Poole. 1993b. Cloning and characterization of the ferric enterobactin receptor gene (*pfeA*) of *Pseudomonas aeruginosa. J. Bacteriol.* **175:**317–324.

Dean, C. R., S. Neshat, and K. Poole. PfeR, an enterobactin-responsive activator of ferric enterobactin receptor gene expression in *Pseudomonas aeruginosa.* Submitted for publication.

Fick, R. B., Jr. (ed.). 1993. *Pseudomonas aeruginosa the Opportunist: Pathogenesis and Disease.* CRC Press, Boca Raton, Fla.

Gensberg, K., K. Hughes, and A. W. Smith. 1992. Siderophore-specific induction of iron uptake in *Pseudomonas aeruginosa. J. Gen. Microbiol.* **138:**2381–2387.

Halle, F., and J.-M. Meyer. 1992. Iron release from ferrisiderophores. A multi-step mechanism involving a NADH/FMN oxidoreductase and a chemical reduction by $FMNH_2$. *Eur. J. Biochem.* **209:**621–627.

Heinrichs, D. E., and K. Poole. 1993. Cloning and sequence analysis of a gene (*pchR*) encoding an AraC family activator of pyochelin and ferripyochelin receptor synthesis in *Pseudomonas aeruginosa. J. Bacteriol.* **175:**5882–5889.

Heinrichs, D. E., and K. Poole. 1996. PchR, a regulator of ferripyochelin receptor gene (*fptA*) expression in *Pseudomonas aeruginosa,* functions both as an activator and as a repressor. *J. Bacteriol.* **178:**2586–2592.

Heinrichs, D. E., L. Young, and K. Poole. 1991. Pyochelin-mediated iron transport in *Pseudomonas aeruginosa:* involvement of a high-molecular-mass outer membrane protein. *Infect. Immun.* **59:**3680–3684.

Heller, K. J., R. J. Kadner, and K. Günther. 1988. Suppression of the *btuB*451 mutation by mutations in the *tonB* gene suggests a direct interaction between TonB and TonB-dependent receptor proteins in the outer membrane of *Escherichia coli. Gene* **64:**147–153.

Hohnadel, D., D. Haas, and J.-M. Meyer. 1986. Mapping of mutations affecting pyoverdine production in *Pseudomonas aeruginosa. FEMS Microbiol. Lett.* **36:**195–199.

Hohnadel, D., and J.-M. Meyer. 1988. Specificity of pyoverdine-mediated iron uptake among fluorescent *Pseudomonas* strains. *J. Bacteriol.* **170:**4865–4873.

Jalal, M. A., M. B. Hossain, D. van der Helm, J. Sanders-Loehr, L. A. Actis, and J. H. Crosa. 1989. Structure of anguibactin, a unique plasmid-related bacterial siderophore from the fish pathogen *Vibrio anguillarum. J. Am. Chem. Soc.* **111:**292–296.

Jeanteur, D., J. H. Lakey, and F. Pattus. 1991. The bacterial porin superfamily: sequence alignment and structure prediction. *Mol. Microbiol.* **5:**2153–2164.

Kilburn, L., K. Poole, and S. Neshat. Manuscript in preparation.

Koebnik, R., and V. Braun. 1993. Insertion derivatives containing segments of up to 16 amino acids identify surface- and periplasm-exposed regions of the FhuA outer membrane receptor of *Escherichia coli* K-12. *J. Bacteriol.* **175:**826–839.

Koester, W. L., L. A. Actis, L. S. Waldbeser, M. E. Tolmasky, and J. H. Crosa. 1991. Molecular characterization of the iron transport system mediated by the pJM1 plasmid in *Vibrio anguillarum* 775. *J. Biol. Chem.* **266:**23829–23833.

Koster, M., W. Ovaa, W. Bitter, and P. Weisbeek. 1995. Multiple outer membrane receptors for uptake of ferric pseudobactins in *Pseudomonas putida* WCS358. *Mol. Gen. Genet.* **248:**735–743.

Koster, M., J. van de Vossenberg, J. Leong, and P. J. Weisbeek. 1993. Identification and characterization of the *pupB* gene encoding an inducible ferric-pseudobactin receptor of *Pseudomonas putida* WCS358. *Mol. Microbiol.* **8:**591–601.

Koster, M., W. van Klompenburg, W. Bitter, J. Leong, and P. Weisbeek. 1994. Role for the outer membrane ferric siderophore receptor PupB in signal transduction across the bacterial cell envelope. *EMBO J.* **13:**2805–2813.

Loper, J. E., C. S. Orser, N. J. Panopoulos, and M. N. Schroth. 1984. Genetic analysis of fluorescent pigment production in *Pseudomonas syringae* pv. *syringae*. *J. Gen. Microbiol.* **130:**1507–1515.

Lundrigan, M. D., and R. J. Kadner. 1986. Nucleotide sequence of the ferrienterochelin receptor FepA in *Escherichia coli:* homology among outer membrane receptors that interact with TonB. *J. Biol. Chem.* **261:**10797–10801.

Marugg, J. D., M. van Spanje, W. P. M. Hoekstra, B. Schippers, and P. J. Weisbeek. 1985. Isolation and analysis of genes involved in siderophore biosynthesis in plant-growth-stimulating *Pseudomonas putida* WCS358. *J. Bacteriol.* **164:**563–570.

McCubbin, M., and R. B. Fick, Jr. 1993. Pathogenesis of *Pseudomonas aeruginosa* lung disease in cystic fibrosis, p. 189–211. *In* R. B. Fick, Jr. (ed.), *Pseudomonas aeruginosa the Opportunist: Pathogenesis and Disease*. CRC Press, Boca Raton, Fla.

Merriman, T. R., M. E. Merriman, and I. L. Lamont. 1995. Nucleotide sequence of *pvdD,* a pyoverdine biosynthetic gene from *Pseudomonas aeruginosa:* PvdD has similarity to peptide synthetases. *J. Bacteriol.* **177:**252–258.

Meyer, J.-M. 1992. Exogenous siderophore-mediated iron uptake in *Pseudomonas aeruginosa:* possible involvement of porin OprF in iron translocation. *J. Gen. Microbiol.* **138:**951–958.

Meyer, J.-M., and M. A. Abdallah. 1978. The fluorescent pigment of *Pseudomonas fluorescens:* biosynthesis, purification and physiochemical properties. *J. Gen. Microbiol.* **107:**319–328.

Meyer, J.-M., D. Hohnadel, A. Khan, and P. Cornelis. 1990. Pyoverdin-facilitated iron uptake in *Pseudomonas aeruginosa:* immunological characterization of the ferripyoverdin receptor. *Mol. Microbiol.* **4:**1401–1405.

Meyer, J.-M., A. Neely, A. Stintzi, C. Georges, and I. A. Holder. 1996. Pyoverdin is essential for virulence of *Pseudomonas aeruginosa*. *Infect. Immun.* **64:**518–523.

Miyazaki, H., H. Kato, T. Nakazawa, and M. Tsuda. 1995. A positive regulatory gene, *pvdS,* for expression of pyoverdin biosynthetic genes in *Pseudomonas aeruginosa*. *Mol. Gen. Genet.* **248:**17–24.

Moores, J. C., M. Magazin, G. S. Ditta, and J. Leong. 1984. Cloning of genes involved in the biosynthesis of pseudobactin, a high-affinity transport agent of a plant growth-promoting *Pseudomonas* strain. *J. Bacteriol.* **157:**53–58.

Morris, J., D. F. Donnelly, E. O'Neill, F. McConnell, and F. O'Gara. 1994. Nucleotide sequence analysis and potential environmental distribution of a ferric pseudobactin receptor gene of *Pseudomonas* sp. strain M114. *Mol. Gen. Genet.* **242:**9–16.

Murphy, C. K., V. I. Kalve, and P. E. Klebba. 1990. Surface topology of the *Escherichia coli* K-12 ferric enterobactin receptor. *J. Bacteriol.* **172:**2736–2746.

Neilands, J. B. 1981a. Microbial iron compounds. *Annu. Rev. Biochem.* **50:**715–731.

Neilands, J. B. 1981b. Iron absorption and transport in microorganisms. *Annu. Rev. Nutr.* **1:**27–46.

Neilands, J. B. 1982. Microbial envelope proteins related to iron. *Annu. Rev. Microbiol.* **36:**285–309.

Neilands, J. B., K. Konopka, B. Schwyn, M. Coy, R. T. Francis, B. H. Paw, and A. Bagg. 1987. Comparative biochemistry of microbial iron assimilation, p. 3–33. *In* G. Winkelmann, D. van der Helm, and J. B. Neilands (ed.), *Iron Transport in Microbes, Plants and Animals*. VCH Verlagsgesellschaft mbH, Weinheim, Germany.

O'Hoy, K., and V. Krishnapillai. 1987. Recalibration of the *Pseudomonas aeruginosa* PAO chromosome map in time units using high-frequency-of-recombination donors. *Genetics* **115:**611–618.

O'Sullivan, D. J., J. Morris, and F. O'Gara. 1990. Identification of an additional ferric-siderophore uptake gene clustered with receptor, biosynthesis, and *fur*-like regulatory genes in fluorescent *Pseudomonas* sp. strain M114. *Appl. Environ. Microbiol.* **56:**2056–2064.

Poole, K., S. Neshat, and D. E. Heinrichs. 1991. Pyoverdine-mediated iron transport in *Pseudomonas aeruginosa:* involvement of a high-molecular-mass outer membrane protein. *FEMS Microbiol. Lett.* **78:**1–5.

Poole, K., S. Neshat, K. Krebes, and D. E. Heinrichs. 1993. Cloning and nucleotide sequence analysis of the ferripyoverdine receptor gene *fpvA* of *Pseudomonas aeruginosa. J. Bacteriol.* **175:**4597–4604.

Poole, K., L. Young, and S. Neshat. 1990. Enterobactin-mediated iron transport in *Pseudomonas aeruginosa. J. Bacteriol.* **172:**6991–6996.

Poole, K., Q. Zhao, S. Neshat, D. E. Heinrichs, and C. R. Dean. The *Pseudomonas aeruginosa tonB* gene encodes a novel TonB protein. *Microbiology,* in press.

Postle, K. 1993. TonB protein and energy transduction between membranes. *J. Bioenerg. Biomembr.* **25:**591–602.

Prince, R. W., C. D. Cox, and M. L. Vasil. 1993. Coordinate regulation of siderophore and exotoxin A production: molecular cloning and sequencing of the *Pseudomonas aeruginosa fur* gene. *J. Bacteriol.* **175:**2589–2598.

Rombel, I. T., and I. L. Lamont. 1992. DNA homology between siderophore genes from fluorescent pseudomonads. *J. Gen. Microbiol.* **138:**181–187.

Sawatzki, G. 1987. The role of iron binding proteins in bacterial infection, p. 477–489. *In* G. Winkelmann, D. van der Helm, and J. B. Neilands (ed.), *Iron Transport in Microbes, Plants and Animals.* VCH Verlagsgesellschaft mbH, Weinheim, Germany.

Schramm, E., J. Mende, V. Braun, and R. M. Kamp. 1987. Nucleotide sequence of the colicin B activity gene *cba:* consensus pentapeptide among TonB-dependent colicins and receptors. *J. Bacteriol.* **169:**3350–3357.

Sexton, R., P. R. Gill, Jr., M. J. Callanan, D. J. O'Sullivan, D. N. Dowling, and F. O'Gara. 1995. Iron-responsive gene expression in *Pseudomonas fluorescens* M114: cloning and characterization of a transcription-activating factor, PbrA. *Mol. Microbiol.* **15:**297–306.

Silver, S., and M. Walderhaug. 1992. Gene regulation of plasmid- and chromosome-determined inorganic ion transport in bacteria. *Microbiol. Rev.* **56:**195–228.

Sokol, P. A., and D. E. Woods. 1983. Demonstration of an iron-siderophore-binding protein in the outer membrane of *Pseudomonas aeruginosa. Infect. Immun.* **40:**665–669.

Sriyosachati, S., and C. D. Cox. 1986. Siderophore-mediated iron acquisition from transferrin by *Pseudomonas aeruginosa. Infect. Immun.* **52:**885–891.

Stintzi, A., P. Cornelis, D. Hohnadel, J. M. Meyer, C. Dean, K. Poole, S. Kourambas, and V. Krishnapillai. Cloning and characterization of a pyoverdine biosynthesis gene cluster in *Pseudomonas aeruginosa* PAO responsible for the synthesis of pseudoverdine, a pyoverdine chromophore-related compound. *Microbiology,* in press.

Teintze, M., M. B. Hossain, C. L. Barnes, J. Leong, and D. van der Helm. 1981. Structure of ferric pseudobactin, a siderophore from a plant growth promoting *Pseudomonas. Biochemistry* **20:**6446–6457.

Tsuda, M., H. Miyazaki, and T. Nakazawa. 1995. Genetic and physical mapping of genes involved in pyoverdin production in *Pseudomonas aeruginosa* PAO. *J. Bacteriol.* **177:**423–431.

Venturi, V., C. Ottevanger, M. Bracke, and P. Weisbeek. 1995a. Iron regulation of siderophore biosynthesis and transport in *Pseudomonas putida* WCS358: involvement of a transcriptional activator and of the Fur protein. *Mol. Microbiol.* **15:**1081–1093.

Venturi, V., P. Weisbeek, and M. Koster. 1995b. Gene regulation of siderophore-mediated iron acquisition in *Pseudomonas:* not only the Fur repressor. *Mol. Microbiol.* **17:**603–610.

Visca, P., A. Ciervo, and N. Orsi. 1994. Cloning and nucleotide sequence of the *pvdA* gene encoding the pyoverdin biosynthetic enzyme L-ornithine N^5-oxygenase in *Pseudomonas aeruginosa. J. Bacteriol.* **176:**1128–1140.

Wolz, C., K. Hohloch, A. Ocaktan, K. Poole, R. W. Evans, N. Rochel, A.-M. Albrecht-Gary, M. A. Abdallah, and G. Doering. 1994. Iron release from transferrin by pyoverdin and elastase from *Pseudomonas aeruginosa. Infect. Immun.* **62:**4021–4027.

Zimmermann, L., K. Hantke, and V. Braun. 1984. Exogenous induction of the iron dicitrate transport system of *Escherichia coli* K-12. *J. Bacteriol.* **159:**271–277.

Molecular Biology of Pseudomonads
Edited by T. Nakazawa et al.

Chapter 34

Molecular Mechanism of Conversion to Mucoidy in *Pseudomonas aeruginosa*

Hongwei Yu, Michael J. Schurr, John C. Boucher, Jaime M. Martinez-Salazar, Daniel W. Martin, and V. Deretic

Chronic endobronchiolitis complicated by infections with *Pseudomonas aeruginosa* is the major cause of high morbidity and mortality in cystic fibrosis (CF) (Pedersen, 1992; Koch and Høiby, 1993). Conversion to the mucoid, exopolysaccharide alginate-overproducing form is associated with the persistence of *P. aeruginosa* in the respiratory tracts of CF patients (Pedersen, 1992). The exopolysaccharide alginate plays several roles in the pathogenesis of the CF lung. For example, alginate inhibits phagocytosis by neutrophils and macrophages (Speert, 1994) and insulates bacterial cells from reactive oxygen intermediates and hypochlorite generated by the phagocytic cells of the host (Learn et al., 1987; Simpson et al., 1989). Alginate also affects leukocyte function (chemotaxis, oxidative burst, interference with opsonization), plays an immunomodulatory role (induction of proinflammatory lymphokines, suppression of lymphocyte transformation), and may have other functions (adhesion, antibiotic resistance in biofilms, etc.) (Pedersen, 1992; Deretic, 1996). Several recent reviews address the wealth of information on the chemistry (Gacesa and Russell, 1990), biochemistry (May et al., 1991), and pathogenic properties (Pedersen, 1992) of alginate. May and Chakrabarty (1994) have recently reviewed several aspects of the molecular biology of alginate production. In this work, we will focus only on the molecular mechanism of conversion to mucoidy.

The known phenomena controlling conversion to mucoidy in *P. aeruginosa* can be summarized as follows: (i) mutations in the *muc* loci cause conversion to mucoidy (Fyfe and Govan, 1980; Martin et al., 1993c); (ii) many of the characterized *muc* mutations in CF isolates or laboratory strains (Fig. 1 and Table 1) are point mutations (nonsense and frameshift) in the *mucA* gene (Martin et al., 1993c; De Vries and Ohman, 1994; Boucher

Hongwei Yu, Michael J. Schurr, John C. Boucher, and V. Deretic • Department of Microbiology and Immunology, 5641 Medical Science Building II, University of Michigan Medical School, Ann Arbor, Michigan 48109-0620. ***Jaime M. Martinez-Salazar*** • Depto. de Genetica Molecular, Centro de Investigacion sobre Fijacion de Nitrogeno, UNAM, Av. Universidad s/n Col Chamilpa, Cuernavaca, Morelos, Mexico 62100. ***Daniel W. Martin*** • Department of Microbiology and Immunology, Stanford University School of Medicine, D052 Fairchild Building, Stanford, California 94305.

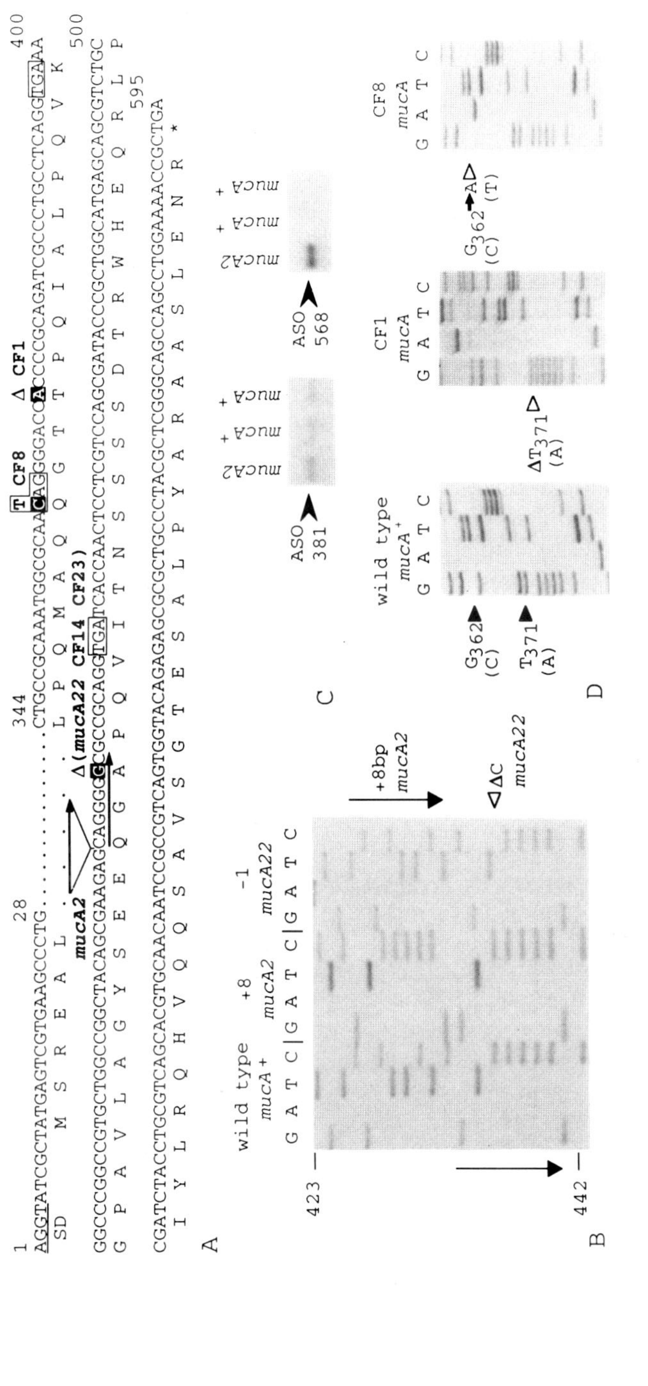

Figure 1. Mutations in the *mucA* gene causing conversion to mucoidy in *P. aeruginosa*. Reproduced with permission from Martin et al. (1993c).

Table 1. Characterized mutations in the *mucA* gene responsible for the conversion to mucoid colony morphology in clinical CF isolates and laboratory strains of *P. aeruginosa*[a]

Group[b]	Strain(s) (genotype)	Mutation (type)	MucA truncation	Reference(s)
I	CF8	C to T 362 (nonsense)	TAG at 362	Martin et al., 1993c
II	CF1	ΔA at 371 (frameshift)	TGA at 396	Martin et al., 1993c
	PAM425 (*muc3739*)	ΔC at 386 (frameshift)		Boucher et al., 1996
III	PAO568 (*mucA2*)	8-bp duplication at 434 (frameshift)	TGA at 450	Martin et al., 1993c
	PAO578 (*mucA22*) CF14, 23, FRD1	ΔG at 440 (frameshift)		Martin et al., 1993a; DeVries and Ohman, 1994

[a]The *mucA* gene is located immediately downstream of *algU*. In the wild-type nonmucoid *P. aeruginosa* PAO1, this gene of 582 bp encodes a polypeptide of 194 amino acids with the predicted M_r of 20,997 and pI of 5.57.
[b]The characterized mutations in the *mucA* gene can be placed into three groups according to the positions of premature termination codons (MucA truncation).

et al., 1996); (iii) as a result of *mucA* inactivation, the alternative sigma factor AlgU (Martin et al., 1993a), also known as AlgT (DeVries and Ohman, 1994; see also Ohman et al., this volume), is available to direct the transcription of alginate-specific biosynthetic and ancillary regulatory genes (Martin et al., 1993a; Martin et al., 1993c; Martin et al., 1994) (Fig. 2); (iv) additional elements located in the *algU mucABCD* gene cluster control AlgU activity, and experimental inactivation of *mucB* (also known as *algN* [Goldberg et al., 1993]) or *mucD* on the *P. aeruginosa* chromosome causes the mucoid phenotype (Martin et al., 1993b; Boucher et al., 1996); (v) AlgU is the *P. aeruginosa* equivalent (Yu et al., 1995) of the extreme heat shock (stress) sigma factor σ^E from enteric bacteria (Hiratsu et al., 1995; Raina et al., 1995; Rouvière et al., 1995); (vi) AlgU is inducible by environmental stress (Schurr et al., 1995a); and (vii) in addition to controlling alginate production, AlgU controls other stress response functions in *P. aeruginosa* (Martin et al., 1994; Yu et al., 1995; Yu et al., in press).

ALGINATE SYNTHESIS IN *P. AERUGINOSA* IS POSITIVELY REGULATED BY AlgU, A STRESS-RELATED ALTERNATIVE SIGMA FACTOR

The *algU* gene (Martin et al., 1993a) is at the 5′ end of the *algU mucABCD* gene cluster located at 67.5 min of the *P. aeruginosa* chromosomal map. Insertional inactivation of *algU* on the chromosome of mucoid cells abrogates transcription of the key alginate biosynthetic gene *algD* and alginate production (Martin et al., 1993a). In the initial report on the *algU* sequence (Martin et al., 1993a), global homology searches indicated that the predicted gene product of *algU* was homologous to the alternative sigma factor σ^H (Spo0H), a stationary-phase and sporulation sigma factor from *Bacillus* spp. Curiously, AlgU displayed only marginal similarity with the σ^{70} family of sigma factors in which σ^H was originally classified (Lonetto et al., 1992). More recent global homology searches (Deretic et al., 1994; Lonetto et al., 1994) have revealed that AlgU is one of the founding members of a novel family of alternative sigma factors (Fig. 3) that is only distantly related to the σ^{70} family. In this new classification, Spo0H shows similarities to both the σ^{70} group on one side and AlgU homologs on the other and is placed between these two large clusters of alternative sigma factors (Lonetto et al., 1994; Deretic et al., 1994; Deretic et al., 1995).

Significantly, the availability of the *algU* sequence and other related σ factors in the GenBank database has facilitated the identification of a large number of AlgU homologs in diverse bacteria. One group of very close AlgU homologs (including only those members with ≥60% identity to AlgU) is designated here the AlgU-RpoE family of alternative sigma factors (Fig. 3). The AlgU-RpoE family includes *rpoE* from *Escherichia coli* (Deretic et al., 1994) and *Salmonella typhimurium* (Martin et al., 1994), *algU* from *Azotobacter vinelandii* (Martinez-Salazar et al., 1996), *rpoE* from *Photobacterium* sp. strain SS9 (Chi and Bartlett, 1995), and *rpoE* from *Haemophilus influenzae* (Fleischmann et al., 1995). The *E. coli rpoE* gene, initially identified on the basis of sequence similarity of its predicted gene product to AlgU (66% identity and 91% overall homology), has

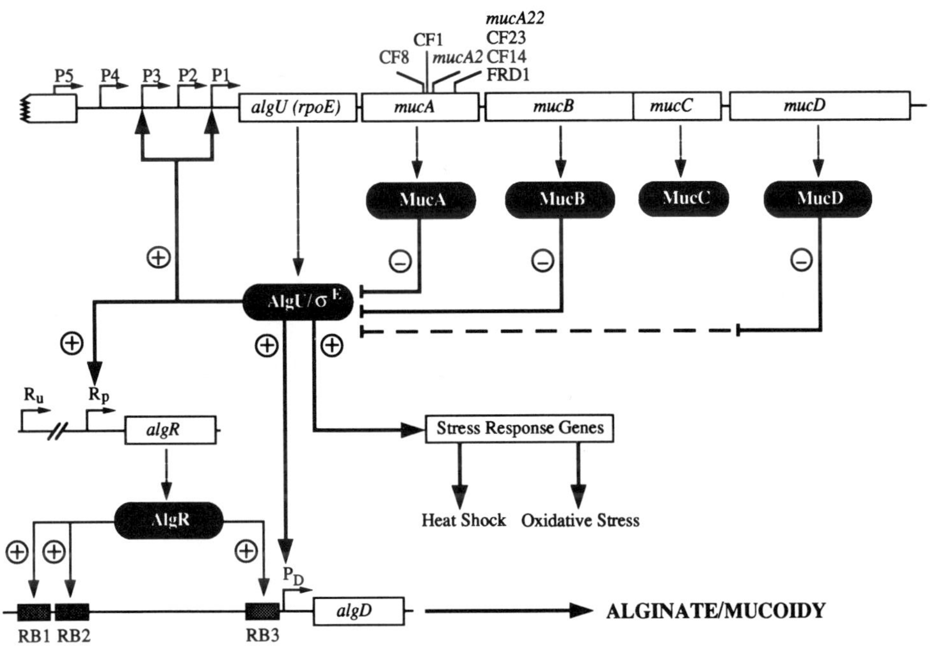

Figure 2. Regulatory circuitry controlling *algD* transcription and expression of the mucoid phenotype. The *algU mucABCD* gene cluster is at the top of the regulatory cascade and controls *algD* expression and conversion to mucoidy. The *algU* gene has five promoters, two of which are AlgU dependent (σ^E promoters). Transcription of *algR* from its R_p (proximal) promoter is AlgU dependent. The *algD* gene appears to be transcribed from a single AlgU-dependent promoter, P_D. Two factors are absolutely required for expression of *algD*: AlgU, an alternative sigma factor directing transcription at P_D, and AlgR, a response regulator which binds to the three sites, RB1, RB2, and RB3, upstream of P_D to further augment transcription of *algD*. MucA, MucB, and MucD are negative regulators of AlgU. Mutations inactivating *mucA*, as detected in CF strains (Fig. 1; Table 1), and experimental mutagenesis of *mucB* and *mucD* result in conversion to mucoidy. Modified from Martin et al. (1994).

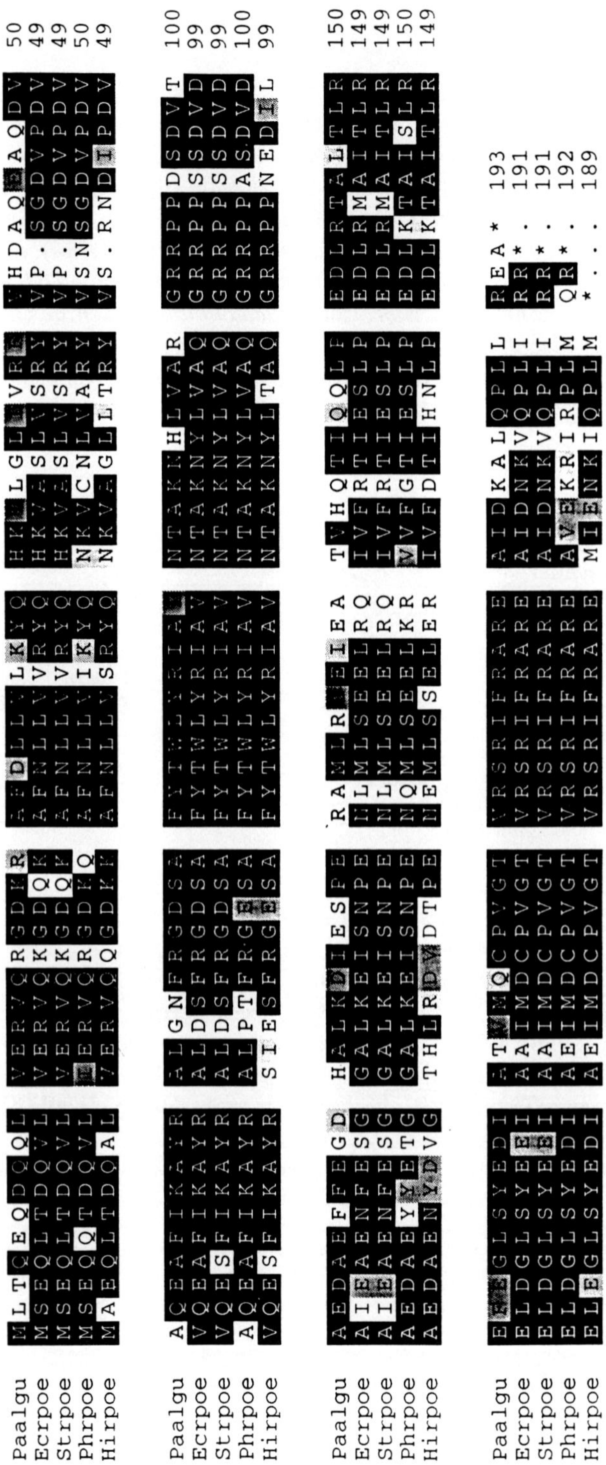

Figure 3. The AlgU-RpoE family of sigma factors. Individual sigma factors are described in the text. Paalgu, *P. aeruginosa* AlgU; Ecrpoe, *E. coli* RpoE (σ^E); Strpoe, *S. typhimurium* RpoE (σ^E); Phrpoe, *Photobacterium* sp. RpoE; Hirpoe, *H. influenzae* RpoE.

been recently demonstrated (Hiratsu et al., 1995; Raina et al., 1995; Rouvière et al., 1995) to encode the previously biochemically characterized alternative sigma factor σ^E (Erickson and Gross, 1989; Wang and Kaguni, 1989). It has been shown that AlgU and σ^E are functionally interchangeable in *P. aeruginosa* (Yu et al., 1995). The *rpoE* gene from *E. coli* can complement mutations in *algU* and restore the mucoid phenotype in *P. aeruginosa* (Yu et al., 1995), thus demonstrating the equivalence of AlgU and σ^E. Recently, Schurr et al. (1995b) purified AlgU, demonstrated its activity in an in vitro transcription runoff assay, and showed its association with RNA polymerase. A similar result was reported by Hershberger et al. (1995), who cloned *algT* (*algU*) by PCR and investigated its activity on one of the previously mapped promoters (Martin et al., 1994; DeVries and Ohman, 1994).

The alternative sigma factor AlgU is responsible for transcription (Martin et al., 1993a; Martin et al., 1994; Wozniak and Ohman, 1994) of the critical alginate biosynthetic gene *algD*, also affecting the expression of the genes located downstream of *algD* (Chitnis and Ohman, 1993), and the response regulator *algR*, which further augments *algD* transcription (Fig. 2). Normally, in the wild-type nonmucoid cells that do not have mutations in their *muc* genes (see later sections), AlgU is active at only a very low level. In mucoid cells, AlgU is no longer under negative control by the *muc* genes, and thus the increased transcription of the genes described above (Fig. 2) brings about increased alginate production and mucoid phenotype.

What is the function of σ^E, the *E. coli* equivalent of AlgU, since this organism does not make alginate? *E. coli* σ^E directs transcription of two genes, *rpoH* (from one of its promoters) and *htrA* (Erickson and Gross, 1989; Lipinska et al., 1988; Wang and Kaguni, 1989). RpoH is the major heat shock sigma factor σ^{32}, which plays a crucial role in bacterial physiology under adverse environmental conditions (Grossman et al., 1984). The second σ^E-dependent gene, *htrA*, was initially isolated as a gene essential for *E. coli* growth at elevated temperatures (Lipinska et al., 1988). It was later shown to affect *S. typhimurium* sensitivity to reactive oxygen intermediates, survival in macrophages, and virulence in mice (Johnson et al., 1991). Thus, it was expected that *rpoE* could play a role in the stress response and bacterial resistance to heat and oxidants, but this idea could not be tested since the *rpoE* gene was not available until very recently and appropriate mutations could not be generated. The *algU* mutants of *P. aeruginosa*, being readily available (Martin et al., 1993a; Martin et al., 1994; Yu et al., 1995), have been used to test this hypothesis. The *algU*::Tc^r *P. aeruginosa* strains were found to be more sensitive to high temperatures and reactive oxygen intermediates than the corresponding parental *algU*$^+$ strains (Martin et al., 1994; Yu et al., 1995). Similar to what was found for *algU* inactivation, *rpoE* mutations were recently shown to cause temperature sensitivity in *E. coli* (Hiratsu et al., 1995; Raina et al., 1995; Rouvière et al., 1995). These analyses and analogies suggest that AlgU may play a broader function in *P. aeruginosa* stress response and adaptation to adverse environmental conditions. Thus, the alginate genes controlled by AlgU may represent only a subset of cellular stress-responsive defense systems in *P. aeruginosa* (Deretic et al., 1994; Martin et al., 1994). In further support of this notion, preliminary results indicate that the *algU* mutants are more susceptible to killing by phagocytic cells even when *algU* is inactivated in a wild-type nonmucoid background such as PAO1 (Yu et al., in press).

CRITICAL *alg* PROMOTERS SHARE CONSERVED GAACTT (–35) AND TCTgA (–10) CANONICAL SEQUENCES

The promoters controlled by AlgU and σ^E are highly conserved (Fig. 4) and display a very tight canonical sequence (GAACTT) in the –35 region and a somewhat relaxed –10 sequence (TCTgA) spaced by 16 or 17 bp (Lipinska et al., 1988; Erickson and Gross, 1989; Deretic et al., 1994; Martin et al., 1994). Recent analyses of the *algD* and *algR* promoters have revealed the presence of σ^E consensus sequences at appropriate positions relative to the mRNA start sites (Deretic et al., 1994; DeVries and Ohman, 1994; Martin et al., 1994; Schurr et al., 1995a). The upstream region of *algU* has five promoters (Schurr et al., 1995a), two of which (P1 and P3) are σ^E promoters (Martin et al., 1994; Schurr et al., 1995a). Inactivation of *algU* on the chromosome causes the disappearance of the P1 and P3 signals, as determined by S1 nuclease protection analyses (Schurr et al., 1995a). The *E. coli rpoE* gene can complement the *algU* mutation and restore transcription from P1 and P3 promoters in *algU*::Tc^r *P. aeruginosa,* confirming that AlgU and σ^E are functionally interchangeable (Schurr et al., 1995a).

INDUCTION OF AlgU, *alg* PROMOTERS, AND ALGINATE PRODUCTION BY HEAT SHOCK

The *algU* transcripts from P1 and P3 can be induced by environmental insults such as heat shock even in the wild-type *muc*$^+$ background (Schurr et al., 1995a). Under conditions of extreme heat shock (shift from 30°C to 50°C), *algU* expression is induced and the increased synthesis or stability of the AlgU protein can be detected by metabolic labeling and analysis of newly synthesized polypeptides on two-dimensional gels (Schurr et al., 1995a). Comparisons of isogenic mutants under inducing conditions have revealed that at least five polypeptides are positively controlled by AlgU (Yu et al., in press). Thus, AlgU appears to be involved in the stress response of *P. aeruginosa* in a more general sense. Interestingly, *algU*-dependent induction of alginate synthesis has been observed in wild-type nonmucoid strains upon exposure to stress factors. Depending on

	-35		-10	+1
σ^E consensus	**GAACTT** —— 16/17 bp —— **TCTgA** 5/6 bp			
Pa algU P1	GA**GAACTT**TTGCAAGAAGCCCGAG**TCT**ATCTTGGCA			
Pa algU P3	TG**GAACTT**TCTTAGACGCATCGGT**TC**CA**A**AGCAGGA			
Pa algR	GG**G**C**ACTT**TTCGGGCCTAAAGCGAG**TCT**C**A**GCGTCG			
Pa algD	CG**GAACTT**CCCTCGCAGAGAAAACA**TC**CT**A**TCACCG			
Pa rpoH	AG**GAACTT**ATACACCCGCTTGCAG**TC**A**GA**TATCCGA			
Ec rpoH	TT**GAACTT**GTGGATAAAATCACGG**TCTGA**TAAAACA			
Ec htrA	CG**GAACTT**CAGGCTATAAAACGAA**TCTGA**AGAACA			
Ec rpoE	CG**GAACTT**TACAAAAACGAGACAC**TCTAA**CCCTTTG			
St rpoE	CG**GAACTT**TACGAAACATAGACAC**TCTAA**CCTGTTG			
St htrA	CG**GAACTT**CGCGTTATAAAATGAA**TCTGA**CGTACAC			

Figure 4. Compilation of σ^E promoters. *Pa, P. aeruginosa; Ec, E. coli; St, S. typhimurium.*

the factors used, this physiological induction can result in a transient but uniform mucoid colony morphology on plates (Boucher et al., 1996; Schurr et al., 1995a).

REGULATION OF *algU* BY THE DOWNSTREAM GENES *mucABCD: muc* MUTATIONS CAUSE CONVERSION TO MUCOIDY

Located immediately downstream of *algU* are four tightly linked genes, *mucABCD* (Fig. 2 and 5), which affect *algU* activity (Martin et al., 1993b; Martin et al., 1993c; Boucher et al., 1996). Genetic evidence indicates that *mucA, mucB,* and *mucD* act as negative regulators of AlgU. The experimental support for the proposed roles comes from the following observations: (i) mutations disrupting the *mucA* coding frame have been found to be present in mucoid strains but absent in nonmucoid parents (Fig. 1), and gene replacements with the mutant *mucA* alleles cause conversion to mucoidy (Martin et al., 1993c); (ii) inactivation of *mucA* or *mucB* significantly increases *algU* activity (Schurr et al., 1994); (iii) insertional inactivation of *mucB* on the chromosome (Martin et al., 1993b) or in experiments carried out with plasmids (Goldberg et al., 1993) results in the mucoid phenotype; and (iv) inactivation of *mucD* on the chromosome also causes conversion of *P. aeruginosa* to the mucoid phenotype (Boucher et al., 1996).

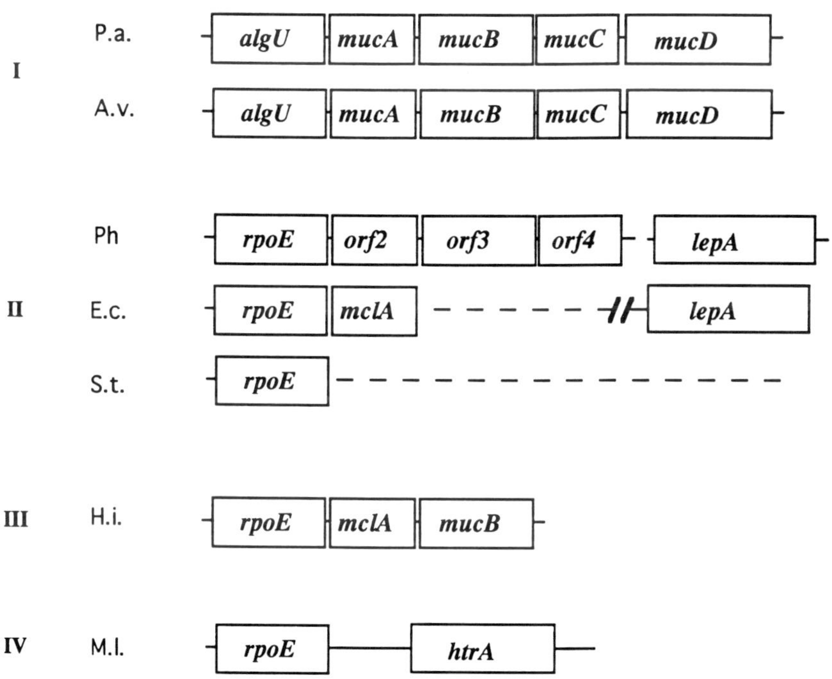

Figure 5. Conservation of *algU* homologs, their cognate negative regulators, and genetic organization of the corresponding gene clusters. Four different cluster organization types (I to IV) have been discerned. Individual genes and functions are described in the text. P.a., *P. aeruginosa;* A.v., *A. vinelandii;* Ph, *Photobacterium* sp. strain SS9; E.c., *E. coli*; S.t., *S. typhimurium;* H.i., *H. influenzae;* M.l., *M. leprae.*

The *algU mucABCD* gene cluster is allelic with a group of previously mapped *muc* mutations (Fyfe and Govan, 1980; Martin et al., 1993a). Mutations in the *mucA* gene are responsible for the conversion to mucoidy in a significant number of clinical mucoid strains isolated from CF patients (Table 1) (Martin et al., 1993a; Martin et al., 1993c). Second-site suppressor mutations in *algU* are epistatic to *mucA* mutations and result in pseudoreversion from mucoid to nonmucoid phenotype (Table 2) (Schurr et al., 1994; DeVries and Ohman, 1994). The known mutations (Martin et al., 1993c; DeVries and Ohman, 1994; Boucher et al., 1996) in the *mucA* gene can be classified into three categories (Table 1). Interestingly, all of the characterized *mucA* alleles in mucoid CF isolates have either frameshift or nonsense mutations. The functions of MucA and other regulators of AlgU are presently under investigation. It has been proposed that MucA may act in a manner analogous to that of anti-sigma factors (Deretic et al., 1994). In support of this idea are the recent findings that AlgU and MucA form a complex, as revealed by cross-linking studies, and that MucA inhibits AlgU activity in vitro (M. J. Schurr, H. Yu, J. M. Martinez-Salazar, J. C. Boucher, and V. Deretic, unpublished data).

CONSERVATION OF THE CLUSTERS ENCODING AlgU-RpoE SIGMA FACTORS AND THEIR REGULATORS

The strong conservation of *algU* and *rpoE* can also be extended to the downstream genes in other members of the AlgU-RpoE family, which by analogy with the *Pseudomonas* system may affect their cognate sigma factors (Fig. 5). The *mucA* homologs have been identified in all gram-negative bacteria studied thus far (Fig. 5): *E. coli* (Yu et al., 1995), *A. vinelandii* (Martinez-Salazar et al., 1996), *Photobacterium* sp. strain SS9 (Chi and Bartlett, 1995), and *H. influenzae* (Fleischmann et al., 1995). Homologs of *mucB* have also been characterized in several of these bacteria. In the cases where the sequencing effort has progressed significantly into the cluster, homologs of *mucC* (also termed *algM;* see Ohman et al., this volume) and *mucD* have also been found. However, there are also exceptions to this rule; in such cases, *mucC* and *mucD* equivalents are missing or are not linked to the first three genes in the cluster (e.g., *H. influenzae rpoE mclA mucB* is not followed by *mucCD;* Fig. 5).

The members of the AlgU-RpoE class of sigma factors are encoded by the first gene in each cluster. Four organizational types of clusters have been recognized thus far (Fig. 5). The *P. aeruginosa algU mucABCD* cluster (Martin et al., 1993a; Martin et al., 1993b; Martin et al., 1993c; Martin et al., 1994; Boucher et al., 1996) and *A. vinelandii algU*

Table 2. Mutations in *algU* causing pseudoreversion to nonmucoidy in *P. aeruginosa*[a]

Parental strain	Nonmucoid derivative	*algU* or *algT* allele	Nucleotide change (mutation type)	Effect at protein level	References
PAO578	PAO578[74]	*algU*[74]	TGG→TGA (nonsense)	Trp-74→stop	Schurr et al., 1994
	PAO578[160]	*algU*[160]	GATA→GAA (frameshift)	Truncation at position 165	Schurr et al., 1994
FRD1	FRD60	*algT*[18]	GAC→GGC (missense)	Asp-18→Gly-18	DeVries and Ohman, 1994
	FRD75	*algT*[29]	TAC→TGC (missense)	Tyr-29→Cys-29	DeVries and Ohman, 1994

[a]Only a fraction of nonmucoid derivatives have mutations in *algU* (*algT*).

mucABCD (Martinez-Salazar et al., 1996) are nearly identical in organization. The last gene in this group is *mucD*, encoding a close homolog of HtrA from enteric bacteria. HtrA is a serine peptidase which is controlled by σ^E in *E. coli* (Lipinska et al., 1988; Raina et al., 1995; Rouvière et al., 1995) and is required for full resistance of enterobacteriaceae to heat and reactive oxygen intermediates. It has been proposed that HtrA removes oxidatively damaged or heat-denatured proteins, which otherwise become toxic to the cell. In keeping with similarities to *htrA*, mutations in *mucD* render *P. aeruginosa* sensitive to hydrogen peroxide and elevated temperatures (Boucher et al., 1996). It is likely that MucD plays a role in *P. aeruginosa* physiology similar or identical to that of HtrA in enteric bacteria.

Other types of clusters are shown in Fig. 5 in diminishing order of similarities to *algU mucABCD*. For example, *Photobacterium* sp. strain SS9 does not have an *htrA* (*mucD*) homolog in its *rpoE orf2 orf3 orf4* cluster. The entire cluster is important for adaptation of this deep-sea bacterium to high pressure and extreme cold. The *orf4* gene encodes a homolog of MucC and is required for the cold-temperature-adapted growth of *Photobacterium* sp. strain SS9 (Chi and Bartlett, 1995). In *E. coli*, only the first gene (*mclA*, for *mucA*-like) following *rpoE* has been identified thus far (Yu et al., 1995). It is likely that once the cluster is completely characterized, it will resemble the one in *Photobacterium* sp. In this organism, the *lepA* gene is located immediately following the cluster (in place of *mucD*), while *rpoE* in *E. coli* is tightly linked to *lepA*. The recent determination of the complete sequence of the *H. influenzae* genome (Fleischmann et al., 1995) has revealed the presence of close homologs of *algU* (*rpoE*), *mucA*, and *mucB*. These genes, termed *rpoE*, *mclA*, and *mucB* (Fleischmann et al., 1995), are followed by an unrelated gene transcribed in the opposite direction. Thus, these three genes may represent the minimal organizational unit of the gene clusters encoding the AlgU-RpoE sigma factors and their regulators.

An even simpler rendition of the cluster (*rpoE htrA*) has been noted in *Mycobacterium leprae* (GenBank accession number U15180), but the gene product of *rpoE* in this case shows only limited homology to AlgU and may not be a bona fide member of the AlgU-RpoE group. Nevertheless, the linkage of *rpoE* and *htrA* in *M. leprae* is reminiscent of the two termini in the *algU mucABCD* cluster. The predicted gene product of *M. leprae rpoE* and a variety of other factors in different organisms show 20 to 28% identity with AlgU. Among members of this family of proteins are HrpL in *Pseudomonas syringae* (Xiao et al., 1994; see also Hutcheson et al., this volume) and CarQ in *Myxococcus xanthus* (McGowan et al., 1993); further homologs in this group, such as FecI, PbrA, and PvdS, are discussed elsewhere in this volume (Dowling et al.). As the membership in this superfamily increases, it is likely that further divisions and classification in separate subgroups will continue within what initially appeared as a relatively homogeneous family of alternative sigma factors (termed extracytoplasmic function [Lonetto et al., 1994] or σ^E-like [Deretic et al., 1995] proteins) of which the AlgU-RpoE group is only a subset.

NEGATIVE REGULATORY FEEDBACK: THE ROLES OF MucD AND AlgW

The presence of *mucD* in the cluster encoding *algU* and its regulators indicates that expression of *mucD* may be coordinated with the expression of the remainder of the cluster. This possibility suggested to us that this linkage may not only reflect coordi-

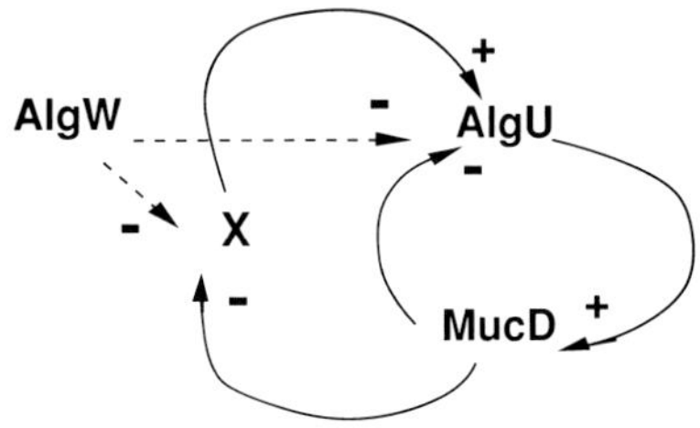

Figure 6. Proposed model of negative feedback regulation of AlgU by AlgW and MucD. AlgW and MucD are homologs of the serine protease HtrA (DegP). X is a putative regulatory factor or signal-generating molecule (oxidatively damaged substances, denatured proteins, etc.). Arrows do not imply direct interactions, and additional intermediate factors cannot be excluded. These regulatory loops include transcriptional events (such as the likely effects of AlgU on *mucD* transcription) and posttranscriptional interactions (such as AlgW and MucD effects on X or AlgU).

nated induction but may extend its effects to the processes which control the return of the system to its baseline level. If *mucD* is one of the functions induced by AlgU activation (e.g., from the P1 and P3 promoters at the beginning of the cluster), its effects may not be limited to removal of denatured proteins or other intended targets. By performing its physiological function, MucD may provide negative feedback control by removing the signals that induce the system (e.g., denatured proteins) or by acting directly on the positive regulators (Fig. 6). In keeping with this prediction, inactivation of *mucD* causes conversion to mucoidy (Boucher et al., 1996). Another *htrA*-like element, *algW*, recently identified at 69 min of the *P. aeruginosa* chromosomal map (Boucher et al., 1996), shows effects similar to those of *mucD*. When *algW* is inactivated, this enhances induction of mucoidy by exposure to mediators of environmental stress (Boucher et al., 1996). The proposed positive and negative feedback loops involving MucD and AlgW are illustrated in Fig. 6.

CONCLUDING REMARKS

The characterization of AlgU (AlgT) and its regulators is the product of investigations by numerous groups (Fyfe and Govan, 1980; MacGeorge et al., 1986; Flynn and Ohman, 1988; May et al., 1991; Woods et al., 1991; Martin et al., 1993a; Martin et al., 1993b) aimed at elucidating the mechanism of conversion to mucoid phenotype in *P. aeruginosa*. Once *algU* and the downstream genes were characterized, it became apparent that functions of AlgU extended beyond the control of mucoidy to other stress-related phenomena in pseudomonads. It also appears that the currently available information on the *algU mucABCD* cluster will provide a useful model for future analyses of the emerging similar systems in other bacteria.

In *P. aeruginosa,* conversion to mucoidy most likely represents only one aspect of stress response phenomena regulated by AlgU. Investigations of other functions controlled by this stress sigma factor may uncover novel aspects of bacterial physiology and stress response while improving our understanding of microbial pathogenesis and host-parasite interactions in CF.

Acknowledgments. This work was supported by grant AI31139 from the National Institute of Allergy and Infectious Diseases, grant G844 from the Cystic Fibrosis Foundation, and a grant from Texas Higher Education Coordinating Board. H.Y. and M.J.S. were Cystic Fibrosis Foundation postdoctoral fellows. J.M.M.-S., permanently affiliated with Instituto de Biotecnología, Universidad Autónoma de México, Cuernavaca, Morelos, Mexico 62271, was on sabbatical leave at the University of Texas Health Science Center at San Antonio.

REFERENCES

Boucher, J. C., J. M. Martinez-Salazar, M. J. Schurr, M. H. Mudd, H. Yu, and V. Deretic. 1996. Two distinct loci affecting conversion to mucoidy in *Pseudomonas aeruginosa* in cystic fibrosis encode homologs of the serine protease HtrA. *J. Bacteriol.* **178:**511–523.

Chi, E., and D. H. Bartlett. 1995. An *rpoE*-like locus controls outer membrane protein synthesis and growth at cold temperatures and high pressures in deep-sea bacterium *Photobacterium* sp. strain SS9. *Mol. Microbiol.* **17:**713–726.

Chitnis, C. E., and D. E. Ohman. 1993. Genetic analysis of the alginate biosynthetic gene cluster of *Pseudomonas aeruginosa* shows evidence of an operonic structure. *Mol. Microbiol.* **8:**583–593.

Deretic, V. 1996. Molecular biology of mucoidy in *Pseudomonas aeruginosa,* p. 223–244. *In* J. A. Dodge, D. J. H. Brock, and J. H. Widdicombe (ed.), *Cystic Fibrosis—Current Topics,* vol. 3. John Wiley & Sons, Chichester.

Deretic, V., M. J. Schurr, J. C. Boucher, and D. W. Martin. 1994. Conversion of *Pseudomonas aeruginosa* to mucoidy in cystic fibrosis: environmental stress and regulation of bacterial virulence by alternative sigma factors. *J. Bacteriol.* **176:**2773–2780.

Deretic, V., M. J. Schurr, and H. Yu. 1995. *P. aeruginosa,* mucoidy and chronic infection phenotype in cystic fibrosis. *Trends Microbiol.* **3:**351–356.

DeVries, C. A., and D. E. Ohman. 1994. Mucoid-to-nonmucoid conversion in alginate-producing *Pseudomonas aeruginosa* often results from spontaneous mutations in *algT,* encoding a putative alternative sigma factor, and shows evidence for autoregulation. *J. Bacteriol.* **176:**6677–6687.

Erickson, J. W., and C. A. Gross. 1989. Identification of the sigma subunit of *Escherichia coli* polymerase: a second sigma factor involved in high-temperature gene expression. *Genes Dev.* **3:**1462–1471.

Fleischmann, R. D., M. D. Adams, O. White, et al. 1995. Whole-genome random sequencing and assembly of *Haemophilus influenzae* RD. *Science* **169:**496–512.

Flynn, J. L., and D. E. Ohman. 1988. Cloning of genes from mucoid *Pseudomonas aeruginosa* which control spontaneous conversion to the alginate-producing phenotype. *J. Bacteriol.* **170:**1452–1460.

Fyfe, J. A. M., and J. R. W. Govan. 1980. Alginate synthesis in mucoid *Pseudomonas aeruginosa:* a chromosomal locus involved in control. *J. Gen. Microbiol.* **119:**443–450.

Gacesa, P., and N. J. Russell. 1990. The structure and properties of alginate, p. 29–49. *In* P. Gacesa and N. J. Russell (ed.), *Pseudomonas Infections and Alginate: Biochemistry, Genetics and Pathology.* Chapman & Hall, Ltd., London.

Goldberg, J. B., W. L. Gorman, J. Flynn, and D. E. Ohman. 1993. A mutation in *algN* permits *trans* activation of alginate production by *algT* in *Pseudomonas* species. *J. Bacteriol.* **175:**1303–1308.

Grossman, A. D., J. W. Erickson, and C. A. Gross. 1984. The *htpR* gene product of *E. coli* is a sigma factor for heat-shock promoters. *Cell* **38:**383–390.

Hershberger, C. D., R. W. Ye, M. R. Parsek, Z. D. Xie, and A. M. Chakrabarty. 1995. The *algT* (*algU*) gene of *Pseudomonas aeruginosa,* a key regulator involved in alginate biosynthesis, encodes an alternative σ factor (σ^E). *Proc. Natl. Acad. Sci. USA* **92:**7941–7945.

Hiratsu, K., M. Amemura, H. Nashimoto, H. Shinagawa, and K. Makino. 1995. The *rpoE* gene of *Escherichia coli,* which encodes σ^E, is essential for bacterial growth at high temperature. *J. Bacteriol.* **177:**2918–2922.

Johnson, K., I. Charles, G. Dougan, D. Pickard, P. O'Gaora, G. Costa, T. Ali, I. Miller, and C. Hormaeche. 1991. The role of a stress-response protein in *Salmonella typhimurium* virulence. *Mol. Microbiol.* **5:**401–407.

Koch, C., and N. Høiby. 1993. Pathogenesis of cystic fibrosis. *Lancet* **341:**1065–1069.

Learn, D. B., E. P. Brestel, and S. Seetharama. 1987. Hypochlorite scavenging by *Pseudomonas aeruginosa* alginate. *Infect. Immun.* **55:**1813–1818.

Lipinska, B., S. Sharma, and C. Georgopoulos. 1988. Sequence analysis and regulation of the *htrA* gene of *Escherichia coli:* a σ^{32}-independent mechanism of heat-inducible transcription. *Nucleic Acids Res.* **16:**10053-10067.

Lonetto, M., M. Gribskov, and C. A. Gross. 1992. The σ^{70} family: sequence conservation and evolutionary relationship. *J. Bacteriol.* **174:**3843–3849.

Lonetto, M. A., K. L. Brown, K. E. Rudd, and M. J. Buttner. 1994. Analysis of the *Streptomyces coelicolor sigE* gene reveals the existence of a subfamily of eubacterial RNA polymerase σ factors involved in the regulation of extracytoplasmic functions. *Proc. Natl. Acad. Sci. USA* **86:**7573–7577.

MacGeorge, J., V. Korolik, A. F. Morgan, V. Asche, and B. W. Holloway. 1986. Transfer of a chromosomal locus responsible for mucoid colony morphology in *Pseudomonas aeruginosa* isolated from cystic fibrosis patients to *P. aeruginosa* PAO. *J. Med. Microbiol.* **21:**331–336.

Martin, D. W., B. W. Holloway, and V. Deretic. 1993a. Characterization of a locus determining the mucoid status of *Pseudomonas aeruginosa:* AlgU shows sequence similarities with a *Bacillus* sigma factor. *J. Bacteriol.* **175:**1153–1164.

Martin, D. W., M. J. Schurr, M. H. Mudd, and V. Deretic. 1993b. Differentiation of *Pseudomonas aeruginosa* into the alginate-producing form: inactivation of *mucB* causes conversion to mucoidy. *Mol. Microbiol.* **9:**497–506.

Martin, D. W., M. J. Schurr, M. H. Mudd, J. R. W. Govan, B. W. Holloway, and V. Deretic. 1993c. Mechanism of conversion to mucoidy in *Pseudomonas aeruginosa* infecting cystic fibrosis patients. *Proc. Natl. Acad. Sci. USA* **90:**8377–8381.

Martin, D. W., M. J. Schurr, H. Yu, and V. Deretic. 1994. Analysis of promoters controlled by the putative sigma factor AlgU regulating conversion to mucoidy in *Pseudomonas aeruginosa:* relationship to stress response. *J. Bacteriol.* **176:**6688–6696.

Martínez-Salazar, J. M., S. Moreno, R. Nájera, J. C. Boucher, G. Espín, G. Soberón-Chávez, and V. Deretic. 1996. Characterization of the genes coding for the putative sigma factor AlgU and its regulators MucA, MucB, MucC, and MucD in *Azotobacter vinelandii* and evaluation of their roles in alginate biosynthesis. *J. Bacteriol.* **178:**1800–1820.

May, T. B., and A. M. Chakrabarty. 1994. *Pseudomonas aeruginosa:* genes and enzymes of alginate synthesis. *Trends Microbiol.* **2:**151–157.

May, T. B., D. Shinabarger, R. Maharaj, J. Kato, L. Chu, J. D. DeVault, S. Roychoudhury, N. A. Zielinski, A. Berry, R. K. Rothmel, T. K. Misra, and A. M. Chakrabarty. 1991. Alginate synthesis by *Pseudomonas aeruginosa:* a key pathogenic factor in chronic pulmonary infections of cystic fibrosis patients. *Clin. Microbiol. Rev.* **4:**191–206.

McGowan, S. J., H. C. Gorham, and D. A. Hodgson. 1993. Light-induced carotenogenesis in *Myxococcus xanthus:* DNA sequence analysis of the *carR* region. *Mol. Microbiol.* **10:**713–725.

Pedersen, S. S. 1992. Lung infection with alginate-producing, mucoid *Pseudomonas aeruginosa* in cystic fibrosis. *APMIS* **100**(Suppl. 28):1–79.

Raina, S., D. Missiakas, and C. Georgopoulos. 1995. The *rpoE* gene encoding the σ^E (σ^{24}) heat shock sigma factor of *Escherichia coli. EMBO J.* **14:**1043–1055.

Rouvière, P. E., A. D. L. Peñas, J. Mecsas, C. Z. Lu, K. E. Rudd, and C. A. Gross. 1995. *rpoE,* the gene encoding the second heat-shock sigma factor, σ^E, in *Escherichia coli. EMBO J.* **14:**1032–1042.

Schurr, M. J., D. W. Martin, M. H. Mudd, and V. Deretic. 1994. Gene cluster controlling conversion to alginate-overproducing phenotype in *Pseudomonas aeruginosa:* functional analysis in a heterologous host and role in the instability of mucoidy. *J. Bacteriol.* **176:**3375–3382.

Schurr, M. J., H. Yu, J. C. Boucher, N. S. Hibler, and V. Deretic. 1995a. Multiple promoters and induction by heat shock of the gene encoding the alternative sigma factor AlgU (σ^E) which controls mucoidy in cystic fibrosis isolates of *Pseudomonas aeruginosa. J. Bacteriol.* **177:**5670–5679.

Schurr, M. J., H. Yu, J. M. Martinez-Salazar, N. S. Hibler, and V. Deretic. 1995b. Biochemical characterization and posttranslational modification of AlgU, a regulator of stress response in *Pseudomonas aeruginosa. Biochem. Biophys. Res. Commun.* **216:**874–880.

Simpson, J. A., S. E. Smith, and R. T. Dean. 1989. Scavenging by alginate of free radicals released by macrophages. *Free Radical Biol. Med.* **6:**347–353.

Speert, D. P. 1994. *Pseudomonas aeruginosa* infections in patients with cystic fibrosis, p. 183–235. *In* A. L. Baltch and R. P. Smith (ed.), *Pseudomonas aeruginosa Infections and Treatment.* Marcel Dekker, Inc., New York.

Wang, Q., and J. M. Kaguni. 1989. A novel sigma factor is involved in expression of the *rpoH* gene of *Escherichia coli. J. Bacteriol.* **171:**4248–4253.

Woods, D. E., P. A. Sokol, L. E. Bryan, D. G. Storey, S. J. Mattingly, H. J. Vogel, and H. Ceri. 1991. *In vivo* regulation of virulence in *Pseudomonas aeruginosa* associated with genetic rearrangement. *J. Infect. Dis.* **163:**143–149.

Wozniak, D. J., and D. E. Ohman. 1994. Transcriptional analysis of the *Pseudomonas aeruginosa* genes *algR*, *algB*, and *algD* reveals a hierachy of alginate gene expression which is modulated by *algT*. *J. Bacteriol.* **176:**6007–6014.

Xiao, Y., S. Heu, J. Yi, Y. Lu, and S. W. Hutcheson. 1994. Identification of putative alternative sigma factor and characterization of a multicomponent regulator cascade controlling the expression of *Pseudomonas syringae* pv. syringae Pss61 *hrp* and *hrmA* genes. *J. Bacteriol.* **176:**1025–1036.

Yu, H., J. C. Boucher, N. S. Hibler, and V. Deretic. 1996. Virulence properties of *Pseudomonas aeruginosa* lacking the extreme-stress sigma factor AlgU (σ^E). *Infect. Immun.* **64:**in press.

Yu, H., M. J. Schurr, and V. Deretic. 1995. Functional equivalence of *Escherichia coli* σ^E and *Pseudomonas aeruginosa* AlgU: *E. coli rpoE* restores mucoidy and reduces sensitivity to reactive oxygen intermediates in *algU* mutants of *P. aeruginosa*. *J. Bacteriol.* **177:**3259–3268.

Molecular Biology of Pseudomonads
Edited by T. Nakazawa et al.

Chapter 35

Metal Resistances in Pseudomonads: Genes and Mechanisms

Carlos Cervantes and Simon Silver

The environmental exposure of bacteria to the toxic ions of metal and metalloid elements selects resistant strains possessing genes encoding highly specific mechanisms of resistance. The ions for which such resistances are known include several lacking any biological function (arsenic, cadmium, chromate, lead, mercury, silver, tellurite, tin, and thallium) as well as essential micronutrients (cobalt, copper, nickel, and zinc). Genetic resistance determinants usually reside on plasmids, only occasionally on transposons, and infrequently on the bacterial chromosome. Genes conferring resistance to metal ions isolated from *Pseudomonas* strains of diverse origins have been cloned and sequenced (Silver and Walderhaug, 1992; Cervantes and Gutierrez-Corona, 1994; Cervantes et al., 1994; Silver and Ji, 1994; Silver and Phung, 1996). In this review, we gather representative information on the genetic and biochemical strategies displayed by pseudomonads and related bacteria in their effort to cope with toxic metal inorganic ions.

MERCURY

Resistance to mercuric ions is the best understood of the bacterial heavy-metal resistances (Silver and Walderhaug, 1992). Plasmid-conferred mercury resistance genes from many sources have been cloned and sequenced, including the first two from *Pseudomonas* transposon Tn*501* and plasmid R100 (containing transposon Tn*21*) from *Shigella* spp. Although the bacterial sources were different, both sequences contained about 62% G+C, suggesting a pseudomonad origin. A single mechanism of mercury resistance is displayed by all systems studied in detail, namely, enzymatic reduction of Hg^{2+} to nontoxic, volatile Hg^0 by the enzyme mercuric reductase encoded by the *merA* gene. All mercury resistance systems also encode proteins that carry out the specific transport of mercury from outside the cell to the intracellular mercuric reductase enzyme.

Carlos Cervantes • Instituto de Investigaciones Químico-Biólogicas, Universidad Michoacana, 58240 Morelia, Mich., Mexico. ***Simon Silver*** • Department of Microbiology and Immunology, University of Illinois College of Medicine, Chicago, Illinois 60612-7344.

However, recent studies, especially with pseudomonads, have shown there is a structural diversity of *mer* determinants (Fig. 1) that had not been appreciated earlier. Most *mer* determinants occur on plasmids, but available sequences include chromosomal determinants from gram-negative *Thiobacillus ferrooxidans* (Inoue et al., 1989) and gram-positive *Bacillus* sp. (Wang et al., 1989), where a low G+C base composition for the *mer* operon indicates a long adaptation to the cellular environment. The first five *mer* deter-

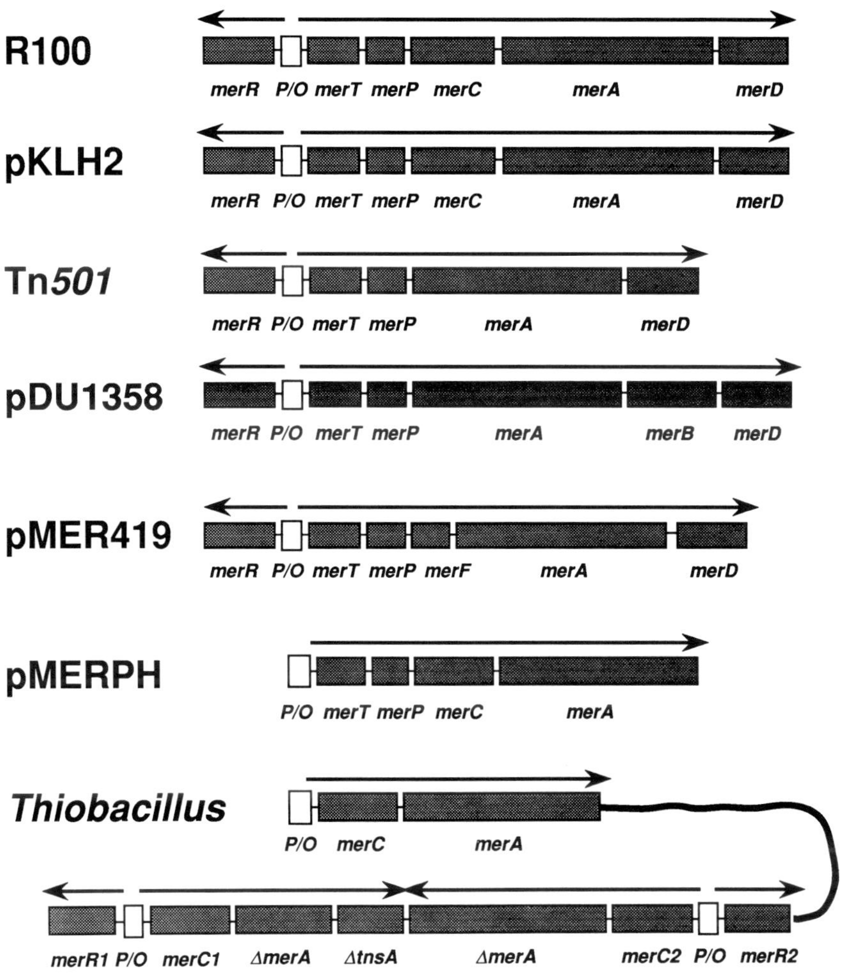

Figure 1. The organization of the *mer* operons of *Pseudomonas* and related gram-negative bacteria: plasmid R100 (transposon Tn*21*: isolated from *Shigella flexneri*), plasmid pKHL2 (isolated from *Acinetobacter* sp.), transposon Tn*501* (plasmid pVS1 from *P. aeruginosa*), plasmids pDU1358 (isolated from *Serratia marcescens*), pMER419 (isolated from *Pseudomonas* sp.), and pMERPH (isolated from *P. putrefaciens*), and the chromosomal *T. ferrooxidans* determinant. Shaded boxes indicate genes, with names below. Open boxes indicate transcriptional operator/promoter sites with mRNA transcripts indicated above with arrows (from Silver and Phung [1996], with permission).

minants shown in Fig. 1 start with a regulatory gene, *merR*, which is transcribed from the strand opposite to that of the remaining *mer* genes (Fig. 1). *merR* genes have been recognized in six of the seven *mer* systems from gram-negative bacteria. The current exception is the recently reported pMERPH system (originally from a *Pseudomonas putrefaciens* isolate; Osborn et al., 1996) for which the *merR* gene probably occurs but has yet to be located. The MerR protein binds as a homodimer to the adjacent operator/promoter site of the *mer* operon (O'Halloran, 1993; O'Halloran et al., 1989; Summers, 1992), functioning both as a repressor (in the absence of mercury) and as an inducer (in the presence of mercury). The MerR protein remains bound to the operator/promoter site even in the absence of mercury. The predicted amino acid sequence of MerR suggests that the DNA-binding region forms a helix-turn-helix motif as do many other regulatory proteins (Silver and Walderhaug, 1992; Summers, 1992). The MerR proteins from the top five gram-negative bacterial systems shown in Fig. 1 share 85% to 94% amino acid identities, but only about 55% identities with the *Thiobacillus* MerR sequences.

Then each *mer* determinant starts with an operator/promoter region followed by genes involved in mercury transport into the cells (Fig. 1). For Tn*501* and plasmid pDU1358, these are the *merT* and *merP* genes which determine, respectively, an inner membrane protein and a periplasmic mercury-binding protein. These are sufficient for mercury transport, but four (of the seven systems shown in Fig. 1) have an additional gene, *merC*, which determines an inner membrane protein that has been shown in the case of *Thiobacillus* to constitute a mercury transport system by itself (Kusano et al., 1990).

The gene encoding mercuric reductase, *merA*, follows in each determinant (Fig. 1). The reductase is a homodimeric, NADPH-dependent, flavin adenine dinucleotide-containing enzyme. The crystal structure for the *Bacillus* form of the enzyme has been solved (Schiering et al., 1991). The active site of mercuric reductase occurs at the subunit interface, including the active site cysteine pair of one subunit and the carboxyl-terminal vicinal cysteine pair of the other subunit (Distefano et al., 1990). It has been postulated that mercuric reducatase functions a bit like an American baseball glove, with an amino-terminal domain (which is sequence homologous to the periplasmic MerP protein) containing a vicinal cysteine pair that catches Hg^{2+} from the membrane MerT protein and then passes Hg^{2+} off to the carboxyl-terminal region (highly conserved in all mercuric reductase sequences) with another cysteine pair, which then shuffles Hg^{2+} to the active site. In this model the intracellular Hg^{2+} would never be free but rather passed on from cysteine pair to cysteine pair, protecting the intracellular environment. Mercuric reductase shows a structural and functional homology to gluthathione reductase of eukaryotic cells including human erythrocytes (Schiering et al., 1991). The gene for a second regulatory protein, MerD, follows the reductase gene in the first four systems shown in Fig. 1. However, *merD* is missing in the remaining three systems shown. Mutations in the *merD* gene reduce slightly the level of mercury resistance, and the MerD protein shows a sequence similarity to MerR, particularly in the helix-turn-helix region (Brown et al., 1986). MerD is a secondary minor regulator of the *mer* operon (Mukhopadhyay et al., 1991) that binds to the same operator region as MerR does.

Only pDU1358 (of the seven systems shown in Fig. 1) has the *merB* gene encoding an organomercurial lyase enzyme. However, we expect this situation to change since organomercurial lyase activity was found with more than half of the *Pseudomonas mer* determinants initially tested (Clark et al., 1977). A *Pseudomonas stutzeri* system with a *merB* gene is under study (Reniero et al., 1995). The *P. stutzeri* plasmid has two mercury resistance operons; one system is broad spectrum (like pDU1358) with a *merB* gene, while the other is narrow spectrum and lacks a *merB* gene. The broad-spectrum mercurial resistance operon of *P. stutzeri* appears to have a gene order similar to the systems at the top of Fig. 1, except for the remarkable placement of *merB* between *merR* and *merT* (rather than after *merA*), with an additional transcriptional start signal before the *merB* gene (P. Barbieri and E. Galli, personal communication; Reniero et al., 1995). Clearly there are variations in gene order and structure among *mer* operons, the significance of which we do not understand.

The mercury-resistant *Pseudomonas* sp. strain K-62 studied by Tonomura and Furukawa 25 years ago has two separate *merB* genes for organomercurial lyase and resistance (Kiyono et al., 1995a; Kiyono et al., 1995b, 1995c). One of the two *Pseudomonas* sp. strain K-62 organomercurial resistance determinants has been mapped on a 26-bp plasmid (Kiyono et al., 1995b), which has also been demonstrated to contain mercury transport activity (MerT and MerP) that determines hyperaccumulation of Hg^{2+} but not CH_3Hg^+ (Kiyono et al., 1995c). This is the first demonstration that an organomercurial does not use the mercury uptake system of inorganic Hg^{2+}. A 6-kb region containing the mercury resistance operon has been sequenced (Kiyono et al., 1995a) and contains the same genes as shown in Fig. 1 for plasmid pDU1358 plus an additional 181-codon open reading frame between *merA* and *merB* that lacks homology to known proteins.

There remain two additional variations of *mer* operon structure seen in Fig. 1. The new plasmid pMER419 mercury resistance determinant has an additional open reading frame, *merF* (Fig. 1), although it has no known function (Hobman et al., 1994). The MerF predicted amino acid sequence shows homology to the longer MerT membrane transport protein. The additional complexity with the *Thiobacillus* chromosomal *mer* determinant includes a region between two oppositely oriented *merR* genes that is occupied by two functional *merC* genes and three partial (and therefore nonfunctional) genes, including two for mercuric reductase (Fig. 1, bottom).

COPPER

Copper is an essential micronutrient for most, if not all, living organisms since it is the constituent of many metalloenzymes and proteins involved in electron transport, redox, and other important reactions (Lontie, 1984). However, copper also is toxic, as it is involved in free radical formation that can damage cellular constituents. High levels of copper exert a pressure on microorganisms that results sometimes in the selection of variants possessing genetic determinants of copper resistance (Trevors, 1987). Genes related to normal copper metabolism in bacteria usually reside on the chromosome (Brown et al., 1994), whereas copper resistance genes are located on plasmids.

Plasmid-determined resistance to copper has been found in diverse gram-negative bacterial species (Trevors, 1987), but only three copper resistance determinants have been analyzed to the molecular level (Silver et al., 1993b; Cooksey, 1994; Silver and Ji, 1994; Brown et al., 1994; Cervantes and Gutierrez-Corona, 1994).

The best-studied bacterial copper resistance determinant comes from plasmid pPT23 identified in a strain of *Pseudomonas syringae* pv. tomato (Bender and Cooksey, 1986).

Four structural genes, arranged in the *cop* operon, were identified: two of them *copA* and *copB*, are necessary for expression of partial copper resistance, while plasmids with deletions in *copC* or *copD* still confer a low level of resistance (Mellano and Cooksey, 1988). From sequence analysis, an octa-peptide containing aspartic acid, histidine, and methionine residues is repeated several times in both CopA and CopB and is proposed to function as a copper-binding motif (Mellano and Cooksey, 1988; Cooksey, 1994; Brown et al., 1994).

Cha and Cooksey (1991) found that CopA and CopC are periplasmic proteins able to bind, respectively, 11 and 1 copper atoms per polypeptide (Fig. 2). CopB is an outer membrane protein which binds additional copper (Cha and Cooksey, 1991) and may be involved in cross-membrane copper transport (Silver et al., 1993b; Cooksey, 1994). Cooksey et al. (1990) found that the *copB* gene from plasmid pPT23 shows homology with plasmid or chromosomal DNA from copper-resistant pathogenic and saprophytic plant-associated pseudomonads. The finding that homology was significant even with DNA from copper-sensitive strains led Cooksey and colleagues to propose that *cop* genes may have a function other than copper resistance and that plasmid *cop* genes might have evolved in pseudomonads from chromosomal genes (Cooksey et al., 1990; Cooksey, 1994). The fourth gene product, CopD, is associated with the inner membrane, where it is thought to participate in copper transport (Cha and Cooksey, 1993; Fig. 2); however, direct data are lacking.

Transcriptional regulation of the *cop* operon is carried out by a *trans*-acting pair of regulatory proteins, CopR, which is a DNA-binding transcriptional regulatory protein, and CopS, which is a membrane-embedded copper sensor protein (Brown et al., 1994; Cooksey, 1994; Silver and Ji, 1994). From proposed protein sequences, this pair of regulator proteins are typical of the two components "sensor" (CopS, with an invariant histidine residue assumed to be the site of autophosphorylation by ATP in the presence of

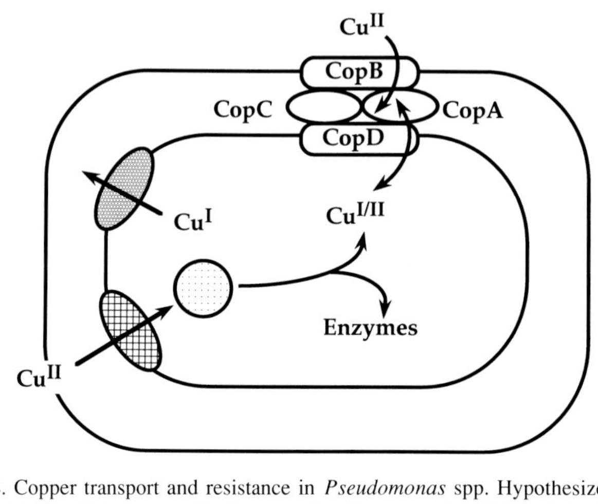

Figure 2. Copper transport and resistance in *Pseudomonas* spp. Hypothesized uptake, efflux, and intracellular copper-binding proteins (Brown et al., 1994) and the CopABCD products of the plasmid-encoded copper resistance system of *P. syringae* (Cooksey, 1994) (modified from Silver and Phung [1996], with permission).

high extracellular copper) and "responder" (CopR, with an invariant aspartate residue assumed to be *trans*-phosphorylated from CopS, resulting in activation to an operator DNA-binding form) (Parkinson and Kofoid, 1992; Cooksey, 1994; Brown et al., 1994). Cooksey (1994) identified an additional regulatory affector of the *copABCDRS* determinant, a chromosomally determined DNA-binding protein called CopM.

Brown et al. (1995) cloned the *pco* copper resistance determinant from *Escherichia coli* plasmid pRJ1004. The *pco* system is the *E. coli* equivalent of *Pseudomonas cop*, and the genes are arranged in the same order: *pcoABCDRSE* (Brown et al., 1994; Brown et al., 1995). The *pco* gene products show significant sequence homology to the *cop* gene products. The amino acid sequence identities of the homologous protein pairs are: PcoA/CopA, 76%; PcoB/CopB, 54%; PcoC/CopC, 66%; and PcoD/CopD, 38% (Silver et al., 1993b). Surprisingly, the *E. coli* system appears to confer copper resistance by an efflux mechanism (Brown et al., 1994; Silver et al., 1993b) and not by increased uptake. We propose that the Cop and Pco systems function in comparable ways, and perhaps efflux across the cellular membrane is a short-term, immediate response to copper toxicity while extracytoplasmic copper sequestration is a long-term solution, functioning only after days. While colonies of the copper-resistant *P. syringae* pv. tomato strain turn bright blue, attributed to copper binding to the CopA, CopB, and CopC proteins, comparable colonies of resistant *Xanthomonas* and *E. coli* strains and most other copper-resistant pseudomonads turn brown over several days of exposure to copper in agar medium (Cooksey, 1994; Brown et al., 1994), again an apparent difference requiring an explanation that is not currently available.

The chromosome of *Xanthomonas campestris* pv. juglandis, a pathogen of walnuts, is the source of the third sequenced copper resistance determinant (Lee et al., 1994). Although of chromosomal origin, the four structural genes, *copABCD*, of the *Xanthomonas* determinant show significant homology with both *cop* and *pco* genes (Silver and Ji, 1994; Lee et al., 1994); surprisingly, the protein sequences were more similar for the *Xanthomonas*/*E. coli* pairs than for the *Xanthomonas* (a pseudomonad)/*Pseudomonas* protein pairs.

Copper resistance has also been encountered in strains of *X. campestris* pv. vesicatoria bearing the large plasmids pXvCu (Stall et al., 1986) or pXV10A (Bender et al., 1990). The DNAs of the copper resistance determinant from plasmids pXV10A and pXvCu showed strong homology with one another but only slight similarity to the *P. syringae cop* copper resistance genes (Bender et al., 1990). Voloudakis et al. (1993), however, found significant homology between copper resistance plasmid DNA from diverse *Xanthomonas* strains and the *copA* gene from *P. syringae*, suggesting a possible common origin for the copper resistance determinants from these plant-associated bacteria. It seems that copper resistance commonly occurs in environmental pseudomonads. The specifics of the physiological and biochemical processes remain, however, to be determined.

Garde and Bender (1991) used a probe from pXV10A to detect copper resistance determinants from a variety of soil bacteria; genomic DNA from copper-sensitive strains failed to hybridize to the pXV10A probe, thus allowing the proposal of a nonendogenous origin of the *Xanthomonas* copper resistance genes. Since the *P. syringae* resistance determinants were postulated to be of chromosomal origin (Garde and Bender, 1991; see above), exchange of plasmid DNA between *Pseudomonas* and *Xanthomonas* spp. is suggested to be responsible for the similarities between the copper resistance determinants of these bacteria (Voloudakis et al., 1993).

CADMIUM

Cadmium is very toxic for bacteria and higher living forms (Trevors et al., 1986). Higham et al. (1984) reported that a cadmium-resistant strain of *Pseudomonas putida* produced low-molecular-weight proteins able to chelate cadmium. These proteins were purified and appeared to be similar to the cysteine-rich metallothioneins of animals (Higham et al., 1984), which are metal-complexing small proteins involved in cation homeostasis and detoxification (Kägi and Kojima, 1988). The in vitro chemical analysis of the *Pseudomonas* metallothioneins was quite convincing (Higham et al., 1984). Bacterial metallothioneins have since been well studied in cyanobacteria (Turner and Robinson, 1995). However, the *Pseudomonas* metallothioneins have proven to be a puzzle. The original work could not be confirmed in the initial laboratory (nor in our own or by others; P. J. Sadler and S. Silver, unpublished results). Therefore the question of *Pseudomonas* metallothionein polypeptides must be taken as unresolved today.

Nevertheless, both gram-negative and gram-positive bacteria have well-understood plasmid-encoded systems for cadmium resistance (Ji and Silver, 1995; Nies and Silver, 1995). Whereas there is a single mechanism for bacterial mercury resistance, the biochemical mechanisms of bacterial plasmid-determined cadmium resistance are more diverse. The best-understood system of cadmium resistance is the *cad* operon from a plasmid of *Staphylococcus aureus* (Nucifora et al., 1989; Silver et al., 1989; Ji and Silver, 1995). Resistance to cadmium in this gram-positive bacterium results from cation efflux by CadA, a plasmid-encoded P-type ATPase (Nucifora et al., 1989; Silver et al., 1989; Ji and Silver, 1995). Gram-negative bacteria have different mechanisms. Plasmid pGU100, from the soil bacterium *P. putida*, confers resistance to cadmium by a mechanism that involves reduced cadmium uptake (Horitsu et al., 1986), apparently by cadmium efflux. Unfortunately, the most recent efforts in cloning this *Pseudomonas* cadmium-resistance determinant in *E. coli* resulted instead in isolation of cadmium-resistant *E. coli* with an insertion sequence element inserted into a chromosomal location (Itoh et al., 1994).

A different form of cadmium resistance, governed by the *czc* operon on *Alcaligenes eutrophus* plasmid pMOL30, couples resistances to cadmium, zinc, and cobalt and has been studied in detail (Nies et al., 1987; Nies et al., 1989; Diels et al., 1995; Nies, 1995; Nies and Silver, 1995). The *czc* operon consists of three structural genes, *czcCBA* plus two or more regulatory genes, concerning which there is no current agreement (Nies, 1992b; Nies and Silver, 1995; Diels et al., 1995). The CzcCBA complex (Fig. 3) is an example of so-called RND systems (for resistance, nodulation, and cell division, since different members are involved in cation resistance, nodulation in *Rhizobium*, and cell division in *E. coli*) (Diels et al., 1995). For the cation efflux examples, the three proteins are the major inner membrane transporter CzcA, the outer membrane protein CzcC, and a "membrane fusion" protein, CzcB, which is considered to bridge the periplasmic space, thus ensuring that the effluxed divalent cation is exported to the outside of the cell and not deposited in the periplasmic space where it might be uneconomically retaken up by the divalent cation uptake transporter (Nies and Silver, 1995; Diels et al., 1995). Although direct data are lacking for the cellular positioning of these proteins, it has become

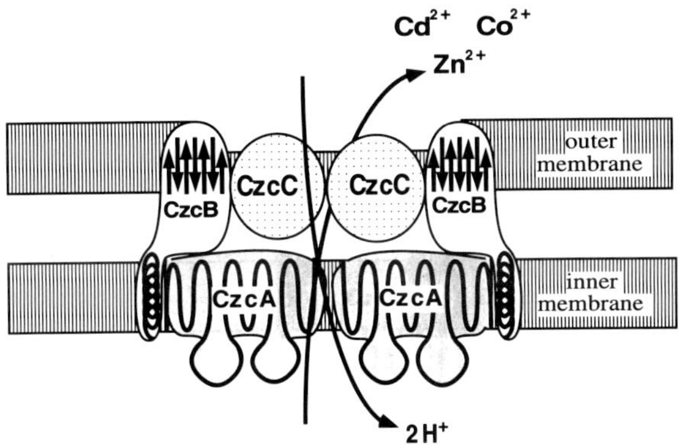

Figure 3. Czc model for cadmium, zinc, and cobalt efflux system functioning as proton/cation antiporter consisting of inner membrane (CzcA), outer membrane (CzcC), and "membrane fusion" (CzcB) proteins (adapted from model of Q. Dong and S. Silver; Diels et al., 1995).

clear that cadmium efflux occurs by a chemiosmotic cation/proton antiporter system (Nies, 1995; Nies and Silver, 1995). CzcA is the central membrane protein during efflux, and the ancillary proteins CzcB and CzcC are needed for full resistance levels and full efflux of all three cations (Nies et al., 1989; Nies, 1992a; Nies and Silver, 1995). The *czcD* gene downstream from the structural genes *czcCBA*, together with one or more upstream regulatory genes (Nies, 1992a; 1992b; Nies and Silver, 1995; Diels et al., 1995), regulates the functioning of the Czc system in a way not currently understood.

A second plasmid from *A. eutrophus* CH34, pMOL28, contains the *cnr* operon which confers resistances to cobalt and nickel, but not cadmium (Liesegang et al., 1993; Silver and Ji, 1994; Ji and Silver, 1995; Diels et al., 1995). A mutation can add zinc resistance to the *cnr* repertoire (Diels et al., 1995), and a third related *Alcaligenes* system is called *ncc* for nickel, cobalt, and cadmium resistances. These distinct systems for divalent cation resistance show sequence homologies for the A, B, and C structural proteins and are thought to all be represented by the model in Fig. 3 for three-component divalent cation/proton antiporters.

ARSENIC

Arsenic toxicity depends on its oxidation state: trivalent arsenicals (arsenite) are about 100 times more toxic than pentavalent derivatives (arsenate) (Nakamuro and Sayato, 1981). Thus, oxidation of As(III) to As(V) represents a potential detoxification process that allows microorganisms to tolerate higher levels of arsenite. Osborne and Ehrlich (1976) and Phillips and Taylor (1976) isolated *Alcaligenes* strains able to oxidize arsenite. Arsenite oxidase was recently purified and shown to be an inner membrane enzyme that uses azurin and cytochrome *c* as electron acceptors (Anderson et al., 1992). Other microbial transformations of arsenic include methylation and demethylation (Summers and Silver, 1978; Craig, 1989), but these processes seem not to be related to resistance mechanisms.

Arsenic resistance plasmids confer tolerance to arsenate and arsenite, as well as to antimony (III), to a wide variety of gram-positive and gram-negative bacteria, including *E. coli* (Silver et al., 1981) and *Pseudomonas aeruginosa* (Cervantes and Chávez, 1992). Resistance to all three ions is inducible, and cross-induction of resistances occurs (Silver et al., 1981; Cervantes and Chávez, 1992).

The arsenic resistance determinant from *E. coli* plasmid R773 was sequenced (Chen et al., 1986; San Francisco et al., 1990), and the products of each gene have been studied in detail. The *ars* operon of plasmid R773 contains five genes, namely, *arsR, arsD, arsA, arsB,* and *arsC,* in order (Rosen et al., 1992; Silver et al., 1993a). A closely related DNA sequence with the same five genes has recently been determined for the *ars* operon of plasmid R46 (Bruhn et al., in press). A chromosomal version of the *ars* operon was sequenced as part of the genome project (ECOUW76 release), and this consists of only the *arsR, arsB,* and *arsC* genes, missing *arsD* and *arsA* (Carlin et al., 1995; Diorio et al., 1995). The *E. coli* chromosomal *ars* operon is sufficiently dissimilar from that of plasmid R773 to be undetectable by Southern blot analysis. However, the chromosomal *ars* operon used as a probe picks up weak hybridization with the *P. aeruginosa* PAO1 chromosomal DNA (Diorio et al., 1995), so we expect that similar chromosomal arsenic resistance systems will be found widely in pseudomonads. A comparable pattern of *arsR, arsB,* and *arsC* without *arsA* and *arsD* has been previously found twice in gram-positive plasmid versions of the *ars* operon (Silver and Ji, 1994; Ji and Silver, 1995). Moderate resistance is conferred by the *E. coli* chromosomal *ars* operon, and a stronger level of resistance is conferred by the plasmid operon (Carlin et al., 1995; Diorio et al., 1995).

The functioning of the three structural proteins, ArsA, ArsB, and ArsC, is diagrammed in Fig. 4 in a manner that explains how ArsB can function as an arsenite efflux transporter with or without ArsA. ArsB is an integral inner membrane protein of 429 amino acids that has been shown in gene fusion experiments to pass through the membrane 12 times with little sequence in either the cytoplasmic or periplasmic space (Wu et al., 1992). Functioning alone, ArsB is a chemiosmotic arsenite efflux

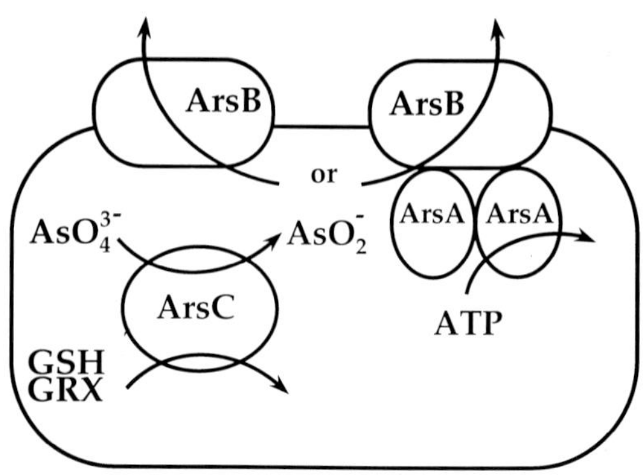

Figure 4. Functioning of the proteins of the *ars* operons of plasmids and the chromosomes of gram-negative cells (from Silver and Phung [1996], with permission). GSH, glutathione; GRX, glutathione reductase.

system that is energized by the cell membrane potential (Bröer et al., 1993; Dey and Rosen, 1995). ArsB also functions as a membrane anchor (Tisa and Rosen, 1990) for the ATPase subunit ArsA, and when ArsA is attached the complex functions exclusively as an efflux ATPase (Fig. 4) (Rosen et al., 1992; Silver et al., 1993a). The ATPase mode confers a higher level of arsenite resistance than the chemiosmotic mode does (Dey and Rosen, 1995). This unique either-or pattern of energy coupling has not been found in any other bacterial membrane transport system (Silver et al., 1993a).

The ArsA protein has been purified and studied in elegant detail in vitro as an arsenite- or antimonite-stimulated ATPase (Karkaria et al., 1990; Karkaria et al., 1991; Kaur and Rosen, 1993). The 583-amino-acid-long ArsA protein from plasmid R773 appears to have resulted from gene duplication and fusion, since the amino and carboxyl half-sequences are closely homologous and each contains a canonical ATP-binding motif (Chen et al., 1986), both of which are required for resistance in vivo and ATPase activity in vitro. The active ArsA ATPase is a homodimer, which therefore would contain four ATP-binding sites. Both ATP-binding sites per chain are required for activity, but complementation studies (Kaur and Rosen, 1993) have shown that the amino and carboxyl half-molecules can complement when produced in vivo as separate polypeptides.

The gene, *arsC*, encodes a soluble arsenate reductase that reduces intracellular arsenate to arsenite. Arsenite is then extruded out of the cells by the ArsB protein (Ji and Silver, 1992) (Fig. 4). The arsenate reductase from gram-positive microbes couples with thioredoxin (but not glutaredoxin) to provide reducing potential for As(V)-to-As(III) conversion and has a high affinity (micromolar affinity constant) for arsenate as substrate (Ji and Silver, 1992; Ji et al., 1994). In contrast, arsenate reductase from plasmid R773 in gram-negative bacteria appears strikingly different. The two ArsC sequences are less than 20% identical, and the gram-positive ArsC has four cysteines as potential active site residues, whereas the gram-negative ArsC has only two cysteines (Silver et al., 1993a; Ji and Silver, 1995) and appears to use only one of the two cysteines in arsenate reduction. Plasmid R773 ArsC uses glutaredoxin (but not thioredoxin) (Gladysheva et al., 1994) and has a rather low affinity for arsenate (8 mM AsO_4^{3-} affinity constant) in vitro. Future efforts will clarify how the same enzymatic reaction, required for arsenate resistance (Chen et al., 1986), can be carried out by apparently quite dissimilar mechanisms.

The *ars* operon is regulated by the ArsR protein, a *trans*-acting repressor, and the operon can be induced by arsenate, arsenite, antimonite, and bismuth in vivo (Wu and Rosen, 1991), but only arsenite and antimony in vitro. Arsenate is reduced inside the cell by the ArsC protein to arsenite, the actual inducer. The ArsR proteins belong to a new class (or maybe a "subclass") of DNA-binding proteins which are proposed to contain helix-turn-helix DNA-binding regions with two arsenite-coordinating cysteines (Bairoch, 1993; Fig. 5). This is in striking contrast to the MerR mercury resistance regulatory protein, which also has a helix-turn-helix DNA-binding region (near the amino end) but in which cysteines that coordinate Hg^{2+} to affect activation are distant (near the carboxyl end; Fig. 5). The two regulatory proteins also differ in that ArsR is a repressor (that dissociates from the DNA in the presence of oxyanion inducer) while MerR is an activator (that alters the conformation of bound DNA in the presence of Hg^{2+}, leading to transcription) (Summers, 1992; O'Halloran, 1993). In addition to ArsR, this new subfamily of helix-turn-helix proteins includes CadC, the repressor of the gram-positive cadmium ATPase system (Endo and Silver, 1995), and SmtB, the repressor of the metallothionein system of cyanobacteria (Turner and Robinson, 1995). The *ars* operon of gram-negative plasmids has a second regulatory gene, *arsD*, which encodes an inducer-independent *trans*-acting regulatory protein that controls the upper level of *ars* gene expression (Wu and Rosen, 1993).

Inducible resistance to arsenic (and antimony) salts conferred by the transferable plasmid pUM310 was found in a clinical *P. aeruginosa* isolate (Cervantes and Chávez, 1992), but the mechanism of resistance has not yet been studied.

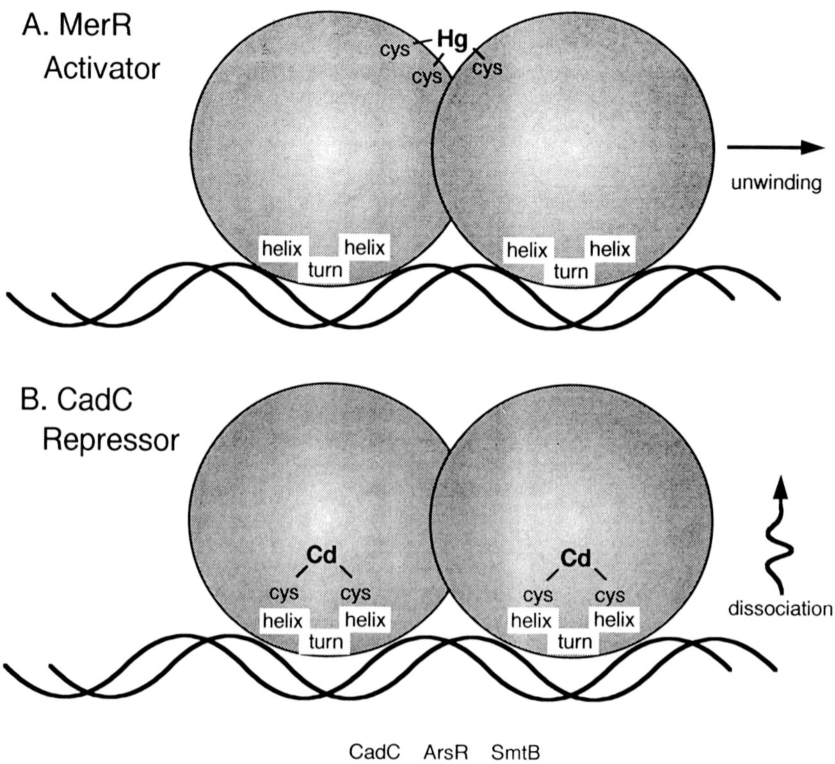

Figure 5. Model for different metal binding by MerR (mercury resistance operon, e.g., of Tn*501*) and CadC (cadmium resistance operon, e.g., of plasmid pI258). Hg^{2+} is bound by three cysteine thiols involving both subunits. The cysteines are amino distal, whereas the predicted helix-turn-helix DNA-binding motif is amino proximal in the sequence. Cd^{2+} is hypothesized to be bound by the two cysteines within the helix-turn-helix motif of CadC, but whether coordination is within a subunit (as shown) or between subunits is not known. The other members of the CadC family are ArsR (repressor of the arsenic resistance operon, e.g., plasmid R773) and SmtB (repressor of the metallothionein system of cyanobacteria).

CHROMIUM

Hexavalent chromium [Cr(VI); chromate] is toxic to cells, whereas trivalent chromium [Cr(III)] is very insoluble and therefore relatively innocuous when found extracellularly (Cary, 1982; Cervantes and Silver, 1992). Chromate is a competitive inhibitor of sulfate transport in *Pseudomonas* (Ohtake et al., 1987; Cervantes and Ohtake, 1988) and *Alcaligenes* (Nies et al., 1990).

Plasmid-determined resistance to chromate has been found in several species of *Pseudomonas* (Summers and Jacoby, 1978; Horitsu et al., 1987; Bopp et al., 1983; Cervantes-Vega et al., 1986; Cervantes and Ohtake, 1988). Resistance results from decreased chromate accumulation by *P. aeruginosa* (Ohtake et al., 1987; Cervantes and Ohtake, 1988). Sulfate transport is not altered by the presence of chromate resistance plasmids (Ohtake et al., 1987). A chromate resistance determinant from *P. aeruginosa* plasmid pUM505 was cloned and sequenced (Cervantes et al., 1990). From sequence analysis, a hydrophobic polypeptide of 416 amino acids, ChrA, was predicted as the principal gene product. ChrA is postulated to play a still-to-be-defined role in chromate membrane transport (Cervantes et al., 1990). A second chromate resistance determinant, cloned from *A. eutrophus* plasmid pMOL28, encodes a polypeptide showing 29% amino acid identity with the *Pseudomonas* ChrA (Nies et al., 1990). Recently, a cyanobacterial version of ChrA was identified that is 62% identical to the *A. eutrophus* ChrA but only 28% identical to the *P. aeruginosa* ChrA (Nicholson and Laudenbach, 1995). We may expect that the chromate resistance system will be found more widely in bacteria. The *Alcaligenes* determinant contains an additional upstream gene, *chrB*, proposed to be responsible for the inducibility of the resistance (Nies et al., 1990). The cloned *Pseudomonas* determinant lacks the *chrB* gene and is constitutive.

The capacity to reduce chromate to Cr(III) is not plasmid mediated (Bopp and Ehrlich, 1988; Ishibashi et al., 1990) and probably is not a primary resistance mechanism (conferring only low-level tolerance to chromate). Chromate reduction has been found with diverse *Pseudomonas* strains (Romanenko and Koren'kov, 1977; Lebedeva and Lyalikova, 1979; Horitsu et al., 1987; Bopp and Ehrlich, 1988; Ishibashi et al., 1990; Suzuki et al., 1992) and appears to be a secondary reaction of a still unknown metabolic pathway (Ishibashi et al., 1990). Nevertheless, bacterial chromate reduction has the potential to become a useful bioremediation technology (Lovley, 1993; Ohtake and Silver, 1994). Soluble NADH-dependent chromate reductases have been partially purified and characterized from *P. putida* (Ishibashi et al., 1990) and *Pseudomonas ambigua* (Suzuki et al., 1992). A distinct, membrane-bound chromate reductase was found in *P. fluorescens* (Bopp and Ehrlich, 1988).

TELLURIUM

Although tellurium is not considered to be a pollutant metal, its oxyanions, Te(IV) (tellurite; TeO_3^{2-}) and Te(VI) (tellurate; TeO_4^{2-}), are highly toxic to gram-negative bacteria (however, gram positives are usually resistant to those compounds). Resistance to tellurium compounds is a common genetic marker on transferable R plasmids of *Pseudomonas* spp. (Summers and Jacoby, 1977), especially plasmids belonging to incompatibility groups IncP-1 and IncP-2 (Jacoby, 1986). A cryptic tellurium resistance determinant was found in the broad-host-range plasmid RP4 (also called RK2), which was originally isolated from a clinical *P. aeruginosa* strain (Walter and Taylor, 1989). Tellurium resistance genes are contained in transposon Tn*521* (Bradley et al., 1988), from which they have been cloned and expressed (Walter and Taylor, 1989). Sequence analysis of the predicted polypeptides, however, gives no insights as to a possible resistance mechanism (Walter et al., 1991).

A different tellurium resistance determinant was cloned and expressed from *E. coli* plasmid pHH1508a, but again the predicted amino acid sequences provided no clues to the tolerance mechanism (Walter and Taylor, 1989). Both *Pseudomonas* and *E. coli* tellurite resistance systems are constitutively expressed. A third, inducible tellurium resistance determinant from *Alcaligenes* plasmid pMER610 was sequenced (Jobling and Ritchie, 1987, 1988). This determinant encodes four polypeptides, but again the mechanism of resistance remains elusive. No relationship was found between the resistance phenotype and tellurite transport (Lloyd-Jones et al., 1991).

Reduction of tellurite [Te(IV)] to innocuous metallic Te(0) seems unrelated to resistance to tellurite or tellurate, since tellurite-sensitive cells can reduce the oxyanions. Thus, tellurite resistance has been the most frustrating case to date of DNA sequencing of several plasmid resistance systems yielding no inkling as to the resistance mechanism.

SILVER

Silver is highly toxic for bacteria, mainly acting as a respiration poison. Silver as a significant environmental pollutant may be limited to mining areas, photographic film processing factories, and hospital discharges (from the use of silver salts in burn treatment wards). Plasmid-conferred silver resistance has been reported in diverse bacteria (Summers et al., 1978; Silver, 1981; Silver and Misra, 1988). In no case is the mechanism of silver resistance known, or even studied sufficiently that one might set a reasonable hypothesis (Slawson et al., 1992b). Belly and Kydd (1982) described a silver-resistant *Pseudomonas* isolate that was suggested to detoxify the metal by reduction or by complexing Ag^+ with cell components. The genetic basis of this resistance has not been reported. A different plasmid silver resistance system, pKK1, was found in a *P. stutzeri* strain isolated from a silver mine (Haefeli et al., 1984). Slawson et al. (1992a) studied silver uptake and resistance of pKK1-containing cells, but failed to solve the resistance mechanism. Silver (1981) reported that resistance to silver ions in an *E. coli* strain harboring a different plasmid (that originated from a *Citrobacter* isolate) could be ascribed to less avid extracting of toxic silver ions from AgCl precipitate in the medium (or alternative organic complexes of silver) by the resistant cells as compared to a silver-sensitive strain lacking the plasmid. Deshpande and Chopade (1994) have recently described a plasmid silver resistance determinant in *Acinetobacter baumannii* that may have a basis of silver efflux from the resistant cell. Chromosomally encoding Ag^+ efflux in the gram-positive bacterium *Enterococcus hirae* was established by uptake measurements with everted membrane vesicles (Solioz and Odermatt, 1995). This is the most advanced understanding for a system of Ag^+ transport. The gene governing efflux determines a P-type ATPase that extrudes Ag^+ and Cu^+, providing low-level resistance to both. The chromosomally encoded P-type ATPase for copper and silver is closely homologous to the cadmium efflux ATPase (governed by plasmids in gram-positive bacteria) (Silver et al., 1989; Silver and Walderhaug, 1992; Silver and Ji, 1994; Ji and Silver, 1995). There is also evidence for an interplay between Ag^+ and copper transport in gram-negative bacteria (Ghandour et al., 1988).

OTHER METAL RESISTANCE SYSTEMS

Resistance to other less-studied metal ions in *Pseudomonas* spp. has been reported, including tolerance to aluminum (Appanna et al., 1994), boron (Summers and Jacoby, 1977), gallium (Al-Aoukaty et al., 1992) , tributyl-tin (Miller et al., 1995), lead (Diels et al., 1995), and thallium (Diels et al., 1995). Plasmid-determined lead resistance in *S. aureus* may be related to intracellular (cytoplasmic) accumulation of lead phosphate crystals (I. Mahler, personal communication). Pb resistance in *Alcaligenes* spp., however, is associated with deposits outside the cytoplasmic membrane in the periplasmic space (Diels et al., 1995).

REFERENCES

Al-Aoukaty, A., V. Appanna, and H. Falter. 1992. Gallium toxicity and adaption in *Pseudomonas fluorescens*. *FEMS Microbiol. Lett.* **92:**265–272.

Anderson, G. L., J. Williams, and R. Hille. 1992. The purification and characterization of arsenite oxidase from *Alcaligenes faecalis*, a molybdenum-containing hydroxylase. *J. Biol. Chem.* **267:**23674–23682.

Appanna, V., M. Kepes, and P. Rochon. 1994. Aluminum tolerance in *Pseudomonas fluorescens* ATCC 13525: involvement of a gelatinous lipid-rich residue. *FEMS Microbiol. Lett.* **119:**295–302.

Bairoch, A. 1993. A possible mechanism for metal-ion induced DNA-protein dissociation in a family of prokaryotic transcriptional regulators. *Nucleic Acids Res.* **21:**2515.

Belly, R. T., and G. C. Kydd. 1982. Silver resistance in microorganisms. *Dev. Ind. Microbiol.* **23:**567–577.

Bender, C. L., and D. A. Cooksey. 1986. Indigenous plasmids in *Pseudomonas syringae* pv. *tomato*: conjugative transfer and role in copper resistance. *J. Bacteriol.* **165:**534–541.

Bender, C. L., D. K. Malvick, K. E. Conway, S. George, and P. Pratt. 1990. Characterization of pXV10A, a copper resistance plasmid in *Xanthomonas campestris* pv. *vesicatoria*. *Appl. Environ. Microbiol.* **56:**170–175.

Bopp, L. H., A. M. Chakrabarty, and H. L. Ehrlich. 1983. Chromate resistance plasmid in *Pseudomonas fluorescens*. *J. Bacteriol.* **155:**1105–1109.

Bopp, L. H., and H. L. Ehrlich. 1988. Chromate resistance and reduction in *Pseudomonas fluorescens* strain LB300. *Arch. Microbiol.* **150:**426–431.

Bradley, D. E., K. K. Grewal, D. E. Taylor, and J. Whelan. 1988. Characterization of RP4 tellurite-resistance transposon Tn*521*. *J. Gen. Microbiol.* **134:**2009–2018.

Bröer, S., G. Ji, A. Bröer, and S. Silver. 1993. Arsenic efflux governed by the arsenic resistance determinant of *Staphlyococcus aureus* plasmid pI258. *J. Bacteriol.* **175:**3480–3485.

Brown, N. L., S. R. Barrett, J. Camakaris, B. T. O. Lee, and D. A. Rouch. 1995. Molecular genetics and transport analysis of the copper-resistance determinant (*pco*) from *Escherichia coli* plasmid pRJ1004. *Mol. Microbiol.* **17:**1153–1166.

Brown, N. L., B. T. O. Lee, and S. Silver. 1994. Bacterial transport of and resistance to copper, p. 405–434. *In* H. Sigel and A. Sigel (ed.), *Metal Ions in Biological Systems*, vol. 30. Marcel Dekker, New York.

Brown, N. L., T. K. Misra, J. N. Winnie, A. Schmidt, M. Seiff, and S. Silver. 1986. The nucleotide sequence of the mercuric resistance operons of plasmid R100 and transposon Tn*501*: further evidence for *mer* genes which enhance the activity of the mercuric ion detoxification system. *Mol. Gen. Genet.* **202:**143–151.

Bruhn, D. F., J. Li, S. Silver, F. Roberto, and B. P. Rosen. The arsenical resistance operon of IncN plasmid R46. *FEMS Microbiol. Lett.*, in press.

Carlin, A., W. Shi, S. Dey, and B. P. Rosen. 1995. The *ars* operon of *Escherichia coli* confers arsenical and antimonial resistance. *J. Bacteriol.* **177:**981–986.

Cary, E. W. 1982. Chromium in air, soil and natural waters, p. 49–64. *In*. S. Langard (ed.) *Biological and Environmental Aspects of Chromium*. Elsevier, Amsterdam.

Cervantes, C., and J. Chávez. 1992. Plasmid-determined resistance to arsenic and antimony in *Pseudomonas aeruginosa*. *Antonie Leeuwenhoek* **61:**333–337.

Cervantes, C., and F. Gutierrez-Corona. 1994. Copper resistance mechanisms in bacteria and fungi. *FEMS Microbiol. Rev.* **14:**121–138.

Cervantes, C., G. Ji, J. L. Ramírez, and S. Silver. 1994. Resistance to arsenic compounds in microorganisms. *FEMS Microbiol. Rev.* **15:**355–367.

Cervantes, C., and H. Ohtake. 1988. Plasmid-determined resistance to chromate in *Pseudomonas aeruginosa*. *FEMS Microbiol. Lett.* **56:**173–176.

Cervantes, C., H. Ohtake, L. Chu, T. K. Misra, and S. Silver. 1990. Cloning, nucleotide sequence, and expression of the chromate resistance determinant of *Pseudomonas aeruginosa* plasmid pUM505. *J. Bacteriol.* **172:**287–291.

Cervantes, C., and S. Silver. 1992. Bacterial chromate resistance and chromate reduction. *Plasmid.* **27:**65–71.

Cervantes-Vega, C., J. Chávez, N. A. Córdova, P. de la Mora, and J. A. Velasco. 1986. Resistance to metals by *Pseudomonas aeruginosa* clinical isolates. *Microbios* **48:**159–163.

Cha, J.-S., and D. A. Cooksey. 1991. Copper resistance in *Pseudomonas syringae* mediated by periplasmic and outer membrane proteins. *Proc. Natl. Acd. Sci. USA* **88:**8915–8919.

Cha, J.-S., and D. A. Cooksey. 1993. Copper hypersensitivity and uptake in *Pseudomonas syringae* containing cloned components of the copper resistance operon. *Appl. Environ. Microbiol.* **59:**1671–1674.

Chen, C.-M., T. K. Misra, S. Silver, and B. P. Rosen. 1986. Nucleotide sequence of the structural genes for an anion pump. The plasmid-encoded arsenical resistance operon. *J. Biol. Chem.* **261:**15030–15038.

Clark, D., A. A. Weiss, and S. Silver. 1977. Mercury and organomercurial resistance determined by plasmids in *Pseudomonas*. *J. Bacteriol.* **132:**186–196.

Cooksey, D. A. 1994. Molecular mechanisms of copper resistance and accumulation in bacteria. *FEMS Microbiol. Rev.* **14:**381–386.

Cooksey, D. A., H. R. Azad, J.-S. Cha, and C.-K. Lim. 1990. Copper resistance gene homologs in pathogenic and saprophytic bacterial species from tomato. *Appl. Environ. Microbiol.* **56:**431–435.

Craig, P. J. 1989. Biological and environmental methylation of metals, p. 437–463. *In* F. R. Hartley (ed.), *The Chemistry of the Metal-Carbon Bond*, vol. 5. John Wiley and Sons, London.

Deshpande, L. M., and B. A. Chopade. 1994. Plasmid mediated silver resistance in *Acinetobacter baumannii*. *BioMetals* **7:**49–56.

Dey, S., and B. P. Rosen. 1995. Dual mode of energy coupling by the oxyanion-translocating ArsB protein. *J. Bacteriol.* **177:**385–389.

Diels, L., Q. Dong, D. van der Lelie, W. Baeyens, and M. Mergeay. 1995. The *czc* operon of *Alcaligenes eutrophus* CH34: from resistance mechanism to the removal of heavy metals. *J. Ind. Microbiol.* **14:**142–153.

Diorio, C., J. Cai, J. Marmor, R. Shinder, and M. S. DuBow. 1995. An *Escherichia coli* chromosomal *ars* operon homolog is functional in arsenic detoxification and is conserved in gram-negative bacteria. *J. Bacteriol.* **177:**2050–2056.

Distefano, M. D., M. J. Moore, and C. T. Walsh. 1990. Active site of mercuric reductase resides at the subunit interface and requires cys_{135} and cys_{140} from one subunit and cys_{558} and cys_{559} from the adjacent subunit: evidence from in vivo and in vitro heterodimer formation. *Biochemistry* **29:**2703–2713.

Endo, G., and S. Silver. 1995. CadC, the transcriptional regulatory protein of the cadmium resistance system of *Staphylococcus aureus* plasmid pI258. *J. Bacteriol.* **177:**4437–4441.

Garde, S., and C. L. Bender. 1991. DNA probes for detection of copper resistance genes in *Xanthomonas campestris* pv. *vesicatoria*. *Appl. Environ. Microbiol.* **57:**2435–2439.

Ghandour, W., J. A. Hubbard, J. A. Deistung, M. N. Hughes, and R. K. Poole. 1988. The uptake of silver ions by *Escherichia coli* K12: toxic effects and interactions with copper ions. *Appl. Microbiol. Biotechnol.* **28:**559–565.

Gladysheva, T. B., K. L. Oden, and B. P. Rosen. 1994. Properties of the arsenate reductase of plasmid R773. *Biochemistry* **33:**7288–7293.

Haefeli, C., C. Franklin, and K. Hardy. 1984. Plasmid-determined silver resistance in *Pseudomonas stutzeri* isolated from a silver mine. *J. Bacteriol.* **158:**389–392.

Higham, D. P., P. J. Sadler, and M. D. Scawen. 1984. Cadmium-resistant *Pseudomonas putida* synthesizes novel cadmium proteins. *Science* **225:**1043–1046.

Hobman, J., G. Kholodii, V. Nikiforov, D. A. Ritchie, P. Strike, and O. Yurieva. 1994. The sequence of the *mer* operon of pMER327/419 and transposon ends of pMER327/419, 330 and 05. *Gene* **146:**73–78.

Horitsu, H., S. Futo, Y. Miyazawa, S. Ogai, and K. Kawai. 1987. Enzymatic reduction of hexavalent chromium by hexavalent chromium tolerant *Pseudomonas ambigua* G-1. *Agric. Biol. Chem.* **51:**2417–2420.

Horitsu, H., K. Yamamoto, S. Wachi, K. Kawai, and A. Fukuchi. 1986. Plasmid-determined cadmium resistance in *Pseudomonas putida* GAM-1 isolated from soil. *J. Bacteriol.* **165:**334–335.

Inoue, C., K. Sugawara, T. Shiratori, T. Kusano, and Y. Kitagawa. 1989. Nucleotide sequence of the *Thiobacillus ferrooxidans* chromosomal gene encoding mercuric reductase. *Gene* **84:**47–54.

Ishibashi, Y., C. Cervantes, and S. Silver. 1990. Chromium reduction in *Pseudomonas putida. Appl. Environ. Microbiol.* **56:**2268–2270.

Itoh, M., T. Suzuki, Y. Kimata, K. Kawai, H. Horitsu, and K. Takamizawa. 1994. Cadmium resistance acquirement by IS*1* transposition into *Escherichia coli* C600. *J. Ferment. Bioeng.* **78:**466–468.

Jacoby, G. A. 1986. Resistance plasmids of *Pseudomonas*, p. 265–293. *In* J. R. Sokatch (ed.), *The Biology of Pseudomonas. The Bacteria*, vol. 10. Academic Press, Orlando, Fla.

Ji, G., E. A. Garber, L. G. Armes, C.-M. Chen, J. A. Fuchs, and S. Silver. 1994. Arsenate reductase of *Staphylococcus aureus* plasmid pI258. *Biochemistry* **33:**7294–7299.

Ji, G., and S. Silver. 1992. Reduction of arsenate to arsenite by ArsC protein of the arsenic resistance operon of *Staphylococcus aureus* plasmid pI258. *Proc. Natl. Acad. Sci. USA* **89:**7974–7978.

Ji, G., and S. Silver. 1995. Plasmid resistance mechanisms for heavy metals of environmental concern. *J. Ind. Microbiol.* **14:**61–75.

Jobling, M. G., and D. A. Ritchie. 1987. Genetic and physical analysis of plasmid genes expressing inducible resistance of tellurite in *Escherichia coli. Mol. Gen. Genet.* **208:**288–293.

Jobling, M. G., and D. A. Ritchie. 1988. The nucleotide sequence of a plasmid determinant for resistance to tellurium anions. *Gene* **66:**245–258.

Kägi, J. H. R., and A. Y. Kojima (ed.). 1988. Metallothionein II. Birkhäuser Verlag, Basel.

Karkaria, C. E., C. M. Chen, and B. P. Rosen. 1990. Mutagenesis of a nucleotide-binding site of an anion-translocating ATPase. *J. Biol. Chem.* **265:**7832–7836.

Karkaria, C. E., R. F. Steiner, and B. P. Rosen. 1991. Ligand interactions in the ArsA protein, the catalytic component of an anion-translocating adenosinetriphosphatase. *Biochemistry* **30:**2625–2628.

Kaur, P., and B. P. Rosen. 1993. Complementation between nucleotide binding domains in an anion-translocating ATPase. *J. Bacteriol.* **175:**351–357.

Kiyono, M., H. Fujimori, and H. Pan-Hou. 1995a. Genetic and physiological analysis of mercurials resistance of *Pseudomonas* K-62, p. 111. *In* Abstracts of the Fifth International Symposium on *Pseudomonas*: Molecular Biology and Biotechnology, Tsukuba, Japan, August, 1995.

Kiyono, M., T. Omura, H. Fujimori, and H. Pan-Hou. 1995b. Organomercurial resistance determinants in *Pseudomonas* K-62 are present on two plasmids. *Arch. Microbiol.* **163:**242–247.

Kiyono, M., T. Omura, H. Fujimori, and H. Pan-Hou. 1995c. Lack of involvement of *merT* and *merP* in methylmercury transport in mercury resistant *Pseudomonas* K-62. *FEMS Microbiol. Lett.* **128:**301–306.

Kusano, T., G. Ji, C. Inoue, and S. Silver. 1990. Constitutive synthesis of a transport function encoded by the *Thiobacillus ferrooxidans merC* gene cloned in *Escherichia coli. J. Bacteriol.* **172:**2688–2692.

Lebedeva, E. V., and N. N. Lyalikova. 1979. Reduction of crocoite by *Pseudomonas chromatophila* sp. nov. *Mikrobiologiya* **48:**517–522.

Lee, Y.-A., M. Hendson, N. J. Panopoulos, and M. N Schroth. 1994. Molecular cloning, chromosomal mapping, and sequence analysis of copper resistance genes from *Xanthomonas campestris* pv. *juglandis*: homology with small blue copper proteins and multicopper oxidase. *J. Bacteriol.* **176:**173–188.

Liesegang, H., K. Lemke, R. A. Siddiqui, and H.-G. Schlegel. 1993. Characterization of the inducible nickel and cobalt resistance determinant *cnr* from pMOL28 of *Alcaligenes euthrophus* CH34. *J. Bacteriol.* **175:**767–778.

Lloyd-Jones, G., D. A. Ritchie, and P. Strike. 1991. Biochemical and biophysical analysis of plasmid pMJ600-encoded tellurite [TeO_3^{2-}] resistance. *FEMS Microbiol. Lett.* **81:**19–24.

Lontie, R. (ed.). 1984. *Copper Proteins and Copper Enzymes.* CRC Press Inc., Boca Raton, Fla.

Lovley, D. R. 1993. Dissimilatory metal reduction. *Annu. Rev. Microbiol.* **47:**263–290.

Mellano, M. A., and D. A. Cooksey. 1988. Nucleotide sequence and organization of copper resistance genes from *Pseudomonas syringae* pv. *tomato. J. Bacteriol.* **170:**2879–2883.

Miller, C. E., S. Wuertz, J. J. Cooney, and R. M. Pfister. 1995. Plasmids in tributyltin-resistant bacteria from fresh and estuarine waters. *J. Ind. Microbiol.* **14:**337–342.

Mukhopadhyay, D., H. Yu, G. Nucifora, and T. K. Misra. 1991. Purification and functional characterization of MerD. A co-regulator of the mercury resistance operon in Gram-negative bacteria. *J. Biol. Chem.* **266:**18538–18542.

Nakamuro, K., and Y. Sayato. 1981. Comparative studies of chromosomal aberration induced by trivalent and pentavalent arsenic. *Mutat. Res.* **88:**73–80.

Nicholson, M. L., and D. E. Laudenbach. 1995. Genes encoded on a cyanobacterial plasmid are transcriptionally regulated by sulfur availability and CysR. *J. Bacteriol.* **177:**2143–2150.

Nies, A., D. H. Nies, and S. Silver. 1990. Nucleotide sequence and expression of a plasmid-encoded chromate resistance determinant from *Alcaligenes eutrophus. J. Biol. Chem.* **265:**5648–5653.

Nies, D., M. Mergeay, B. Friedrich, and H. G. Schlegel. 1987. Cloning of plasmid genes encoding resistance to cadmium, zinc, and cobalt in *Alcaligenes eutrophus* CH34. *J. Bacteriol.* **169:**4865–4868.

Nies, D. H. 1992a. Resistance to cadmium, cobalt, zinc, and nickel in microbes. *Plasmid* **27:**17–28.

Nies, D. H. 1992b. CzcR and CzcD, gene products affecting regulation of cobalt, zinc, and cadmium resistance (*czc*) in *Alcaligenes eutrophus. J. Bacteriol.* **174:**8102–8110.

Nies, D. H. 1995. The cobalt, zinc, and cadmium efflux system CzcABC from *Alcaligenes eutrophus* functions as a cation-proton antiporter in *Escherichia coli. J. Bacteriol.* **177:**2707–2712.

Nies, D. H., A. Nies, L. Chu, and S. Silver. 1989. Expression and nucleotide sequence of a plasmid-determined divalent cation efflux system from *Alcaligenes eutrophus. Proc. Natl. Acad. Sci. USA* **86:**7351–7355.

Nies, D. H., and S. Silver. 1989. Metal ion uptake by a plasmid-free metal-sensitive *Alcaligenes eutrophus* strain. *J. Bacteriol.* **171:**4073–4075.

Nies, D. H., and S. Silver. 1995. Ion efflux systems involved in bacterial metal resistances. *J. Ind. Microbiol.* **14:**186–199.

Nucifora, G., L. Chu, T. K. Misra, and S. Silver. 1989. Cadmium resistance from *Staphylococcus aureus* plasmid pI258 *cadA* gene results from a cadmium-efflux ATPase. *Proc. Natl. Acad. Sci. USA* **86:**3544–3548.

O'Halloran, T. V. 1993. Transition metals in control of gene expression. *Science* **261:**715–725.

O'Halloran, T. V., B. Frantz, M. K. Shin, D. M. Ralston, and J. G. Wright. 1989. The MerR heavy metal receptor mediates positive activation in a topologically novel transcription complex. *Cell* **56:**119–129.

Ohtake, H., C. Cervantes, and S. Silver. 1987. Decreased chromate uptake in *Pseudomonas fluorescens* carrying a chromate resistance plasmid. *J. Bacteriol.* **169:**3853–3856.

Ohtake, H., and S. Silver. 1994. Bacterial reduction of toxic chromate, p. 403–415. *In* G. R. Chaudhry (ed.), *Biological Degradation and Bioremediation of Toxic Chemicals*. Chapman and Hall, London.

Osborn, A. M., K. D. Bruce, D. A. Ritchie, and P. Strike. 1996. Nucleotide sequence, regulation and evolutionary analysis of the novel mercury resistance operon of the *Inc*J plasmid pMERPH. *Microbiology* **83:**in press.

Osborne, F. H., and H. L. Ehrlich. 1976. Oxidation of arsenite by a soil isolate of *Alcaligenes. J. Appl. Bacteriol.* **41:**295–305.

Parkinson, J. S., and E. C. Kofoid. 1992. Communication modules in bacterial signaling proteins. *Annu. Rev. Genet.* **26:**71–112.

Phillips, S. E., and M. L. Taylor. 1976. Oxidation of arsenite to arsenate by *Alcaligenes faecalis. Appl. Environ. Microbiol.* **32:**392–399.

Reniero, D., E. Galli, and P. Barbieri. 1995. Cloning and comparison of mercury- and organomercurial-resistance determinants from a *Pseudomonas stutzeri* plasmid. *Gene* **166:**77–82.

Romanenko, V. I., and V. W. Koren'kov. 1977. A pure culture of bacteria utilizing chromates and bichromates as hydrogen acceptors in growth under anaerobic conditions. *Mikrobiologiya* **46:**414–417.

Rosen, B. P., S. Dey, D. Dou, G. Ji, P. Kaur, M. Y. Ksenzenko, S. Silver, and J. Wu. 1992. Evolution of an ion-translocating ATPase. *Ann. N. Y. Acad. Sci.* **671:**257–272.

San Francisco, M. J. D., C. L. Hope, J. B. Owolabi, L. S. Tisa, and B. P. Rosen. 1990. Identification of the metalloregulatory element of the plasmid-encoded arsenical resistance operon. *Nucleic Acids Res.* **18:**619–624.

Schiering, N., W. Kabsch, M. J. Moore, M. D. Distefano, C. T. Walsh, and E. F. Pai. 1991. Structure of the detoxification catalyst mercuric ion reductase from *Bacillus* sp. strain RC607. *Nature* (London) **352:**168–171.

Silver, S. 1981. Mechanisms of plasmid-determined heavy metal resistance, p. 179–189. *In* S. B. Levy, R. C. Clowes, and E. L. Koening (ed.), *Molecular Biology, Pathogenicity and Ecology of Bacterial Plasmids*. Plenum Press, New York.

Silver, S. Bacterial resistance to toxic metal ions—a review. *Gene*, in press.

Silver, S., K. Budd, K. M. Leahy, W. V. Shaw, D. Hammond, R. P. Novick, G. R. Willsky, M. H. Malamy, and H. Rosenberg. 1981. Inducible plasmid-determined resistance to arsenate, arsenite, and antimony(III) in *Escherichia coli* and *Staphylococcus aureus*. *J. Bacteriol.* **146:**983–996.

Silver, S., and G. Ji. 1994. Newer systems for bacterial resistances to toxic heavy metals. *Environ. Health Perspect.* **102**(Suppl. 3):107–113.

Silver, S., G. Ji, S. Bröer, S. Dey, D. Dou, and B. P. Rosen. 1993a. Orphan enzyme or patriarch of a new tribe: the arsenic resistance ATPase of bacterial plasmids. *Mol. Microbiol.* **8:**637–642.

Silver, S., B. T. O. Lee, N. L. Brown, and D. A. Cooksey. 1993b. Bacterial plasmid resistances to copper, cadmium and zinc, p. 38–53. *In* A. J. Welch and S. K. Chapman (ed.), *The Chemistry of the Copper and Zinc Triads*. Royal Society of Chemistry, London.

Silver, S., and T. K. Misra. 1988. Plasmid-mediated heavy metal resistance. *Annu. Rev. Microbiol.* **42:**717–743.

Silver, S., G. Nucifora, L. Chu, and T. K. Misra. 1989. Bacterial resistance ATPases: primary pumps for exporting toxic cations and anions. *Trends Biochem. Sci.* **14:**76–80.

Silver, S., and L. T. Phung. 1996. Bacterial plasmid-mediated heavy metal resistances: new surprises. *Annu. Rev. Microbiol.* **50:**in press.

Silver, S., and M. Walderhaug. 1992. Gene regulation of plasmid- and chromosomal-determined inorganic ion transport in bacteria. *Microbiol. Rev.* **56:**195–228.

Slawson, R. M., J. T. Trevors, and H. Lee. 1992a. Silver accumulation and resistance in *Pseudomonas stutzeri*. *Arch. Microbiol.* **158:**398–404.

Slawson, R. M., M. I. van Dyke, H. Lee, and J. T. Trevors. 1992b. Germanium and silver resistance, accumulation, and toxicity in microorganisms. *Plasmid* **27:**72–79.

Solioz, M., and A. Odermatt. 1995. Copper and silver transport by CopB-ATPase in membrane vesicles of *Enterococcus hirae*. *J. Biol. Chem.* **270:**9217–9221.

Stall, R. E., D. C. Loschke, and J. B. Jones. 1986. Linkage of copper resistance and avirulence loci on a self-transmissible plasmid in *Xanthomonas campestris* pv. *vesicatoria*. *Phytopathology* **76:**240–243.

Summers, A. O. 1992. Untwist and shout: a heavy metal-responsive transcriptional regulator. *J. Bacteriol.* **174:**3097–3101.

Summers, A. O., and G. A. Jacoby. 1977. Plasmid-determined resistance to tellurium compounds. *J. Bacteriol.* **129:**276–281.

Summers, A. O., and G. A. Jacoby. 1978. Plasmid-determined resistance to boron and chromium compounds in *Pseudomonas aeruginosa*. *Antimicrob. Agents Chemother.* **13:**637–640.

Summers, A. O., G. A. Jacoby, M. N. Swartz, G. McHugh, and L. Sutton. 1978. Metal cation and oxyanion resistances in plasmids of gram-negative bacteria, p.128–131. *In*. D. Schlessinger (ed.), *Microbiology—1978*. American Society for Microbiology, Washington, D.C.

Summers, A. O., and S. Silver. 1978. Microbial transformations of metals. *Annu. Rev. Microbiol.* **32:**637–672.

Suzuki, T., N. Miyata, H. Horitsu, K. Kawai, K. Takamizawa, Y. Tai, and M. Okazaki. 1992. NAD(P)H-dependent chromium(VI) reductase of *Pseudomonas ambigua* G-1: a Cr(V) intermediate is formed during the reduction of Cr(VI) to Cr(III). *J. Bacteriol.* **174:**5340–5345.

Tisa, L. S., and B. P. Rosen. 1990. Molecular characterization of an anion pump: the ArsB protein is the membrane anchor for the ArsA protein. *J. Biol. Chem.* **265:**190–194.

Trevors, J. T. 1987. Copper resistance in bacteria. *Microbiol. Sci.* **4:**29–31.

Trevors, J. T., G. W. Stratton, and G. M. Gadd. 1986. Cadmium transport, resistance and toxicity in bacteria, algae, and fungi. *Can. J. Microbiol.* **32:**447–464.

Turner, J. S., and N. J. Robinson. 1995. Cyanobacterial metallothioneins: biochemistry and molecular genetics. *J. Ind. Microbiol.* **14:**119–125.

Voloudakis, A. E., C. L. Bender, and D. A. Cooksey. 1993. Similarity between copper resistance genes from *Xanthomonas campestris* and *Pseudomonas syringae*. *Appl. Environ. Microbiol.* **59:**1627–1634.

Walter, E. G., and D. E. Taylor. 1989. Comparison of tellurite resistance determinants from the IncPα plasmid RP4Te^r and the IncHII plasmid pHH1508a. *J. Bacteriol.* **171:**2160–2165.

Walter, E. G., C. M. Thomas, J. P. Ibbotson, and D. E. Taylor. 1991. Transcriptional analysis, translational analysis, and sequence of the *kilA*-tellurite resistance region of plasmid RK2Te^r. *J. Bacteriol.* **173:**1111–1119.

Wang, Y., M. Moore, H. S. Levinson, S. Silver. C. Walsh, and I. Mahler. 1989. Nucleotide sequence of a chromosomal mercury resistance determinant from a *Bacillus* sp. with broad-spectrum mercury resistance. *J. Bacteriol.* **171:**83–92.

Wu, J., and B. P. Rosen. 1991. The ArsR protein is a trans-acting regulatory protein. *Mol. Microbiol.* **5:**1331–1336.

Wu, J., and B. P. Rosen. 1993. The *arsD* gene encodes a second *trans*-acting regulatory protein of the plasmid-encoded arsenical resistance operon. *Mol. Microbiol.* **8:**615–623.

Wu, J., L. S. Tisa, and B. P. Rosen. 1992. Membrane topology of the ArsB protein, the membrane subunit of an anion-translocating ATPase. *J. Biol. Chem.* **267:**12570–12576.

Molecular Biology of Pseudomonads
Edited by T. Nakazawa et al.

Chapter 36

Common Steps in Extracellular Protein Secretion and Biogenesis of Pili in *Pseudomonas aeruginosa*

Stephen Lory, Hong-Mei Lu, and Jeffrey C. Pepe

Extracellular protein localization by gram-negative pathogenic microorganisms is an essential component of their virulence characteristics. Accordingly, these bacteria have evolved elaborate systems to ensure that proteins which are important in pathogenesis are correctly targeted to the sites of action. During the past 5 years, work from a number of laboratories has shown that secretion across the outer membrane is a complex process, with a rather substantial number of components dedicated to the secretion of one or a limited number of proteins. In contrast, all signal peptide-containing proteins, numbering several hundred, are secreted by a pathway which requires a machinery consisting of approximately half a dozen components. Moreover, some bacteria can have several independent extracellular secretion pathways functioning simultaneously. The fundamental principles that are applicable to protein secretion from gram-negative bacteria are very likely reproduced in other biological processes as well. This notion is supported by the fact that homologs of individual components of the extracellular secretion machinery are required for assembly of filamentous bacteriophages and for the uptake of DNA into gram-positive bacteria (Russell, 1994; Albano et al., 1989).

Systems for extracellular protein secretion have been categorized into three general types on the basis of secretion apparatus homologies and conservation of information within the secreted proteins themselves (reviewed by Salmond and Reeves [1993]). *Pseudomonas aeruginosa* possesses all three pathways, each dedicated to the export of a different protein or a group of proteins. The first class is called the type I secretion system, and it forms the signal peptide-independent secretion pathway, initially identified as the export system for the *Escherichia coli* hemolysin. The type I secretion system decodes information within the carboxyl terminus of the protein to be secreted. From the evidence available to date, this translocation pathway appears to bypass completely the periplasmic compartment of the bacterial cell envelope. The example for type I secretion in *P. aeruginosa* is the extracellular release of alkaline protease, the product of the *aprA* gene (Guzzo et al., 1991). The

Stephen Lory, Hong-Mei Lu, and Jeffrey C. Pepe • Department of Microbiology, Box 357242, University of Washington, Seattle, Washington 98195.

machinery is encoded by three genes, *aprD, aprE*, and *aprF*, and AprA appears to be the sole substrate secreted by this pathway.

The second pathway for extracellular secretion is the type II secretion system, which is an extension of the general secretory pathway (Pugsley, 1993). This pathway was initially described as a surface localization system, dedicated solely to secretion of *Klebsiella oxytoca* pullulanase (Pugsley et al., 1990). However, it is now recognized that the type II pathway operates in a wide range of bacteria, and in many instances it directs the export of more than a single protein from the same bacterium. In *P. aeruginosa*, the determinants of the type II pathway are encoded in a gene cluster containing 11 genes, *xcpP, xcpQ, xcpR, xcpS, xcpT, xcpU, xcpV, xcpW, xcpX, xcpY*, and *xcpZ* (reviewed by Tommassen et al. [1992]), as well as an additional gene linked to the type IV pilus biogenesis cluster, called *pilD* (also called *xcpA*) (Nunn et al., 1990; Bally et al., 1991). A relatively heterogeneous set of proteins is secreted by this type of mechanism, including exotoxin A, elastase, alkaline phosphatase, and phospholipase C. Like many secreted proteins, those utilizing the type II pathway are synthesized with typical secretion signal peptides which direct them first into the periplasm. It is in this compartment that the type II machinery identifies the extracellularly destined proteins and directs their subsequent translocation across the outer membrane.

The type III secretion system is found in a number of pathogenic microorganisms with intracellular life cycles, including *Yersinia, Shigella*, and *Salmonella* species. The existence of a type III secretion system in *P. aeruginosa* is assumed from the observed homology between *P. aeruginosa* exoenzyme S (ExoS) and the *Yersinia* sp. YopE protein (Yahr et al., 1995). More significantly, a *P. aeruginosa* gene cotranscribed with the *exoS* gene is homologous to the *Yersinia sycE/yerA*, which encodes a YopE chaperone and is required for YopE secretion.

SHARED DETERMINANTS OF BIOGENESIS OF TYPE IV PILI AND THE MACHINERY OF THE TYPE II SECRETION PATHWAY

P. aeruginosa produces a class of appendages called pili, which play a role in several important biological processes including adhesion to epithelial cells during infection (reviewed by Strom and Lory [1993]). Additionally, pili are receptors for bacteriophages, and they are involved in a form of translocation referred to as twitching motility (Bradley, 1973, 1980). The subunits that make up the pilus filament belong to the type IV family of related pilins that are expressed by a number of different gram-negative microorganisms. The type IV family of bacterial pili is characterized by the lack of typical N-terminal hydrophobic signal peptides, which implies a novel mechanism for secretion of these subunits and their assembly into pili (Strom and Lory, 1987). This contrasts with the basic mechanism of secretion of subunits and assembly of *E. coli* pili, which are initially synthesized with typical signal peptides and then are secreted from the periplasm by the general secretion pathway (Dodd and Eisenstein, 1984).

Work from several laboratories has identified genes that encode determinants required for expression of type IV pili by *P. aeruginosa*, most of which apparently encode assembly functions (Nunn et al., 1990; Alm and Mattick, 1995; Russell and Darzins, 1994; Martin et al., 1993; Martin et al., 1995; Whitchurch and Mattick, 1994). Sequence analysis of these genes revealed a striking homology with the determinants of the type II secretion systems. This relationship is based almost exclusively on sequence homologies, which implies that these proteins may function similarly as well. However, complementation of *xcp* genes with those encoding homologous pilus biogenesis functions has not been successful.

The related proteins required for pilus biogenesis and for the type II secretion pathway belong to three categories. The largest group of homologous proteins are related to the pilin subunits, mainly by sequence similarities at their respective amino termini (Strom and Lory, 1993; Russell and Darzins, 1994; Alm and Mattick, 1995). The maturation of these proteins requires the activity of a common enzyme, product of the *pilD* gene (Lory, 1995; also see below). The second group of related proteins is represented by XcpQ and PilQ (Akrim et al., 1993; Martin et al., 1993). These are synthesized with typical signal peptides, and they are very likely localized in the bacterial outer membrane. Mutations in *xcpQ* lead to periplasmic accumulation of extracellularly secreted enzymes (S. Lory, unpublished data), and mutants of *P. aeruginosa* with a *pilQ* mutation are nonpiliated (Martin et al., 1993). Products of genes *pilB, pilT*, and *pilU* are related to the XcpR component of the type II secretion system by sequence similarities, and each of these proteins contains a nucleotide binding site (Walker sequence). Lack of functional XcpR, due to the mutation in the Walker sequence, results in a pleiotropic extracellular secretion defect (Turner et al., 1993). Bacteria with transposon insertions in the *pilB* gene, or Walker sequence mutations in PilB, are defective in assembly of pili (Nunn et al., 1990). In contrast, mutations in either *pilU* or *pilT* result in hyperpiliation; however, these mutants are incapable of twitching motility (Whitchurch and Mattick, 1994).

The only protein which functions simultaneously in the biogenesis of pili and the type II secretion pathway is the product of the *pilD* (*xcpA*) gene. This gene was discovered independently as being required for assembly of pili (Nunn et al., 1990) and secretion of exoenzymes (Bally et al., 1991; Strom et al., 1991). The complete purification and biochemical characterization of PilD led to the elucidation of its function, which is shared by all of its homologs in other bacteria. PilD is responsible for two consecutive post-translational modifications of its substrates: cleavage of the leader peptide and methylation of the mature protein (Nunn and Lory, 1991; Strom et al., 1993b). All PilD substrates are members of the type IV pilin family (Nunn and Lory, 1992; Bally et al., 1992), with the highest conservation of sequence being near the processing site (Fig. 1). This homology very likely defines a recognition site for PilD. The activity of PilD leads to the removal of the short N-terminal leader peptide by hydrolysis of the peptide bond between glycine and phenylalanine, followed by N-methylation of the phenylalanine using *S*-adenosylmethionine as a methyl donor (Fig. 2). Presently, PilD remains the sole component of the type II secretion machinery, and of the pilus biogenesis apparatus, that has an identified biochemical activity. While the cleavage of the leader peptide is required for assembly of pilin and pilin-like proteins into a functional pilus or secretion apparatus, the requirement for the N-methylation of these proteins has yet to be established.

The conservation of protein sequences among certain components of pilus biogenesis apparatus and the machinery of extracellular protein secretion implies that these two processes may be mechanistically related. Alternatively, the functional relatedness may be limited to the initial step of assembly of two similar structures: the extracellular secretion machinery, in the form of an organelle within the gram-negative cell envelope,

```
                          ↓
PilA             mkAQKG   FTLIELMIVVAIIGILAAIAIPQyqnyvarsegasa 42
PilE            mrtRQKG   FTLLEMVVVVAVIGILLGIAIPSyqnyvirsnrteg 43
PilV     mllksrhrslHQSG   FSMIEVLVALLLISIGVLGMIAMqgktiqytadsve 50

XcpT           mqrrQQSG   FTLIEIMVVVVILGILAALVVPQvmsrpdqakvtva 44
XcpU             mrASRG   FTLIELMVVMVIISVLIGLAVLStgfastsreldse 42
XcpV             mkRARG   FTLLEVLVALAIFAMVAASVLSAsarslqnasrled 42
XcpW             mrLQRG   FTLLELLIAIAIFALLALATYRMfdsvmqtdqatrv 42
```

Figure 1. Alignment of the N-terminal regions of *P. aeruginosa* proteins involved in biogenesis of type IV pili (Pil) and in extracellular protein secretion (Xcp). The shaded area shows the regions of the highest sequence conservation; arrow indicates the peptide bond cleaved by the leader peptidase. Sources for sequences used for the alignments: PilA, Johnson et al. (1986); PilE, Russell and Darzins (1994); PilV, Alm and Mattick (1995); XcpT through XcpW, Bally et al. (1992).

and the pilus filament protruding from the outer membrane. It is unclear which of the many products function directly in facilitating export of a particular protein and which are required for assembly of a functional apparatus. PilD is an example of the latter, in which it functions in the maturation of pilin monomers or the pilin-like proteins. Presumably, after processing of its substrates (precursor forms of pilin and XcpT through XcpW), it is not further required for subsequent assembly of pili or for secretion of extracellular enzymes from the bacterial periplasm.

STRUCTURE-FUNCTION RELATIONSHIP OF THE PREPILIN PEPTIDASE-METHYL TRANSFERASE

Given the critical role of PilD in the biogenesis of pili and maturation of components of the extracellular secretion machinery, several attempts were made to understand the relationship of the two reactions catalyzed by this enzyme. The effort was greatly aided by the availability of sequences of PilD homologs from several different bacteria, which served as a guide for the selection of amino acids for site-directed mutagenesis. The alignment of one of the most conserved regions of these proteins is shown in Fig. 3.

A very striking feature within this conserved stretch of amino acids is the presence of 4 cysteine residues in a pairwise arrangement. Substitution of serine or glycine residues for any one of these cysteines resulted in a significant reduction of both leader peptidase and methyl transferase activities (Strom et al., 1993a). It is not clear whether these cysteines compose the enzymatic center of the enzyme, where they are shared by both the peptidase and methyl transferase active sites, or whether the mutations alter the overall structural integrity of the enzyme. Alternatively, the cysteines may play a role in catalyzing proteolysis and in methylation by binding a common cofactor. Several lines of evidence suggest that the protease site is distinct from the methyl donor binding site, since competitive inhibition of pilin methylation has no effect on pilin's proteolytic activity. Clearly more extensive mutagenesis and elucidation of the three-dimensional structure of PilD are essential to make precise assignments of the catalytic sites.

A second region of PilD, potentially important for its methyl transferase activity, is amino acids 93 through 98 (Fig. 3), which shares homology with the active sites of

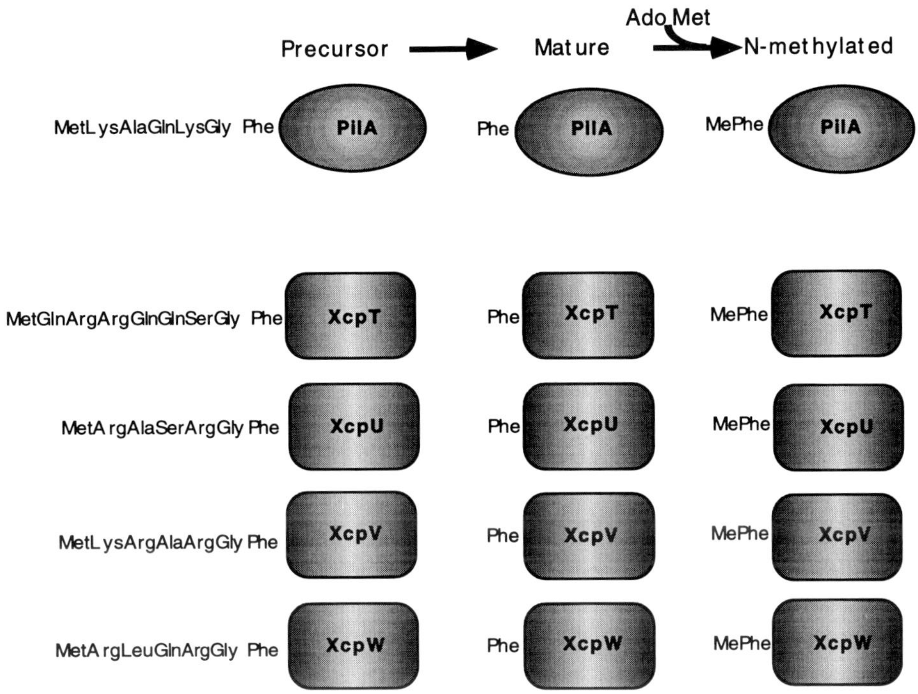

Figure 2. Posttranslational modifications of the pilin subunits and components of the extracellular secretion machinery catalyzed by PilD.

*Eco*RI and *Eco*RII methyl transferases (Strom et al., 1993a). This region includes amino acids which are conserved in all PilD homologs: glycine at 95 and a charged, usually basic residue at 96 (lysine in PilD). Systematic mutagenesis of the codons for these amino acids revealed that these two residues play a critical role in the methyl transferase reaction and a partial to negligible role in the proteolysis of prepilin. These mutants therefore, for the first time, separate the two activities and are further evidence for distinct active sites for the two reactions catalyzed by PilD. Figure 4 compares the relative rates of cleavage and methylation of prepilin by the wild-type PilD, as well as by several mutants with substitutions at position 95 or 96. Substitutions of serine for glycine at position 95 resulted in a variant that had a leader peptidase activity identical to that of the wild-type enzyme; however, its methyl transferase activity was almost undetectable. Substitutions for lysine at position 96 had variable effects. A conservative substitution (arginine for lysine) had no effect on either prepilin cleavage or its subsequent methylation. This is not surprising, since arginine is found at this position in five other PilD homologs, including the *Klebsiella pneumoniae* PulO, shown in Fig. 3. A substitution of a glutamic acid for arginine, which results in introduction of an oppositely charged residue, had a moderate effect, with rates of prepilin cleavage and methylation reduced by approximately 45% and 70%, respectively. The substitution of a leucine for lysine yielded an enzyme that showed 42% of the wild-type leader peptidase activity, but the methyl

```
           •  •                               •  •
BfpP     50  KCNNCGKKIRWYYLIPVLGYFLCRGECGYCH    80

PulO     59  FCPQCREPIAWRDNIPLLGFLFLKGRSRCCG    89

TcpJ     47  MCPKCGNKISWYDNVPLLSYLLLHGKCRHCD    77

PilD-Ng  69  CCPKCRVPIRAWQNIPIVSYLLLRGKCASCQ    99

PilD-Pa  71  ACPRCGHEIRPWENIPLVSYLALGGKCSSCK    101
                                      / \
                                     S   E
                                         L
                                         R
```

Figure 3. Alignment of conserved regions of selected prepilin leader peptidase-methyl transferases. Specific amino acid residues indicated are: conserved cysteines (dots), invariant glycines (shaded), and the region of homology with the *Eco*RI and *Eco*RII methyl transferases (boxed). Also indicated are the amino acid substitutions resulting in the mutant forms of the *P. aeruginosa* PilD (PilD-Pa). Sources for sequences: *E. coli* BfpP, Zhang et al., (1994); *K. oxytoca* PulO, Pugsley and Reyss (1990); *Vibrio cholerae* TcpJ, Kaufman et al. (1991); *Neisseria gonorrhoeae* PilD-Ng, Lauer et al. (1993); *P. aeruginosa* PilD-Pa, Nunn et al. (1990).

transferase activity was severely reduced, to approximately 5% of the wild type. Clearly, this region is critical for the methyl transferase reaction of PilD and could represent the binding site for *S*-adenosylmethionine, or it may be involved in the transfer of the methyl group onto the phenylalanine acceptor residue.

TARGETING SIGNALS ON EXOTOXIN A ARE RESPONSIBLE FOR ITS EXTRACELLULAR LOCALIZATION

The sequences and structural features of proteins targeted to the extracellular space and recognized by the Xcp machinery have been investigated by genetic methods. It is accepted that secretion via the type II secretion pathway is a process involving protein sorting from a periplasmic pool, which occurs after the initial translocation across the cytoplasmic membrane and the concomitant cleavage of signal peptide. Therefore, the mature proteins destined for the external space contain information that periplasmic proteins lack and that the export machinery can decode. Extracellular proteins of *P. aeruginosa* comprise a group of polypeptides without any obvious sequence homologies, suggesting that the Xcp machinery very likely recognizes a conformational signal, assembled after folding of the polypeptide in the periplasm.

One of the interesting features of secretion of extracellular proteins via the *P. aeruginosa* type II pathway is the extensive variation in the rate of transit through the periplasm. While some proteins such as elastase, which require an activation step during secretion, reside relatively long in the periplasm, others, such as exotoxin A, are virtually undetectable in this compartment. This raised the question as to whether exotoxin A bypasses the periplasm altogether. This possibility was investigated, using mutant forms of exotoxin A that are retarded in their secretion across the cytoplasmic membrane and subsequent

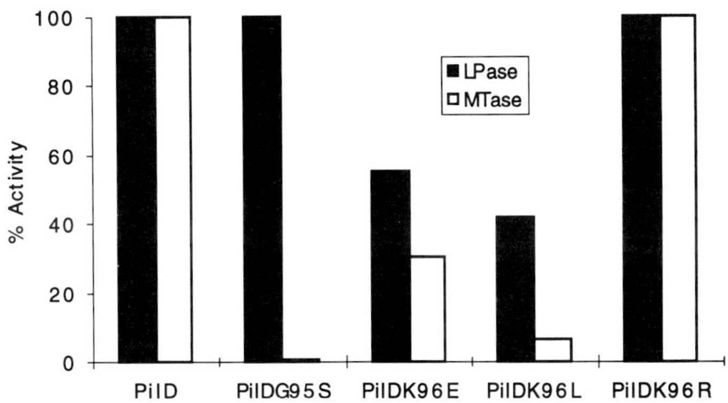

Figure 4. Cleavage and methylation catalyzed by PilD and selected mutants. Relative rates of leader peptide cleavage from prepilin (LPase) and methylation of mature pilin (MTase) are compared.

folding in the periplasm (Lory et al., 1983). Fractionation of bacterial lysates into extracellular, periplasmic, and cell-associated compartments showed that a portion of the mutant exotoxin A is retained in the periplasm, and following inhibition of further synthesis, this pool is eventually translocated across the outer membrane (Lu et al., 1993). This experiment demonstrated that the pathway for extracellular secretion of exotoxin A is identical to that of the other secreted proteins utilizing the type II secretion pathway.

It was shown that mutations that alter the acidic nature of the amino terminus of the mature exotoxin A resulted in a delay in its secretion from the periplasm. This observation raised the possibility that targeting signals may be contained in this domain. Alternatively, the adverse effect of mutations on secretion across the outer membrane could be the consequence of an overall perturbation of the targeting signal at a different portion of the molecule. To identify such a targeting signal in exotoxin A, a deletion-fusion approach was taken. A series of deletions of the exotoxin A gene were generated and then fused to the gene for the periplasmic enzyme β-lactamase to give exotoxin A–β-lactamase hybrids. Figure 5 shows schematically the structure of the hybrid proteins and the secretability of these proteins from *P. aeruginosa*. The hybrid consisting of the full-length exotoxin A fused to β-lactamase was secreted almost as efficiently as exotoxin A alone, implying that the passenger proteins in these constructs do not significantly influence the interaction of the targeting signal with the secretion machinery. Furthermore, fusion of the eukaryotic protein interleukin-4 to exotoxin A resulted in a protein which was efficiently secreted. The extent of secretion of other exotoxin A–β-lactamase fusions varied with the individual construct; however, in each case at least 50% of the synthesized product was secreted from *P. aeruginosa*. Furthermore, secretion of the hybrid proteins depended on a functional type II secretion pathway, since the exotoxin A–β-lactamase fusions were not secreted from *xcp* mutants of *P. aeruginosa*. Occasionally, a severe stability problem was encountered, and some hybrid proteins were poorly expressed. Presumably this was the consequence of slow translocation across the periplasm, where the proteins could be degraded by proteases.

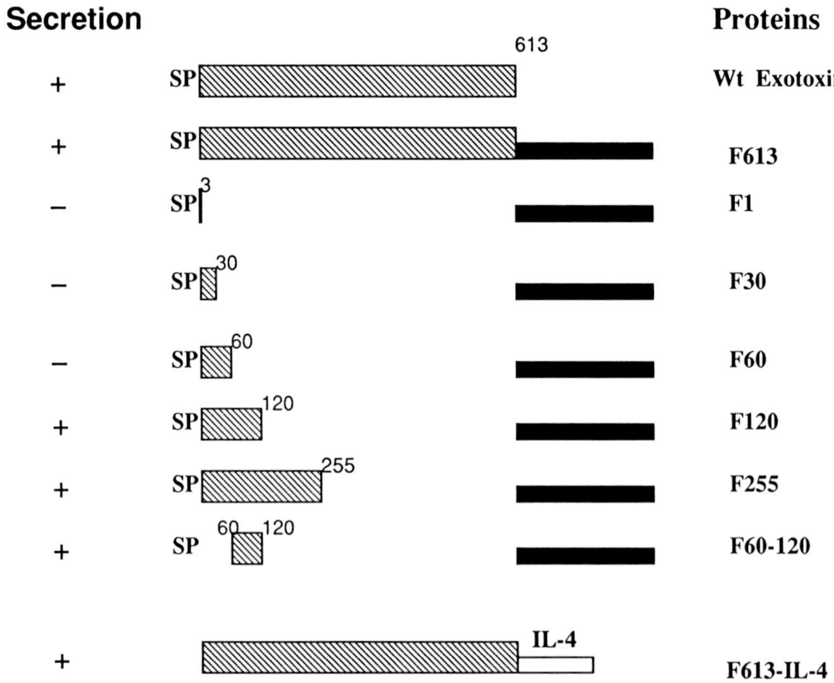

Figure 5. Schematic representation of the fusions between exotoxin A and β-lactamase or interleukin-4. SP, signal peptide of exotoxin A; hatched boxes, mature region of exotoxin A; solid boxes, mature region of *E. coli* β-lactamase; open box, mature region of murine interleukin-4 (IL-4).

The deletion-fusion studies resulted in delineation of the minimal exotoxin A sequence that is recognized by the Xcp machinery. It was found between amino acids 60 and 120 of the mature polypeptide. Presumably, this region contains the extracellular targeting signal. The sequence itself is unremarkable with respect to its amino acid composition, which is characterized by a series of β-sheets, interrupted by turns. The crystal structure of exotoxin A is known (Allured et al., 1986), and this toxin is apparently secreted in its final conformation (Strom et al., 1991). Thus the 60-amino-acid domain was examined in the context of its three-dimensional structure. Amino acids 60 to 120 are found largely on the surface of the folded toxin, in a domain previously identified as containing the portion of the exotoxin A responsible for its interaction with eukaryotic cells during the cellular intoxication process (Guidi-Rontani and Collier, 1987).

Identification of a relatively short (60-amino-acid) targeting sequence in exotoxin A implies that a similar sequence should exist on all other *P. aeruginosa* secreted proteins utilizing the type II secretion pathway. Inspection of phospholipase C and elastase, which are known to utilize the same secretion pathway as exotoxin A, failed to identify sequences homologous with the region 60–120 of exotoxin A. Furthermore, phospholipase C and elastase lack a region rich in predicted β-strands interrupted by turns. If there is a sequence motif part of the secretion signal, it is very likely represented in all of these proteins by a complex tertiary structure.

CONCLUDING REMARKS

A great deal of information on extracellular protein secretion and biogenesis of pili in *P. aeruginosa* has been derived from genetic studies. Characterization of mutants with defined phenotypes resulted in isolation of genes. Sequence analysis revealed a remarkable conservation of the various proteins in taxonomically diverse bacterial species. It is clear that *P. aeruginosa*, having a well-developed genetic system and being a good source of abundant amounts of material for biochemical studies, will continue to be the major model system in studies of protein secretion and pilus biogenesis.

Acknowledgments. These studies were supported by NIH grant AI 21495. J.C.P. has a postdoctoral fellowship from the Cystic Fibrosis Foundation.

REFERENCES

Akrim, M., M. Bally, G. Ball, J. Tommassen, H. Teerink, A. Filloux, and A. Lazdunski. 1993. Xcp-mediated protein secretion in *Pseudomonas aeruginosa*: evidence for regulation of *xcp* gene expression. *Mol. Microbiol.* **10:**431–443.

Albano, M., R. Breitling, and D. A. Dubnau. 1989. Nucleotide sequence and genetic organization of the *Bacillus subtilis comG* operon. *J. Bacteriol.* **171:**5386–5404.

Allured, V. S., R. J. Collier, S. F. Carroll, and D. B. McKay. 1986. Structure of exotoxin A of *Pseudomonas aeruginosa* at 3.0-Angstrom resolution. *Proc. Natl. Acad. Sci. USA* **83:**1320–1324.

Alm, R. A., and J. S. Mattick. 1995. Identification of a gene, *pilV*, required for the type 4 fimbrial biogenesis in *Pseudomonas aeruginosa*, whose product possesses a prepilin-like leader sequence. *Mol. Microbiol.* **16:**485–496.

Bally, M., G. Ball, A. Badere, and A. Lazdunski. 1991. Protein secretion in *Pseudomonas aeruginosa*: the *xcpA* gene encodes an integral inner membrane protein homologous to *Klebsiella pneumoniae* secretion function protein PulO. *J. Bacteriol.* **173:**479–486.

Bally, M., A. Filloux, M. Akrim, G. Ball, A. Lazdunski, and J. Tommassen. 1992. Protein secretion in *Pseudomonas aeruginosa*: characterization of seven *xcp* genes and processing of secretory apparatus components by prepilin peptidase. *Mol. Microbiol.* **6:**1121–1132.

Bradley, D. E. 1973. Basic characterization of a *Pseudomonas aeruginosa* pilus-dependent bacteriophage with a non-contractile tail. *J. Virol.* **12:**1139–1148.

Bradley, D. E. 1980. A function of *Pseudomonas aeruginosa* PAO pili: twitching motility. *Can. J. Microbiol.* **26:**146–154.

Dodd, D. C., and B. I. Eisenstein. 1984. Dependence of secretion and assembly of type 1 fimbrial subunits of *Escherichia coli* on normal protein export. *J. Bacteriol.* **159:**1077–1079.

Guidi-Rontani, C., and R. J. Collier. 1987. Exotoxin A of *Pseudomonas aeruginosa*: evidence that domain I functions in receptor binding. *Mol. Microbiol.* **1:**67–72.

Guzzo, J., F. C. Duong, M. Wandersman, M. Murgier, and A. Lazdunski. 1991. The secretion genes of *Pseudomonas aeruginosa* are alkaline protease functionally related to those of *Erwinia chrysanthemi* proteases and *Escherichia coli* alpha hemolysin. *Mol. Microbiol.* **5:**447–453.

Johnson, K., M. L. Parker, and S. Lory. 1986. Nucleotide sequence and transcriptional initiation site of two *Pseudomonas aeruginosa* pilin genes. *J. Biol. Chem.* **261:**15703–15706.

Kaufman, M. R., J. M. Seyer, and R. K. Taylor. 1991. Processing of TCP pilin by TcpJ typifies a common step intrinsic to a newly recognized pathway of extracellular protein secretion by Gram-negative bacteria. *Genes Dev.* **5:**1834–1846.

Lauer, P., N. H. Albertson, and M. Koomey. 1993. Conservation of genes encoding components of a type IV pilus assembly/two-step protein export pathway in *Neisseria gonorrhoeae*. *Mol. Microbiol.* **9:**357–368.

Lory, S. 1995. Leader peptidases of Type IV prepilins and related proteins, p. 31–48. *In* G. von Heijne (ed.), *Signal Peptidases*. R. G. Landis Company, Austin, Tex.

Lory, S., P. C. Tai, and B. D. Davis. 1983. Mechanism of excretion of proteins by Gram-negative bacteria: *Pseudomonas aeruginosa* exotoxin A. *J. Bacteriol.* **156:**695–702.

Lu, H.-M., S. Mizushima, and S. Lory. 1993. Periplasmic intermediate in the extracellular secretion pathway of *Pseudomonas aeruginosa* exotoxin A. *J. Bacteriol.* **175:**7453–7467.

Martin, P. R., M. Hobbs, P. D. Free, Y. Jeske, and J. S. Mattick. 1993. Characterization of *pilQ*, a new gene required for the biogenesis of type 4 fimbriae in *Pseudomonas aeruginosa*. *Mol. Microbiol.* **9:**857–868.

Martin, R. M., A. A. Watson, T. F. McCaul, and J. S. Mattick. 1995. Characterization of a five-gene cluster for the biogenesis of the type 4 fimbriae in *Pseudomonas aeruginosa*. *Mol. Microbiol.* **16:**497–508.

Nunn, D., P. Bergman, and S. Lory. 1990. Products of three accessory genes, *pilB*, *pilC* and *pilD*, are required for biogenesis of *Pseudomonas aeruginosa* pili. *J. Bacterol.* **172:**2911–2919.

Nunn, D. N., and S. Lory. 1991. Product of the *Pseudomonas aeruginosa* gene *pilD* is a prepilin leader peptidase. *Proc. Natl. Acad. Sci. USA* **88:**3281–3285.

Nunn, D. N., and S. Lory. 1992. Components of the protein-excretion apparatus of *Pseudomonas aeruginosa* are processed by the type IV prepilin peptidase. *Proc. Natl. Acad. Sci. USA* **89:**47–51.

Pugsley, A. P. 1993. The complete general protein secretory pathway in Gram-negative bacteria. *Microbiol. Rev.* **57:**50–108.

Pugsley, A. P., C. d'Enfert, and M. G. Kornacker. 1990. Genetics of extracellular protein secretion by Gram-negative bacteria. *Annu. Rev. Genet.* **24:**67–90.

Pugsley, A. P., and I. Reyss. 1990. Five genes at the 3′ end of the *Klebsiella pneumoniae pulC* operon are required for pullulanase secretion. *Mol. Microbiol.* **4:**365–379.

Russell, M. 1994. Phage assembly: a paradigm for bacterial virulence factor export? *Science* **265:**612–614.

Russell, M. A., and A. Darzins. 1994. The *pilE* gene product of *Pseudomonas aeruginosa*, required for the pilus biogenesis, shares amino acid sequence identity with the N-termini of type 4 prepilin proteins. *Mol. Microbiol.* **13:**973–985.

Salmond, G. P. C., and P. J. Reeves. 1993. Membrane traffic wardens and protein secretion in Gram-negative bacteria. *Trends Biochem. Sci.* **18:**7–12.

Strom, M., P. Bergman, and S. Lory. 1993a. Identification of active-site cysteines in the conserved domain of PilD, the bifunctional leader peptidase/N-methyl transferase of *Pseudomonas aeruginosa* pilins. *J. Biol. Chem.* **268:**15788–15794.

Strom, M. S., and S. Lory. 1987. Mapping of export signals of *Pseudomonas aeruginosa* pilin with alkaline phosphatase fusions. *J. Bacteriol.* **169:**3181–3188.

Strom, M. S., and S. Lory. 1993. Structure-function and biogenesis of the type IV pili. *Annu. Rev. Microbiol.* **47:**565–596.

Strom, M. S., D. Nunn, and S. Lory. 1991. Multipe roles of the pilus biogenesis protein *pilD:* involvement of *pilD* in excretion of enzymes from *Pseudomonas aeruginosa*. *J. Bacteriol.* **173:**1175–1180.

Strom, M. S., D. N. Nunn, and S. Lory. 1993b. A single bifunctional enzyme, PilD, catalyzes cleavage and N-methylation of proteins belonging to the type IV pilin family. *Proc. Natl. Acad. Sci. USA* **90:**2404–2408.

Tommassen, J. A., A. Filloux, M. Bally, M. Murgier, and A. Lazdunski. 1992. Protein secretion in *Pseudomonas aeruginosa*. *FEMS Microbiol. Rev.* **103:**73–90.

Turner, L. R., J. C. Lara, D. N. Nunn, and S. Lory. 1993. Mutations in the consensus ATP-binding sites of XcpR and PilB eliminate extracellular protein secretion and pilus biogenesis in *Pseudomonas aeruginosa*. *J. Bacteriol.* **175:**4962–4969.

Whitchurch, C. B., and J. S. Mattick. 1994. Characterization of a gene, *pilU*, required for twitching motility but not phage sensitivity in *Pseudomonas aeruginosa*. *Mol. Microbiol.* **13:**1079–1091.

Yahr, T. L., A. K. Hovey, S. M. Kulich, and D. W. Frank. 1995. Transcriptional analysis of exoenzyme S structural gene. *J. Bacteriol.* **177:**1169–1178.

Zhang, H. Z., S. Lory, and M. S. Donnenberg. 1994. A plasmid-encoded prepilin peptidase gene from enteropathogenic *Escherichia coli*. *J. Bacteriol.* **176:**6885–6891.

Molecular Biology of Pseudomonads
Edited by T. Nakazawa et al.

Chapter 37

The General Secretion Pathway in *Pseudomonas aeruginosa*: Molecular Mechanisms and Regulation

Andrée Lazdunski, Alain Filloux, Gérard Michel, Maryline Foglino, Maryse Murgier, Amel Latifi, Virginie Chapon, Sophie Bléves, and Marc Bally

Many gram-negative bacteria can secrete proteins to the extracellular medium. Exoproteins produced by these species have to cross the cell envelope, which includes two membranes, making the secretion mechanisms of particular interest. Two main pathways have been identified (Pugsley, 1993). The exoproteins following the first of these two pathways have direct access to the external medium and thus bypass the periplasm. Translocation through this pathway does not involve a classical signal sequence. The best-characterized secretion systems of this type are those of *Escherichia coli* α-hemolysin (Kenny et al., 1991) and *Erwinia chrysanthemi* proteases (Létoffé et al., 1990). The second translocation pathway is signal sequence dependent: an N-terminal signal sequence directs the protein to the periplasm, from where it is translocated across the outer membrane in a second, independent step requiring the expression of several genes. Many gram-negative bacteria possess a system of this type (called the general secretion pathway) by which proteins with signal peptides are secreted. The best-characterized system of this type is the secretion of *Klebsiella oxytoca* pullulanase, for which 14 *pul* genes appear to be required (Pugsley, 1993).

Pseudomonas aeruginosa produces a large number of extracellular proteins, most of which are virulence factors. Both types of secretion pathway are used by *P. aeruginosa* (Lazdunski et al., 1992; Tommassen et al., 1992). Alkaline protease is secreted by the one-step mechanism, and three membrane proteins are required: AprD, AprE, and AprF. The genes encoding these proteins are clustered adjacent to the alkaline protease structural gene *aprA* (Guzzo et al., 1991b). Sequence data indicate that AprD, AprE and AprF are homologous to the accessory proteins required for the secretion of proteases B and C from *Erwinia chrysanthemi* and α-hemolysin from *E. coli* (Duong et al., 1992). Other

Andrée Lazdunski, Alain Filloux, Gérard Michel, Maryline Foglino, Maryse Murgier, Amel Latifi, Virginie Chapon, Sophie Bléves, and Marc Bally • Laboratoire d'Ingénierie et Dynamique des Systèmes Membranaires, Centre National de la Recherche Scientifique UPR 9027, 31 Chemin Joseph Aiguier, B.P. 71, 13402 Marseille Cedex 20, France.

proteins secreted from *P. aeruginosa* (elastase, lipase, exotoxin A, phospholipases, alkaline phosphatase) follow the signal peptide-dependent pathway, the second step of which (translocation across the outer membrane) involves 12 *xcp* genes (Tommassen et al., 1992).

This review summarizes our current knowledge of the general secretion pathway in gram-negative bacteria, with particular emphasis on *P. aeruginosa*. We will try to define the functions, as far as they are known, of the various proteins involved in the secretion machinery and, more briefly, the genetic regulation of the corresponding genes.

GENETIC ANALYSIS OF THE GENERAL SECRETION PATHWAY IN *P. AERUGINOSA*

xcp Mutations

Most *P. aeruginosa* exoproteins are synthesized as precursors, that is, proteins with signal sequences. *P. aeruginosa* exoproteins produced from the genes expressed in *E. coli* (exotoxin A, elastase, and phospholipase) are exported to the periplasm, confirming that they are recognized by the Sec export machinery. This suggests that the first step in the secretion of these extracellular proteins is the same as the pathway followed by cell envelope proteins. In *P. aeruginosa xcp* mutants (extracellular protein deficient), the exoproteins accumulate in the periplasm (Filloux et al., 1987). Thus, these mutants are affected in the common process that translocates signal sequence-containing proteins across the outer membrane. Only the alkaline protease is secreted from these mutants, providing further evidence that this enzyme uses an independent secretion mechanism (Guzzo et al., 1991a). Most of the *xcp* mutations map at 40 min on the chromosomal map. The DNA sequence of a 12-kb region has been determined, and 11 genes have thereby been identified (named *xcpP* to *-Z*) (Filloux et al., 1990; Bally et al., 1992; Akrim et al., 1993). They appear to be organized into two operons in diverging orientations (Fig. 1). A single independent *xcp* secretion gene, *xcpA*, has been identified, mapping at 70 min on the chromosome (Bally et al., 1991). Some major characteristics of the Xcp proteins are listed in Fig. 2.

Gram-Negative Bacteria Have a Conserved Secretion System

The 12 Xcp proteins appear to be homologous to the Pul proteins involved in the specific secretion of pullulanase from *K. oxytoca* (Fig. 2) (Tommassen et al., 1992). Hybridization experiments have also revealed sequences similar to *xcp* genes in other *Pseudomonas* species (De Groot et al., 1991). Furthermore, corresponding genes have been identified or cloned over recent years from a variety of gram-negative bacteria, including *Erwinia, Xanthomonas, Aeromonas*, and *Vibrio* spp. (for a review, see Pugsley [1993]). Mutations in these *out, xps, exe*, and *eps* genes, respectively, are pleiotropic and result in the accumulation of numerous (normally secreted) proteins in the periplasm. This confirms that secretion of these exoproteins involves passage through the periplasm and that the secretion system is widely conserved among gram-negative bacteria. However, despite the homology between the various systems, no cross-functioning has been demonstrated.

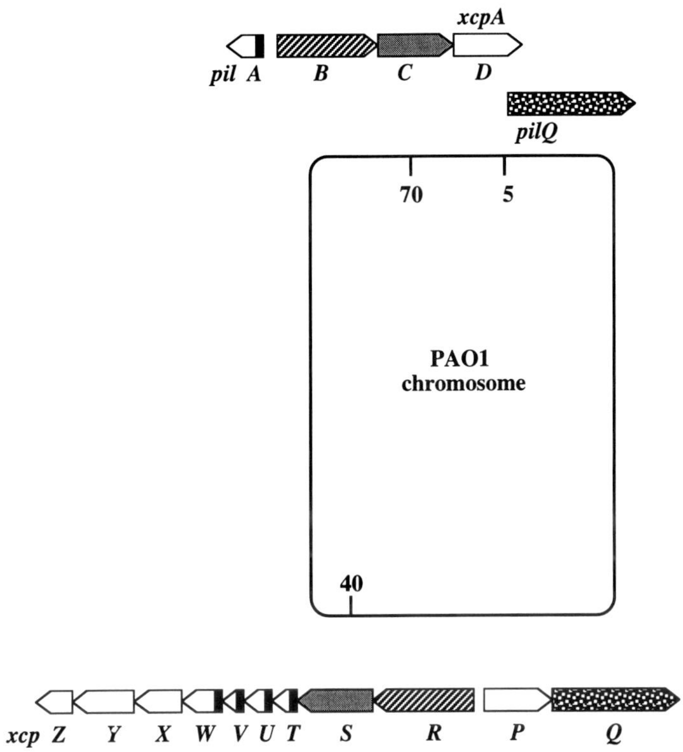

Figure 1. Genetic organization and localization of genes involved in the general protein secretion pathway (*xcp*) and pili biogenesis (*pil*) on the chromosomal map of *P. aeruginosa* PAO1. Homologous proteins are represented by the same symbols.

Are There Other Secretion Genes in *P. aeruginosa*?

No sequences similar to two of the *pul* genes (*pulS* and *pulN*) have been found in *P. aeruginosa*. However, the *P. aeruginosa* secretion system has not been reconstituted in *E. coli*, and thus it has not been demonstrated that all the genes involved have been identified. Similarly, there has been no systematic study replacing genes in one species with their homologs from other species, although some combinations have been tested: e.g., *pulE*, *pulL*, and *pulM* do not complement mutations of the genes *xcpR*, *xcpY*, or *xcpZ* (De Groot et al., 1991; M. Bally, unpublished data). However, *Xanthomonas campestris* and *Erwinia chrysanthemi* mutants can be complemented by the entire secretion operons of *P. aeruginosa* or *Erwinia carotova* (De Groot et al., 1991; Murata et al., 1990). These studies are consistent with the existence of functional blocks of genes, encoding complexes the components of which are not interchangeable even where there are only minor differences, because of the requirements for interaction. The only proteins demonstrated to be interchangeable are XcpA in *P. aeruginosa* and PulO in *K. oxytoca* (Bally et al., 1992). These proteins have an enzymatic function, which could be the reason for their interchangeability.

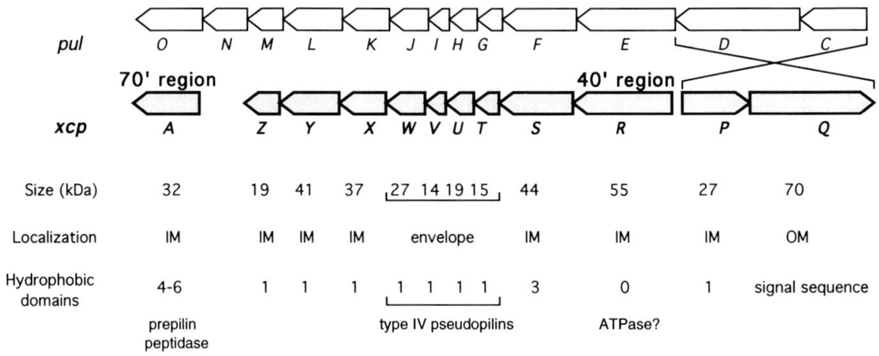

Figure 2. Characteristics of proteins encoded by the *xcp* genes at 40 and 70 min. The *pul* genes are shown at the top according to their order on the *K. oxytoca* chromosome.

FUNCTIONS OF THE INDIVIDUAL Xcp PROTEINS

XcpA, XcpT, XcpU, XcpV, and XcpW

XcpA, a protein of 34 kDa with four to six hydrophobic domains, is associated with the cytoplasmic membrane (Bally et al., 1991). Its role in secretion was elucidated when it was identified as PilD, a protein involved in pilus biogenesis (Nunn and Lory, 1991; Strom et al., 1993). *P. aeruginosa* has polar pili which contribute to both adhesion and flagellum-independent (or twitching) motility (Strom and Lory, 1993). They are built from a single type of subunit of 15 kDa, PilA. The primary structure of PilA is similar to that of the pilus subunits in other bacterial species which are pathogenic for mammals, including *Neisseria gonorrhoeae, Moraxella bovis*, and *Bacteroides nodosus*. All these homologous pilins (type IV pilins) have a conserved N-terminal domain: a short, positively charged sequence followed by a stretch of about 25 hydrophobic residues. Despite the general similarity with signal sequences, only the extreme N-terminal charged residues are cleaved during pilus biogenesis. The *pilD/xcpA* gene encodes the peptidase responsible for this N-terminal cleavage. Besides the *pilD* gene, the *pilC* and *pilB* genes have also been implicated in the assembly of the PilA subunits (Nunn and Lory, 1991).

Four of the proteins encoded by *xcp* genes at the locus at 40 min, XcpT, -U, -V, and -W, have N termini similar to those of the IV pilins (Bally et al., 1992), suggesting that XcpA is involved in their maturation. Specific expression of cloned *xcpT* in an *xcpA* mutant and a wild-type control confirmed that XcpA (or pilin peptidase) is indeed involved in the cleavage of the presequence of XcpT (Bally et al., 1992). The role of pilin peptidase was similarly confirmed for XcpU, -V, and -W by Nunn and Lory (1993), who also demonstrated that the phenylalanine in position +1 of these mature proteins is methylated, as is the corresponding phenylalanine in mature pilin subunits. The pilin peptidase has been purified and its properties have been investigated in vitro using prepilins (Strom et al., 1993). It is a bifunctional enzyme with both cleavage and methylation functions. While type IV pilins and their secretion homologs are methylated, the role of methylation in pilus biogenesis and secretion of proteins is unknown. Both events, cleavage and methylation, take place on the internal face of the cytoplasmic membrane.

The cellular localization of XcpT, also known as a "pseudo-pilin," has been investigated in *P. aeruginosa* PAO1. Under physiological conditions, the protein is associated with both cytoplasmic and outer membrane vesicles (V. Chapon, unpublished data). Its *K. oxytoca* homolog, PulG, has a similar distribution when produced in *E. coli* but is relatively enriched in the outer membrane fractions. Cleavage of pre-PulG by PulO (which removes six residues) does not affect this localization (Pugsley and Possot, 1993). In *P. aeruginosa* PAK, most of the precursor form of XcpT is found in the inner membrane (Nunn and Lory, 1993). These proteins do not have the general features characteristic of outer membrane proteins, despite being recovered in part in outer membrane fractions. Possibly these proteins are constituents of a complex in the cell envelope, interacting with both membranes. This may explain the somewhat confusing finding with classic cell envelope fractionation techniques. The structure of PulG and XcpT was therefore investigated in vivo using permeating, bifunctional reagents. PulG produced in *E. coli* was reported to form homodimers (Pugsley and Possot, 1993), and the apparent association of these units in the membrane was independent of the expression of other *pul* genes. The PulG homolog, XcpT, behaves similarly: a homodimer-sized complex has been identified immunologically after in vivo cross-linking with dithio-*bis*(succimidylpropionate) (Chapon, unpublished). The maturation of PulG or XcpT is not required for this dimerization. It is thus likely that the proteins form dimers before the assembly of larger complexes. Interestingly, purified pili dissociated by octylglucoside give a mixture of subunit monomers and dimers (Watts et al., 1983).

XcpR and XcpS

XcpR and XcpS are homologous to the proteins encoded by the genes *pilB* and *pilC*, which map close to *pilD* (Fig. 1) (Bally et al., 1992). *pilB* and *pilC* are involved in the morphogenesis of pili, and similar genes are found in numerous species (Hobbs and Mattick, 1993). XcpR and its homologs are the only proteins in these secretion systems which do not have a hydrophobic domain. XcpR and its homolog from *K. oxytoca*, PulE, have been produced in *E. coli*, where they are cytoplasmic. However, immunodetection of the *xcpR* gene product in *P. aeruginosa* leads to a different conclusion: XcpR was found associated with inner membrane vesicles (Bally, unpublished). The nature of the association was clearly different from that of an integral membrane protein like XcpZ: XcpR but not XcpZ is dissociated from the membrane by high-ionic-strength solution or treatment with mild denaturing agents or alkali. XcpR thus displays the characteristics of a peripheral membrane protein associated to the membrane via interaction with another protein. Indeed, we recently found that XcpY, which is an integral membrane protein, is involved in the association of XcpR with the inner membrane (Bally, unpublished).

All members of the XcpR family contain a sequence conforming to the Walker A ATP-binding motif: GX_4GKS/T. The Walker B motif ($RX_{6\text{-}8}Y_4D$, where Y = hydrophobic residue) is less well conserved (Pugsley, 1993). Mutations affecting the Walker A motifs in XcpR or PilB render the proteins defective for secretion and piliation, respectively (Turner et al., 1993). The region between these two blocks is well conserved among XcpR homologs, a feature not observed in transport ATPases. XcpR has been partially purified from inclusion bodies obtained following overproduction in *E. coli*. It was not found to efficiently bind ATP after renaturation (G. Michel, unpublished data).

The similarity between PilB-PilC and XcpR-XcpS suggests that XcpR and XcpS are involved in pseudo-pilin translocation and/or morphogenesis. We tested the possible role of the ATP-binding protein XcpR by growing *P. aeruginosa* cells in the presence of an ATPase inhibitor (sodium azide). In these conditions, when we looked at XcpT processing as an indicator of inner membrane insertion and translocation, a strong inhibition of XcpT maturation was observed. However, the level of processing in a *P. aeruginosa* secretion-defective *xcpR* mutant was comparable to that of the wild type. Those apparently contradictory results suggested either that XcpR is not required or that alternative abortive pathways exist. Inner membrane translocation in *E. coli* is supported by the Sec machinery, including the SecA ATPase. Interestingly, we could show that pseudo-pilin maturation is *sec* dependent in *E. coli* and that this dependence could be partially relieved by the expression of the other *xcp* genes (A. Filloux, unpublished data). Thus Xcp proteins, including XcpR and XcpS, may be able to replace the activity of the Sec proteins for the insertion of pseudo-pilins into the cytoplasmic membrane. We could hypothesize that, in the absence of a functional Xcp machinery, the *P. aeruginosa* Sec homologs support translocation of pseudo-pilins but do not assemble them properly in the cell envelope. Xcp proteins, such as XcpR, could have this particular additional function in promoting both translocation and assembly of pseudo-pilin subunits into cell envelope polymeric structures.

XcpQ

XcpQ is the only Xcp protein with a classic N-terminal signal sequence. By analogy with its homolog PulD, it is expected to be localized in the outer membrane (Akrim et al., 1993). XcpQ and PulD belong to a large family, the other members of which are involved in a variety of biological processes (Hobbs and Mattick, 1993). PulD, OutD (*Erwinia chrysanthemi*), and XpsD (*X. campestris*) participate in *sec*-dependent secretion. YscC (*Yersinia enterocolitica*), MxiD (*Shigella flexneri*), HrpH (*Pseudomonas syringae*), and probably HrpA (*Pseudomonas solanacearum*) are involved in the secretion of proteins which do not have classic signal sequences. This pathway differs from that of the secretion of α-hemolysin from *E. coli* and thus is a third type of mechanism for the secretion of pathogenicity determinants from bacteria that are pathogenic for plants and animals (Van Gijsegem et al., 1993). Another member of this family, gpIV from the filamentous phage M13, is associated with the biogenesis of the phage particles and their secretion once assembled (Kazmierczak et al., 1994). These various members of the family display differing degrees of similarity with each other, reflecting their different functions in diverse systems. The common element to all these systems appears to be the requirement for a porelike structure in the outer membrane. pIV has recently been shown to form multimers of probably 10 to 12 subunits (Kazmierczak et al., 1994). These structures could form gated channels in the outer membrane that allow passage of assembling phages or secreted proteins to the external medium.

XcpP, XcpX, XcpY, and XcpZ

Each of the four proteins XcpP, -X, -Y, and -Z has a hydrophobic domain which could be a potential transmembrane segment. Indeed, it has been demonstrated that XcpY and XcpZ and their homologs PulL and PulM are inner membrane proteins (Filloux et al.,

1990; Pugsley, 1993). The topology of XcpP, -X, -Y, and -Z shows the existence of a large periplasmic domain which could interact at the outer membrane level (S. Bléves, unpublished data). By analogy with the Ton system in *E. coli* (Postle, 1993), the role of these four proteins may be to form an energetic link between the two membranes. In the current model for the Ton system, TonB, ExbB, and ExbD may interact in the inner membrane forming a proton channel which energizes siderophore transport systems in the outer membrane by transducing the electrochemical gradient. Consistent with this model, Wong and Buckley (1989) described the involvement of the electron motive force in the translocation of aerolysin across the outer membrane of *Aeromonas salmonicida* by the Exe proteins.

INTRAGENIC INFORMATION

Various different approaches have been used to try to identify secretion signals in proteins secreted from *P. aeruginosa* and other gram-negative bacteria. They include deletions, construction of hybrid proteins, and mutagenesis. No common sequence has been identified. This suggests that the secretion signal may involve a structure made up of nonconsecutive amino acids brought together by protein folding in the periplasm. The importance of the conformation in recognition by the secretion machinery is illustrated by *E. coli dsb* mutants. DsbA catalyzes the formation of disulfide bridges in proteins and is required for the rapid secretion of the periplasmic form of pullulanase (Pugsley, 1992). Similarly, its homolog in *Vibrio cholerae*, TcpG, is required for secretion of proteases and cholera toxin (Peek and Taylor, 1992). Thus, stabilization of the tertiary structure by DsbA or its homologs may be necessary for secretion, but other proteins may also be involved in such structure stabilization. For example, the *P. aeruginosa* elastase has a propeptide which remains associated with the mature enzyme in the periplasm as a specific chaperone and is lost as elastase is translocated across the outer membrane (Braun et al., 1996). Another example is LipB, which is required for lipase to fold into an active conformation and is also required for its secretion (Frenken et al., 1993). LipB is associated with the inner membrane and has a large periplasmic domain. These chaperones may be directly or indirectly involved in recognition by the secretion machinery.

GENETIC REGULATION OF *xcp* GENES

Many virulence factors secreted by *P. aeruginosa* follow the Xcp general secretion pathway. The production of these various factors is controlled by a variety of environmental signals (including for example iron or phosphate starvation, ionic strength of the medium, and growth phase). Perhaps surprisingly, in view of these numerous different situations triggering exoprotein production, secretion does not depend on constitutive expression of the *xcp* genes.

The 11 *xcp* genes mapping at 40 min on the chromosome are organized into two divergent operons 219 bp apart (Fig. 1). In a dot-blot analysis of *xcp* mRNA, we showed that expression of these operons in coordinated and varies according to the growth phase: *xcp* expression increases at the onset of stationary phase, when several exoproteins are synthesized and secreted. Thus, the two processes coincide (Akrim et al., 1993).

The synthesis of three proteases (elastase, alkaline protease, and LasA staphylolytic protease) and of toxin A is controlled by the transcriptional activator LasR (Gambello and Iglewski, 1991). We have shown that the expression of the *xcp* genes is also regulated by *lasR*, and they are thus part of a regulon which coordinates the synthesis of both virulence factors and components of the general secretion pathway (Chapon, unpublished). LasR is thought to be activated by the binding of a small molecule derived from homoserine lactone (*N*-oxohexanoyl-L-homoserine lactone [ODDHL]), and the production of ODDHL involves *lasI* gene expression. LasR and LasI are homologous to LuxR and LuxI, which are involved in the regulation of *Vibrio fischeri* bioluminescence (Passador et al., 1993). The Lux system is the archetype of a regulatory mechanism which has been increasingly studied in recent years (Fuqua et al., 1994). It involves an environmental sensing system which signals the bacterial population density via small membrane diffusible molecules (autoinducers). All autoinducers described to date are derived from homoserine lactone. Their accumulation in the medium, an indicator of increasing cell density, induces a variety of late-growth-phase processes. This regulation mechanism by "quorum sensing" is found in many bacterial species including *Agrobacterium, Erwinia, Yersinia*, and *Rhizobium*. All these systems present two elements, the putative autoinducer synthase (the I protein) and the transcription regulator (the R protein) (Fuqua et al., 1994; Williams et al., this volume).

Recently, we obtained evidence for a second general regulation system by autoinduction in *P. aeruginosa*. The *vsmR* and *vsmI* genes (virulence and secondary metabolism genes) were cloned by complementation of an autoinducer-deficient mutant (Latifi et al., 1995). These genes are very similar to the *rhlR* and *rhlI* genes, identified as regulators of rhamnolipid synthesis (Ochsner et al., 1994). Thus, the same genes have been found in

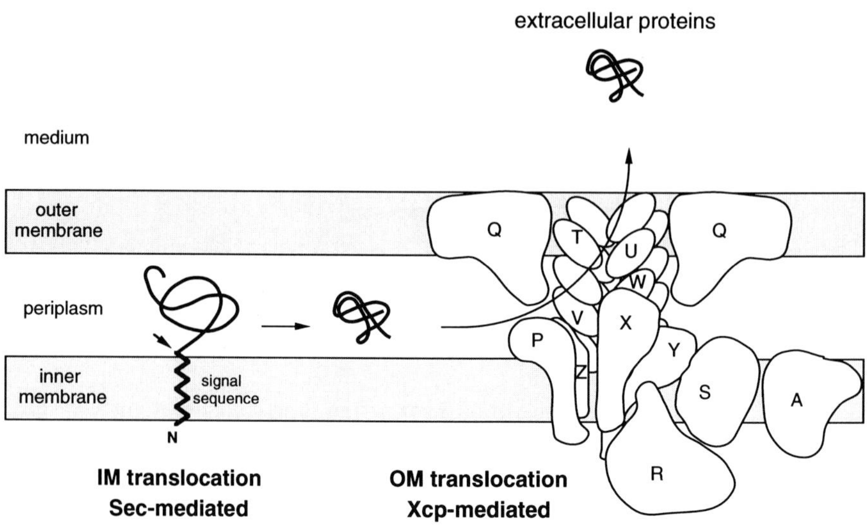

Figure 3. Model for the two-step secretion pathway. Exoproteins are translocated across the inner membrane via the Sec machinery, and the signal sequence is removed by the leader peptidase. The exoproteins are subsequently targeted to the Xcp secretion apparatus and translocated across the outer membrane.

two independent investigations of different phenomena. We showed that this system also regulates the synthesis of elastase, alkaline protease, pyocyanine, and cyanide (Latifi et al., 1995). It also controls the production of Xcp proteins (Chapon, unpublished). The *vsmR/I* (*rhlR/I*) system interacts with the *lasR/I* regulation system. The autoinducers in the *vsmR/I* system have been characterized as the novel *N*-acyl homoserines *N*-butanoyl-L-homoserine lactone and *N*-hexanoyl-L-homoserine lactone (Winson et al., 1995).

Therefore, at least two general systems of regulation by autoinduction appear to be responsible for the physiological coordination of the synthesis of various virulence factors with their secretion.

CONCLUSION

The secretion pathway constituted by the Xcp proteins in *P. aeruginosa* and their homologs in other gram-negative species appears to be an extension of the Sec system: the Sec system translocates proteins across the inner membrane, and the Xcp system translocates products across the outer membrane (Fig. 3). The similarities with systems for the release of phages suggest that there is no restriction on either the size or the type of molecule translocated by the Xcp pathway. This characteristic in particular indicates that this translocation across the outer membrane is fundamentally different from the mechanisms described for translocation across the inner membrane.

Acknowledgments. We thank G. Ball and C. Soscia for expert technical assistance. This work was supported in part by the Ministère de la Recherche et de la Technologie and by the Association Française de Lutte contre la Mucoviscidose.

REFERENCES

Akrim, M., M. Bally, G. Ball, J. Tommassen, H. Teerink, A. Filloux, and A. Lazdunski. 1993. Xcp-mediated protein secretion in *Pseudomonas aeruginosa*: identification of two additional genes and evidence for regulation of *xcp* gene expression. *Mol. Microbiol.* **10:**431–443.

Bally, M., G. Ball, A. Badère, and A. Lazdunski. 1991. Protein secretion in *Pseudomonas aeruginosa*: the *xcpA* gene encodes an integral inner membrane protein homologous to *Klebsiella pneumoniae* secretion function protein PulO. *J. Bacteriol.* **173:**479–486.

Bally, M., A. Filloux, M. Akrim, G. Ball, A. Lazdunski, and J. Tommassen. 1992. Processing of components of the secretory apparatus of *Pseudomonas aeruginosa* by prepilin peptidase. *Mol. Microbiol.* **6:**1121–1131.

Braun, P., J. Tommassen, and A. Filloux. 1996. Role of the propeptide in folding and secretion of elastase of *Pseudomonas aeruginosa*. *Mol. Microbiol.* **19:**297–306.

De Groot, A., A. Filloux, and J. Tommassen. 1991. Conservation of *xcp* genes, involved in the two-step protein secretion process, in different *Pseudomonas* species and other Gram-negative bacteria. *Mol. Gen. Genet.* **229:**278–284.

Duong, F., A. Lazdunski, B. Cami, and M. Murgier. 1992 Sequence of a cluster of genes controlling synthesis and secretion of alkaline protease in *Pseudomonas aeruginosa*: relationships to other secretory pathways. *Gene* **121:**47–54.

Filloux, A., M. Bally, G. Ball, M. Akrim, J. Tommassen, and A. Lazdunski. 1990. Protein secretion in Gram-negative bacteria: transport across the outer membrane involves common mechanisms in different bacteria. *EMBO J.* **9:**4323–4329.

Filloux, A., M. Murgier, B. Wretlind, and A. Lazdunski. 1987. Characterization of two *P. aeruginosa* mutants with defective secretion of extracellular proteins and comparison with other mutants. *FEMS Microbiol. Lett.* **40:**159–163.

Frenken, L. G. J., A. de Groot, J. Tommassen, and C. T. Verrips. 1993. Role of the *lipB* gene product in the folding of the secreted lipase of *Pseudomonas glumae*. *Mol. Microbiol.* **9:**591–599.

Fuqua, W. C., S. C. Winans, and E. P. Greenberg. 1994. Quorum sensing in bacteria: the LuxR-LuxI family of cell-density-responsive transcriptional regulators. *J. Bacteriol.* **176:**269–275.

Gambello, M. I., and B. H. Iglewski. 1991. Cloning and characterization of the *Pseudomonas aeruginosa lasR* gene, a transcriptional activator of elastase expression. *J. Bacteriol.* **173:**3000–3009.

Guzzo, J., F. Duong, C. Wandersman, M. Murgier, and A. Lazdunski. 1991a. The secretion genes of *Pseudomonas aeruginosa* alkaline protease are functionally related to those of *Erwinia chrysanthemi* proteases and *Escherichia coli* α-haemolysin. *Mol. Microbiol.* **5:**447–453.

Guzzo, J., J. M. Pagès, F. Duong, A. Lazdunski, and M. Murgier. 1991b. *Pseudomonas aeruginosa* alkaline protease: evidence for secretion genes and study of secretion mechanism. *J. Bacteriol.* **173:**5290–5297.

Hobbs, M., and J. S. Mattick. 1993. Common components in the assembly of type 4 fimbriae, DNA transfer systems, filamentous phage and protein secretion apparatus; a general system for the formation of surface-associated protein complexes. *Mol. Microbiol.* **10:**233–243.

Kazmierczak, B. I., D. L. Mielke, M. Russel, and P. Model. 1994. pIV, a filamentous phage protein that mediates phage export across the bacterial cell envelope, forms a multimer. *J. Mol. Biol.* **238:**187–198.

Kenny, B., R. Haigh, and I. B. Holland. 1991. Analysis of the haemolysin transport process through the secretion from *E. coli* of PCM, CAT or β-galactosidase fused to the Hly-C-terminal signal domain. *Mol. Microbiol.* **5:**2557–2568.

Latifi, A., M. K. Winson, M. Foglino, B. W. Bycroft, G. S. Stewart, A. Lazdunski, and P. W. Williams. 1995. Multiple homologues of LuxR and LuxI control expression of virulence determinants and secondary metabolites through quorum sensing in *Pseudomonas aeruginosa. Mol. Microbiol.* **17:**333–343.

Lazdunski, A., M. Murgier, M. Bally, A. Filloux, J. Guzzo, M. Akrim, F. Duong, and J. Tommassen. 1992. Secretion of extracellular proteins in *Pseudomonas aeruginosa*: existence of two pathways that are wide-spread among Gram-negative bacteria, p. 83–93. *In* E. Galli, S. Silver, and B. Witholt (ed.), *Pseudomonas: Molecular Biology and Biotechnology*. American Society for Microbiology, Washington, D.C.

Létoffé, S., P. Delepelaire, and C. Wandersman. 1990. Protease secretion by *Erwinia chrysanthemi*: the specific secretion functions are analogous to those of *Escherichia coli* α-haemolysin. *EMBO J.* **9:**1375–1382.

Murata, H., M. Fons, A. Chatterjee, A. Collmer, and A. K. Chatterjee. 1990. Characterization of transposon insertion Out$^-$ mutants of *Erwinia carotovora* subsp. *carotovora* defective in enzyme export and of a DNA segment that complements *out* mutations in *E. carotovora* subsp. *carotovora*, *E. carotovora* subsp. *atroseptica*, and *Erwinia chrysanthemi*. *J. Bacteriol.* **172:**2970–2978.

Nunn, D. N., and S. Lory. 1991. Product of the *Pseudomonas aeruginosa* gene *pilD* is a prepilin leader peptidase. *Proc. Natl. Acad. Sci. USA* **88:**3281–3285.

Nunn, D. S., and S. Lory. 1993. Cleavage, methylation and localization of the *Pseudomonas aeruginosa* export proteins XcpT, -U, -V, and -W. *J. Bacteriol.* **175:**4375–4382.

Ochsner, U. A., A. K. Koch, A. Fiechter, and J. Reiser. 1994. Isolation and characterization of a regulatory gene affecting rhamnolipid biosurfactant synthesis in *Pseudomonas aeruginosa. J. Bacteriol.* **176:**2044–2054.

Passador, L., J. M. Cook, M. J. Gambello, L. Rust, and B. H. Iglewski. 1993. Expression of *Pseudomonas aeruginosa* virulence genes requires cell-to-cell communication. *Science* **260:**1127–1130.

Peek, J. A., and R. K. Taylor. 1992. Characterization of a periplasmic thiol: disulfide interchange protein required for the functional maturation of secreted virulence factors of *Vibrio cholerae*. *Proc. Natl. Acad. Aci. USA* **89:**6210–6214.

Postle, K. 1993. TonB protein and energy transduction between membranes. *J. Bioenerg. Biomembr.* **25:**591–601.

Pugsley, A. P. 1992. Translocation of a folded protein across the outer membrane in *Escherichia coli*. *Proc. Natl. Acad. Sci. USA* **89:**12058–12062.

Pugsley, A. P. 1993. The complete general secretory pathway in gram-negative bacteria. *Microbiol. Rev.* **57:**50–108.

Pugsley, A. P., and O. Possot. 1993. The general secretory pathway of *Klebsiella oxytoca*: no evidence for relocalization or assembly of pilin-like PulG protein into a multiprotein complex. *Mol. Microbiol.* **10:**665–674.

Strom, M. S., and S. Lory. 1993. Structure-function and biogenesis of the type IV pili. *Annu. Rev. Microbiol.* **47:**565–596.

Strom, M. S., D. N. Nunn, and S. Lory. 1993. A single bifunctional enzyme, PilD, catalyzes cleavage and N-methylation of proteins belonging to the type IV pilin family. *Proc. Natl. Acad. Sci. USA* **90:**2404–2408.

Tommassen, J., A. Filloux, M. Bally, M. Murgier, and A. Lazdunski. 1992. Protein secretion in *Pseudomonas aeruginosa. FEMS Microbiol. Rev.* **103:**73–90.

Turner, L. R., J. C. Lara, D. N. Nunn, and S. Lory. 1993. Mutations in the consensus ATP-binding sites of XcpR and PilB eliminate extracellular protein secretion and pilus biogenesis in *Pseudomonas aeruginosa. J. Bacteriol.* **175:**4962–4969.

Van Gijsegem, F., S. Genin, and C. Boucher. 1993. Conservation of secretion pathways for pathogenicity determinants of plant and animal bacteria. *Trends Microbiol.* **1:**175–180.

Watts, T. H., C. M. Kay, and W. Paranchych. 1983. Spectral properties of three quaternary arrangements of *Pseudomonas* pilin. *Biochemistry* **22:**3640–3646.

Winson, M. K., M. Camara, A. Latifi, M. Foglino, S. R. Chhabra, M. Daykin, M. Bally, V. Chapon, G. P. C. Salmond, B. W. Bycroft, A. Lazdunski, G. S. A. B. Stewart, and P. Williams. 1995. Multiple N-acyl-L-homoserine lactone signal molecules regulate production of virulence determinants and secondary metabolites in *Pseudomonas aeruginosa. Proc. Natl. Acad. Sci. USA* **92:**9427–9431.

Wong, K. R., and J. T. Buckley. 1989. Proton motive force involved in proteins transport across the outer membrane of *Aeromonas salmonicida. Science* **246:**654–655.

Section VIII

MEDICAL ASPECTS AND PATHOGENESIS

Molecular Biology of Pseudomonads
Edited by T. Nakazawa et al.

Chapter 38

Cationic Peptides: a Class of Antibiotics Able To Access the Self-Promoted Uptake Pathway across the *Pseudomonas aeruginosa* Outer Membrane

Robert E. W. Hancock, Kevin Piers, Melissa Brown, Tim Falla, Monisha Gough, Manhong Wu, and Shafique Fidai

Pseudomonas aeruginosa has been a major target for antibiotic drug discovery programs in large pharmaceutical companies. However, as each succeeding "antipseudomonal" antibiotic has hit the market, it has been rapidly followed by the development of serious resistance. For example, the antipseudomonal penicillins and third-generation cephalosporins have been plagued by resistance due to depressed chromosomal β-lactamases; the carbapenem β-lactam, imipenem, rapidly induced mutations lacking the imipenem-specific porin OprD; and the use of the fluoroquinolones has been restricted by DNA gyrase and multiple-antibiotic resistance (efflux) mutations. Each of these newer groups of antibiotics is a variation on a theme, a compound that has a structure and mode of action that are related to previously introduced antibiotics. Thus bacteria can adapt existing mechanisms (through mutation) to develop resistance to these variant antibiotics. This is an even greater problem with *P. aeruginosa*, which has high intrinsic resistance to antibiotics due to a large extent to the low permeability of its outer membrane (Hancock and Bell, 1989). Thus a relatively small decrease in susceptibility to a given antibiotic is sufficient to make this organism clinically untreatable by this antibiotic. For this reason there is considerable rationale for investigating novel classes of antimicrobial agents.

One of the more reliable classes of antipseudomonal antibiotics is the aminoglycosides. Resistance rates have been fairly steady at around 10% of isolates over the past decade. In the course of studying the mechanisms of uptake of antibiotics across the *P. aeruginosa* outer membrane, we discovered that the aminoglycosides utilized a fundamentally different mechanism (Hancock, 1984; Hancock and Bell, 1989; Hancock et al., 1981) compared to the β-lactams, which in general pass through the water-filled channels of pro-

Robert E. W. Hancock, Kevin Piers, Melissa Brown, Tim Falla, Monisha Gough, Manhong Wu, and Shafique Fidai • Department of Microbiology and Immunology, University of British Columbia, Vancouver, B.C. V6T 1Z3, Canada.

teins termed porins. We termed this mechanism self-promoted uptake (Hancock, 1984). The property of aminoglycosides that permits them to use this pathway is their positively charged nature, with three to five positive charges appended to a trisaccharide backbone. Subsequently we demonstrated that self-promoted uptake occurred in *Escherichia coli* (Hancock and Farmer, 1993) and *Enterobacter cloacae* (Piers et al., 1994) and was the major uptake mechanism for the polymyxins (Hancock, 1984; Hancock et al., 1981), azithromycin (Farmer et al., 1992), and deglucoteichoplanins (Hancock and Farmer, 1993). The latter two represented interesting situations in which traditional classes of gram-positive specific antibiotics were derivatized to give them a charge of +2 such that they acquired useful activity against gram-negative bacteria due to their ability to access self-promoted uptake across the outer membrane (which excluded the parent antibiotics).

For this reason, we started to look for polycationic molecules that would have the ability to utilize self-promoted uptake. The cationic peptides, one of nature's most common answers to microbial infections, represent such a class.

SELF-PROMOTED UPTAKE

Self-promoted uptake involves the interaction of polycationic antibiotics with the divalent cation (Ca^{2+}/Mg^{2+})-binding sites on cell surface lipopolysaccharide (LPS) (Fig. 1). These cationic antibiotics have an affinity for such sites that is two to four orders of magnitude higher than that of the divalent cations that normally occupy them. Therefore they competitively displace the divalent cations in a highly cooperative manner. This results in an increase in the surface area of the outer membrane (see, e.g., Sawyer et al.,

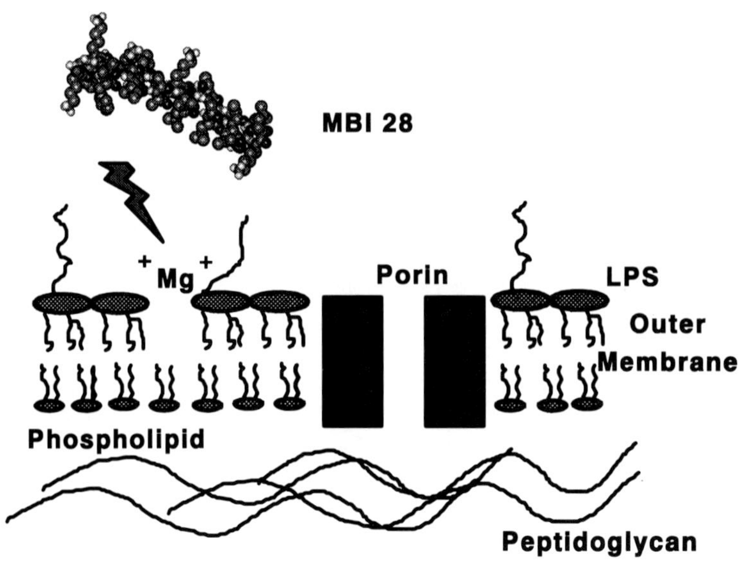

Figure 1. Diagram of self-promoted uptake across the outer membrane. See text for explanation. MBI 28 (formerly termed CEMA [Piers et al., 1994]) has the sequence KWKLFKKIGIGAVLKVLTTGLPALKLTK.

1988), since the antibiotics are much bulkier than the divalent cations they displace, and a dramatic change in its physiochemical and electrostatic properties. Biochemically, we have observed cooperative permeabilization of the outer membrane to such probe molecules as the small basic protein lysozyme, the chromogenic β-lactam nitrocefin, and the hydrophobic fluorophor 1-*N*-phenyl naphthylamine (NPN). Thus, we have proposed that the outer membrane becomes more permeable to the cationic antibiotic itself. The relevance of self-promoted uptake is evidenced by aminoglycoside-supersusceptible mutants of *P. aeruginosa* which have LPS changes resulting in enhanced affinity of these aminoglycosides for LPS binding and outer membrane permeabilization (Rivera et al., 1988), as well as polymyxin-resistant mutants of *P. aeruginosa* and *E. coli* for which the inverse is true (Hancock et al., 1991; Young et al., 1992). Thus we can say that self-promoted uptake leads directly to cell killing.

There is, however, considerable heterogeneity in the ways such cationic antibiotics interact with the outer membrane. For example, some cationic antibiotics permeabilize outer membranes to probe molecules at concentrations well below the MIC, whereas others are only effective at the MIC. This clearly depends on the killing potency of the antibiotic, since, e.g., polymyxin B only permeabilizes at the MIC (0.5 μg/ml) and is able at this concentration to cause membrane perturbations (which would equate to loss of cytoplasmic membrane integrity in cells). In contrast, deacylated polymyxin B can permeabilize outer membranes at a similar concentration (Vaara and Vaara, 1983) but is ineffective in perturbing phospholipid bilayer membranes (Schroder et al., 1992).

A second indication of heterogeneity resides in the differential effects of mutants. Thus, a *tolA* mutant (Rivera et al., 1988) of *P. aeruginosa* has a dramatic (16- to 32-fold) effect on susceptibility to aminoglycosides but a minimal influence on polymyxin susceptibility (around 2-fold). Similarly, a *pmx* mutant of *E. coli* induces a 64-fold increase in polymyxin resistance but only a 2- to 4-fold increase in gentamicin and azithromycin resistance. These data may reflect differences in the preferred interaction sites of polymyxin and the aminoglycosides (possibly due to LPS heterogeneity [Hancock et al., 1994] and differences in the structures of these molecules). Consistent with this idea, the number of binding sites per LPS molecule is different for polymyxin and the aminoglycosides.

CATIONIC PEPTIDES FROM NATURE

Cationic peptide antimicrobial agents have been discovered in many living things. They are produced by bacteria, fungi, plants, insects, crustaceans, amphibians, mammals, and humans (Boman et al., 1991; Hancock et al., 1995; Lehrer et al., 1993; Zasloff, 1987). In each case they are a major contributor to defense against microbes. For example, when insects acquire a bacterial infection, they induce the production of one or several peptides which are antibacterial in nature. The skin of frogs virtually never becomes infected even when damaged in the presence of highly contaminated water because cationic peptides are induced to destroy any bacteria introduced. Similarly, the most abundant proteinaceous molecules in the neutrophil, a dedicated microbe-killing cell in humans and mammals, are the defensins, which are antimicrobial cationic peptides present at a level of 5 to 18% of neutrophil protein (Lehrer et al., 1993). Other abundant species of cationic peptides are found at mucosal membrane surfaces in the mammalian upper intestine and trachea (Hancock et al., 1995). Indeed, some feel that such cationic peptides represent the "missing link" in muscosal immunity. (Of interest to *Pseudomonas* sp. researchers is the possibility that the prevalence of *P. aeruginosa* infections in cystic fibrosis patients could possibly result from a defect in secretion across the lung mucosa of as-yet-unidentified antimicrobial cationic peptides.)

Cationic peptides show marked structural variations despite thematic similarities. Thus there are at least four classes of cationic peptides (Hancock et al., 1995), including β-stranded peptides with two or three antiparallel β-strands connected by disulfides (e.g., neutrophil defensins, crab tachyplesins); α-helical peptides that may contain a kink or turn in the middle of two α-helical regions (e.g., insect cecropins); loops which are stabilized by a single disulfide (e.g., neutrophil bactenicins); and peptides of unknown structure with predominating amino acid such as proline, tryptothan, or histidine (e.g., indolicidins). These peptides all have two strongly preserved properties. First, they contain multiple positive charges due to a number of lysines and/or arginines. Second, the peptides are amphipathic, with a hydrophilic face (containing the positive charges) and a hydrophobic face. In light of these strongly conserved properties and functions, despite variant secondary structure, we consider this to be the finest argument for convergent evolution, in which a variety of peptides have converged to acquire a common function.

ANTIPSEUDOMONAL ACTIVITIES OF CATIONIC PEPTIDES

Cationic peptides in nature vary from gram-positive selective to gram-negative selective to broad spectrum. For example, insect cecropins are considered to be preferentially active against gram-negative bacteria, nisin is selective for gram-positive bacteria, and magainins are effective against both classes. In addition, selected peptides can have antifungal, antiviral (against enveloped viruses), or antiparasite (Hancock et al., 1995; Lehrer et al., 1993) activities.

There are no known peptides that are specific for *P. aeruginosa*, but the gram-negative selective peptides can include *Pseudomonas* spp. as part of their antibacterial spectrum. Studies on cecropin variants have indicated that the precise determinants of antipseudomonal activity are different from the determinants of activity against other gram-negative bacteria. For example, a Lys-6→Leu-6 mutation of cecropin A virtually abolished activity against *P. aeruginosa* while not affecting activity against *E. coli* (Andreu et al., 1985).

Table 1 shows the comparative activities of several cationic peptides against *P. aeruginosa* compared with activities against *E. coli* and *Staphylococcus aureus*. These MICs are never exceptionally low. However, they are competitive with MICs of many antibiotics against these organisms. Furthermore, these MICs do not appear to vary much between different strains of a given species, and they appear unaffected by most clinically important antibiotic resistance mechanisms (Piers et al., 1994; R. E. W. Hancock, unpublished data). Furthermore, attempts to isolate mutants resistant to cationic peptides have been unsuccessful to date.

The *P. aeruginosa* supersusceptible mutant Z61 has a defect in its barrier properties due to multiple mutations (at least three) which affect antibiotic efflux (Li et al., 1994) and possibly also outer membrane permeability (Angus et al., 1987). This mutant has enhanced susceptibility to all classes of antibiotic, with MICs that are 4-fold to 10,000-

Table 1. Activity of selected cationic peptides against *P. aeruginosa*, *E. coli*, and *S. aureus*

Peptide or antibiotic	Class	MIC (μg/ml)[a]							
		P. aeruginosa			*E. coli*			*S. aureus*	
		SS	S	R	SS	S	R	S	R
Melittin	α-Helical	8.0	8.0	8.0	4.0	8.0	8.0	8.0	8.0
CEME	α-Helical	1.2	2.4	4.8	0.6	1.2	2.4	9.6	9.6
MBI-28	α-Helical	1.4	2.8	2.8	0.7	1.4	2.8	>64.0	>64.0
Bactenecin	Loop	2.0	32.0		4.0	64.0		>64.0	>64.0
Polymyxin B	Cationic lipopeptide	0.06	0.5	0.5	0.06	0.5	32.0	>64.0	>64.0
Gentamicin	Aminoglycoside	0.25	1.0	200	0.5	1.0	4.0	2.0	>64.0
Ceftazidime	Cephalosporin	0.03	0.5	200	0.06	0.5	0.5	8.0	>64.0

[a] All MICs were determined in Luria broth (0.8% tryptone, 0.5% yeast extract) using the microtiter broth dilution assay as described by Piers et al. (1994) or in unpublished laboratory data. The Mg^{2+} content of this medium is recognized to be lower than that of serum. Abbreviations: SS, supersusceptible mutant (*P. aeruginosa* Z61, *E. coli* DC2); S, normally susceptible strain (*P. aeruginosa* H103, *E. coli* UB1005); R, resistant variant (*P. aeruginosa* H103/RP1, *E. coli* SC9252, *S. aureus* SAP0017).

fold lower than those of the parent strain K799. Interestingly, the decrease in MIC for the cationic peptides appeared minimal for the more potent α-helical peptides (Table 1; Piers and Hancock, 1994), indicating that these efflux systems are irrelevant for this class of peptides.

An important feature of these cationic peptides is their rapid killing of bacteria (Piers and Hancock, 1994) as compared with other antibiotics at the MIC. This is probably related to their ability to selectively form channels in bacterial membranes (Hancock et al., 1995; Skerlavaj et al., 1990).

RECOMBINANT PRODUCTION OF CATIONIC PEPTIDES

It is extremely difficult to produce large quantities of cationic peptides from nature. For example, for the rabbit defensins, only 200 mg of purified peptide can be obtained from a single animal. An alternative methodology involves protein chemical synthesis using a peptide synthesizer. However, this is relatively expensive and difficult to scale up. Magainin Sciences Inc. have had some success using solution-phase chemical synthesis, but this still tends to be relatively expensive.

With this in mind, we set out to devise a recombinant DNA methodology for production of cationic peptides in bacteria. It soon became apparent that the two challenges we were facing were (i) protecting the producing bacterium from the antibacterial peptide and (ii) protecting the peptide from bacterial proteases during synthesis. We will not discuss all of the approaches that did not work (Piers et al., 1993), but rather the general approach that did. The cationic peptides were produced as a four-component fusion protein comprising, from the N terminus, an affinity binding segment (to permit downstream affinity purification), an anionic protective segment (to bind to the cationic peptide protein and protect it from proteases), a methionine (to permit removal of the peptide by cyanogen bromide), and a cationic peptide antibiotic segment. Two basic variations were devised. For *S. aureus* expression, the affinity binding and anionic protective segments were fused as a protein A binding domain, resulting in secretion of the fusion protein. In *E. coli* a separate anionic binding domain had to be included, and the resultant protein was produced cytoplasmically as inclusion bodies. However, a broad range of affinity binding regions and cationic peptide regions could be synthesized, and especially in the latter case, since the peptide expressing region was synthesized on a DNA synthesizer, virtually any sequence could be produced. The resultant peptide, after purification, was indistinguishable from chemically synthesized peptide (Piers et al., 1993; Piers and Hancock, 1994). This recombinant DNA technology provides a basic platform for isolation of variant peptides through screening of combinatorial libraries.

INTERACTION OF CATIONIC PEPTIDES WITH THE OUTER MEMBRANE

Cationic peptides interact with cells in a manner consistent with their being taken up by self-promoted uptake (Fig. 1). Dansyl polymyxin displacement experiments have indicated that they interact both with purified LPS (Fig. 2) and with LPS in the context of intact cells (Piers et al., 1994; Piers and Hancock, 1994). The affinities of MBI-28 (formerly CEMA), polymyxin B, rabbit defensin 1 (MCP-1), CEME, and gentamicin for *P. aeruginosa* LPS were, respectively, 1,214-, 914-, 800-, 654-, and 71-fold higher than the affinity for Mg^{2+} (see Piers et al. [1994] for the structures of CEME and CEMA). The actual I_{50} values (concentration resulting in 50% displacement of dansyl polymyxin from the LPS) were as low as 0.7 μM, indicating an interaction with an affinity as high as that of most transport systems in *P. aeruginosa.*

Interaction of the cationic peptides with intact *P. aeruginosa* cells resulted in permeabilization of these cells to lysozyme and NPN (Table 2). Lysozyme is a 14,000-Da basic protein which is able to destroy the peptidoglycan and lyse cells. However, it is normally denied access to the periplasmic peptidoglycan by the outer membrane. Thus one can follow outer membrane permeabilization by monitoring enhanced lysis as a function of cationic peptide concentration and derive an EC_{50} as the concentration leading to 50% of maximal lysis by lysozyme. In contrast, NPN is a small (219-Da) hydrophobic probe which fluo-

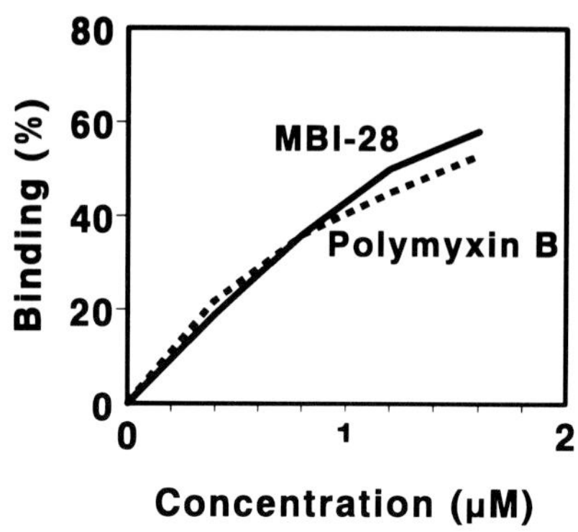

Figure 2. Level of binding of MBI-28 and polymyxin B to *P. aeruginosa* LPS, assessed as the percentage of dansyl polymyxin displaced by the given compound.

Table 2. I_{50} values for permeabilization of intact *P. aeruginosa* cells to lysozyme and NPN

Peptide	EC_{50} (μg/ml)[a]	
	Lysozyme	NPN
MCP-1	ND	15
CEME	0.7	0.7
MBI-28	0.3	0.2
Polymyxin B	1.5	0.2
Melittin	5.5	0.9

[a]EC_{50}, concentration of peptide leading to 50% maximal cell lysis (in the case of lysozyme) or 50% maximum uptake of the fluorophor NPN (as revealed by enhanced fluorescence as the NPN enters the cell membrane interior). Data are excerpted and rearranged from Piers et al. (1994). In the absence of peptide, no lysis was seen and only background fluorescence was observed since neither lysozyme nor NPN is taken up. The experiments were performed in 5 mM sodium HEPES (*N*-2-hydroxyethylpiperazine-*N′*-2-ethanesulfonic acid) buffer (pH 7.5) with 1 mM KCN to permit observation of rapid kinetics. Divalent cations were highly antagonistic. ND, not done.

resces strongly in a hydrophobic environment (e.g., a membrane interior) but weakly in a hydrophilic environment (the extracellular solution). The intact outer membrane of wild-type cells normally excludes NPN and other hydrophobic probes. However, when cells are permeabilized by cationic peptides they take up NPN proportionally with the extent of outer membrane damage. It should be noted that there is an energized efflux system for NPN (Loh et al., 1984), and energy inhibitors must be added to permit NPN to remain in the cell, where the cellular concentration can be assessed by enhanced fluorescence.

It is of interest that there is a substantial difference (eightfold) in the concentration of polymyxin B required to enhance uptake of NPN as opposed to lysozyme, an observation that presumably reflects the relatively small size and/or hydrophobicity of the former. In contrast, CEME and MBI-28 cause enhanced permeability to both at similar concentrations, suggesting that these cationic peptides cause more extreme perturbations of the outer membrane at their minimal effective concentrations than does polymyxin B. Other results indicated that peptides can be designed for enhanced access to self-promoted uptake, since MBI-28, which differs from CEME by the addition of two extra positively charged amino acids at the carboxyl terminus, is a more effective outer membrane permeabilizer.

In contrast to many cationic antibiotics, the cationic peptides are unaffected by polymyxin resistance mutations in *E. coli* (Piers et al., 1994) and *P. aeruginosa* (unpublished data). However, they are more effective against an *S. typhimurium phoP/phoQ* mutant than against its parent strain, a result consistent with data for other cationic peptides including defensins (Piers et al., 1994). Furthermore, their activities were antagonized by addition of 1 mM Mg^{2+} but not by 80 mM Na^{+}, a result consistent with competition for Mg^{2+} binding sites on LPS (Piers et al., 1994; Piers and Hancock, 1994). Thus these data are generally consistent with the utilization of the self-promoted uptake pathway by the cationic peptides.

CONSEQUENCES OF SELF-PROMOTED UPTAKE

One of the immediate consequences of accessing the self-promoted uptake pathway is that cationic peptides bind to LPS (Fig. 3). We have recently demonstrated

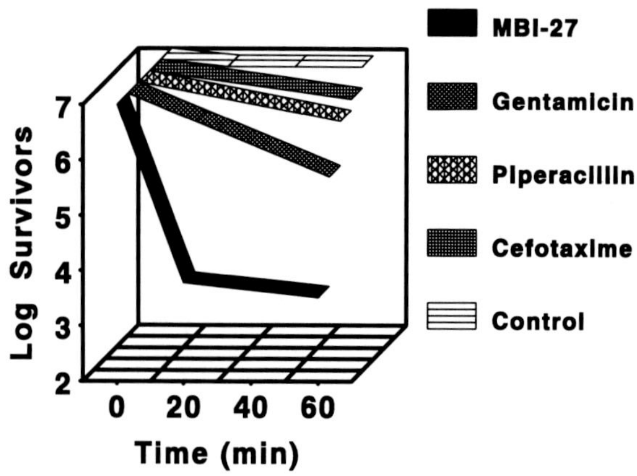

Figure 3. Kinetics of killing of *P. aeruginosa* by the cationic peptide MBI-27 (=CEME) and by other antipseudomonal antibiotics at the MIC. Data are from Piers et al. (1993) and the literature.

that cationic peptides neutralize the ability of LPS (endotoxin) to induce tumor necrosis factor in macrophage cell lines and in intact animals, and they prevent death from endotoxic shock in galactosamine-sensitized mice (N. M. Kelly, M. Gough, and R. E. W. Hancock, unpublished). Thus these peptides actually prevent endotoxic shock, whereas other antibiotics promote LPS release (Goto and Nakamura, 1980) and consequent endotoxemia.

A second consequence is that cationic peptides increase the permeability of the outer membrane (Table 2). Thus, since the outer membrane barrier of *P. aeruginosa* limits uptake of conventional antibiotics, the cationic peptides have the clear potential to work in synergy with these antibiotics. One caveat should be observed when the outer-membrane-permeabilizing and inner-membrane-perturbing concentrations of these molecules are quite similar. Under these circumstance, one would not necessarily expect synergy. However, we have been able to design peptides with lower or no antibiotic activity which are still competent outer membrane permeabilizers and which do show synergy with conventional antibiotics (data not shown).

CONCLUSIONS

There have been no new classes of antibiotics in the past 23 years since the introduction of the quinolones. We believe that the cationic peptides represent a breakthrough in this respect. While there are many barriers to overcome prior to demonstration of clinical efficacy, the good antibiotic activities, apparent lack of resistance problems, potential for synergy with conventional antibiotics, and antiendotoxic activity of cationic peptides, as well as their use as natural antibiotics throughout nature, indicate that they are worthy of consideration. Our ability to make these peptides by recombinant DNA technology makes these the first recombinant antibiotics.

Acknowledgments. Financial assistance from the Canadian Bacterial Diseases Network and, more recently, Micrologix Biotech Inc. is gratefully acknowledged. K.P. was the recipient of a Medical Research Council (MRC) predoctoral studentship; M.B. and T.F. received Canadian Cystic Fibrosis Foundation Fellowships; S.F. was an MRC/Industry Fellow.

REFERENCES

Andreu, D., R. B. Merrifield, H. Steiner, and H. G. Boman. 1985. N-terminal analogues of cecropin A: synthesis, antibacterial activity, and conformational properties. *Biochemistry* **24:**1683–1688.

Angus, B. L., J. Fyfe, and R. E. W. Hancock. 1987. Mapping and characterization of two mutations to antibiotic supersusceptibility in *Pseudomonas aeruginosa. J. Gen. Microbiol.* **133:**2905–2914.

Boman, H. G., I. Faye, G. H. Gudmundsson, J.-Y. Lee, and D.-A. Lidholm. 1991. Cell-free immunity in *Cecropia*. A model system for antibacterial proteins. *Eur. J. Biochem.* **201:**23–31.

Farmer, S., Z. Li, and R. E. W. Hancock. 1992. Influence of outer membrane mutations on susceptibility of *Escherichia coli* to the dibasic macrolide azithromycin. *J. Antimicrob. Chemother.* **29:**27–33.

Goto, H., and S. Nakamura. 1980. Liberation of endotoxin from *Escherichia coli* by antibiotics. *Jpn. J. Exp. Med.* **50:**35–43.

Hancock, R. E. W. 1984. Alterations in outer membrane permeability. *Annu. Rev. Microbiol.* **38:**237–264.

Hancock, R. E. W., and A. Bell. 1989. Antibiotic uptake into Gram-negative bacteria, p. 21–28. *In* G. G. Jackson, H. D. Schlumberger, and H. J. Zeiler (ed.), *Perspectives in Anti-Infective Therapy*. Vieweg und Sohn, Braunschweig, Germany.

Hancock, R. E. W., C. Egli, and N. Karunaratne. 1994. Molecular organization and structural role of outer membrane macromolecules, p. 263–279. *In* J. M. Ghuysen and R. Hakenbeck (ed.), *Bacterial Cell Wall*. Elsevier Science B. V., Amsterdam.

Hancock, R. E. W., T. Falla, and M. H. Brown. 1995. Cationic bacterial peptides. *Adv. Microb. Physiol.*, **37:**135–175.

Hancock, R. E. W., and S. W. Farmer. 1993. Mechanism of uptake of deglucoteichoplanin amide derivatives across outer membranes of *Escherichia coli* and *Pseudomonas aeruginosa. Antimicrob. Agents Chemother.* **37:**453–456.

Hancock, R. E. W., S. Farmer, Z. Li, and K. Poole. 1991. Interaction of aminoglycosides with the outer membranes and purified lipopolysaccharide and OmpF porin of *Escherichia coli. Antimicrob. Agents Chemother.* **35:**1309–1314.

Hancock, R. E. W., V. J. Raffle, and T. I. Nicas. 1981. Involvement of the outer membrane in gentamicin and streptomycin uptake and killing in *Pseudomonas aeruginosa. Antimicrob. Agents Chemother.* **19:**777–785.

Lehrer, R. I., A. K. Lichtenstein, and T. Ganz. 1993. Defensins: antimicrobial and cytotoxic peptides of mammalian cells. *Annu. Rev. Immunol.* **11:**105–128.

Li, X., D. M. Livermore, and H. Nikaido. 1994. Role of efflux pumps in intrinsic resistance of *Pseudomonas aeruginosa*: resistance of tetracycline, chloramphenicol, and norfloxacin. *Antimicrob. Agents Chemother.* **38:**1732–1741.

Loh, B., C. Grant, and R. E. W. Hancock. 1984. Use of the fluorescent probe 1-*N*-phenylnaphthylamine to study the interactions of aminoglycoside antibiotics with the outer membrane of *Pseudomonas aeruginosa. Antimicrob. Agents Chemother.* **26:**546–551.

Piers, K. L., M. B. Brown, and R. E. W. Hancock. 1993. Recombinant DNA procedures for producing small antimicrobial cationic peptides in bacteria. *Gene* **134:**7–13.

Piers, K. L., M. B. Brown, and R. E. W. Hancock. 1994. Improvement of outer membrane-permeabilizing and lipopolysaccharide-binding activities of an antimicrobial cationic peptide by C-terminal modification. *Antimicrob. Agents Chemother.* **38:**2311–2316.

Piers, K. L., and R. E. W. Hancock. 1994. The interaction of recombinant cecropin/melittin hybrid peptide with the outer membrane of *Pseudomonas aeruginosa. Mol. Microbiol.* **12:**951–958.

Rivera, M., R. E. W. Hancock, J. G. Sawyer, A. Haug, and E. J. McGroarty. 1988. Enhanced binding of polycationic antibiotics to lipopolysaccharide from an aminoglycoside-supersusceptible *tolA* mutant strain of *Pseudomonas aeruginosa. Antimicrob. Agents Chemother.* **32:**649–655.

Sawyer, J. G., N. L. Martin, and R. E. W. Hancock. 1988. Interaction of macrophage cationic proteins with the outer membrane of *Pseudomonas aeruginosa. Infect. Immun.* **56:**693–698.

Schroder, G., K. Brandenburg, and U. Seydel. 1992. Polymyxin B induces transient permeability fluctuations in asymmetric planar lipopolysaccharide phospholipid bilayers. *Biochemistry.* **31:**631–638.

Skerlavaj, B., D. Romeo, and R. Gennaro. 1990. Rapid membrane permeabilization and inhibition of vital functions of gram-negative bacteria by bactenecins. *Infect. Immun.* **58:**3724–3730.

Vaara, M., and T. Vaara. 1983. Polycations sensitize enteric bacteria to antibiotics. *Antimicrob. Agents Chemother.* **24:**107–113.

Young, M. L., M. Bains, A. Bell, and R. E. W. Hancock. 1992. Role of *Pseudomonas aeruginosa* outer membrane protein OprH in polymyxin and gentamicin resistance: isolation of an OprH-deficient mutant by gene replacement techniques. *Antimicrob. Agents Chemother.* **36:**2566–2568.

Zasloff, M. 1987. Magainins, a class of antimicrobial peptides from *Xenopus* skin: isolation, characterization of two active forms and partial cDNA sequence of a precursor. *Proc. Natl. Acad. Sci. USA* **84:**5449–5453.

Molecular Biology of Pseudomonads
Edited by T. Nakazawa et al.

Chapter 39

Genes Involved in the Biosynthesis of *Pseudomonas aeruginosa* Lipopolysaccharide

Joseph S. Lam, Teresa R. de Kievit, and Heather L. Currie

Lipopolysaccharide (LPS) molecules of *Pseudomonas aeruginosa* are the predominant antigens found in the outer membrane, anchored to the outer leaflet via lipid A. The core oligosaccharide and the long-chain O-antigen polymer extend outward, and these surface-exposed regions have been visualized by electron microscopy to form a hydrophilic fibrous coat that becomes the first barrier between the bacterium and its environment (Lam et al., 1992). LPS of *P. aeruginosa* is heterogeneous in size, due to variations in the amount of O-side-chain polymer substituted on the core, as well as in the types of constituent O-side-chain sugars. Several studies have provided evidence that most *P. aeruginosa* strains can simultaneously express an A-band form and a B-band form of LPS (Lam et al., 1989; Rivera et al., 1988; Rivera and McGroarty, 1989). Structurally, A-band LPS is a common antigen among *P. aeruginosa* strains, consisting primarily of a short-chained neutral polysaccharide of $\alpha1\rightarrow2,\alpha1\rightarrow3,\alpha\rightarrow3$-linked D-rhamnose (Arsenault et al., 1991). In contrast, B-band is the O-antigen-containing LPS; differences in the chemistry and structure of its O-repeat units distinguish this species into 17 serotypes (Liu et al., 1983). Recently, three additional serotypes were introduced (Liu and Wang, 1990).

As well as being structurally distinct from one another, several lines of evidence suggest that A-band and B-band LPS are separate molecules. These two forms of LPS can be separated from one another using gel filtration chromatography under conditions that employ a very slow flow rate and deoxycholate in the buffers (Rivera et al., 1988; Handelsman, 1990). In addition, two A-band-specific monoclonal antibodies, N1C9 (Lam et al., 1989) and E87 (Yokota et al., 1990), reacted to identical LPS bands in Western immunoblots when LPS was prepared from either a wild-type strain (A^+B^+) or a B-band-deficient strain (A^+B^-) (Lam et al., 1989; McGroarty and Rivera, 1990). That the presence or absence of B-band O antigen has no effect on the relative mobility of A-band LPS in sodium dodecyl sulfate-polyacrylamide gels indicates that the two are in fact distinct molecules.

Joseph S. Lam, Teresa R. de Kievit, and Heather L. Currie • Department of Microbiology, University of Guelph, Guelph, Ontario, N1G 2W1, Canada.

In addition to the lipid A-associated endotoxic activity, B-band O antigen contributes to the virulence of *P. aeruginosa. P. aeruginosa* rough mutants lacking long B-band polymers were more susceptible to phagocytosis (Engels et al., 1985), gave a higher 50% lethal dose (LD_{50}) value in mouse challenge experiments (Cryz et al., 1984), and were serum sensitive (Schiller and Hatch, 1983; Dasgupta et al., 1994). In contrast, A-band LPS did not contribute to serum resistance (Dasgupta et al., 1994). However, either A-band LPS or A-band polysaccharide may contribute to the inflammatory response by virtue of a chemotactic effect on human polymorphonuclear leukocytes. These A-band-containing antigens were as effective as a control chemotactic reagent (f-Met-Leu-Phe) in causing the migration of polymorphonuclear leukocytes (H. L. Currie, A. Kharazmi, and J. S. Lam, unpublished data).

Recent studies have indicated that an antigenic shift occurs in which B-band is replaced by A-band as the predominant LPS antigen on the surface of *P. aeruginosa* isolates from cystic fibrosis (CF) patients. During the course of pulmonary infection, *P. aeruginosa* CF isolates become either polytypeable (agglutinate with more than one serotyping serum due to the shortening of B-band O antigen) or nontypeable (no agglutination with any serotyping sera due to the lack of B-band polymer) and large amounts of a mucoid substance, alginate, are produced (Hancock et al., 1983; Penketh et al., 1983; Pitt et al., 1986). In a longitudinal study performed by our laboratory, examining serial CF isolates from individual patients, a progressive decrease in B-band LPS production was observed while A-band LPS remained unchanged (Lam et al., 1989). The apparent antigenic shift between B-band and A-band LPS, along with the emergence of alginate production, should be further examined to understand how this bacterium reorganizes its cell surface in the chronically infected lungs of CF patients.

While the genetics and metabolic pathways of LPS synthesis in members of the family *Enterobacteriaceae* are relatively well understood, little is known about LPS synthesis in *P. aeruginosa*. To understand the synthesis and regulation of *P. aeruginosa* A-band and B-band LPS, our first objective was to isolate genes involved in these processes. We will discuss results collected to date on the identification, characterization, and map locations of three LPS genes of *P. aeruginosa* PAO1 (serotype O5), namely, *rfbA, rfc,* and *psaA* (formerly called *gca*).

LPS MUTANTS AND ISOLATION OF A-BAND AND B-BAND GENE CLUSTERS

As a first step in isolating LPS genes of *P. aeruginosa*, transposon Tn*5*-751 mutagenesis of strain PAO1 was performed to generate a B-band-minus mutant called ge6. Similarly, by chemical mutagenesis of strain AK1401 using ethyl methanesulfate, an A-band-minus mutant, rd7513, was isolated. The relevant properties of these and other serotype O5-derived LPS mutants discussed in this chapter are listed in Table 1.

Following isolation of these mutants, a PAO1 genomic library was generated in cosmid vector pCP13. This library was mated independently into both rd7513 (A^- mutant) and ge6 (B^- mutant), and transconjugants were screened for complementation using monoclonal antibodies N1C9 (specific for A-band) and MF15-4 (specific for B-band), respectively. A cosmid clone was isolated that was able to restore A-band synthesis in mutant rd7513. This recombinant cosmid was designated pFV3 and was shown to contain a 27-

Table 1. *P. aeruginosa* serotype O5-derived LPS mutants

Strain	Phenotype and relevant properties	Reference and/or source
PAO1	Wild-type serotype O5, A^+B^+	Hancock and Carey, 1979
AK44	Rough, A^+B^-, complete core	Kropinski et al., 1979
ge6	Rough, A^+B^-, complete core	Lightfoot and Lam, 1993
AK14O1	Semirough (SR), A^+, B-band contains core-plus-one O-repeat unit	Berry and Kropinski, 1986; Lam et al., 1989
rd7513	SR, A^-, derived from AK14O1, B-band contains core-plus-one O-repeat unit	Lightfoot and Lam, 1991
OP5.2	SR, chromosomal *rfc* knockout mutant, A^+, B-band contains core-plus-one O-repeat unit	de Kievit et al., 1995
OP5.3	SR, chromosomal *rfc* knockout mutant, A^+, B-band contains core-plus-one O-repeat unit	de Kievit et al., 1995
OP5.5	SR, chromosomal *rfc* knockout mutant, A^+, B-band contains core-plus-one O-repeat unit	de Kievit et al., 1995
JL-*rfbA*-M1[a]	Rough, chromosomal *rfbA* knockout mutant	Dasgupta and Lam, 1995
JL-*rfbA*-M2	Rough, chromosomal *rfbA* knockout mutant	Dasgupta and Lam, 1995

[a] JL-*rfbA*-M1 and JL-*rfbA*-M2 were formerly referred to as M1 and M2, respectively (Dasgupta and Lam, 1995).

kb insert (Lightfoot and Lam, 1991). B-band synthesis was complemented in mutant ge6 by a cosmid clone called pFV100 containing a 26-kb insert (Lightfoot and Lam, 1993). Restriction enzyme site analysis of both pFV3 and pFV100 was performed, and the restriction maps of these two cosmid clones are shown in Fig. 1.

rfbA

To identify individual genes involved in O-antigen biosynthesis, several subclones of pFV100 were generated. These subclones were mobilized into various O5 rough mutants which were then analyzed for B-band synthesis. Complementation studies using the B-band-minus mutant AK44 allowed the isolation of a relatively small construct that was able to restore O-antigen synthesis. This subclone contained a 1.4-kb *Xba-Hin*dIII insert and was designated pFV110 (Dasgupta and Lam, 1995) (Fig. 1). The nucleotide sequence of the pFV110 insert was determined, and one open reading frame was identified that could code for a polypeptide of 303 amino acids with a predicted size of 33 kDa (Dasgupta and Lam, 1995). Because this is the first report of a gene that is involved in *P. aeruginosa* O-antigen biosynthesis, it was designated *rfbA*. In gene expression experiments using *Escherichia coli* maxicells, a protein band with an apparent molecular mass of 32.5 kDa was observed. This observed size coincided well with that calculated from the nucleotide sequence (33 kDa) (Dasgupta and Lam, 1995).

To confirm the involvement of *rfbA* in O-antigen synthesis, gene replacement experiments were performed. The pFV110 insert, containing *rfbA*, was cloned into suicide vector pEX100T (Schweizer and Hoang, 1995). An 875-bp Gm^r cassette was then inserted within the coding region, generating a mutation in *rfbA*. The resulting plasmid was subsequently allowed to undergo homologous recombination with the PAO1 chromosome. By using a sucrose-sensitivity selection system, it was possible to isolate transconjugants that had exchanged the wild-type gene for the mutant allele. This selec-

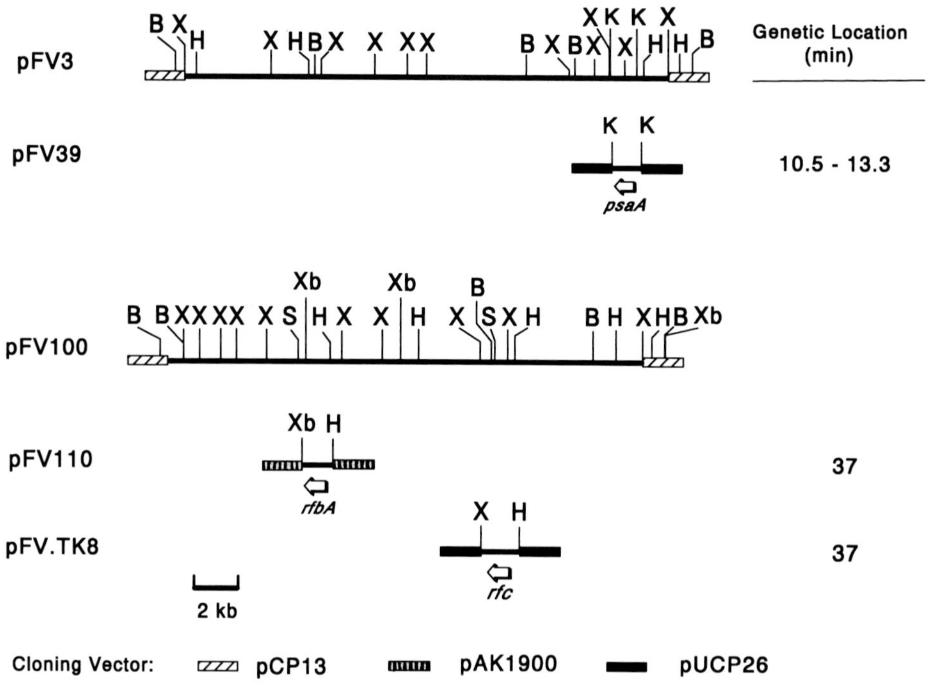

Figure 1. Restriction maps and chromosomal locations of cosmid clones pFV3 (*psa* gene cluster) and pFV100 (*rfb* gene cluster). pFV39 contains the *psaA* gene and complements A-band synthesis in the mutant rd7513. Subclones pFV110 (*rfbA*) and pFV.TK8 (*rfc*) complement B-band synthesis in mutants AK44 and AK1401, respectively. Arrows indicate the open reading frames and the direction of transcription of *psaA*, *rfbA*, and *rfc*. Restriction enzymes: B, *Bam*HI; H, *Hin*dIII; K, *Kpn*I; S, *Spe*I; Xb, *Xba*I; X, *Xho*I.

tion is based on the fact that the gene replacement vector pEX100T contains a copy of the *sacB* gene which renders gram-negative organisms sensitive to sucrose. By plating transconjugants on media containing sucrose it is possible to separate true recombinants from merodiploids. True recombinants were easily identified as sucrose-resistant colonies, since they had lost the vector-associated *sacB* gene, whereas merodiploids contain a copy of *sacB* and cannot grow on a sucrose-containing medium. Sucrose-resistant PAO1 *rfbA* mutants, JL-*rfbA*-M1 and JL-*rfbA*-M2, were isolated that exhibited the same rough phenotype as AK44, indicating that *rfbA* is essential for O-antigen production.

Homology searches of the nucleic acid and amino acid sequences of *rfbA* revealed that the gene product, RfbA, is highly homologous to TrsF of *Yersinia enterocolitica* serotype O:3 (Skurnik et al., 1995). The TrsF protein is apparently involved in the synthesis of D-fucosamine, which is a residue in the *Y. enterocolitica* LPS outer core region (GenBank accession no. Z47767; Skurnik et al., 1995). Therefore, it is likely that TrsF and RfbA have a similar function in the synthesis of the outer core region and the O-repeat units of *Y. enterocolitica* and *P. aeruginosa*, respectively. Further work is under way to determine the exact function of RfbA and to see whether RfbA and TrsF are functionally interchangeable.

rfc

The *rfc* gene is frequently found within the *rfb* clusters of gram-negative organisms. *rfc* is believed to code for an O-polymerase enzyme which polymerizes individual O-repeat units in long-chain O antigen. Mutants containing a defective copy of this gene produce LPS with a complete core substituted by one O-repeat unit, but lack long O-antigen polymers. Such mutants are described as having a semirough (SR) phenotype. When pFV100 was mobilized into *P. aeruginosa* SR mutant AK14O1, long-chain O-antigen synthesis was restored. These results suggested that an *rfc* gene was located within the O5 *rfb* cluster (de Kievit et al., 1995). Subcloning and Tn*1000* mutagenesis experiments localized the putative *rfc* gene to a 1.9-kb *Xho*I-*Hin*dIII fragment of pFV100. This fragment was cloned, and the resulting plasmid was designated pFV.TK8 (Fig. 1). To confirm that pFV.TK8 codes for an O-polymerase enzyme, gene replacement experiments were performed. PAO1 *rfc* mutants were generated using the gene replacement strategy described above for *rfbA*. Several knockout mutants, OP5.2, OP5.3, and OP5.5, were isolated that expressed that typical SR phenotype, indicating that they were no longer producing a functional O-polymerase enzyme (de Kievit et al., 1995).

Sequence analysis of the 1.9-kb fragment, containing the *rfc* coding region, revealed one open reading frame that could code for a protein of 438 amino acids with a predicted mass of 48.9 kDa. Although there are a number of enterobacterial *rfc* genes reported in the literature, a homology search of the *P. aeruginosa rfc* nucleotide and amino acid sequences did not yield any significant homology. Structural data have shown that the sugar composition of the PAO1 O antigen differs significantly from that of enterobacterial O antigens (Knirel, 1990). Therefore, considering the unique specificity of an enzyme for its substrate, in this case the O-repeat unit, it is not surprising that the *P. aeruginosa rfc* showed little homology with enterobacterial *rfc* genes. The *P. aeruginosa rfc* gene product does, however, have several features in common with other Rfc proteins. For example, hydropathy analysis suggests that the *P. aeruginosa* Rfc contains 11 putative membrane-spanning domains, while those of enteric organisms have been reported to have between 11 and 13 membrane-spanning domains (Morona et al., 1994). In addition, the *P. aeruginosa* Rfc protein has an amino acid composition and codon usage similar to those reported for other Rfc proteins. Last, the *rfc* coding region has a lower moles percent G+C (44.8 mol%) than the *P. aeruginosa* chromosomal average (67.2 mol%) (Palleroni, 1984). A low G+C content is common among other *rfc* genes (Collins and Hackett, 1991; Brown et al., 1992; Klena and Schnaitman, 1993; Morona et al., 1994) and has also been observed in the *rfb* clusters so far analyzed. Consistent with this latter point, the G+C content of *rfbA* was found to be 54.4 mol% (Dasgupta and Lam, 1995), which is significantly lower than the chromosomal average of *P. aeruginosa.*

To determine whether a similar *rfc* gene was present in each of the 20 O serotypes, Southern DNA-DNA hybridization analysis was performed using an O5 *rfc*-specific probe. The probe hybridized to a common 1.5-kb *Xho*I fragment of serotypes O2, O5, O16, O18, and O20, suggesting that they contain a similar O-polymerase gene (de Kievit et al., 1995). In these same five *P. aeruginosa* serotypes, an O5 *rfbA*-specific probe was found to hybridize to a common 4.6-kb *Xho*I fragment (Dasgupta and Lam, 1995). These hybridization results were expected since serotypes O2, O5, O16, and O20 share a similar O-repeat backbone structure (Knirel, 1990). Although the O-antigen structure of serotype O18 has not yet been determined, O18 exhibits cross-reactivity with polyclonal antisera raised against serotype O5, suggesting that its O-repeat unit is structurally similar to that of O5.

psaA

A second cosmid clone, pFV3, was isolated from the PAO1 library because of its ability to complement A-band LPS synthesis in the A-band-minus mutant rd7513. Various subclones were constructed, and Tn*1000* mutagenesis was performed to identify the region responsible for the restoration of A-band LPS production in rd7513. The smallest subclone capable of restoring A-band LPS synthesis in rd7513 contained a 1.6-kb *Kpn*I fragment. This recombinant plasmid was designated pFV39 (Lightfoot and Lam, 1993). Maxicell and sequence analyses were performed to identify the gene product encoded by pFV39. In addition, a functional assay determined the role played by this protein in A-band LPS synthesis. Maxicell analysis in *E. coli* CSR603 demonstrated the production of a 37-kDa protein from pFV39 (Lightfoot and Lam, 1993). Yokota et al. (1990) showed that *P. aeruginosa* strains which expressed a D-rhamnan polysaccharide similar to A-band LPS contained enzymes responsible for the conversion of GDP–D-mannose to GDP–D-rhamnose. To determine if this 37-kDa protein displayed similar activity, supernatants of whole-cell lysates from rd7513 and rd7513(pFV39) were incubated with ^{14}C-labeled GDP–D-mannose. Supernatant from rd7513(pFV39) synthesized ^{14}C-labeled GDP-rhamnose from ^{14}C-labeled GDP–D-mannose, whereas supernatant from rd7513 did not (Lightfoot and Lam, 1993). Thus the protein was designated as Gca (GDP–D-mannose conversion protein for A-band polysaccharide) (Lightfoot, 1993; Currie et al., 1995). However, we have recent evidence suggesting that the *gca* gene is part of an operon, and we therefore propose to change the name of this gene to *psaA* (*P. aeruginosa* A-band LPS) in anticipation of naming other genes that are also involved in the synthesis of A-band LPS.

Nucleotide sequence analysis revealed that the 1.6-kb insert of pFV39 contained an open reading frame coding for the 36.5-kDa PsaA protein (Currie et al., 1995). The PsaA protein was homologous to YefA of *E. coli* and RfbD of *Vibrio cholerae* (Currie et al., 1995). YefA is postulated to be a GDP–D-mannose dehydratase involved in fucose biosynthesis, and RfbD is thought to be a dehydratase, oxidoreductase, or epimerase functioning in the production of the O-antigen sugar perosamine from GDP–D-mannose (Manning et al., 1994). The enzymatic steps required for the conversion of GDP–D-mannose to GDP–D-rhamnose involve a GDP–D-mannose dehydrase (equivalent to a dehydratase) and a GDP-4-keto-D-rhamnose reductase (Markovitz, 1964). Therefore, on the basis of sequence homology between PsaA and the two proteins YefA and RfbD, and considering the steps required to convert GDP–D-mannose to GDP–D-rhamnose, we propose that the PsaA protein functions either as a dehydratase or as a bifunctional enzyme facilitating the conversion of GDP–D-mannose to GDP–D-rhamnose (Currie et al., 1995).

To determine if the *psaA* gene was conserved in all 20 *P. aeruginosa* O serotypes, Southern hybridizations were performed using the *psaA* gene as a DNA probe. *psaA* was conserved on a 1.6-kb *Kpn*I fragment in each of the 20 O serotypes, with the exception of serotype O12 which hybridized to a 7.0-kb fragment (Currie et al., 1995). Other pseudomonads were also examined to ascertain the presence of this gene among different species (Table 2). Four of the six pseudomonads screened showed the same 1.6-kb *Kpn*I probe-reactive fragment observed for *P. aeruginosa* (Currie et al., 1995). Of the four pseudomonads which were found to contain *psaA*, only *Pseudomonas acidovorans* and *Pseudomonas putida* showed reactivity with the A-band-specific monoclonal antibody N1F10 in Western immunoblots (Currie et al., 1995). These two organisms may express either A-band common antigen or a different LPS molecule with similar antigenic epitopes (Currie et al., 1995). *Pseudomonas cepacia* (recently reclassified as *Burkholderia cepacia*) and *Pseudomonas syringae* were also shown to contain the *psaA* gene. However, both failed to react with the A-band-specific antibody (Currie et al., 1995). These strains displayed a rough LPS phenotype on sodium dodecyl sulfate-polyacrylamide gels, which likely accounts for their lack of reactivity on Western immunoblots. Therefore it remains unclear whether A-band LPS is in fact expressed in other isolates of *B. cepacia* and *P. syringae*.

Once the presence and conservation of the *psaA* gene had been established, it was of interest to determine if a region of this gene could be amplified from the 20 *P. aeruginosa* O serotypes by PCR. Primers were designed from the *psaA* gene sequence, and PCR amplification of a 700-bp product was detected from each of the serotypes (Currie et al., 1995). Due to the cross-reactivity of the *psaA* gene probe with other *Pseudomonas* species, PCR amplification of genomic DNA from these species may generate a similar product. In the CF lung, the only *psaA*-cross-reactive species of clinical significance is *B. cepacia*. Since rapid clinical identification of both *P. aeruginosa* and *B. cepacia* is essential, PCR amplification using a combination of primers specific for conserved genes such as *psaA* may prove to be useful in the identification of these organisms from clinical isolates. Primers specific for either *P. aeruginosa* or *B. cepacia* could then be employed to differentiate between these two organisms.

CHROMOSOMAL MAPPING

To map the A-band and B-band LPS genes of *P. aeruginosa*, chromosomal DNA from strain PAO1 was digested with restriction enzymes *Spe*I and *Dpn*I and separated using

Table 2. Reactivity of non-*aeruginosa* pseudomonads with the *psaA* gene probe and monoclonal antibody N1F10[a]

Strain	Size (kb) of Southern probe-reactive fragments	Western reactivity with N1F10	Source[b]
Pseudomonas acidovorans	1.6	+	T. Warren
Pseudomonas cepacia 92-449	1.6	–	W. Johnson
Pseudomonas fluorescens PF5	NR[c]	–	D. Cuppel
Pseudomonas putida PUG-1	1.6	+	D. Cuppel
Pseudomonas stutzeri H364 (ATCC 17588)	NR	–	R. E. W. Hancock
Pseudomonas syringae H365 (ATCC 19310)	1.6	–	R. E. W. Hancock

[a]Southern hybridizations performed by *Kpn*I digest; Western immunoblots performed with the A-band LPS-specific monoclonal antibody N1F10.
[b]T. Warren and R. E. W. Hancock, University of British Columbia, Vancouver, British Columbia, Canada; W. Johnson, Laboratory Centre for Disease Control, Ottawa, Ontario, Canada; D. Cuppel, Agriculture Canada, London, Ontario, Canada.
[c]NR, no reaction with the *psaA* gene probe.

pulsed-field gel electrophoresis. Southern hybridizations were then carried out. The A-band LPS genes on pFV3 mapped between positions 5.75 and 5.89 Mbp on the 5.9-Mbp chromosome, corresponding to between 10.5 and 13.3 min on the 75-min linkage map (Lightfoot and Lam, 1993). The insert in pFV100, which contains the B-band LPS genes, mapped at 1.9 Mbp (or 37 min) (Lightfoot and Lam, 1991, 1993). The map position of the B-band genes was confirmed by Southern analysis using *rfbA* as a probe. This smaller B-band-specific probe bound to the same *Dpn*I fragment, but only hybridized to a single *Spe*I band, differing from the larger pFV100 probe which reacted with three *Spe*I fragments (T. Dasgupta and J. A. Lam, unpublished). These results confirm the chromosomal map position of the *rfb* cluster at 37 min.

The chromosomal mapping results provide evidence that *rfbA* and *rfc* are located within the O5 *rfb* cluster, which is 22 min downstream of the *psaA* gene. Other researchers have also provided information that suggests that the chromosomal regions, aside from the ones we have localized, may contain genes which play a role in *P. aeruginosa* LPS synthesis. In an earlier study by Matsumoto and Tazaki (1975), conjugation and transduction were used to identify a chromosomal locus called *som* (for somatic antigen) in several Habs serotypes (the Habs typing scheme contains 16 of the 17 serotypes that were adopted as the International Antigenic Typing Scheme for *P. aeruginosa*) (Liu et al., 1983). This *som* gene was capable of conferring O-specificity of a donor strain to a recipient strain. The same genetic determinant was also found in *P. aeruginosa* PAO1 as two markers, *somA* and *somB*, both of which mapped at 40 min on the PAO1 chromosome (Holloway and Matsumoto, 1984; Holloway et al., 1994). It is possible that *somA* and *somB* fall within the O5 *rfb* cluster. However, since their map position was determined using different methods from those used to map the *rfb* genes, their exact location remains unclear. More recently, Goldberg and coworkers (1993) have reported that the *algC* gene, which maps at 12 min (Shortridge et al., 1991), was able to restore smooth LPS synthesis in the *P. aeruginosa* mutant AK1012. *algC* has been shown to encode a bifunctional enzyme with both phosphomannomutase and phosphoglucomutase activities (Coyne et al., 1994; Ye et al., 1994). Previously, it had been shown that phosphomannomutase is involved in the synthesis of mannuronic acid residues, which are the components of the exopolysaccharide alginate (Zielinski et al., 1991). Strain AK1012 is a core-deficient mutant which is devoid of L-rhamnose and D-glucose in its outer core region (Dasgupta et al., 1994; de Kievit and Lam, 1994). The presence of complete core is an essential prerequisite for the attachment of the O-antigen polymer. Therefore, *algC* likely restores a mutation in a gene required for outer core biosythesis in AK1012.

In addition to the O5 *rfb* cluster, O-antigen biosynthetic genes from *P. aeruginosa* serotype O11 have been isolated (Goldberg et al., 1992). In this study a cosmid clone containing serotype O11 *rfb* genes was mobilized into an *E. coli* strain and the recombinant *E. coli* cells were found to express *P. aeruginosa* O antigen on their surface. However, individual genes involved in serotype O11 O-antigen biosynthesis were not identified.

CONCLUDING REMARKS

In conclusion, three LPS genes of *P. aeruginosa* PAO1 have been identified and characterized in our laboratory. Mapping of these LPS genes has revealed that they are organized into two separate clusters, *rfb* (B-band LPS synthesis) and *psa* (A-band LPS synthesis), which are located in different regions of the chromosome. Several other genes have been identified in both *rfb* and *psa* gene clusters, and studies are under way to characterize the precise role these genes play in *P. aeruginosa* LPS biosynthesis.

Acknowledgments. This work is supported by grants from the Canadian Bacterial Diseases Network, the Medical Research Council of Canada (MT-12881), and the Canadian Cystic Fibrosis Foundation (CCFF). T.R.de K. and H.L.C. are recipients of studentships from the CCFF.

REFERENCES

Arsenault, T. L., D. W. Hughes, D. B. MacLean, W. A. Szarek, A. M. B. Kropinski, and J. S. Lam. 1991. Structural studies on the polysaccharide portion of "A-band" lipopolysaccharide from a mutant (AK14O1) of *Pseudomonas aeruginosa* strain PAO1. *Can. J. Chem.* **69:**1273–1280.

Berry, D., and A. M. Kropinski. 1986. Effects of lipopolysaccharide mutations and temperature on plasmid transformation efficiency in *Pseudomonas aeruginosa*. *Can. J. Microbiol.* **32:**436–438.

Brown, P. K., L. K. Romana, and P. R. Reeves. 1992. Molecular analysis of the *rfb* gene cluster of *Salmonella* serovar *muenchen* (strain M67), the genetic basis of the polymorphism between groups C2 and B. *Mol. Microbiol.* **6:**1385–1394.

Collins, L. V., and J. Hackett. 1991. Molecular cloning, characterization, and nucleotide sequence of the *rfc* gene, which encodes an O-antigen polymerase of *Salmonella typhimurium*. *J. Bacteriol.* **173:**2521–2529.

Coyne, M. J., Jr., K. S. Russell, C. L. Coyle, and J. B. Goldberg. 1994. The *Pseudomonas aeruginosa algC* gene encodes phosphoglucomutase, required for the synthesis of a complete lipopolysaccharide core. *J. Bacteriol.* **176:**3500–3507.

Cryz, S. J., Jr., T. L. Pitt, E. Fürer, and R. Germanier. 1984. Role of lipopolysaccharide in virulence of *Pseudomonas aeruginosa*. *Infect. Immun.* **44:**508–513.

Currie, H. L., J. Lightfoot, and J. S. Lam. 1995. Prevalence of *gca*, a gene involved in synthesis of A-band common antigen polysaccharide in *Pseudomonas aeruginosa*. *Clin. Diagn. Lab. Immunol.* **2:**554–562.

Dasgupta, T., T. R. de Kievit, H. Masoud, E. Altman, J. C. Richards, I. Sadovskaya, D. P. Speert, and J. S. Lam. 1994. Characterization of lipopolysaccharide-deficient mutants of *Pseudomonas aeruginosa* derived from serotypes O3, O5, and O6. *Infect. Immun.* **62:**809–817.

Dasgupta, T, and J. S. Lam. 1995. Identification of *rfbA*, involved in B-band lipopolysaccharide biosynthesis in *Pseudomonas aeruginosa* serotype O5. *Infect. Immun.* **63:**1674–1680.

de Kievit, T. R., T. Dasgupta, H. Schweizer, and J. S. Lam. 1995. Molecular cloning and characterization of the *rfc* gene of *Pseudomonas aeruginosa* (serotype O5). *Mol. Microbiol.* **16:**565–574.

de Kievit, T. R., and J. S. Lam. 1994. Monoclonal antibodies that distinguish inner core, outer core, and lipid A regions of *Pseudomonas aeruginosa* lipopolysaccharide. *J. Bacteriol.* **176:**7129–7139.

Engels, W., J. Endert, M. A. F. Kamps, and C. P. A. vanBoven. 1985. Role of lipopolysaccharides in opsonization and phagocytosis of *Pseudomonas aeruginosa*. *Infect. Immun.* **49:**182–189.

Goldberg, J. B., K. Hatano, G. S. Meluleni, and G. B. Pier. 1992. Cloning and surface expression of *Pseudomonas aeruginosa* O-antigen in *Escherichia coli*. *Proc. Natl. Acad. Sci. USA* **89:**10716–10720.

Goldberg, J. B., K. Hatano, and G. B. Pier. 1993. Synthesis of lipopolysaccharide O-side chains by *Pseudomonas aeruginosa* PAO1 requires the enzyme phosphomannomutase. *J. Bacteriol.* **175:**1605–1611.

Hancock, R. E. W., and A. M. Carey. 1979. Outer membrane of *Pseudomonas aeruginosa:* heat- and 2-mercaptoethanol-modifiable proteins. *J. Bacteriol.* **140:**902–910.

Hancock, R. E. W., L. M. Mutharia, L. Chan, R. P. Darveau, D. P. Speert, and G. B. Pier. 1983. *Pseudomonas aeruginosa* isolates from patients with cystic fibrosis: a class of serum-sensitive, nontypeable strains deficient in lipopolysaccharide O-side chains. *Infect. Immun.* **42:**170–177.

Handelsman, M. Y. L. 1990. An ultrastructural and immunochemical study of the lipopolysaccharide of *Pseudomonas aeruginosa*. Ph. D. thesis. University of Guelph, Guelph, Ontario, Canada.

Holloway, B. W., and H. Matsumoto. 1984. *Pseudomonas aeruginosa*, p. 1194–1198. *In* S. J. O'Brien (ed.), *Genetic Maps 1984: Compilation of Linkage and Restriction Maps of Genetically Studied Organisms*. Cold Spring Harbor Laboratory Press, Cold Spring Harbor, N.Y.

Holloway, B. W., U. Römling, and B. Tümmler. 1994. Genomic mapping of *Pseudomonas aeruginosa* PAO. *Microbiology* **140:**2907–2929.

Klena, J. D., and C. A. Schnaitman. 1993. Function of the *rfb* gene cluster and the *rfe* gene in the synthesis of O-antigen by *Shigella dysenteriae* 1. *Mol. Microbiol.* **9:**393–402.

Knirel, Y. A. 1990. Polysaccharide antigens of *Pseudomonas aeruginosa. Crit. Rev. Microbiol.* **17:**273–304.

Kropinski, A. M., L. C. Chan, and F. H. Milazzo. 1979. The extraction and analysis of lipopolysaccharide from *Pseudomonas aeruginosa* strain PAO and three rough mutants. *Can. J. Microbiol.* **25:**390–398.

Lam, J. S., L. L. Graham, J. Lightfoot, T. Dasgupta, and T. J. Beveridge. 1992. Ultrastructural examination of the lipopolysaccharide of *Pseudomonas aeruginosa* strains and their isogenic rough mutants by freeze substitution. *J. Bacteriol.* **174:**7159–7167.

Lam, M. Y., E. J. McGroarty, A. M. Kropinski, L. A. Macdonald, S. S. Pedersen, N. Høiby, and J. S. Lam. 1989. Occurrence of a common lipopolysaccharide antigen in standard and clinical strains of *Pseudomonas aeruginosa. J. Clin. Microbiol.* **27:**962–967.

Lightfoot, J. 1993. Molecular cloning of genes involved with expression of lipopolysaccharides in *Pseudomonas aeruginosa*. Ph. D. thesis. University of Guelph, Guelph, Ontario, Canada.

Lightfoot, J., and J. S. Lam. 1991. Molecular cloning of genes involved with expression of A-band lipopolysaccharide, an antigenically conserved form, in *Pseudomonas aeruginosa. J. Bacteriol.* **173:**5624–5630.

Lightfoot, J., and J. S. Lam. 1993. Chromosomal mapping, expression and synthesis of lipopolysaccharide in *Pseudomonas aeruginosa*—a role for guanosine diphospho (GDP)-D-mannose. *Mol. Microbiol.* **8:**771–782.

Liu, P. V., H. Matsumoto, H. Dusama, and T. Bergan. 1983. Survey of heat-stable major somatic antigens of *Pseudomonas aeruginosa. Int. J. Syst. Bacteriol.* **33:**256–264.

Liu, P. V., and S. P. Wang. 1990. Three new major somatic antigens of *Pseudomonas aeruginosa. J. Clin. Microbiol.* **28:**922–925.

Manning, P. A., U. H. Stroeher, and R. Morona. 1994. Molecular basis for O-antigen biosynthesis in *Vibrio cholerae* O1: Ogawa-Inaba switching, p. 77–94. *In* I. K. Wachsmuth, P. A. Blake, and O. Olsvik (ed.), *Vibrio cholerae and Cholera: Molecular to Global Prespectives*. American Society for Microbiology, Washington, D.C.

Markovitz, A. 1964. Biosynthesis of guanosine diphosphate D-rhamnose and guanosine diphosphate D-talomethylose from guanosine diphosphate α-D-mannose. *J. Biol. Chem.* **239:**2091–2098.

Matsumoto, H., and T. Tazaki. 1975. Serotypic recombination in *Pseudomonas aeruginosa*, p. 281–290. *In* S. Mitsuhashi and H. Hashimoto (ed.), *Microbial Drug Resistance*. University of Tokyo Press, Tokyo.

McGroarty, E. J., and M. Rivera. 1990. Growth-dependent alterations in production of serotype-specific and common antigen lipopolysaccharides in *Pseudomonas aeruginosa* PAO1. *Infect. Immun.* **58:**1030–1037.

Morona, R., M. Mavris, A. Fallarino, and P. A. Manning. 1994. Characterization of the *rfc* region of *Shigella flexneri. J. Bacteriol.* **176:**733–747.

Palleroni, N. J. 1984. Genus I. Pseudomonas, p. 141–199. *In* N. R. Krieg and J. C. Holt (ed.), *Bergey's Manual of Systematic Bacteriology*, vol. 1. The Williams and Wilkins Co., Baltimore.

Penketh, A., T. Pitt, D. Roberts, M. E. Hodson, and J. C. Batten. 1983. The relationship of phenotype changes in *Pseudomonas aeruginosa* to the clinical condition of patients with cystic fibrosis. *Am. Rev. Respir. Dis.* **127:**605–608.

Pitt, T. L., J. MacDougall, A. R. L. Penketh, and E. M. Cooke. 1986. Polyagglutinating and non-typable strains of *Pseudomonas aeruginosa* in cystic fibrosis. *J. Med. Microbiol.* **21:**179–186.

Rivera, M., L. E. Bryan, R. E. W. Hancock, and E. J. McGroarty. 1988. Heterogeneity of lipopolysaccharide from *Pseudomonas aeruginosa*: analysis of lipopolysaccharide chain length. *J. Bacteriol.* **170:**512–521.

Rivera, M., and E. J. McGroarty. 1989. Analysis of a common-antigen lipopolysaccharide from *Pseudomonas aeruginosa. J. Bacteriol.* **171:**2244–2248.

Schiller, N. L., and R. A. Hatch. 1983. The serum sensitivity, colonial morphology, serogroup specificity, and outer membrane protein of *Pseudomonas aeruginosa* isolated from several clinical sites. *Diagn. Microbiol. Infect. Dis.* **1:**145–157.

Schweizer, H. P., and T. T. Hoang. 1995. An improved system for gene replacement and *xylE* fusion analysis in *Pseudomonas aeruginosa. Gene* **158:**15–22.

Shortridge, V. D., M. L. Pato, A. I. Vasil, and M. L. Vasil. 1991. Physical mapping of virulence-associated genes in *Pseudomonas aeruginosa* by transverse alternating-field electrophoresis. *Infect. Immun.* **59:**3596–3603.

Skurnik, M., R. Venho, P. Toivanen, and A. Al-Hendy. 1995. A novel locus of *Yersinia enterocolitica* serotype O:3 involved in lipopolysaccharide outer core biosynthesis. *Mol. Microbiol.* **17:**575–594.

Ye, R. W., N. A. Zielinski, and A. M. Chakrabarty. 1994. Purification and characterization of phosphomannomutase/phosphoglucomutase from *Pseudomonas aeruginosa* involved in biosynthesis of both alginate and lipopolysaccharide. *J. Bacteriol.* **176:**4851–4857.

Yokota, S., S. Kaya, Y. Araki, E. Ito, T. Kawamura, and S. Sawada. 1990. Occurrence of D-rhamnan as the common antigen reactive against monoclonal antibody-E87 in *Pseudomonas aeruginosa* IFO–3080 and other strains. *J. Bacteriol.* **172:**6162–6164.

Zielinski, N. A., A. M. Chakrabarty, and A. Berry. 1991. Characterization and regulation of the *Pseudomonas aeruginosa* gene *algC* encoding phosphomannomutase. *J. Biol. Chem.* **266:**9754–9763.

Molecular Biology of Pseudomonads
Edited by T. Nakazawa et al.

Chapter 40

Pathogenesis of *Burkholderia cepacia* and Export of Protease by the General Secretory Pathway Involving Disulfide Bond Formation in the Periplasm

Teruko Nakazawa and Mitsuko Abe

Burkholderia cepacia (formerly *Pseudomonas cepacia*) (Yabuuchi et al., 1992) has been recognized as an agent for biodegradation of environmental pollutants (Folsom and Chapman, 1991) and for biological control of plant diseases (Burkhead et al., 1994). On the other hand, because of its ubiquitous occurrence and resistance to disinfectants and antibiotics, this microorganism is an opportunistic pathogen of humans. *B. cepacia* colonization of the lungs of patients with cystic fibrosis can lead to severe pneumonia and death (Tablan et al., 1987). In Japan, *B. cepacia* infection is mostly nosocomial and found among immunocompromised patients with no cystic fibrosis background.

MOLECULAR ANALYSIS OF STRAINS OF *B. CEPACIA* ASSOCIATED WITH NOSOCOMIAL INFECTIONS

We have analyzed strains of *B. cepacia* associated with two cases of nosocomial outbreaks in Japan.

Case 1 (Ouchi et al., 1995)

An outbreak of *B. cepacia* infection in a hospital began in 1977 and peaked in 1984. We obtained 100 isolates from various sources such as sputum, pus, blood, urine, and cerebrospinal fluid from inpatients at several wards from March 1983 to February 1984. These isolates were classified into 12 groups by a biochemical typing scheme on the basis of the production of nitrate reductase, β-glucosidase, β-galactosidase, protease, lipase, phospholipase C, and hemolysin. Thirty-three strains from the 12 groups were

Teruko Nakazawa and Mitsuko Abe • Department of Microbiology, Yamaguchi University School of Medicine, Ube, Yamaguchi 755, Japan.

further characterized by DNA fingerprinting by pulsed-field gel electrophoresis, ribotyping, and plasmid profile analysis. Although the results of biochemical typing and the plasmid profiles of the isolates were variable, genomic typing identified the majority of the isolates (32 of 33) as derivatives of a single strain. During the period of the outbreak, chlorhexidine was commonly used in the hospital as a disinfectant. After extensive survey, a solution of chlorhexidine supplied in the hospital was found to be contaminated with chlorhexidine-resistant *B. cepacia*. After this, the disinfectant was autoclaved before distribution to each ward, resulting in a dramatic decrease in the isolation rate of *B. cepacia*. However, a follow-up study after a decade suggests that the derivatives of the previous strain persisted (Ouchi et al., 1995). These results indicate that the outbreak of *B. cepacia* infection was presumably associated with contamination of the chlorhexidine solution by a single strain that produced a variety of derivatives after distribution.

Case 2 (Takigawa et al., 1993)

During the early 1990s, patients admitted to a single hospital ward with hematological malignancies or solid tumors developed respiratory colonization with *B. cepacia*. Among 36 patients colonized, 16 patients developed pneumonia (Yamagishi et al., 1993b). Extensive survey of the hospital environment and equipment revealed *B. cepacia* in nebulizer devices used in the ward, which had been routinely soaked in sodium hypochlorite solution for disinfection. Strains isolated from the pneumonia patients and the nebulizer devices were indistinguishable in regard to biochemical characteristics and DNA fingerprinting by pulsed-field gel electrophoresis and ribotyping. When the chambers of nebulizer devices were routinely autoclaved, *B. cepacia* colonization was eliminated.

Discussion

The above two cases clearly indicate that *B. cepacia* causes nosocomial infection in immunocompromised patients without cystic fibrosis background. However, characteristics associated with the infection of the *B. cepacia* strains are not understood. We have been studying the pathogenesis of *B. cepacia* KF1, which was isolated from a pneumonia patient with acute leukemia who was involved in the case 2 outbreak. This strain produces protease and lipase, but neither phospholipase C nor hemolysin.

PROTEASE AS A POTENTIAL VIRULENCE FACTOR OF *B. CEPACIA*

Bacterial proteases are thought to be involved in pathogenesis. *B. cepacia* 715j, isolated from a cystic fibrosis patient, produces a metalloprotease (Kooi et al., 1994) and causes bronchopneumonia in rat lung when instilled intratracheally (McKevitt et al., 1989). Strain KF1, isolated from non-cystic fibrosis patients, produces a metalloprotease which is enzymatically and immunologically very similar to that produced by strain 715j (Abe and Nakazawa, submitted). The quantities of protease produced by these strains are significantly higher than those produced by other *B. cepacia* strains of environmental or plant origin. Furthermore, *B. cepacia* KF1 produced lung infections in mice when inoculated intratracheally (Yamagishi et al., 1993a).

GENETIC ANALYSIS OF *B. CEPACIA*

Lack of understanding of *B. cepacia* pathogenesis results in part from lack of genetic analysis of this intrinsically multi-drug-resistant bacterium. We have developed a genetic analysis system for *B. cepacia* which includes transposon mutagenesis and complementation of mutations with cloned genes of interest (Abe et al., in press).

Transposon Mutagenesis and Isolation of Protease-Deficient Mutants

To deliver the transposon, pSUP2021 (Simon et al., 1983) was modified to construct pKN31 carrying a Tn*5* derivative containing *neo* and *dhfrII*, which encode neomycin phosphotransferase and trimethoprim-resistant dihydrofolate reductase, respectively (Fig. 1). The transposon was mobilized to *B. cepacia* KF1 by the transfer genes of plasmid RP4 integrated in the chromosome of *Escherichia coli* S17-1. Colonies of *B. cepacia* were isolated on L agar plates containing trimethoprim and kanamycin as selecting agents and tetracycline as a counterselecting agent.

Approximately 5,000 derivatives of *B. cepacia* KF1 were isolated from about 50 separate matings. Among these, 14 isolates had acquired stable protease-deficient mutations. Southern hybridization analysis was performed with *Cla*I and *Mlu*I digests of the mutant strain DNA using the *neo* gene of Tn*5* as a probe. All 14 mutants contained single marker insertions into the chromosome (Fig. 2). Among the 14 mutants, 13 strains were also

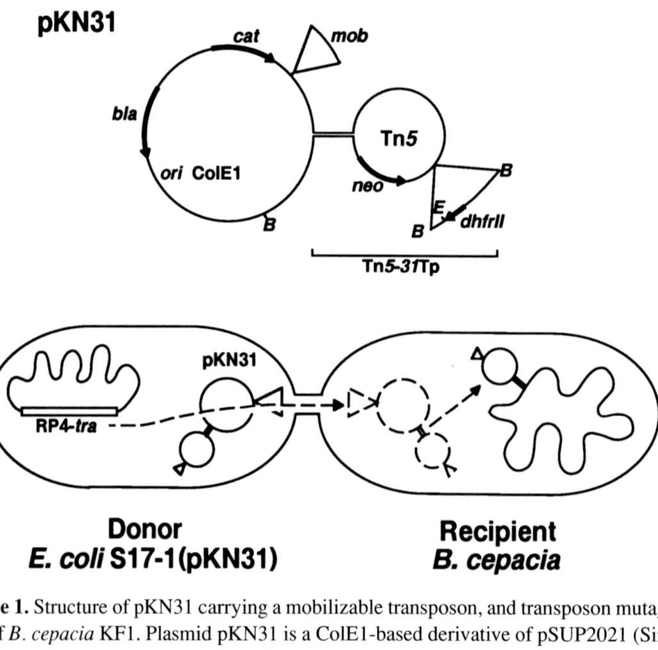

Figure 1. Structure of pKN31 carrying a mobilizable transposon, and transposon mutagenesis of *B. cepacia* KF1. Plasmid pKN31 is a ColE1-based derivative of pSUP2021 (Simon et al., 1983) with transposon Tn*5-31*Tp containing the *neo* and *dhfrII* genes encoding neomycin phosphotransferase and trimethoprim-resistant dihydrofolate reductase, respectively. The plasmid in *E. coli* S17-1 is mobilized to *B. cepacia* by the action of the chromosomal *tra* gene (Simon et al., 1983). The resulting *B. cepacia* clones carrying the transposon on the chromosome were selected on L agar containing trimethoprim (10 μg/ml).

lipase deficient. The 14 mutants were classified into eight groups on the basis of production of protease and lipase in addition to Southern hybridization profiles (Table 1).

Cloning Vector of *B. cepacia*

The *Escherichia-Burkholderia* shuttle plasmid vector pTS1209 (Fig. 3) (Abe et al., in press) consists of the replication origins of ColE1 and an IncW plasmid, pSa (Valentine

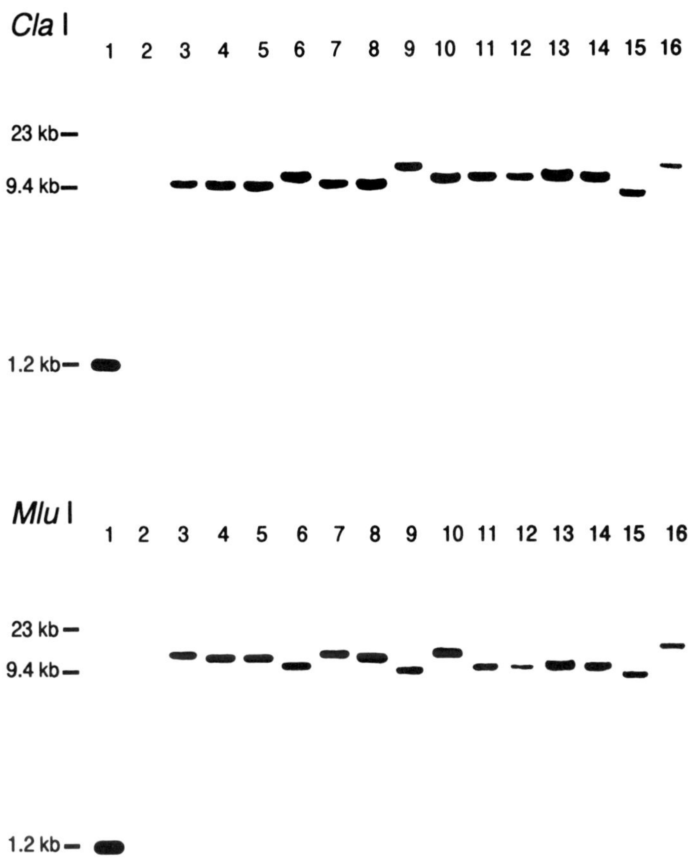

Figure 2. Southern hybridization of *B. cepacia* DNA digested with *Cla*I (upper panel) and *Mlu*I (lower panel) using the *neo* gene of Tn*5* as a probe. Samples (and Southern hybridization types of the *Cla*I and *Mlu*I digests): lane 1, 1.2-kb *Bgl*II-*Sal*I fragment containing the *neo* gene; lane 2, KF1 (negative control); lane 3, KFT1001 (*Cla*I, C; *Mlu*I, B); lane 4, KFT1002 (*Cla*I, C; *Mlu*I, B); lane 5, KFT1003 (*Cla*I, C; *Mlu*I, B); lane 6, KFT1004 (*Cla*I, B; *Mlu*I, C); lane 7, KFT1005 (*Cla*I, C; *Mlu*I, B); lane 8, KFT1006 (*Cla*I, C; *Mlu*I, B); lane 9, KFT1007 (*Cla*I, A; *Mlu*I, C); lane 10, KFT1008 (*Cla*I, B; *Mlu*I, B); lane 11, KFT1011 (*Cla*I, B; *Mlu*I, C); lane 12, KFT1012 (*Cla*I, B; *Mlu*I, C); lane 13 KFT1013 (*Cla*I, B; *Mlu*I, C); lane 14, KFT1014 (*Cla*I, B; *Mlu*I, C); lane 15, KFT1015 (*Cla*I, D; *Mlu*I, D); lane 16, KFT1016 (*Cla*I, A; *Mlu*I, A). Size markers are shown at left.

Table 1. Protease-deficient mutants of *B. cepacia* KF1

Strain[a]	Protease[b]	Lipase[b]	Southern hybridization[c]		Type
			*Cla*I	*Mlu*I	
KFT1001	–	+	C	B	I
KFT1002	–	–	C	B	II
KFT1003	–	–	C	B	II
KFT1004	–	–	B	C	III
KFT1005	–	–	C	B	IV
KFT1006	–	–	C	B	II
KFT1007	–	+++	A	C	V
KFT1008	+	–	B	B	VI
KFT1011	–	–	B	C	III
KFT1012	–	–	B	C	III
KFT1013	–	–	B	C	III
KFT1014	–	–	B	C	III
KFT1015	–	+	D	D	VII
KFT1016	+	–	A	A	VIII
KF1	+++	+++			Wild type

[a]The growth of KFT1001, KFT1005, KFT1015, and KFT1016 was poor.
[b]Activities were determined by the plate assay (Nakazawa et al., 1987) and expressed as: +++, similar to the wild type; +, less than the wild type; –, no activity.
[c]Classified according to the Southern hybridization profiles in Fig. 2.

et al., 1994), and the *bla* and *catII* genes, encoding β-lactamase and the type II chloramphenicol acetyltransferase, respectively. The plasmid has several unique restriction sites which were successfully employed for cloning the genes involved in protease production in *B. cepacia*.

PROTEASE IS SECRETED BY THE GENERAL SECRETORY PATHWAY

Mutant KFT1008, obtained by transposon mutagenesis, produces only 5% of protease as compared to the wild-type strain (Table 1). To isolate a gene complementing the KFT1008 mutation, pTS1209 DNA was purified from *B. cepacia*, digested with *Bam*HI, and ligated with *Bam*HI fragments of chromosomal DNA from strain KF1. The recombinant molecules were introduced into *B. cepacia* KFT1008 by electroporation, and transformants were selected for protease production on skim-milk agar plates (Nakazawa et al., 1987) containing chloramphenicol. A clone showing a halo on the plate was found to carry a plasmid with a 5.6-kb *Bam*HI insert. Subcloning and sequencing identified a 1.4-kb *Eco*47III-*Sal*I fragment that carries a gene, designated *gspF*, that was disrupted by the transposon in KFT1008 (M. Abe and T. Nakazawa, unpublished results). The *gspF* product, GspF, is a 405-amino-acid polypeptide that is highly homologous (47.5% identity) (Bally et al., 1992) to *Pseudomonas aeruginosa* XcpS, an inner membrane protein involved in secretion of extracellular proteins such as elastase, lipase, alkaline phosphatase, and exotoxin. A homolog of *P. aeruginosa xcpR* was found in the upstream region of *gspF* of *B. cepacia* and was designated *gspE*. The XcpR protein of *P. aeruginosa* is thought to be a cytoplasmic protein and has a consensus ATP binding site. In addition

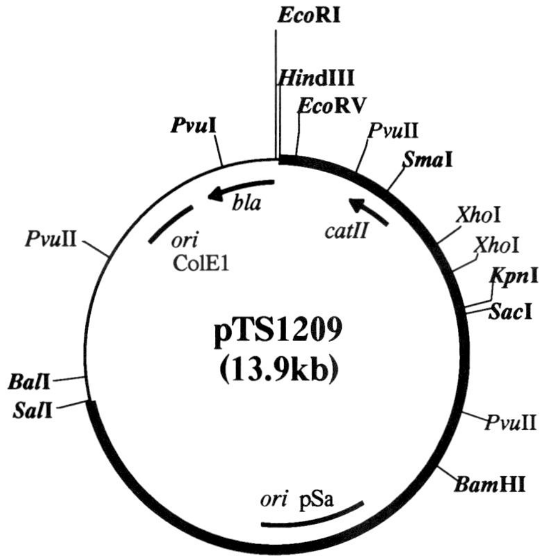

Figure 3. Physical and genetic map of pTS1209, a shuttle plasmid of *E. coli* and *B. cepacia* (Abe et al., in press). The plasmid consists of *ori*ColE1 and *ori*pSa, an IncW plasmid (Valentine et al., 1994), and contains the *bla* and *catII* genes encoding β-lactamase and type II chloramphenicol acetyltransferase, respectively.

to these homologs, *B. cepacia* has genes encoding membrane proteins for the general secretory pathway which have potential cleavage sites for type IV prepilin peptidase (Abe and Nakazawa, unpublished results).

DsbB IS INVOLVED IN PROTEASE SECRETION

Mutant KFT1007 does not produce protease at all, whereas its lipase production is normal (Table 1). The mutation of KFT1007 was complemented (Fig. 4) by a clone carrying recombinant plasmid pMA24, which has a 1.3-kb *Mlu*I fragment of *B. cepacia* KF1 in pTS1209 (Abe and Nakazawa, submitted).

Sequence analysis of the 1.3-kb *Mlu*I fragment of pMA24 revealed an open reading frame, designated *dsbB*, that was disrupted in strain KFT1007 (Abe and Nakazawa, submitted). The 170-amino-acid polypeptide encoded by this open reading frame shows a significant homology (26.5% identity, 52% similarity) with that of *E. coli* DsbB (176 amino acids), which is involved in the formation of disulfide bonds of periplasmic proteins (Missiakas et al., 1993). Two pairs of cysteine residues which are essential for the periplasmic activity of *E. coli* DsbB (Jander et al., 1994) are conserved in *B. cepacia* DsbB. No signal-peptide-like sequence was found at the N terminus. DsbB of *B. cepacia* is a very hydrophobic protein. The protein has four predicted membrane-spanning regions and arginine-rich sequences at the N and C termini, suggesting that the termini are in the cytoplasmic side of the membrane (Jander et al., 1994). L-Cystine, but not L-cysteine, was effective in restoring protease production in *B. cepacia* KFT1007 (Fig. 4).

Strain KFT1007 is also defective in motility, which was restored by the introduction of pMA24 or by the addition of L-cystine to the medium (Abe and Nakazawa,

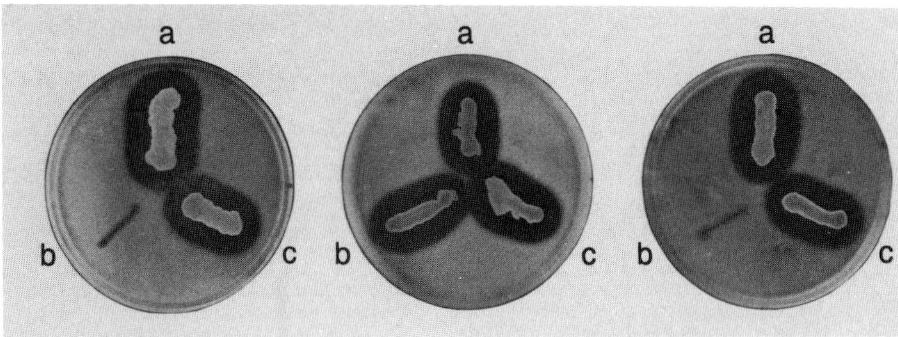

Figure 4. Protease production by *B. cepacia* strains. Bacteria were inoculated on skim-milk agar (left plate), skim-milk agar supplemented with 0.1 mM L-cystine (middle plate), and skim-milk agar supplemented with 1 mM L-cysteine (right plate), followed by incubation at 28°C for 24 h. Strains: a, *B. cepacia* KF1; b, *B. cepacia* KFT1007; c, *B. cepacia* KFT1007(pMA24).

submitted). A mutant of *E. coli dsbB* is nonmotile due to a failure to assemble functional flagella, ascribed to an inability to form disulfide bonds in the P-ring protein of the flagella (Dailey and Berg, 1993). The motility of *E. coli* carrying a mutation in *dsbB* was restored by the introduction of *B. cepacia dsbB* (Abe and Nakazawa, submitted), indicating that *B. cepacia* DsbB is active in the heterologous host. These results suggest that *B. cepacia* also has a disulfide-bond formation system consisting of DsbA and DsbB.

GENERAL SECRETORY PATHWAY OF EXTRACELLULAR METALLOPROTEASE

Elastase encoded by the chromosomal gene *lasB* of *P. aeruginosa* is a zinc protease consisting of 301 amino acid residues with two disulfide bonds (Thayer et al., 1991). It is secreted by a two-step mechanism: first it crosses the inner membrane in a signal sequence-dependent way, and then elastase is translocated across the outer membrane by the Xcp-mediated general secretory pathway (Bally et al., 1992). The DsbB homolog of *P. aeruginosa* is found in databases (Kato et al., 1989) and is highly homologous to *B. cepacia* DsbB. Thus elastase production by *P. aeruginosa* may also be DsbB dependent.

In a sodium dodecyl sulfate-polyacrylamide gel electrophoresis immunoblot with polyclonal antibody raised against purified *B. cepacia* KF1 protease, the culture supernatant of the *dsbB* mutant, KFT1007, showed a 43-kDa immunoreactive band, whereas the wild-type strain and KFT1007 carrying the *dsbB* plasmid showed a 37-kDa band corresponding to the mature metalloprotease (Abe and Nakazawa, submitted). It should be noted that the wild-type strain additionally produced a small amount of the 43-kDa polypeptide. Similar findings are reported by Kooi et al. (1994), suggesting that the 43-kDa protein is a precursor form of the protease.

On the basis of the above results, we propose that metalloprotease of *B. cepacia* is secreted by the general secretory pathway of extracellular protein in gram-negative bacteria. The most extensively studied model of this pathway involves *Klebsiella oxytoca* pullulanase production (Pugsley, 1993). The first step involves translocation of the unfolded proenzyme across the inner membrane, followed by disulfide bond formation and folding in the periplasm. This step may be *sec* and *dsbB* dependent. The second step involves translocation of the folded polypeptide from the periplasm to the outside, across the outer membrane. Proteins encoded by *gspE* and *gspF* and those with the prepilin-like signal sequence are required for the latter step in *B. cepacia* as in *P. aeruginosa* (Bally et al., 1992). Processing of the proenzyme to produce mature and active protease may occur during this step (Kawamoto et al., 1993).

The *lipA* gene of *B. cepacia* DSM3959 encodes a prelipase from which a signal peptide is cleaved during secretion. In the periplasm, prelipase is folded into the active state by a molecular chaperone, Lim, encoded by *limA* (Hobson et al., 1993). The disulfide bond formation system described above is not required for this process, since the *dsbB*-defective mutant strain KFT1007 showed a lipase-positive phenotype. On the other hand, all the other protease-deficient mutants we have isolated (Table 1) were lipase deficient, suggesting common steps in the excretion of both extracellular protein.

Proteases secreted by gram-negative bacteria might attack cellular constituents of the host bacterium if they were produced as an active form within the cells. To avoid such a disadvantage, bacteria produce protease as an inactive form in the cytoplasm and then activate it during the process of secretion. Bacteria utilize one of two systems for secretion of metalloproteases. One is the general secretory pathway, utilized for proteins such as elastase and lipase of *P. aeruginosa* and metalloprotease and lipase of *B. cepacia,* and the other is a one-step secretory pathway, the ABC (ATP-binding cassette) ATPase exporter for proteins such as the alkaline protease of *P. aeruginosa* and the metalloproteases of *Erwinia chrysanthemi* (Fath and Kolter, 1993, Häse and Finkelstein, 1993). Proteases utilizing the general secretory pathway contain more than two cysteine residues, whereas those utilizing the ABC ATPase exporter have none (Table 2). In the general secretory pathway, inactive precursors are secreted into the periplasm and then activated by the help of the disulfide bond formation system for extracellular translocation. On the other hand, the metalloproteases secreted via the ABC ATPase exporter bypass the periplasm, since disulfide bond formation is not involved in the activation process of these proteins.

Table 2. Number of cysteine residues and secretory pathways of metalloproteases of gram-negative bacteria[a]

Metalloprotease	No. of cysteine residues	Secretory pathway
Pseudomonas aeruginosa LasB	4	General secretory pathway
Erwinia carotovora	3	General secretory pathway
Vibrio cholerae	6	General secretory pathway
Serratia marcescens Smp	4	General secretory pathway
Pseudomonas aeruginosa AprA	0	ABC exporter
Erwinia chrysanthemi EC16 PrtC	0	ABC exporter
Erwinia chrysanthemi B374 PrtA	0	ABC exporter
Erwinia chrysanthemi B374 PrtB	0	ABC exporter
Erwinia chrysanthemi B374 PrtC	0	ABC exporter

[a]Metalloproteases listed by Häse and Finkelstein (1993) were analyzed by the GENETYX 7.2 software.

Acknowledgment. This work was supported in part by a Grant-in-Aid for Scientific Research from Ministry of Education, Science and Culture, Japan.

REFERENCES

Abe, M., and T. Nakazawa. The *dsbB* gene product is essential for protease production of *Burkholderia (Pseudomonas) cepacia*. Submitted for publication.

Abe, M., M. Tsuda, M. Kimoto, S. Inouye, A. Nakazawa, and T. Nakazawa. A genetic analysis system of *Burkholderia (Pseudomonas) cepacia*: construction and use of mobilizable transposons and a cloning vector. *Gene*, in press.

Bally, M., A. Filloux, M. Akrim, G. Ball, A. Lazdunski, and J. Tommassen. 1992. Protein secretion in *Pseudomonas aeruginosa;* characterization of seven *xcp* genes and processing of secretory apparatus components by prepilin peptidase. *Mol. Microbiol.* **6:**1121–1131.

Burkhead, K. D., D. A. Schisler, and P. J. Slininger. 1994. Pyrrolnitrin production by biological control agent *Pseudomonas cepacia* B37w in culture and in colonized wounds of potatoes. *Appl. Environ. Microbiol.* **60:**2031–2039.

Dailey, F., and H. C. Berg. 1993. Mutants in disulfide bond formation that disrupt flagellar assembly in *Escherichia coli. Proc. Natl. Acad. Sci. USA* **90:**1043–1047.

Fath, M.J., and R. Kolter. 1993. ABC transporters: bacterial exporters. *Microbiol. Rev.* **57:**995–1017.

Folsom, B. R., and P. J. Chapman. 1991. Performance characterization of a model bioreactor for the biodegradation of trichloroethylene by *Pseudomonas cepacia* G4. *Appl. Environ. Microbiol.* **57:**1602–1608.

Häse, C. C., and R. A. Finkelstein. 1993. Bacterial extracellular zinc-containing metalloproteases. *Microbiol. Rev.* **57:**823–837.

Hobson, A. H., C. M. Buckley, J. L. Aamand, S. T. Jørgensen, B. Diderichsen, and D. J. McConnell. 1993. Activiation of a bacterial lipase by its chaperon. *Proc. Natl. Acad. Sci. USA* **90:**5682–5686.

Jander, G., N. L. Martin, and J. Beckwith. 1994. Two cysteines in each periplasmic domain of the membrane protein DsbB are required for its function in protein disulfide bond formation. *EMBO J.* **13:**5121–5127.

Kato, J., L. Chu, K. Kitano, J. D. DeVault, K. Kimbara, and A. M. Chakrabarty. 1989. Nucleotide sequence of a regulatory region controlling alginate synthesis in *Pseudomonas aeruginosa. Gene* **84:**31–38.

Kawamoto, S., Y. Shibano, J. Fukushima, N. Ishii, K. Morihara, and K. Okuda. 1993. Site-directed mutagenesis of Glu-141 and His-223 in *Pseudomonas aeruginosa* elastase: catalytic activity, processing, and protective activity of the elastase against *Pseudomonas* infection. *Infect. Immun.* **61:**1400–1405.

Kooi, C., A. Cox, P. Darling, and P. A. Sokol. 1994. Neutralizing monoclonal antibodies to an extracellular *Pseudomonas cepacia* protease. *Infect. Immun.* **62:**2811–2817.

McKevitt, A. I., S. Bajaksouzian, J. D. Klinger, and D. E. Woods. 1989. Purification and characterization of an extracellular protease from *Pseudomonas cepacia. Infect. Immun.* **57:**771–778.

Missiakas, D., C. Georgopoulos, and S. Raina. 1993. Identification and characterization of the *Escherichia coli* gene *dsbB*, whose product is involved in the formation of disulfide bonds *in vivo. Proc. Natl. Acad. Sci. USA* **90:**7084–7088.

Nakazawa, T., Y. Yamada, and M. Ishibashi. 1987. Characterization of hemolysin in extracellular products of *Pseudomonas cepacia. J. Clin. Microbiol.* **25:**195–198.

Ouchi, K., M. Abe, M. Karita, T. Oguri, J. Igari, and T. Nakazawa. 1995. Analysis of strains of *Burkholderia* (formerly *Pseudomonas*) *cepacia* isolated in a nosocomial outbreak by biochemical and genomic typing. *J. Clin. Microbiol.* **33:**2353–2357.

Pugsley, A. P. 1993. The complete general secretory pathway in gram-negative bacteria. *Microbiol. Rev.* **57:**50–108.

Simon, R., U. Priefer, and A. Pühler. 1983. A broad host range mobilization system for in vivo genetic engineering: transposon mutagenesis in Gram-negative bacteria. *Bio/Technology* **1:**784–791.

Tablan, O. C., W. J. Martone, C. F. Doershuk, R. C. Stern, M. J. Thomassen, J. D. Klinger, J. W. White, L. A. Carson, and W. R. Jarvis. 1987. Colonization of the respiratory tract with *Pseudomonas cepacia* in cystic fibrosis: risk factors and outcomes. *Chest* **91:**527–532.

Takigawa, K., J. Fujita, K. Negayama, Y. Yamagishi, Y. Yamaji, K. Ouchi, K. Yamada, M. Abe, T. Nakazawa, K. Kawanishi, and J. Takahara. 1993. Nosocomial outbreak of *Pseudomonas cepacia* respiratory infection in immunocompromised patients associated with contaminated nebulizer devices. *J. Jpn. Assoc. Infect. Dis.* **67:**1115–1125.

Thayer, M. M., K. M. Flaherty, and D. B. McKay. 1991. Three-dimensional structure of the elastase of *Pseudomonas aeruginosa* at 1.5-Å resolution. *J. Biol. Chem.* **266:**2864–2871.

Valentine, C. R., M. J. Heinrich, S. L. Chissoe, and B. A. Roe. 1994. DNA sequence of one-kilobase direct repeats of the *sulI* gene of plasmid pSa. *Plasmid* **32:**222–227.

Yabuuchi, E., Y. Kosako, H. Oyaizu, I. Yano, H. Hotta, Y. Hashimoto, T. Ezaki, and M. Arakawa. 1992. Proposal of *Burkholderia* gen. nov. and transfer of seven species of the genus *Pseudomonas* Homology Group II to the new genus, with the type species *Burkholderia cepacia* (Palleroni and Holmes 1981) comb. nov. *Microbiol. Immunol.* **36:**1251–1275.

Yamagishi, Y., J. Fujita, K. Takigawa, H. Miyawaki, J. Takahara, I. Yamadori, K. Negayama, K. Fujimaki, and T. Nakazawa. 1993a. Experimental pneumonia produced by clinical isolates of *Pseudomonas cepacia* in mice. *J. Jpn. Assoc. Infect. Dis.* **67:**816–822.

Yamagishi, Y., J. Fujita, K. Takigawa, K. Negayama, T. Nakazawa, and J. Takahara. 1993b. Clinical features of *Pseudomonas cepacia* pneumonia in an epidemic among immunocompromised patients. *Chest* **103:**1706–1709.

Molecular Biology of Pseudomonads
Edited by T. Nakazawa et al.

Chapter 41

Regulation of the Alginate (*algD*) Operon in *Pseudomonas aeruginosa*

Dennis E. Ohman, Kalai Mathee, Craig J. McPherson, Caroline A. DeVries, Sheng Ma, Daniel J. Wozniak, and Michael J. Franklin

PATHOGENESIS AND ALGINATE

Pseudomonas aeruginosa can cause severe and life-threatening infections in immunosuppressed hosts such as patients with respiratory diseases, burns, cancers undergoing chemotherapy, and cystic fibrosis (CF). Virulence factors produced by *P. aeruginosa* include numerous extracellular toxins, proteases, hemolysins, and exopolysaccharides that play a role depending upon the type of infection. The overproduction of one particular virulence factor, the exopolysaccharide alginate, appears to allow *P. aeruginosa* to persist in the lungs of CF patients and cause chronic bronchopulmonary infection (Govan and Harris, 1986). Alginate overproduction confers a mucoid phenotype (Alg$^+$) due to synthesis of copious amounts of the exopolysaccharide. Production of alginate provides an adherence mechanism, confers increased resistance to the host immune response, and may thwart antibiotic therapy, considering that infection with mucoid *P. aeruginosa* is seldom eradicated in patients with CF.

ALGINATE BIOSYNTHESIS

Alginate is a linear copolymer of β-1,4-linked D-mannuronate and its C-5 epimer L-guluronate. The alginate biosynthetic pathway in *P. aeruginosa* begins with fructose 6-phosphate, which is recruited from central metabolic pathways to form the sugar nucleotide GDP-mannose (Fig. 1). This occurs via the action of the gene products AlgA (phosphomannose isomerase/GDP-mannose pyrophosphorylase) and AlgC (phosphomannose isomerase) (May et al., 1991). GDP-mannose is oxidized by the action of AlgD (GDP-mannose dehydrogenase) and NAD$^+$ to form GDP-mannuronate (Roychoudhury et al., 1989). The mannuronate moiety is polymerized and exported across

Dennis E. Ohman, Kalai Mathee, Craig J. McPherson, Caroline A. DeVries, Sheng Ma, and Michael J. Franklin • Department of Microbiology and Immunology, University of Tennessee and VA Medical Center, Memphis, Tennessee 38163. ***Daniel J. Wozniak*** • Department of Microbiology and Immunology, Wake Forest University, Bowman Gray School of Medicine, Winston-Salem, North Carolina 27157-1064.

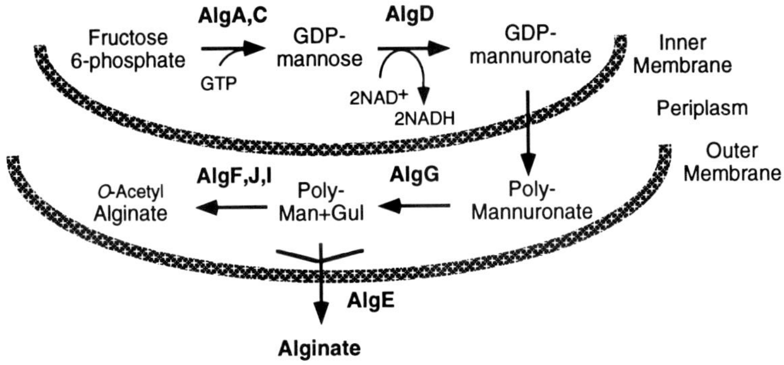

Figure 1. Model for the pathway of alginate biosynthesis in *P. aeruginosa.* Gene products involved at each step are indicated as well as their cellular localization. Note that export of polymer from the cell can occur at the poly-mannuronate stage, with or without epimerization or acetylation. Poly-Man+Gul, poly-mannuronate plus poly-guluronate.

the inner membrane to form poly-D-mannuronate by unknown mechanisms. Candidates for the reaction include AlgL and the gene products represented by mutants defective in *alg-8, alg-44,* and *alg-60* (Maharaj et al., 1993; May et al., 1991; Schiller et al., 1993). Periplasmic AlgG (C5-mannuronate epimerase) converts variable amounts of the D-mannuronate residues to L-guluronate at the polymer level but without forming blocks of adjacent guluronates in the polymer (Chitnis and Ohman, 1990; Franklin et al., 1994). Through an undefined mechanism, alginate is modified by the addition of *O*-acetyl groups to some mannuronate residues by the activities of periplasmic AlgF (Franklin et al., 1993; Shinabarger et al., 1993) as well as AlgJ and AlgI (Franklin and Ohman, 1996). Extrusion of alginate through the outer membrane has been reported to require the gene product AlgE (Chu et al., 1991), which has also been shown to have porin-like activity (Rehm et al., 1994). The polymer does not remain attached to the cell, and its release to the medium may involve the lyase activity of periplasmic AlgL. Alginate accumulates in the culture medium to as much as 2 g/liter, thus generating a highly viscous aqueous environment.

THE ALGINATE GENE CLUSTER FORMS AN OPERON

Most of the genes encoding enzymes for alginate biosynthesis are clustered at 34 min on the *P. aeruginosa* chromosome. A known exception is *algC,* located at about 10 min, encoding an enzyme (phosphomannoglucomutase) that is also used in lipopolysaccharide biosynthesis (Coyne et al., 1994). The main alginate biosynthetic gene cluster, which begins with *algD* and ends with *algA,* appears to form an operon of approximately 18 kb in length (Chitnis and Ohman, 1993). Evidence for this operonic structure comes from studies on polar mutations. A Northern (RNA) hybridization analysis of transcripts from the alginate gene cluster has shown that a polar transposon (Tn*501,* 8.2 kb) insertion in the chromosomal gene cluster, located about 4 kb upstream of *algG* and about 8.5 kb upstream of *algA,* is blocked in the transcription of both *algG* and *algA* without affecting transcription of the upstream gene *algD* (Fig. 2A). Also, a strain with a Tn*501* insertion in *algD* can only be complemented back to Alg⁺ if the complementing plasmid contains the entire alginate cluster (Fig. 2B). If the last gene, *algA*, is truncated from the complementing clone, then the strain retains the Alg⁻ phenotype (Fig. 2B). However, the polar nature of the transposon can be alleviated by forming a merodiploid. For instance, integrating a promoter-proximal segment of the operon on a nonreplicating plasmid into the chromosome downstream of the transposon restores a complete operon which confers the mucoid phenotype (Fig. 2C). The polar nature of transposon insertions in the alginate biosynthetic operon was used to map the location of *algL*, encoding an enzyme with alginate lyase activity (Schiller et al., 1993). Tn*501* insertions downstream of *algL* confer an Alg⁻ phenotype, but the strain still produces alginate lyase. However, insertions from *algD* to *algL* block both alginate production and alginate lyase activity (Fig. 2D).

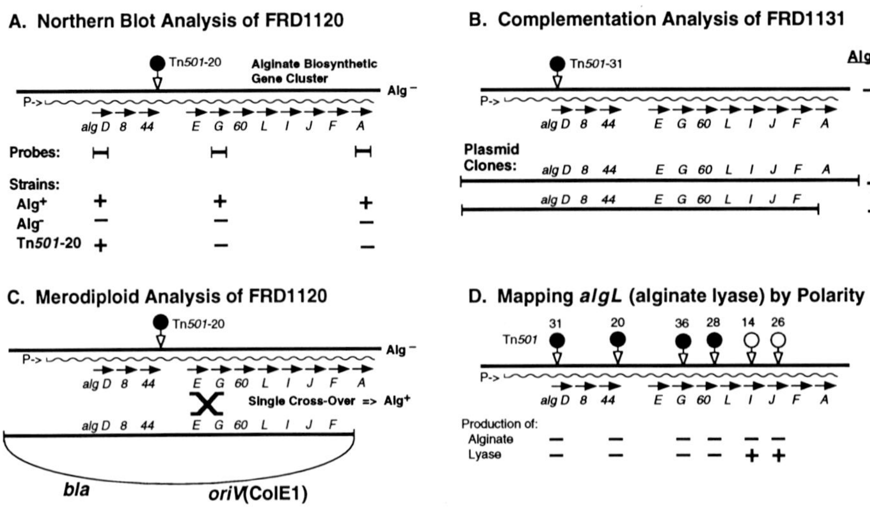

Figure 2. Evidence for the operon structure of the alginate biosynthetic gene cluster at 34 min on the *P. aeruginosa* chromosome. (A) Schematic representation of a Northern (RNA) blot analysis of Alg⁺ strain FRD1, spontaneous Alg⁻ (i.e., *algT18*) strain FRD2, and FRD1120 with a transposon Tn*501*-20 insertion in the alginate biosynthetic gene cluster. Probes shown detected (+ or −) transcripts from *algD, algG,* and *algA* of the alginate biosynthetic operon in the above strains. Note that the Tn*501*-20 insertion showed polar effects on downstream genes (e.g., *algG, algA*). (B) Complementation analysis of strain FRD1131 with the *algD*::Tn*501*-31 polar insertion. FRD1131 can be complemented, thus restoring alginate production (+), only by the entire cluster in *trans*. Note that a clone missing only the last gene (*algA*) does not restore alginate production (−). (C) Merodiploid analysis of strain FRD1120 with Tn*501*-20 in the alginate biosynthetic gene cluster. The Alg⁻ phenotype resulting from the polar effects of the transposon on downstream genes was converted to Alg⁺ by formation of a merodiploid that restores a complete operon. (D) Mapping *algL* in the operon. Alg⁻ strains with mapped Tn*501* insertions in the chromosomal 18-kb alginate gene cluster were tested for the ability (+ or −) to produce the *algL* product (which has alginate lyase activity). Note that transposons upstream of *algL* (numbers 31, 20, 36, and 28) had polar effects on its expression, but those downstream (numbers 14 and 26) did not block lyase activity.

High transcriptional activity of the alginate biosynthetic operon correlates with alginate overproduction and the mucoid phenotype (i.e., Alg⁺). This operon is under complex control, and its expression is subject to a number of regulators (Mohr et al., 1990; Wozniak and Ohman, 1994). Several positive regulatory genes have been identified and include *algRQP* (*algR,2,3*), *algB,* and *algT*(*algU*). To bypass the need for regulators which control the operon, an *algD′* merodiploid was constructed to replace the native promoter with a regulated *trp-lac* (*trc*) promoter (Fig. 3). In this P*trc-algD* merodiploid of the CF strain FRD, alginate was overproduced only in the presence of isopropyl-β-D-thiogalactopyranoside (IPTG).

algT(algU) ENCODES AN ALTERNATE SIGMA FACTOR

The alginate regulatory system is complex and consists of a cascade of factors (Fig. 4). At the head of the hierarchy is a cluster of modulatory genes in the 68-min region of the chromosome, containing *algT-mucA-algN-algM-algY*. Upstream of *algT*(*algU*) is the divergently transcribed gene *nadB*, encoding L-aspartate oxidase presumably for de novo NAD biosynthesis (DeVries et al., 1995). The *algT* gene encodes a positive regulator (of alginate biosynthesis) that is essential for alginate production (Flynn and Ohman, 1988a, 1988b). The cloned *algT* gene from the CF-associated mucoid strain FRD1 activates the Alg⁺ (alginate-overproducing, mucoid) phenotype in otherwise nonmucoid strains (Flynn and Ohman, 1988a, 1988b; Goldberg et al., 1993; Wozniak and Ohman, 1993).

AlgT has sequence similarity to a number of minor sigma factors of RNA polymerase (DeVries and Ohman, 1994). Biochemical evidence that purified AlgT can function as a

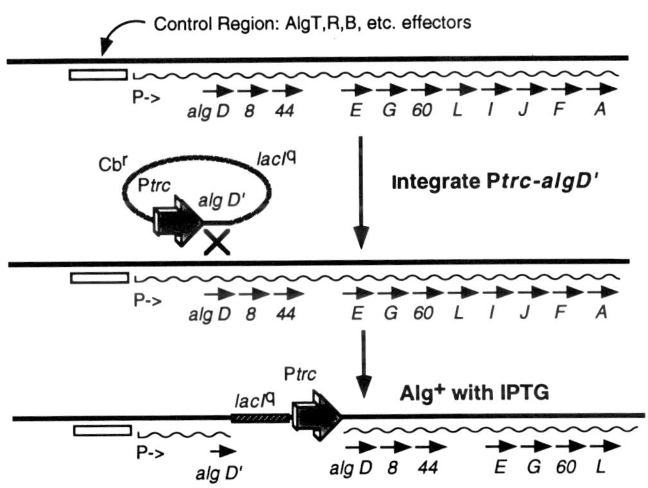

Figure 3. Constructions to bypass the regulators of the alginate biosynthetic gene cluster. A *trc* promoter before an *algD′* DNA fragment was cloned into a narrow-host-range plasmid containing *lacI*^{q}. A merodiploid of the Alg⁺ strain FRD was constructed by integrating the plasmid into the chromosome by homologous recombination, putting the chromosomal alginate operon under the *trc* promoter and with the Alg⁺ phenotype dependent upon IPTG induction.

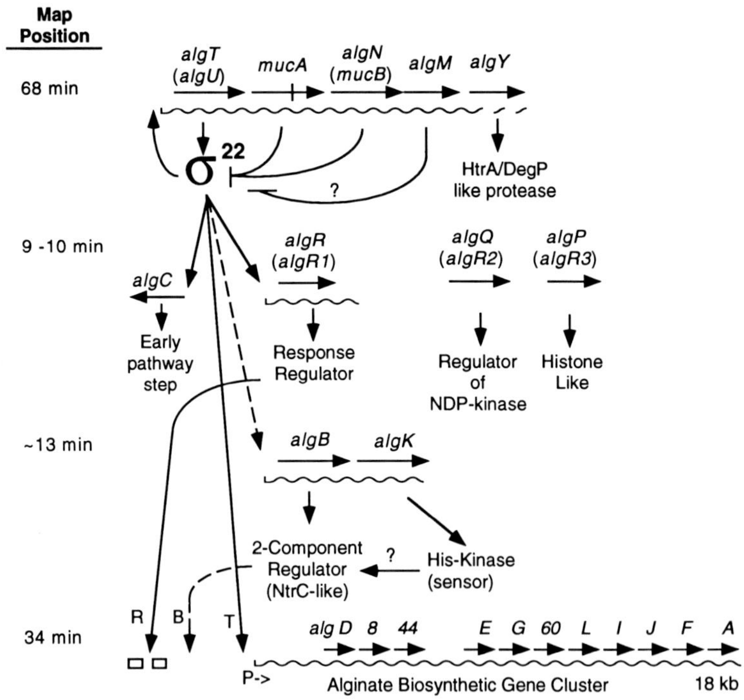

Figure 4. Model for alginate gene regulation. The effects of regulators, either direct (solid lines) or indirect (dashed lines), on specific promoters are indicated with arrows. Chromosomal map positions are shown on the left.

sigma factor was recently obtained (Hershberger et al., 1995). AlgT shows high sequence similarity (66% identity) to sigma-E (σ^E) of *Escherichia coli* (Deretic et al., 1994; DeVries and Ohman, 1994; Lonetto et al., 1994) (Fig. 5). σ^E is a 24-kDa protein and was identified by its involvement in high-temperature expression of σ^{32}, the heat shock sigma factor in *E. coli* (Erickson and Gross, 1989). σ^E and AlgT belong to a new subfamily of eubacterial RNA polymerase sigma factors that typically regulate extracytoplasmic functions (Lonetto et al., 1994). Using sigma sequence conservation analysis (Lonetto et al., 1992), the locations (Fig. 5) in AlgT of the predicted polymerase core binding region (AlgT residues 21 to 38), RpoD box (i.e., for −10 recognition; AlgT residues 68 to 83), and 20-mer (i.e., for −35 recognition; AlgT residues 164 to 184) were observed in approximately the same relative locations as in σ^E (DeVries and Ohman, 1994).

MECHANISM OF MUCOID-TO-NONMUCOID CONVERSION

The mucoid (Alg$^+$) phenotype of *P. aeruginosa* strains from CF patients is typically unstable in the laboratory. This is true of the CF strain FRD1, and its mucoid phenotype is especially unstable when cultures are not maintained under highly aerated conditions (Ohman and Chakrabarty, 1981). Early studies showed that the genetic alterations re-

```
                             core binding
                   *          *
AlgT   MLTQEQDQQLVERVQRGDKRAFDLLVLKYQHKILGLIVRFVHDAQEAQDV    50
       |  |  || ||||||:|| :|| |||::||||:  |: |:|  : :  ||
SigE   MSEQLTDQVLVERVQKGDQKAFNLLVVRYQHKVASLVSRYVPSG-DVPDV    49

                            RpoD box
AlgT   AQEAFIKAYRALGNFRGDSAFYTWLYRIAINTAKNHLVARGRRPPDSDVT   100
        |||||||||||  |||||||||||||||:||||| ||| ||||| |||
SigE   VQEAFIKAYRALDSFRGDSAFYTWLYRIAVNTAKNYLVAQGRRPPSSDVD    99

AlgT   AEDAEFFEGDHALKDIESPERAMLRDEIEATVHQTIQQLPEDLRTALTLR   150
       | :|| ||   |||:|  ||  ||  :|:   |  ||  |||||| |:|||
SigE   AIEAENFESGGALKEISNPENLMLSEELRQIVFRTIESLPEDLRMAITLR   149

                             20mer box
AlgT   EFEGLSYEDIATVMQCPVGTVRSRIFRAREAIDKALQPLLREA          193
       | :|||||:|| :| ||||||||||||||||||  :|||:|
SigE   ELDGLSYEEIAAIMDCPVGTVRSRIFRAREAIDNKVQPLIRR           191
```

Figure 5. Sequence alignment of AlgT (also called AlgU) from *P. aeruginosa* and σ^E (SigE) of *E. coli*, indicated with identities (|) and similarities (:). The approximate regions of AlgT and σ^E that are presumed to be responsible for core binding, −10 recognition (RpoD box), and −35 recognition (20-mer box) are indicated. Also shown are the locations (indicated with *) where amino acid substitutions often occur in spontaneous nonmucoid derivatives in the CF-associated Alg^+ strain FRD.

sponsible for spontaneous Alg^- conversion were closely linked to *algT*, and the genetic "switch" was previously called *algS* (Flynn and Ohman, 1988a, 1988b). Subsequently, spontaneous Alg^- variants were shown to arise due to mutations in the *algT* locus itself. Gene replacement with $algT^+$ DNA was used to provide evidence that the mutations in *algT* were indeed responsible for loss of alginate production (DeVries and Ohman, 1994; Flynn and Ohman, 1988a, 1988b). Over 30 spontaneous Alg^- variants of mucoid strain FRD were isolated by incubation in nonaerated cultures. Sequence analysis revealed two common single-base-pair changes that resulted in missense mutations in *algT* (shown as * in Fig. 5). The spontaneous *algT18* mutant allele changed codon 18 from GAC (Asp) in Alg^+ strains to GGC (Gly) in Alg^- strains. The spontaneous *algT29* mutant allele changed codon 29 from TAC (Tyr) to TGC (Cys) (DeVries and Ohman, 1994). It is curious that among the many independently isolated nonmucoid variants, these two missense mutations in *algT* were so common, and that both resulted in changes in or near the region encoding the core binding region of this sigma factor. Thus, there may be a mechanism which controls this specificity in the base pair alterations observed. Others have also reported mutations in *algT*(*algU*) that resulted in spontaneous nonmucoid conversion; these studies, done in mucoid strain PAO578, revealed a nonsense mutation in the codon for Trp-74 which formed a stop codon, and a frameshift mutation in the codon specifying Asp-160 (Schurr et al., 1994). Perhaps the nature of the mutation (i.e., missense or null) is affected by the strain background or the conditions used to obtain spontaneous nonmucoids.

REGULATION OF AlgT

The *algT* gene is the first in a cluster of genes that appears to form an operon encoding products that may be involved in the control of AlgT activity. Immediately downstream of *algT* is *mucA*. It has been shown that mutation in this gene is often the mechanism of conversion to mucoidy in *P. aeruginosa* infecting CF patients (Martin et al., 1993b). In corroboration, the CF strain FRD has a defective *mucA* allele, suggesting that loss of this gene's function is responsible for the strain's mucoid phenotype (Goldberg et al., 1993; Martin et al., 1993b). The next gene, *algN*(*mucB*), prevents *trans* complementation of *algT*, and its mutation also leads to a mucoid phenotype (Goldberg et al., 1993; Martin et al., 1993a). MucA and AlgN(MucB) are negative regulators of alginate production and appear to play a role as antagonists (or anti-sigma factors) of AlgT. In contrast, the next gene, *algM*, encodes a positive regulator for alginate production (McPherson et al., submitted for publication). The *algY* gene follows in the gene cluster, and its product has high homology with HtrA(DegP), a periplasmic serine protease associated with resistance to heat shock in *E. coli*. AlgY appears to be a negative regulator for alginate production (McPherson et al., submitted). Interestingly, σ^E in *E. coli* directly controls the expression of *htrA* (Erickson and Gross, 1989).

Roles for the gene products of the *algT* gene cluster were proposed based on their effects in *trans* in the typical nonmucoid strain PAO1, which carries *algT-mucA-algN-algM-algY* (wild type). A plasmid clone of the FRD genome (defective in *mucA*) containing *algT-mucA22-mucA-algN-algM* confers the mucoid phenotype, apparently because its presence in multicopy without a *mucA*$^+$ allele overrides the single copy of wild-type *mucA* in the chromosome (Fig. 6). However, loss of *algM* from this clone restores the nonmucoid phenotype, which suggests that AlgM antagonizes the effects of MucA and/or AlgN on AlgT. A clone containing only *algT* confers the mucoid phenotype, suggesting that increasing the stoichiometric amount of AlgT relative to MucA and AlgN allows for sufficient AlgT activity to permit the transcriptional activation of alginate biosynthetic genes.

Our working hypothesis is that the proteins in the *algT*-associated gene cluster form a signal transduction system that modulates AlgT activity, perhaps in response to environmental stress. This is consistent with the notion that the AlgT family of sigma factors typically regulate extracytoplasmic functions (Lonetto et al., 1994). Apparently, the wild-type control of AlgT activity is too stringent in the CF lung. Perhaps under these conditions, full AlgT activity is advantageous and readily achieved by mutation affecting an antagonist (e.g., MucA or AlgN/MucB). When mucoid CF strains are manipulated in the laboratory, selection for strains with reduced AlgT activity occurs, resulting in mutations in *algT* (DeVries and Ohman, 1994). The occurrence of suppressor mutations in *algT* to overcome mutations in *mucA* (to restore the wild-type Alg$^-$ phenotype) provides genetic evidence that AlgT and MucA proteins interact.

TRANSCRIPTIONAL ANALYSIS OF *algT*

The spontaneous *algT* missense mutants have provided valuable tools toward understanding *algT* regulation. RNase protection assays were performed to quantitate *algT* transcripts in the mucoid strain FRD (DeVries and Ohman, 1994). A 300-bp *algT* antisense

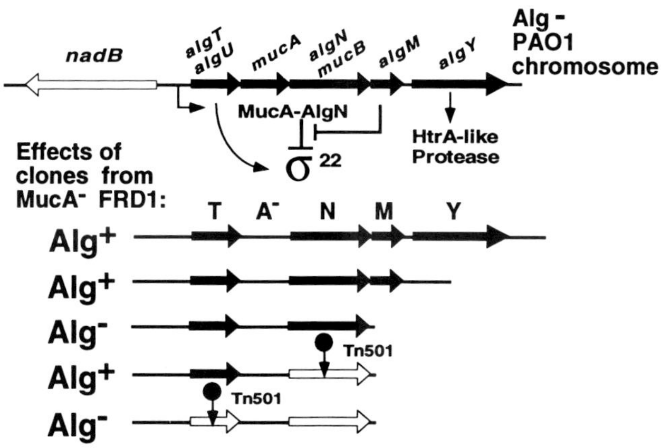

Figure 6. Effect of plasmids containing fragments of the *algT* gene cluster from Alg⁺ strain FRD1 on the alginate-producing phenotype in strain PAO1. Shown is the chromosome of Alg⁻ strain PAO1, which is the *algT mucA algN algM algY* wild type (with alternative designations also shown). The current model suggests that MucA and AlgN proteins antagonize AlgT (σ^{22}) activity and that this is modulated by AlgM. Plasmid-borne DNA fragments from Alg⁺ strain FRD1 (*mucA)* carrying *algT- - -algN-algM-algY* or *algT - - - algN-algM* conferred the Alg⁺ phenotype on PAO1 unless *algM* was removed, thus providing evidence that *algM* encodes a positive regulator. Plasmids carrying *algT - - - algN* did not confer the Alg⁺ phenotype unless *algN* was inactivated, suggesting that *algN* encodes a negative regulator of alginate production.

RNA probe of *algT* was used in hybridizations with RNA from strains containing wild-type *algT* and mutant alleles (*algT18*, *algT29*). A strong band representing *algT* transcripts was observed in the Alg⁺ strain, whereas mutants with the *algT18* and *algT29* alleles showed a four- to fivefold reduction in the accumulation of *algT* transcripts. Likewise, a plasmid-borne *algT-cat* transcriptional fusion was about 3-fold less active in the *algT* missense mutant backgrounds and 20-fold less active in an *algT*::Tn*501* null strain as compared with the mucoid background of strain FRD (DeVries and Ohman, 1994). This suggests that AlgT autoregulates *algT* transcription (see Fig. 4). The RNase protection assay showed that *algT* also controls transcription of the adjacent gene, *algN*. This is consistent with the possibility of an operon containing *algT-mucA-algN-algM* and possibly *algY,* where AlgT acts as an alternative sigma factor for expression of its own promoter (DeVries and Ohman, 1994). Recently, it was shown that AlgT interacts directly with RNA polymerase core as a sigma factor to activate the *algT* promoter (Hershberger et al., 1995).

ANALYSIS OF AlgT-DEPENDENT PROMOTERS

The initiation site of *algT* transcription was determined by primer extension analysis, and a major band was detected starting at about 54 nucleotides upstream of the predicted translation initiation codon of *algT*. The extension product from the *algT* transcript was not readily detected in an *algT* missense mutant, which was consistent with the results obtained in the RNase protection and *algT-cat* fusion assays (DeVries and Ohman, 1994).

The upstream region preceding the transcriptional initiation site of *algT* showed little similarity to the consensus −10 (TATAATG) or −35 (TTGACA) regions in promoters recognized by RNA polymerase containing an *E. coli*-like vegetative σ^{70}. However, the region is similar to promoters recognized by σ^{E} (Erickson and Gross, 1989; Lonetto et al., 1994). An alignment of the σ^{E}-dependent promoters and the promoter (P1) of *algT* showed a match in the −10 (TCTNA) and −35 (GAACTT) regions (Fig. 7). Based on sequence analysis, *algT* may have a second promoter (P2) further upstream (Fig. 7). A recent transcriptional analysis of *algR, algB,* and *algD* revealed a hierarchy of alginate gene expression under *algT* control (Wozniak and Ohman, 1994). In FRD strains containing an *algT*::Tn*501* mutation, transcription from *algD* was undetectable, suggesting that the *algD* promoter also requires AlgT(AlgU) as a sigma factor as well as for expression of the regulators AlgR and AlgB (see Fig. 4). An examination of the *algR* and *algD* promoters shows that they also bear resemblance to the *algT* promoter (Fig. 7). However, this similarity in the *algC* and *algB* promoter is less striking. A transcriptional start (+1) for *algB* starts 300 bp upstream of the ATG initiating AlgB translation (Wozniak and Ohman, 1993) and defines a promoter (P*algB*) which has a −10/−35 region that by its sequence appears to be a σ^{70} promoter. Based on sequence and gel shift analyses, there is also an integration host factor binding site overlapping this promoter which plays a role in its regulation (Wozniak and Ohman, 1993). P*algB* shows a two- to threefold stimulation under Alg^{+} conditions as measured by a *cat* transcriptional fusion (i.e., CAT/intracellular protein) on a low-copy-number (IncP1) vector (Wozniak and Ohman, 1993). DNA upstream of the *Eco*RI site is required for complementation of an *algB* chromosomal mutation, and so P*algB* is apparently important for expression of AlgB. Thus, the control of AlgT on *algB* expression may be indirect (shown as a dashed arrow in Fig. 4).

σ^{E} Dependent Promoters in *E. coli*

```
rpoH P3    CTTGCATTGAACTTGTGGATAAAATCACGGTCTGATAAAACAGT
htrA P     TTTAGTTCGAACTTCAGGCTATAAAACGAATCTGAAGAACACAG
rpoE P2    GCGTTACGGAACTTTACAAAAACGAGACACTCTAACCCTT
Consensus:         -35                   -10
                 GAACTT                 TCTNA
```

AlgT Dependent Promoters in *P. aeruginosa*

```
algT P1    GGAGGGGAGAACTTTTGCAAGA-AGCCCGAGTCTATCTTGGCAAG
algT P2    TAGTGCTGGAACTTTCTTAGAC-GCATCGGTTCCAAAGCAGGATG
algR P     GACTTGGGGCACTTTTCGGGCCTAAAGCGAGTCTCAGCGTCGAGC
algD P     AACGGCCGGAACTTCCCTCGCAGAGAAAACATCCTATCACCG
algC P      TCTTCAGGAACTCGGCGGGCA-ACGCACTGCCAAACCCCCTG
algB P      AATAAAAACACTTTTAATTCA-ATAAGTTATAAAACAACCCAGGTAG
Consensus:         -35                     -10
                 GAACTT                   TCTNA
```

Figure 7. Alignment of σ^{E}-dependent promoters in *E. coli* and AlgT-dependent promoters in *P. aeruginosa*. Note that both appear to utilize the same consensus −10 and −35 promoter sequences.

AlgR AND AlgB CONTROL OF THE ALGINATE BIOSYNTHETIC (*algD*) OPERON

Located at 9 min on the chromosome are the alginate regulatory genes *algR* (*algR1*), *algQ* (*algR2*), and *algP* (*algR3*), and at about 13 min is *algB*, all of which are required for optimal expression of the *algD* operon (for review, see May et al. [1991]). AlgT is required for the transcription of *algB* and *algR* (Wozniak and Ohman, 1991, 1993, 1994). Transcription of *algD* in *P. aeruginosa* was recently analyzed with a low-copy-number, plasmid-borne *algD-cat* operon fusion and by primer extension to the transcription initiation site (366 nucleotides upstream of the ATG translation codon) (Wozniak and Ohman, 1994). In defined *algB*::Tn*501* and *algR*::Sm^r (i.e., streptomycin resistance cartridge) insertion mutants, *algD* expression was reduced 28- and 17-fold, respectively. Thus, the regulatory genes *algT, algR,* and *algB* are all required for *algD* transcription. Initiation of *algR* transcription was absent in *algT* mutants but unaffected in *algB*::Tn*501* and *algR*::Sm^r strains. Thus, neither AlgB nor AlgR appears to be required for autoexpression or alloexpression (Wozniak and Ohman, 1994). The *algR* gene product has been shown to be directly involved in the binding of *algD* upstream sequences (Kato and Chakrabarty, 1991; Mohr et al., 1992). Although *algB* positively regulates *algD* expression (Wozniak and Ohman, 1991), it has not been possible to show a direct interaction of AlgB with the *algD* promoter (Wozniak and Ohman, 1994).

AlgR and AlgB are both response regulators of the two-component regulatory superfamily, which serve as signal transduction systems in bacteria and contain a conserved N-terminal domain typical of response regulators (Hoch and Silhavy, 1995). AlgR has a unique C-terminal domain (Deretic et al., 1989), whereas AlgB belongs to the NtrC subfamily (Wozniak and Ohman, 1991). A sensory component interacting with AlgR, commonly present in other two-component systems, has not been positively identified. However, immediately downstream of *algB* is *algK,* which encodes the cognate histidine protein kinase (Ma and Wozniak, 1995). The conserved amino acid residues of AlgK include a His in the known autophosphorylation domain and the conserved N-(27 amino acids)-DXGXG-(23 amino acids)-GXG in the carboxy terminus. Thus, AlgK is probably an environmental sensor for AlgB (Ma and Wozniak, 1995) (see Fig. 4).

CONCLUSIONS

Regulation of the alginate biosynthetic (*algD*) gene cluster in *P. aeruginosa* appears to be remarkably complex, involving an alternate sigma factor (AlgT) with its control elements (MucA, AlgN, AlgM, AlgY), other regulators (AlgP, AlgQ), two sets of response regulators (AlgR, AlgB) with at least one sensor kinase (AlgK), and also the integration host factor protein. Although expression of alginate genes is involved in pathogenesis (pulmonary infection of CF patients), it is certain that this complex regulon evolved as a stress-response system for more general environmental stimuli. AlgT(AlgU) is a member of a new family (ECF) of alternative sigma factors that appear to play a role in the regulation of extracytoplasmic functions, and alginate production certainly falls into this category. The complexity and nature of the components involved also suggest that alginate biosynthesis may be part of a global stress sensory system. Interestingly, the gene organization in the ECF subfamily is often conserved in nature, suggesting a common mechanism of interaction between the sigma factor and its control elements. Future studies to discern the nature of the interactions between AlgT and its control elements may have broad application to the different systems.

Acknowledgments. We thank the Molecular Resources Center of the University of Tennessee, Memphis, for oligonucleotide synthesis and DNA sequence analysis. This work was supported by Public Health Service grant AI-19146 from the National Institute of Allergy and Infectious Diseases (D.E.O.) and in part by Veterans Administration Medical Research Funds (D.E.O.).

REFERENCES

Chitnis, C. E., and D. E. Ohman. 1990. Cloning of *Pseudomonas aeruginosa algG,* which controls alginate structure. *J. Bacteriol.* **172:**2894–2900.

Chitnis, C. E., and D. E. Ohman. 1993. Genetic analysis of the alginate biosynthetic gene cluster of *Pseudomonas aeruginosa* shows evidence of an operonic structure. *Mol. Microbiol.* **8:**583–590.

Chu, L., T. B. May, A. M. Chakrabarty, and T. K. Misra. 1991. Nucleotide sequence and expression of the *algE* gene involved in alginate biosynthesis by *Pseudomonas aeruginosa. Gene* **107:**1–10.

Coyne, M. J., Jr., K. S. Russell, C. L. Coyle, and J. B. Goldberg. 1994. The *Pseudomonas aeruginosa algC* gene encodes phosphoglucomutase, required for the synthesis of a complete lipopolysaccharide core. *J. Bacteriol.* **176:**3500–3507.

Deretic, V., R. Dikshit, M. Konyecsni, A. M. Chakrabarty, and T. K. Misra. 1989. The *algR* gene, which regulates mucoidy in *Pseudomonas aeruginosa,* belongs to a class of environmentally responsive genes. *J. Bacteriol.* **171:**1278–1283.

Deretic, V., M. J. Schurr, J. C. Boucher, and D. W. Martin. 1994. Conversion of *Pseudomonas aeruginosa* to mucoidy in cystic fibrosis: environmental stress and regulation of bacterial virulence by alternate sigma factors. *J. Bacteriol.* **176:**2773–2780.

DeVries, C. A., D. J. Hassett, J. L. Flynn, and D. E. Ohman. 1995. Genetic linkage in *Pseudomonas aeruginosa* of *algT* and *nadB:* mutation in *nadB* does not affect NAD biosynthesis or alginate production. *Gene* **156:**63–67.

DeVries, C. A., and D. E. Ohman. 1994. Mucoid-to-nonmucoid conversion in alginate-producing *Pseudomonas aeruginosa* often results from spontaneous mutations in *algT,* encoding a putative alternative sigma factor, and shows evidence for autoregulation. *J. Bacteriol.* **176:**6677–6687.

Erickson, J. W., and C. A. Gross. 1989. Identification of the σ^E subunit of *Escherichia coli* RNA polymerase: a second alternate σ factor involved in high-temperature gene expression. *Genes Dev.* **3:**1462–1471.

Flynn, J. L., and D. E. Ohman. 1988a. Cloning of genes from mucoid *Pseudomonas aeruginosa* which control spontaneous conversion to the alginate production phenotype. *J. Bacteriol.* **170:**1452–1460.

Flynn, J. L., and D. E. Ohman. 1988b. Use of a gene replacement cosmid vector for cloning alginate conversion genes from mucoid and nonmucoid *Pseudomonas aeruginosa* strains: *algS* controls expression of *algT. J. Bacteriol.* **170:**3228–3236.

Franklin, M. J., C. E. Chitnis, P. Gacesa, A. Sonesson, D. C. White, and D. E. Ohman. 1994. *Pseudomonas aeruginosa* AlgG is a polymer level alginate C5-mannuronan epimerase. *J. Bacteriol.* **176:**1821–1830.

Franklin, M. J., and D. E. Ohman. 1993. Identification of *algF* in the alginate biosynthetic gene cluster of *Pseudomonas aeruginosa* which is required for alginate acetylation. *J. Bacteriol.* **175:**5057–5065.

Franklin, M. J., and D. E. Ohman. 1996. Identification of *algI* and *algJ* in the *Pseudomonas aeruginosa* alginate biosynthetic gene cluster which are required for alginate O acetylation. *J. Bacteriol.* **178:**2186–2195.

Goldberg, J. B., W. L. Gorman, J. L. Flynn, and D. E. Ohman. 1993. A mutation in *algN* permits transactivation of alginate production by *algT* in *Pseudomonas* species. *J. Bacteriol.* **175:**1303–1308.

Govan, J. R. W., and G. S. Harris. 1986. *Pseudomonas aeruginosa* and cystic fibrosis: unusual bacterial adaptation and pathogenesis. *Microbiol. Sci.* **3:**302–308.

Hershberger, C. D., R. W. Ye, M. R. Parsek, Z.-D. Xie, and A. M. Chakrabarty. 1995. The *algT* (*algU*) gene of *Pseudomonas aeruginosa,* a key regulator involved in alginate biosynthesis, encodes an alternative sigma factor (σ^E). *Proc. Natl. Acad. Sci. USA* **92:**7941–7945.

Hoch, J. A., and T. J. Silhavy (ed.). 1995. *Two-Component Signal Transduction.* American Society for Microbiology, Washington, D.C.

Kato, J., and A. M. Chakrabarty. 1991. Purification of the regulatory protein AlgR1 and its binding in the far upstream region of the *algD* promoter in *Pseudomonas aeruginosa*. *Proc. Natl. Acad. Sci. USA* **88:**1760–1764.

Lonetto, M., M. Gribskow, and C. A. Gross. 1992. The σ^{70} family: sequence conservation and evolutionary relationships. *J. Bacteriol.* **174:**3843–3849.

Lonetto, M. A., K. L. Brown, K. E. Rudd, and M. J. Buttner. 1994. Analysis of *Streptomyces coelicolor sigE* gene reveals the existence of a subfamily of eubacterial RNA polymerase σ factors involved in the regulation of extracytoplasmic functions. *Proc. Natl. Acad. Sci. USA* **91:**7573–7577.

Ma, S., and D. Wozniak. 1995. Identification of a gene *algK* adjacent to the alginate regulatory gene *algB* in *Pseudomonas aeruginosa* which encodes a putative histidine protein kinase of prokaryotic two-component regulation systems, abstr. B76, p. 178. *Abstr. Annu. Meet. Am. Soc. Microbiol. 1995.*

Maharaj, R., T. B. May, S. K. Wang, and A. M. Chakrabarty. 1993. Sequence of the *alg8* and *alg44* genes involved in the synthesis of alginate by *Pseudomonas aeruginosa*. *Gene* **136:**267–269.

Martin, D. W., M. J. Schurr, M. H. Mudd, and V. Deretic. 1993a. Differentiation of *Pseudomonas aeruginosa* into the alginate-producing form: inactivation of *mucB* causes conversion to mucoidy. *Mol. Microbiol.* **9:**497–506.

Martin, D. W., M. J. Schurr, M. H. Mudd, J. R. W. Govan, B. W. Holloway, and V. Deretic. 1993b. Mechanism of conversion to mucoidy in *Pseudomonas aeruginosa* infecting cystic fibrosis patients. *Proc. Natl. Acad. Sci. USA* **90:**8377–8381.

May, T. B., D. Shinabarger, R. Maharaj, J. Kato, L. Chu, J. D. DeVault, S. Roychoudhury, N. A. Zielinski, A. Berry, R. K. Rothmel, T. K. Misra, and A. M. Chakrabarty. 1991. Alginate synthesis by *Pseudomonas aeruginosa:* a key pathogenic factor in chronic pulmonary infections of cystic fibrosis patients. *Clin. Microbiol. Rev.* **4:**191–206.

McPherson, C., K. Mathee, and D. E. Ohman. Regulation of alginate production in *Pseudomonas aeruginosa* by *algM* and *algY*. Submitted for publication.

Mohr, C. D., J. H. J. Leveau, D. P. Krieg, N. S. Hibler, and V. Deretic. 1992. AlgR-binding sites within the *algD* promoter make up a set of inverted repeats separated by a large intervening segment of DNA. *J. Bacteriol.* **174:**6624–6633.

Mohr, C. D., D. W. Martin, W. M. Konyecsni, J. R. W. Govan, S. Lory, and V. Deretic. 1990. Role of the far-upstream sites of the *algD* promoter and the *algR* and *rpoN* genes in environmental modulation of mucoidy in *Pseudomonas aeruginosa*. *J. Bacteriol.* **172:**6576–6580.

Ohman, D. E., and A. M. Chakrabarty. 1981. Genetic mapping of chromosomal determinants for the production of the exopolysaccharide alginate in a *Pseudomonas aeruginosa* cystic fibrosis isolate. *Infect. Immun.* **33:**142–148.

Rehm, B. H., G. Boheim, J. Tommassen, and U. K. Winkler. 1994. Overexpression of *algE* in *Escherichia coli:* subcellular localization, purification, and ion channel properties. *J. Bacteriol.* **176:**5639–5647.

Roychoudhury, S., T. B. May, J. F. Gill, S. K. Singh, D. S. Feingold, and A. M. Chakrabarty. 1989. Purification and characterization of guanosine diphospho-D-mannose dehydrogenase. A key enzyme in the biosynthesis of alginate by *Pseudomonas aeruginosa*. *J. Biol. Chem.* **264:**9380–9385.

Schiller, N. L., S. R. Monday, C. M. Boyd, N. T. Keen, and D. E. Ohman. 1993. Characterization of the *Pseudomonas aeruginosa* alginate lyase gene (*algL*): cloning, sequencing, and expression in *Escherichia coli*. *J. Bacteriol.* **175:**4780–4789.

Schurr, M. J., D. W. Martin, M. H. Mudd, and V. Deretic. 1994. Gene cluster controlling conversion of alginate-overproducing phenotype in *Pseudomonas aeruginosa:* functional analysis in a heterologous host and role in the instability of mucoidy. *J. Bacteriol.* **176:**3375–3382.

Shinabarger, D., T. B. May, A. Boyd, M. Ghosh, and A. M. Chakrabarty. 1993. Nucleotide sequence and expression of the *Pseudomonas aeruginosa algF* gene controlling acetylation of alginate. *Mol. Microbiol.* **9:**1027–1035.

Wozniak, D. J., and D. E. Ohman. 1991. *Pseudomonas aeruginosa* AlgB, a two-component response regulator of the NtrC family, is required for *algD* transcription. *J. Bacteriol.* **173:**1406–1413.

Wozniak, D. J., and D. E. Ohman. 1993. Involvement of the alginate *algT* gene and integration host factor in the regulation of the *Pseudomonas aeruginosa algB* gene. *J. Bacteriol.* **175:**4145–4153.

Wozniak, D. J., and D. E. Ohman. 1994. Transcriptional analysis of the *Pseudomonas aeruginosa* genes *algR*, *algB*, and *algD* reveals a hierarchy of alginate gene expression which is modulated by *algT*. *J. Bacteriol.* **176:**6007–6014.

Molecular Biology of Pseudomonads
Edited by T. Nakazawa et al.

Chapter 42

Regulation of Elastase and Alkaline Proteinase Gene Expression in *Pseudomonas aeruginosa*

Jun Fukushima, Zhiying You, Minoru Kurata, Susumu Kawamoto, Takashi Shigematsu, and Kenji Okuda

CELL DENSITY-DEPENDENT TRANSCRIPTIONAL REGULATION

Pseudomonas aeruginosa produces high levels of extracellular elastase and alkaline proteinase which play roles in the pathogenesis of *Pseudomonas* infection (Morihara and Homma, 1985). We have developed antibody-based assay systems for determination of elastase, alkaline proteinase, and exotoxin A levels to study the regulatory mechanisms and virulence of strains (in preparation). The elastase structural gene *lasB* (Yamamoto et al., 1988; Fukushima et al., 1989; Bever and Iglewski, 1988) and the alkaline proteinase gene *aprA* (Atsumi et al., 1989; Okuda et al., 1990; Guzzo et al., 1991) have been cloned from *P. aeruginosa,* and the structures of these genes and proteins were investigated. The regulation of *lasB* and *aprA* expression is cell density dependent and relies on a complex regulatory mechanism involving the interaction of small diffusible signal molecules with transcriptional regulator proteins (Gambello and Iglewski, 1991; Jones et al., 1993; Passador et al., 1993; Pearson et al., 1994; Latifi et al., 1995; Winson et al., 1995). The first signal molecule to be purified and chemically characterized from *P. aeruginosa* cell-free supernatants was *N*-(3-oxohexanoyl)-L-homoserine lactone (OHHL; Bainton et al., 1992). OHHL was previously known as the "*lux* autoinducer," since in *Photobacterium (Vibrio) fischeri* it is required for the cell density-dependent activation of the luminescence (*lux*) genes (Meighen, 1991). In this marine symbiont, LuxI directs the synthesis of OHHL which interacts with LuxR so that the LuxR-OHHL complex stimulates transcription of the *lux* operon (*luxICDABE*). This leads to increased levels of LuxI and thus more OHHL, which further activates LuxR, setting up an autoinduction cascade. Since OHHL is freely diffusible in the medium (Kaplan and Greenberg, 1985), the induction of a single cell leads directly to induction of neighboring cells, creating a positive feedback circuit that generates a large and rapid response to the initial stimulus. This mechanism,

Jun Fukushima, Zhiying You, Minoru Kurata, Susumu Kawamoto, Takashi Shigematsu, and Kenji Okuda • Department of Bacteriology, Yokohama City University School of Medicine, 3-9 Fukuura, Kanazawa-ku, Yokohama 236, Japan.

now termed "quorum sensing" (Fuqua et al., 1994), constitutes a chemical communication system which enables the organism to sense its population density and respond accordingly. Quorum sensing systems have been identified in diverse gram-negative bacteria, where they regulate expression of virulence determinants and genes for secondary metabolites and conjugation (for reviews see Fuqua et al. [1994], Swift et al. [1994], and Salmond et al. [1995]).

In *P. aeruginosa* PAO1, two LuxR homologs (LasR [Gambello and Iglewski, 1991; Fukushima et al., 1994] and VsmR [Latifi et al., 1995; Winson et al., 1995]) and two LuxI homologs (LasI [Passador et al., 1993] and VsmI [Latifi et al., 1995; Winson et al., 1995]) have been identified. RhlR, which is 98% identical to VsmR, was described in *P. aeruginosa* DSM2659 (Ochsner et al., 1994). LasI directs the synthesis primarily of *N*-(3-oxododecanoyl)-L-homoserine lactone (OdDHL) (Pearson et al., 1994), while VsmI is responsible for the synthesis of *N*-butanoyl-L-homoserine lactone (BHL) together with small amounts of *N*-hexanoyl-L-homoserine lactone (HHL) (Winson et al., 1995). OHHL is also present in very low concentrations and appears to be generated via LasI (Bainton et al., 1992; Pearson et al., 1994). Both LasR-OdDHL and VsmR-BHL are involved in the regulation of expression of two genes, *lasB* and *aprA*, since mutations in either locus abolish both elastase and alkaline proteinase production. The nature of these regulatory mechanisms has not been fully investigated (Gambello and Iglewski, 1991; Ochsner et al., 1994; Latifi et al., 1995; Winson et al., 1995). We are studying the molecular basis of these regulatory systems.

UPSTREAM SEQUENCES FOR ELASTASE REGULATION

The *lasB* promoter contains a region of dyad symmetry similar to the *Photobacterium fischeri lux* box, a 20-bp palindrome sequence located around –40 from the transcription start site (Fig. 1, region III) which is the target site for LuxR (Gray et al., 1994). A similar *lux* box is found in the *vsmI* (Latifi et al., 1995) promoter region. Thus, in *P. aeruginosa,* it is possible that the *lasB lux* box-like element is the target for both LasR-OdDHL and VsmR-BHL.

To define the autoinducer-mediated transcriptional activation of *lasB,* we constructed a series of transcriptional fusions. Various lengths of *lasB* upstream regions were fused to the chloramphenicol acetyltransferase (CAT) structural gene on a *Pseudomonas* plasmid, pME294 (Itoh et al., 1988). Then *Escherichia coli* transcription terminator (*rrnB*) was introduced to inhibit readthrough transcription from the vector (pMETCAT series; Fig. 2) (Fukushima et al., submitted). First, we analyzed the expression pattern during different growth phases. Transcriptional activity was measured by monitoring CAT activity at certain time points over a growth curve in cells harboring pMET6-4CAT(–212), which contains an upstream promoter sequence (–212 to +123) of the elastase gene fused to the *cat* structural gene at a position corresponding to +124 of *lasB*. When the cells were grown in JD synthetic medium (Jensen et al., 1980) there was a rapid increase in CAT activity until the culture reached late-logarithmic growth phase; the increase stopped in the post-logarithmic phase. These results suggested that the activity of this promoter-operator sequence of the elastase genc depends on the extent of population growth or growth phase. It has been demonstrated that the appearance of elastase activity in culture fluid was maximal in the post-logarithmic phase (Whooley and McLaughlin, 1983) and

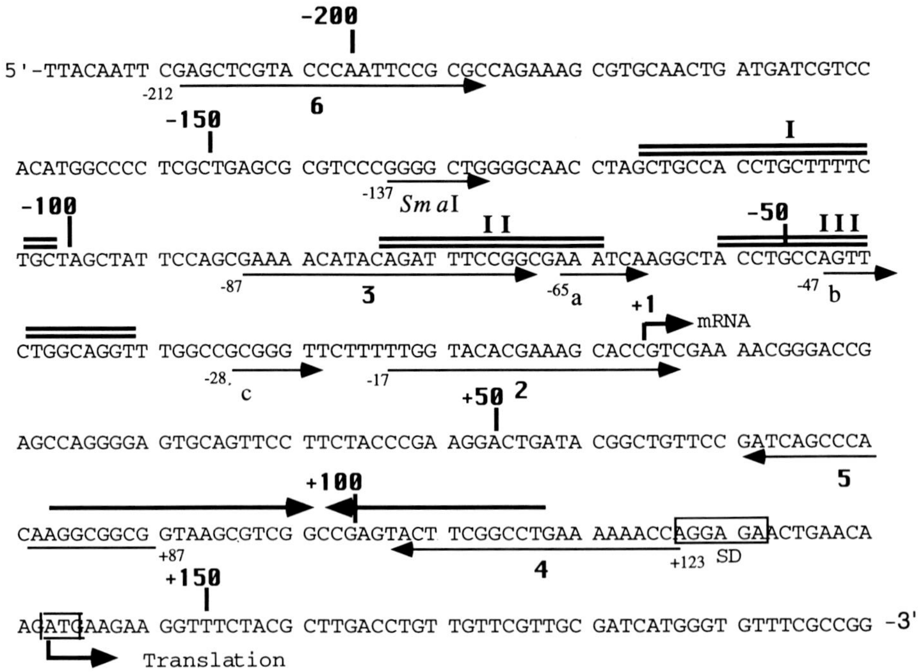

Figure 1. Nucleotide sequence of the 5′ upstream region of *P. aeruginosa* IFO3455 *lasB*. The transcription start site (Mohr et al., 1990) was designated as +1 and the other nucleotides were numbered in relation to it. The Shine-Dalgarno (SD)-like sequence and the translation initiation ATG codon are boxed. A potential stem-loop structure is indicated by convergent overlined half-arrows at position around +100. Regions I and II, which share homology with the *lasA* gene (Freck-O'Donnell and Darzins, 1993) and *aprA* upstream sequences (unpublished observation), and region III, which represents the *lux* box-like sequence, are doubly overlined. Rightward and leftward thin arrows below the nucleotide sequence line represent, respectively, the starting and ending points of each promoter fragment inserted into the CAT vector. Promoter-containing DNA fragments were amplified by PCR using combinations of the rightward three primers (numbers 6, 3, and 2) and the leftward two primers (numbers 5 and 4), which are represented by long thin arrows. The SD sequence containing the *cat* gene was fused to the promoter fragments at a position corresponding to +73 or +124 of *lasB*. Other 5′-deleted fragments (designated by rightward thin arrows marked a, b, and c) were made by BAL 31 exonuclease digestion of the PCR fragment which was generated by using primers 3 and 4. The PCR fragments made by using primers 6 and 4 were also digested by *Sma*I endonuclease, and the promoter-containing fragment (from −137 to +123) was fused to the *cat* gene at a position corresponding to +124 (designated by *Sma*I).

the elastase protein was produced in late- to post-logarithmic phase (Fukushima et al., submitted).

To determine the upstream region required for efficient elastase expression, we used the pMETCAT series plasmids (Fig. 2 and 3) to measure promoter activities. Our findings indicated that the −137 to −88-bp and −65 to −29-bp regions are involved in efficient elastase transcription. The −137 to −88 region includes the sequences (Fig. 1, region I) with similarity to a part of the upstream promoter sequence of *lasB*; the *lasA* gene, which encodes another protease called LasA (Freck-O'Donnell and Darzins, 1993); and an alkaline proteinase gene (our unpublished observation). The –65 to –29 region contains the *lux* box-like element. These two regions may play important roles in *lasB* expression.

Next, we analyzed the enhancement of CAT activity by adding the autoinducers to a culture supernatant of *P. aeruginosa* PAO1 containing various promoter-CAT plasmids. All of the synthetic autoinducers, OHHL, OdDHL, BHL, and HHL, activated elastase gene transcription. BHL seemed to be the most effective for the activation of elastase transcription, and an autoinducer-responsive sequence exists in the region between –65 and –29 bp (unpublished data). Since the –65 to –29-bp region (Fig. 1, III) of the *lasB* promoter contains a *lux* box-like element, we presume that this element is likely to be the target for either or both of the LasR and VsmR transcriptional activators.

The function of the –137 to –88-bp region remains to be elucidated, but it is interesting that in *P. aeruginosa* PAO1, elastase and alkaline proteinase production are all regulated by a cell density-dependent mechanism and small diffusible molecules (Gambello et al., 1993; Latifi et al., 1995).

AUTOINDUCER CASCADE

Gray et al. (1994) previously reported that in the presence of LasR, OdDHL but not OHHL could activate a *lasB*::*lacZ* promoter fusion in an *E. coli* background. However, OHHL can partially restore elastase synthesis in the pleiotropic *P. aeruginosa* mutant PAN067 (Jones et al., 1993; Latifi et al., 1995) and activate a *vsmR vsmI'*::*lux* reporter fusion in *E. coli* (Winson et al., 1995). This discrepancy can now be explained since Pearson et al. (1995) have demonstrated that although OdDHL is able to activate a *lasB*::*lacZ* fusion with functional LasR in *P. aeruginosa,* it does not activate the *lasR* promoter in *P. aeruginosa*. In fact, BHL appears to be necessary for the expression of *lasR* in *P. aeruginosa* (Pearson et al., 1995). Thus it appears that VsmR activates *vsmI* such that BHL (and HHL) is produced, setting up the first autoinduction cascade (Winson et al., 1995). BHL, probably in conjunction with VsmR, activates *lasR,* setting up a second autoinduction cascade which generates OdDHL via LasI (Seed et al., 1995). LasR-OdDHL in turn then activates transcription of *lasB* (Gray et al., 1994). It is likely that the same system contributes to the *aprA* expression. However, there seems to be a discrepancy in that the *lux* box-like sequence is not observed in the *aprA* upstream region. Moreover, since VsmR activates *vsmI* via a *lux* box similar to that located within the *lasB* promoter (Latifi et al., 1995; Winson et al., 1995), it is not apparent why VsmR does not activate the *lasB* promoter directly in a *lasR*-negative background. Clearly there are additional layers of regulatory complexity which remain still to be elucidated.

ALKALINE PROTEINASE REGULATION BY IRON

There are reports on the regulation of alkaline proteinase expression. However, little information is available on the transcriptional regulation of the alkaline proteinase gene. We now know *P. aeruginosa* produces at least four types of proteases including LasA, elastase, LasD, and alkaline proteinase. It is therefore very complicated to attempt to analyze regulation of alkaline proteinase expression by measuring protease activity us-

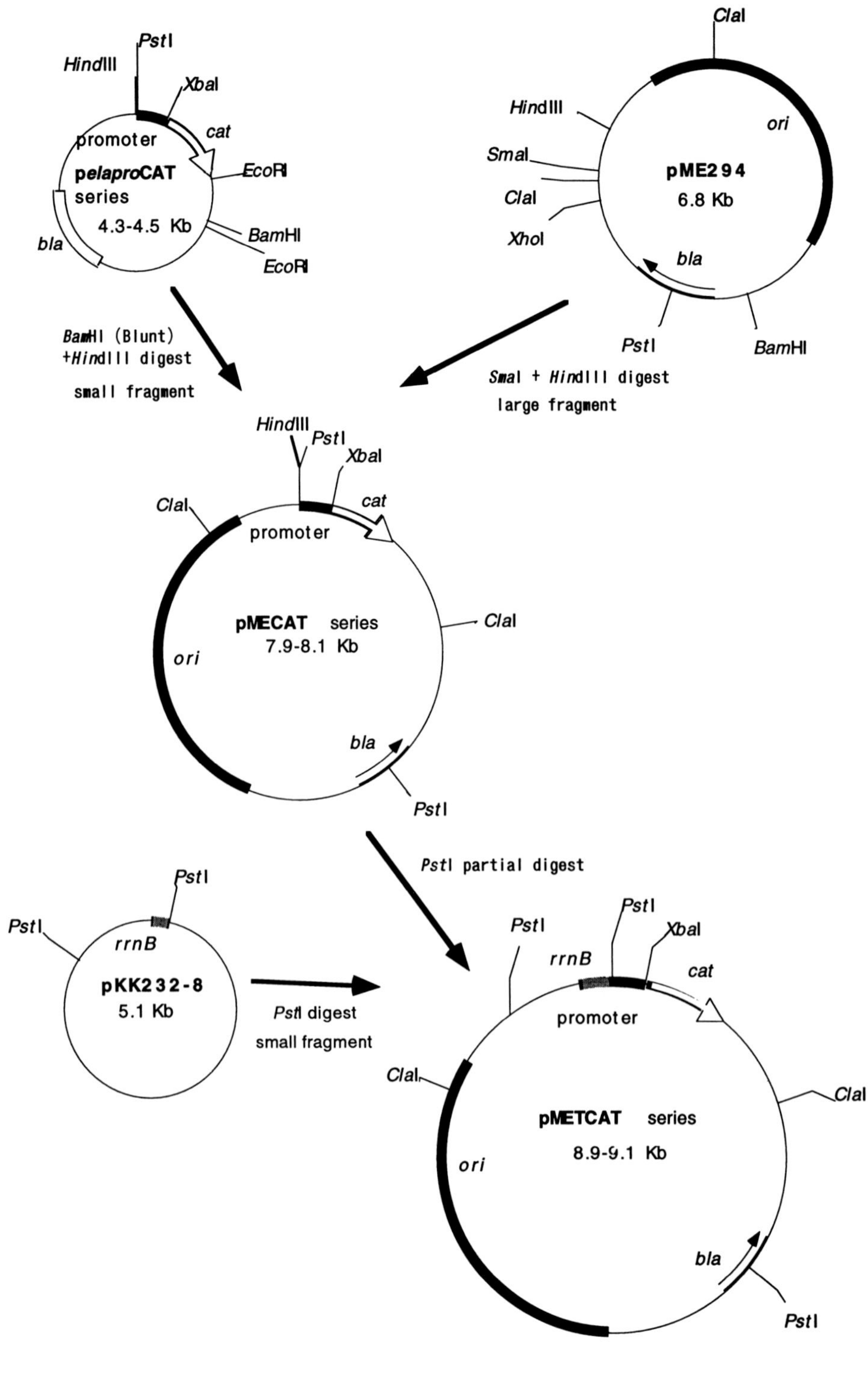
PstI
HindIII
XbaI
cat
promoter
pelaproCAT
series
4.3-4.5 Kb
EcoRI
BamHI
EcoRI
bla
ClaI
HindIII
ori
SmaI
pME294
6.8 Kb
ClaI
XhoI
bla
PstI
BamHI
BamHI (Blunt)
+HindIII digest
small fragment
SmaI + HindIII digest
large fragment
HindIII
PstI
XbaI
ClaI
cat
promoter
pMECAT series
7.9-8.1 Kb
ClaI
ori
bla
PstI
PstI partial digest
PstI
PstI
rrnB
pKK232-8
5.1 Kb
PstI digest
small fragment
PstI
PstI
XbaI
rrnB
cat
promoter
ClaI
ClaI
pMETCAT series
8.9-9.1 Kb
ori
bla
PstI

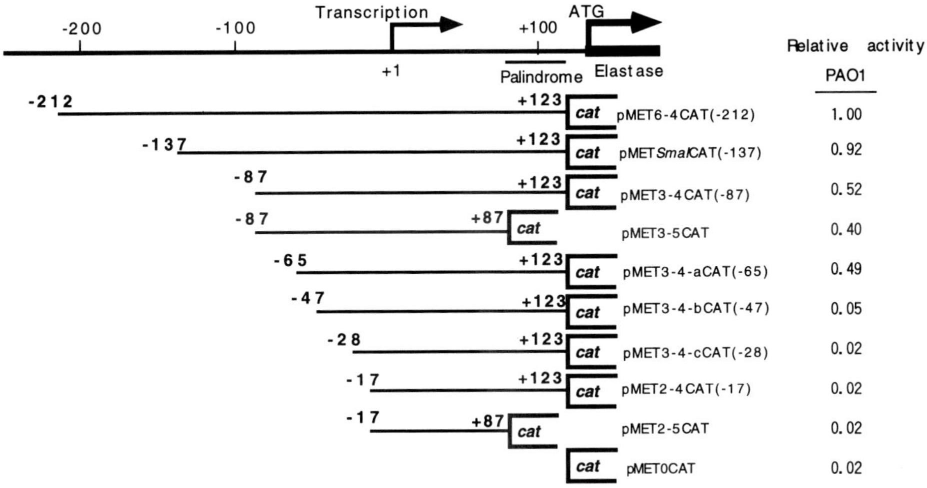

Figure 3. CAT assay of various fragments of the *lasB* fused to the CAT reporter gene: a schematic representation of PCR fragment constructs of the *lasB* upstream region fused to the *cat* reporter gene in pMETCAT. The nucleotide scale is shown with respect to the transcription start site. All constructs, as indicated in the figure, were introduced into *P. aeruginosa* PAO1 cells and sampled for the CAT assay at the same protein content (0.02 μg). The relative CAT activity of the *lasB* promoter constructs is represented in the right column (1.0 value represents the activity of 3.5 nmol/min per μg of protein).

ing complex proteins such as caseine as substrate. For this reason, we have used an immunological enzyme-linked immunosorbent assay (ELISA) system to determine alkaline proteinase protein. One regulatory factor for alkaline proteinase expression is iron availability. Iron has been observed to have a regulatory effect on protease activity expressed in the culture supernatant (Bjorn et al., 1978). Using ELISA assays, primer extension analysis, and Northern (RNA) blotting, we have observed that 10 μM Fe^{2+} completely shuts down alkaline proteinase transcription (manuscript in preparation). In general, a Fur protein-mediated repression mechanism is involved in this type of regulation by iron (for a review see Litwin and Calderwood [1993]). Indeed, a sequence homologous with the Fur repressor binding motif (Fur box) occurs in the region around –50 from the transcription start site of the alkaline proteinase upstream region.

Figure 2. Schematic construction of a series of pMETCAT reporter transcriptional fusions utilizing upstream regions of the *lasB* gene fused to the *cat* reporter gene. PCR products were inserted into the *Pst*I and *Xba*I restriction sites of pCAT-basic (Promega), generating a series of p*elapro*CAT plasmids in *E. coli*. These plasmids were digested with *Bam*HI, blunt-ended, and then digested with *Hin*dIII, providing a fragment containing *lasB-cat* fusions. These fragments were ligated into *Hin*dIII and *Sma*I restriction sites of pME294 (Itoh et al., 1988), generating a series of pMECAT plasmids in *P. aeruginosa* IFO3455. In addition, pKK232-8 (Pharmacia) was digested with *Pst*I, yielding an approximately 1-kb fragment containing the transcription terminator *rrnB*. Insertion of this DNA fragment into the *Pst*I site upstream of the elastase promoter in pMECAT generated the pMETCAT series of *lasB-cat* fusions in *P. aeruginosa* IFO3455. *bla*, β-lactamase gene; *ori*, replication origin and stabilizing region in *P. aeruginosa; cat*, CAT gene.

In addition to the Fur system, we have found an additional locus that affects *aprA* expression. This locus was first identified as an activator region (termed *pvdS*) required for pyoverdin (a siderophore) biosynthesis (Tsuda et al., 1995; Miyazaki et al., 1995). Since *aprA* expression decreased in a *pvdS* mutant isogenic strain of PAO1 at low iron concentrations, PvdS enhances *aprA* transcription (manuscript in preparation). It has been shown that *pvdS* expression is repressed by the Fur repressor itself (Miyazaki et al., 1995; Cunliffe et al., 1995). Iron represses activation factor expression and produces active Fur repressor for *aprA*, resulting in the shutdown of *aprA* expression in a high-iron environment.

SUMMARY

Among the various quorum sensing systems, elastase and alkaline proteinase regulation in *P. aeruginosa* is one of the most complicated. *P. aeruginosa* produces at least four kinds of autoinducers and two types of intracellular receptor-transcription factors. In addition, both Fur and PvdS proteins are responsible for *aprA* regulation, and one more locus in the *lasB* upstream region contributes to efficient expression of elastase. Although autoinducer-mediated regulation has been extensively studied, the role of each member remains unclear. To address this issue, molecular biological and biochemical methodology was introduced. In the first step of this research, we defined the upstream sequences required for efficient elastase transcription and autoinducer-mediated activation by using PCR-cloned and nuclease-digested promoter sequences in a *P. aeruginosa* background. These experiments suggested the hierarchy of transcription factors and autoinducer association; however, they also revealed clearly that additional unknown mechanisms still exist. To identify those systems and the molecular interaction of activation complexes, we are investigating the binding and activation of promoters by using isolated components in in vitro assay systems.

REFERENCES

Atsumi, Y., S. Yamamoto, K. Morihara, J. Fukushima, H. Takeuchi, N. Mizuki, S. Kawamoto, and K. Okuda. 1989. Cloning and expression of the alkaline proteinase gene from *Pseudomonas aeruginosa* IFO3455. *J. Bacteriol.* **171:**5173–5175.

Bainton, N. J., B. W. Bycroft, S. R. Chhabra, P. Stead, L. Gledhill, P. J. Hill, C. E. D. Rees, M. K. Winson, G. P. C. Salmond, G. S. A. B. Stewart, and P. Williams. 1992. A general role for the *lux* autoinducer in bacterial cell signalling: control of antibiotic biosynthesis in *Erwinia*. *Gene* **116:**87–91.

Bever, R. A., and B. H. Iglewski. 1988. Molecular characterization and nucleotide sequence of the *Pseudomonas aeruginosa* elastase structural gene. *J. Bacteriol.* **170:**4309–4314.

Bjorn, M. J., B. H. Iglewski, S. K. Ives, J. C. Sadoff, and M. L. Vasil. 1978. Effect of iron on yields of exotoxin A in cultures of *Pseudomonas aeruginosa* PA103. *Infect. Immun.* **19:**785–791.

Cunliffe, H. E., T. R. Merriman, and I. L. Lamont. 1995. Cloning and characterization of *pvdS*, a gene required for pyoverdine synthesis in *Pseudomonas aeruginosa:* PvdS is probably an alternative sigma factor. *J. Bacteriol.* **177:**2744–2750.

Freck-O'Donnell, L. C., and A. Darzins. 1993. *Pseudomonas aeruginosa lasA* gene: determination of the transcription start point and analysis of the promoter/regulatory region. *Gene* **129:**113–117.

Fukushima, J., T. Ishiwata, M. Kurata, Z. You, and K. Okuda. 1994. Intracellular receptor-type transcription factor, LasR, contains a highly conserved amphipathic region which precedes the putative helix-turn-helix DNA binding motif. *Nucleic Acids Res.* **22:**3706–3707.

Fukushima, J., T. Ishiwata, Z. You, T. Ishii, T. Shigematsu, M. Kurata, S. Chikumaru-Fujita, B. W. Bycroft, P. Williams, G. S. A. B. Stewart, K. Morihara, S. Kawamoto, and K. Okuda. Dissection of the operator region and evaluation of *N*-acylhomoserine lactone mediated transcriptional regulation of elastase expression in *Pseudomonas aeruginosa*. Submitted for publication.

Fukushima, J., S. Yamamoto, K. Morihara, Y. Atsumi, H. Takeuchi, S. Kawamoto, and K. Okuda. 1989. Structural gene and complete amino acid sequence of *Pseudomonas aeruginosa* IFO 3455 elastase. *J. Bacteriol.* **171:**1698–1704.

Fuqua, W. C., S. C. Winans, and E. P. Greenberg. 1994. Quorum sensing in bacteria: LuxR-LuxI family of cell density responsive transcriptional activators. *J. Bacteriol.* **176:**269–275.

Gambello, M. J., and B. H. Iglewski. 1991. Cloning and characterization of the *Pseudomonas aeruginosa lasR* gene, a transcriptional activator of elastase expression. *J. Bacteriol.* **173:**3000–3009.

Gambello, M. J., S. Kaye, and B. H. Iglewski. 1993. LasR of *Pseudomonas aeruginosa* is a transcriptional activator of the alkaline protease gene (*apr*) and an enhancer of exotoxin A expression. *Infect. Immun.* **61:**1180–1184.

Gray, K. M., L. Passador, B. H. Iglewski, and E. P. Greenberg. 1994. Interchangeability and specificity of components from the quorum-sensing regulation systems of *Vibrio fischeri* and *Pseudomonas aeruginosa*. *J. Bacteriol.* **176:**3076–3080.

Guzzo, J., J.-M. Pages, F. Duong, A. Lazdunski, and M. Murgier. 1991. *Pseudomonas aeruginosa* alkaline protease: evidence for secretion genes and study of secretion mechanism. *J. Bacteriol.* **173:**5290–5297.

Itoh, Y., K. Soldati, T. Leisinger, and D. Haas. 1988. Low- and intermediate-copy-number cloning vectors based on the *Pseudomonas* plasmid pVS1. *Antonie Leeuwenhoek* **54:**567–573.

Jensen, S. E., I. T. Fecycz, and J. N. Campbell. 1980. Nutritional factors controlling exocellular protease production by *Pseudomonas aeruginosa*. *J. Bacteriol.* **144:**844–847.

Jones, S., B. Yu, N. J. Bainton, M. Birdsall, B. W. Bycroft, S. R. Chhabra, A. J. R. Cox, P. Golby, P. J. Reeves, S. Stephens, M. K. Winson, G. P. C. Salmond, G. S. A. B. Stewart, and P. Williams. 1993. The *lux* autoinducer regulates the production of exoenzyme virulence determinants in *Erwinia carotovora* and *Pseudomonas aeruginosa*. *EMBO J.* **12:**2477–2482.

Kaplan, H. B., and E. P. Greenberg. 1985. Diffusion of autoinducer is involved in regulation of the *Vibrio fischeri* luminescence system. *J. Bacteriol.* **163:**1210–1214.

Latifi, A., M. K. Winson, M. Foglino, B. W. Bycroft, G. S. A. B. Stewart, A. Lazdunski, and P. Williams. 1995. Multiple homologues of LuxR and LuxI control expression of virulence determinants and secondary metabolites through quorum sensing in *Pseudomonas aeruginosa* PAO1. *Mol. Microbiol.* **17:**333–343.

Litwin, C. M., and S. B. Calderwood. 1993. Role of iron in regulation of virulence genes. *Clin. Microbiol. Rev.* **6:**137–149.

Meighen, E. A. 1991. Molecular biology of bacterial bioluminescence. *Microbiol. Rev.* **55:**123–142.

Miyazaki, H., H. Kato, T. Nakazawa, and M. Tsuda. 1995. A positive regulatory gene, *pvdS*, for expression of pyoverdin biosynthetic genes in *Pseudomonas aeruginosa* PAO. *Mol. Gen. Genet.* **248:**17–24.

Mohr, C. D., L. Rust, A. M. Albus, B. H. Iglewski, and V. Deretic. 1990. Expression patterns of genes encoding elastase and controlling mucoidity: co-ordinate regulation of two virulence factors in *Pseudomonas aeruginosa* isolates from cystic fibrosis. *Mol. Microbiol.* **4:**2103–2110.

Morihara, K., and J. Y. Homma. 1985. *Pseudomonas* protease, p. 41–79. *In* I. A. Holder (ed.), *Bacterial Enzymes and Virulence*. CRC Press, Boca Raton, Fla.

Ochsner, U. A., A. K. Koch, A. Fiechter, and J. Reiser. 1994. Isolation and characterization of a regulatory gene affecting rhamnolipid biosurfactant synthesis in *Pseudomonas aeruginosa*. *J. Bacteriol.* **176:**2044–2054.

Okuda, K., K. Morihara, Y. Atsumi, H. Takeuchi, S. Kawamoto, H. Kawasaki, K. Suzuki, and J. Fukushima. 1990. Complete nucleotide sequence of the structural gene for alkaline proteinase from *Pseudomonas aeruginosa*. *Infect. Immun.* **58:**4083–4088.

Passador, L., J. M. Cook, M. J. Gambello, L. Rust, and B. H. Iglewski. 1993. Expression of *Pseudomonas aeruginosa* virulence gene requires cell-to-cell communication. *Science* **260:**1127–1130.

Pearson, J. P., K. M. Gray, L. Passador, K. D. Tucker, A. Eberhard, B. H. Iglewski, and E. P. Greenberg. 1994. Structure of the autoinducter required for expression of *Pseudomonas aeruginosa* virulence genes. *Proc. Natl. Acad. Sci. USA* **91:**197–201.

Pearson, J. P., L. Passador, B. H. Iglewski, and E. P. Greenberg. 1995. A second *N*-acylhomoserine lactone signal produced by *Pseudomonas aeruginosa*. *Proc. Natl. Acad. Sci. USA* **92:**1490–1494.

Salmond, G. P. C., B. W. Bycroft, G. S. A. B. Stewart, and P. Williams. 1995. The bacterial "enigma": cracking the code of cell-cell communication. *Mol. Microbiol.* **16:**615–624.

Seed, P. C., L. Passador, and B. H. Iglewski. 1995. Activation of the *Pseudomonas aeruginosa lasI* gene by LasR and *Pseudomonas* autoinducer PAI: an autoinduction regulatory hierarchy. *J. Bacteriol.* **177:**654–659.

Swift, S., N. J. Bainton, and M. K. Winson. 1994. Gram-negative bacterial communication by *N*-acyl-homoserine lactones: a universal language? *Trends Microbiol.* **2:**193–198.

Tsuda, M., H. Miyazaki, and T. Nakazawa. 1995. Genetic and physical mapping of genes involved in pyoverdin production in *Pseudomonas aeruginosa. J. Bacteriol.* **177:**423–431.

Whooley, M. A., and A. J. McLaughlin. 1983. The proton motive force in *Pseudomonas aeruginosa* and its relationship to exoprotease production. *J. Gen. Microbiol.* **129:**989–996.

Winson, M. K., M. Camara, A. Latifi, M. Foglino, S. R. Chhabra, M. Daykin, M. Bally, V. Chapon, G. P. C. Salmond, B. W. Bycroft, A. Lazdunski, G. S. A. B. Stewart, and P. Williams. 1995. Multiple *N*-acyl-L-homoserine lactone signal molecules regulate production of virulence determinants and secondary metabolites in *Pseudomonas aeruginosa. Proc. Natl. Acad. Sci. USA* **92:**9427–9431.

Yamamoto, S., J. Fukushima, Y. Atsumi, Y. Takeuchi, Y., S. Kawamoto, K. Okuda, and K. Morihara. 1988. Cloning and characterization of elastase structural gene from *Pseudomonas aeruginosa* IFO 3455. *Biochem. Biophys. Res. Commun.* **152:**1117–1122.

Section IX

PLANT-BACTERIAL INTERACTIONS

Molecular Biology of Pseudomonads
Edited by T. Nakazawa et al.

Chapter 43

Bacterial Ice Nucleation as a Tool in the Study of the Determinants of Epiphytic Fitness in Bacterial Plant Pathogens

Steven E. Lindow

EPIPHYTIC BACTERIA AND THEIR ADAPTATIONS TO LIFE ON LEAVES

The leaves and flowers of healthy plants are normally colonized by large numbers of bacteria, including plant-pathogenic bacteria. Fluorescent *Pseudomonas* species, particularly strains of *Pseudomonas syringae,* are often prominent constituents of the epiphytic microflora (Gross et al., 1983; Hirano and Upper, 1983, 1990; Lindow, 1982, 1985; Lindow et al., 1978a; Lindow et al., 1978b). Nearly all plant-pathogenic bacteria, and particularly *P. syringae,* occur as epiphytes before initiating disease in plants (Hirano and Upper, 1983, 1990). In fact, initiation of disease by plant-pathogenic bacteria is unlikely unless relatively large epiphytic population sizes of these bacteria develop. The probability of disease has been shown to be proportional to the logarithm of the epiphytic population size of *P. syringae* (Rouse et al., 1985). Thus individual cells of pathogens such as *P. syringae* appear to have a low but finite probability of initiating infection. For this reason, factors that influence the epiphytic population size of phytopathogenic bacteria are important in determining the likelihood of disease.

The relatively hostile nature of the leaf surface environment has probably selected for bacterial adaptations, so-called epiphytic fitness traits, that are required for bacterial growth and/or survival in this habitat (Beattie and Lindow, 1995). The leaf surface is subject to relatively high fluxes of UV radiation, which can be deleterious to all microorganisms (Burrage, 1971, 1976). The leaf surface also frequently undergoes rapid changes in the availability of free moisture, often wetting and drying several times in each day (Burrage, 1971, 1976). Nutrients required for epiphytic growth of bacteria on leaves are often limiting (Morgan and Tukey, 1964; Morris and Rouse, 1985; Tukey, 1970; Wilson and Lindow, 1994a, 1994b). Unfortunately, little is known of the adaptive traits that bacteria have evolved to exploit leaf surfaces. While there has been considerable conjecture as to traits that might contribute to colonization of leaves (Dickinson, 1986; Henis

Steven E. Lindow • Department of Environmental Science, Policy, and Management, University of California, Berkeley, California 94720-3110.

and Bashan, 1986; Beattie and Lindow, 1995; Lindow, 1991), relatively few critical tests of the contribution of particular traits to epiphytic fitness have been reported.

In one such study, mobility was found to benefit the survival of *P. syringae* strains on leaves (Haefele and Lindow, 1987). A significantly higher percentage of the cells of a motile parental strain and a motile revertant strain than of a nonmotile mutant were recovered from leaves that were surface sterilized with UV radiation (Haefele and Lindow, 1987). The population size of the nonmotile mutant strain decreased more than that of the motile strain when leaves were exposed to prolonged dry conditions. These observations suggest that motile cells have an advantage over nonmotile cells on leaf surfaces, since they can find refuges in or on the leaf where they can avoid physical environmental stresses. In contrast, the production of pyoverdine siderophores by *P. syringae* strains appeared not to be a major epiphytic fitness factor. A siderophore-producing parental strain and several nonproducing mutants exhibited similar population sizes after growth under different conditions on leaves both in the greenhouse and under field conditions (Loper and Lindow, 1987). The production of the plant growth regulator 3-indoleacetic acid (IAA) appeared to make a minor contribution to the fitness of *P. syringae* pv. savastanoi. Strains of this pathogen which were cured of a plasmid carrying IAA biosynthetic genes exhibited slightly less ability than the parental strain to survive in mixtures for long periods of time in gall tissues (Silverstone et al., 1993). It is possible that other plasmid-borne genes in addition to those conferring IAA biosynthesis also contributed to the altered behavior of the mutant and parental strains. The effects of most bacterial phenotypes on epiphytic fitness have not, however, been studied.

There is strong evidence that many epiphytic fitness traits are plant inducible. For example, strains of *P. syringae* exhibit considerable phenotypic differences when grown in laboratory cultures and on leaves. The survival of *P. syringae* cells when applied to the surface of plants in the greenhouse or in the field and incubated under dry conditions was substantially greater when the cells were first grown on plants than when they were grown in any of several different liquid or solid culture media (Wilson and Lindow, 1993). These results suggest that when *P. syringae* is grown on plants rather than in culture, it expresses a subset of genes which contribute to its ability to survive stresses associated with the leaf surface environment. The use of random genomic *lux* fusions revealed that 2% of the genes of *P. syringae* are expressed on plants but not in culture, and vice versa (Cirvilleri and Lindow, 1994). Some of these plant-inducible genes likely contribute to epiphytic fitness and are probably associated with the considerable phenotypic plasticity seen in this species (Wilson and Lindow, 1993). An approach to identifying potential fitness genes or those that are not expressed in culture is therefore needed.

BACTERIAL ICE NUCLEATION

Many strains of *P. syringae*, as well as some strains of *Pseudomonas fluorescens*, *Erwinia herbicola*, *Pseudomonas viridiflava*, and *Xanthomonas campestris*, are able to catalyze the formation of ice at temperatures as warm as −2°C (Gurian-Sherman and Lindow, 1993; Lindow, 1983; Lindow et al., 1982). In all ice nucleation-active (Ice$^+$) bacterial species, ice nucleation activity is conferred by a single gene which encodes a unique membrane-associated protein of about 130 kDa in mass (Lindow et al., 1989; Warren and Corotto, 1989; Warren and Wolber, 1991; Wolber, 1992; Wolber and Warren, 1989). As much as 85% of the internal portion of ice nucleation genes encodes a highly conserved, tandemly repeated 48-amino-acid sequence (Warren and Wolber, 1991). Molecular modeling of the three-dimensional structure of this family of proteins reveals that they likely form extended structures composed largely of paired β-hairpins (Kajava and Lindow, 1993). Each 48-amino-acid repeating unit is proposed to form three paired β-hairpins which alternate in position on opposite sides of the longitudinal axis of the protein. The ice proteins are thought to be nearly planar and to interact with the surface constituents of the outer membrane of bacteria (Kajava and Lindow, 1993). The surface of the repetitive units apparently provides numerous hydrogen-bonding groups that orient water molecules into a structure very close to that of ice (Kajava and Lindow, 1993). Ice proteins also can apparently form aggregates of unlimited size by antiparallel interdigitation of the 48-amino-acid repeating units (Kajava and Lindow, 1993); such large aggregates are apparently required for ice nucleation activity at temperatures above −10°C (Burke and Lindow, 1990; Govindarajan and Lindow, 1988). Thus, ice nucleation activity apparently is conferred by these unique proteins that may have evolved specifically for this phenotype.

The bacterial ice nucleation phenotype is useful in at least two ways in exploring epiphytic fitness traits in bacteria. The supercooling temperature of a leaf, the coldest temperature to which a leaf can be cooled before ice nucleation occurs, increases proportionally with the logarithm of the number of Ice$^+$ bacteria. For example, as the population size of an Ice$^+$ *P. syringae* strain increases from 10^2 to 10^6 cells per leaf, the supercooling temperature increases from about −4 to about −2°C (Hirano et al., 1985; Lindow, 1993) (Fig. 1). Thus measurements of the supercooling temperature of leaves are an easy way to estimate the population size of Ice$^+$ bacteria on a given leaf. Because the population sizes of Ice$^+$ and other bacteria vary greatly from leaf to leaf, accurate estimates of mean bacterial population size require measurement of bacterial numbers on large num-

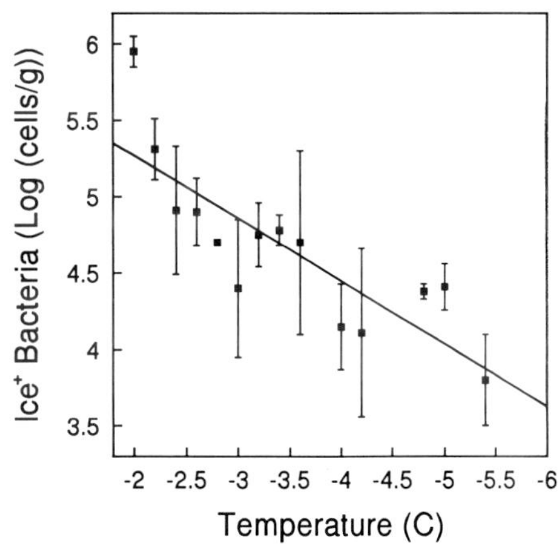

Figure 1. Relationship between the population size of *P. syringae* Cit7 on spinach leaves and the supercooling temperature of the leaves. The vertical bars represent the standard error of the determination of mean log-transformed bacterial population size normalized per gram (fresh weight) of leaf. The line represents the regression $y = 0.41x + 6.09$ ($r^2 = 0.68$; $p = 0.0003$).

bers of individual leaves (Hirano et al., 1982). Measurements of the supercooling temperature of leaves allow estimates of bacterial population size to be made on a large number of leaves and therefore provide a good estimate of the mean population size of bacteria (Lindow, 1993).

The ice nucleation gene from *P. syringae* is also useful as a reporter gene. In order to be useful for bacteria growing on leaves or in other natural habitats, a reporter gene must confer a phenotype that is easy to quantify, has little or no background activity, and can be measured in samples containing relatively few bacterial cells. Bacterial ice nucleation activity is a sensitive reporter gene system that has been used to estimate the transcription of bacterial genes to which it has been fused, when these genes are present in bacteria grown on plants and in other habitats (Georgakopoulos et al., 1994; Huynh et al., 1989; Lindgren et al., 1989; Loper and Lindow, 1994; Rahme et al., 1992). Leaves, soil, and other natural constituents contain few if any ice nuclei active at temperatures of –5°C or higher (Lindow et al., 1982); background ice nucleation activity, therefore, is generally quite low. Ice nucleation activity is measured by a droplet freezing assay which is quick and easy to accomplish without the need for expensive, dedicated equipment. In this assay, drops of appropriate dilutions of bacterial suspensions, leaf macerates, or soil suspensions are placed on the surface of a paraffin-coated aluminum foil "raft," which is floated on the surface of a refrigerated circulating bath. Such refrigerated baths are common in most laboratories, and most maintain liquid temperatures to within 0.05°C. This degree of temperature stability is suitable for ice nucleation measurements. Since single ice nucleation events can be readily detected by the droplet freezing assay, ice nucleation is a relatively sensitive phenotype for use in reporter gene systems. Ice nucleation from *inaZ* gene fusions has been estimated to be more than 1,000-fold more sensitive than the measurements of light from *luxAB* gene fusions and about 10^6-fold more sensitive than measurements of β-galactosidase from *lacZ* fusions (Lindgren et al., 1989). Ice nucleation activity increases approximately with the square root of the content of ice nucleation protein in bacterial cells (Lindgren et al., 1989). Measurements of ice nucleation activity therefore provide amplified signals of the transcription of genes to which a promoterless ice nucleation gene is fused. Fusions of a cloned gene to a promoterless *inaZ* can be easily made by using the reporter transposon Tn*3*-Spice (Lindgren et al., 1989). In addition, *inaZ* is available on stable plasmids such as pVSP61 which provide upstream cloning sites (Loper and Lindow, 1994).

IDENTIFYING EPIPHYTIC FITNESS DETERMINANTS BY USING ICE NUCLEATION ASSAYS

The ice nucleation phenotype has been instrumental in identifying novel epiphytic fitness genes in *P. syringae*. The population sizes of random Tn*5* mutants of an Ice$^+$ *P. syringae* strain were estimated by using a tube nucleation test (Lindow, 1993). Random Tn*5* mutants were selected on a basis of deficiencies in epiphytic growth or survival on plants rather than deficiencies in predetermined phenotypes exhibited in culture (Lindow et al., 1993; Beattie and Lindow, 1994a). The tube freezing procedure was used to measure the population sizes of 5,300 mutants of *P. syringae* exposed to alternating wet and dry conditions on bean leaves (Lindow et al., 1993). The population sizes of 82 mutants were found to be reduced under these conditions. Of these mutants, over half exhibited a reduced ability to survive the stresses associated with dry leaves, while others grew more slowly or attained reduced stationary-phase population sizes on leaves. While some epiphytic fitness mutants were altered in phenotypes that could be measured in culture, many mutants were not altered in any in vitro phenotype examined. Only three of the epiphytic fitness mutants were auxotrophs, and none had catabolic deficiencies for any of 31 organic compounds tested. Other mutants that exhibited reductions in one or more of the following were identified: flagellar motility, osmotolerance, desiccation tolerance, growth rate in batch culture, and extracellular polysaccharide production. All of the mutants retained the ability to produce disease symptoms on the compatible host plant, bean, to incite a hypersensitive response on the nonhost plant, tobacco, and to produce a fluorescent pyoverdine siderophore (Lindow et al., 1993; Beattie and Lindow, 1994a).

The behaviors of the epiphytic fitness mutants identified above were also compared in the field and in growth chambers to evaluate the relative fitness of the strains in these two conditions and to determine the significance of the altered survival seen in growth chamber environments. The mutants that were evaluated under both conditions differed from the parental strain more under field conditions than under laboratory conditions with respect to survival immediately following inoculation onto bean leaves and the size of the epiphytic populations that they established, demonstrating that their fitness is reduced more under field conditions than in the laboratory (Beattie and Lindow, 1994b). As under growth chamber conditions, the four mutants that were evaluated exhibited distinctive behaviors in the field.

The expression of the individual loci required for each of the four mutant strains described above to survive on dry leaf surfaces has been investigated by fusing a promoterless *inaZ* gene downstream of the putative promoter region of each locus (unpublished data). The expression of one locus, *estA*, was similarly expressed under different conditions in culture and on plants (G. Andersen and S. E. Lindow, unpublished data). In all cases, this locus, also required for methionine biosynthesis in culture, appeared to exhibit moderate levels of transcription that were nearly constant, irrespective of the external environment of the cells. Other loci involved in epiphytic fitness that were identified by Tn*5* insertions are being isolated, and their regulation is being assessed by using ice nucleation reporter gene fusions.

Because the ice nucleation phenotype can be conferred on most other gram-negative bacteria by introduction of cloned ice nucleation genes, the benefits of this easily measured and unique phenotype can be exploited in other systems. For example, the regulation of genes involved in the hypersensitive response and pathogenicity (*hrp* genes) was readily measured in *P. syringae* pv. phaseolicola, which is normally devoid of ice nucleation activity (Lindgren et al., 1989; Rahme et al., 1992). There would appear to be many opportunities to evaluate gene expression and population sizes by using nucleation in other systems.

REFERENCES

Beattie, G. A., and S. E. Lindow. 1994a. Survival, growth, and localization of epiphytic fitness mutants of *Pseudomonas syringae* on leaves. *Appl. Environ. Microbiol.* **60:**3790–3798.

Beattie, G. A., and S. E. Lindow. 1994b. Comparison of the behavior of epiphytic fitness mutants of *Pseudomonas syringae* under controlled and field conditions. *Appl. Environ. Microbiol.* **60:**3799–3808.

Beattie, G. A., and S. E. Lindow. 1995. Epiphytic fitness of phytopathogenic bacteria: physiological adaptations for growth and survival, p. 1–28. *In* J. L. Dangl (ed.), *Bacterial Pathogenesis of Plants and Animals: Molecular and Cellular Mechanisms.* Springer-Verlag, Berlin.

Burke, M. J., and S. E. Lindow. 1990. Surface properties and size of the ice nucleation site in ice nucleation active bacteria: theoretical considerations. *Cryobiology* **27:**80–84.

Burrage, S. W. 1971. The micro-climate at the leaf surface, p. 91–101. *In* T. F. Preece and C. H. Dickinson (ed.), *Ecology of Leaf Surface Micro-Organisms.* Academic Press, New York.

Burrage, S. W. 1976. Aerial microclimate around plant surfaces, p. 173–183. *In* C. H. Dickinson and T. F. Preece (ed.), *Microbiology of Aerial Plant Surfaces.* Academic Press, San Francisco.

Cirvilleri, G., and S. E. Lindow. 1994. Differential expression of genes of *Pseudomonas syringae* on leaves and in culture evaluated with random genomic *lux* fusions. *Mol. Ecol.* **3:**249–257.

Dickinson, C. H. 1986. Adaptations of micro-organisms to climatic conditions affecting aerial plant surfaces, p. 77–100. *In* N. J. Fokkema and J. van den Heuvel (ed.), *Microbiology of the Phyllosphere.* Cambridge University Press, New York.

Georgakopoulos, D. G., M. Hendson, N. J. Panopoulos, and M. N. Schroth. 1994. Analysis of expression of a phenazine biosynthesis locus of *Pseudomonas aureofaciens* pgs12 on seeds with a mutant carrying a phenazine biosynthesis locus ice nucleation reporter gene fusion. *Appl. Environ. Microbiol.* **60:**4573–4579.

Govindarajan, A. G., and S. E. Lindow. 1988. Size of bacterial ice nucleation sites measured *in situ* by gamma radiation inactivation analysis. *Proc. Natl. Acad. Sci. USA* **85:**1334–1338.

Gross, D. C., Y. S. Cody, E. L. Proebsting, G. K. Radamaker, and R. A. Spotts. 1983. Distribution, population dynamics, and characteristics of ice nucleation active bacteria in deciduous fruit tree orchards. *Appl. Environ. Microbiol.* **46:**1370–1379.

Gurian-Sherman, D., and S. E. Lindow. 1993. Bacterial ice nucleation: significance and molecular basis. *FASEB J.* **9:**1338–1343.

Haefele, D. M., and S. E. Lindow. 1987. Flagellar motility confers epiphytic fitness advantages to *Pseudomonas syringae. Appl. Environ. Microbiol.* **53:**2528–2533.

Henis, Y., and Y. Bashan. 1986. Epiphytic survival of bacterial leaf pathogens, p. 252–268. *In* N. J. Fokkema and J. van den Heuvel (ed.), *Microbiology of the Phyllosphere.* Cambridge University Press, New York.

Hirano, S. S., L. S. Baker, and C. D. Upper. 1985. Ice nucleation temperature of individual leaves in relation to population sizes of ice nucleation active bacteria and frost injury. *Plant Physiol.* **77:**259–265.

Hirano, S. S., E. V. Nordheim, D. C. Arny, and C. D. Upper. 1982. Lognormal distribution of epiphytic bacterial populations on leaf surfaces. *Appl. Environ. Microbiol.* **44:**695–700.

Hirano, S. S., and C. D. Upper. 1983. Ecology and epidemiology of foliar bacterial plant pathogens. *Annu. Rev. Phytopathol.* **21:**243–269.

Hirano, S. S., and C. D. Upper. 1990. Population biology and epidemiology of *Pseudomonas syringae. Annu. Rev. Phytopathol.* **28:**155–177.

Huynh, T. V., D. Dahlbeck, and B. J. Staskawicz. 1989. Bacterial blight of soybean: regulation of a pathogen gene determining host cultivar specificity. *Science* **245:**1374–1377.

Kajava, A., and S. E. Lindow. 1993. A molecular model of the three-dimensional structure of bacterial ice nucleation proteins. *J. Mol. Biol.* **232:**709–717.

Lindgren, P. B., R. Frederick, A. G. Govindarajan, N. J. Panopoulos, B. J. Staskawicz, and S. E. Lindow. 1989. An ice nucleation reporter system: identification of inducible pathogenicity genes in *Pseudomonas syringae* pv. *phaseolicola. EMBO J.* **8:**1291–1301.

Lindow, S. E. 1982. Population dynamics of epiphytic ice nucleation active bacteria on frost sensitive plants and frost control by means of antagonistic bacteria, p. 395–416. *In* P. H. Li and A. Sakai (ed.), *Plant Cold Hardiness.* Academic Press, New York.

Lindow, S. E. 1983. The role of bacterial ice nucleation in frost injury to plants. *Annu. Rev. Phytopathol.* **21:**363–384.

Lindow, S. E. 1985. Integrated control and role of antibiosis in biological control of fireblight and frost injury, p. 83–115. *In* C. Windels and S. E. Lindow (ed), *Biological Control on the Phylloplane.* American Phytopathological Society Press, St. Paul, Minn.

Lindow, S. E. 1991. Determinants of epiphytic fitness in bacteria, p. 295–314. *In* S. S. Hirano and J. Andrews (ed.), *Microbiology of the Phyllosphere.* Springer-Verlag, New York.

Lindow, S. E. 1993. Novel method for identifying bacterial mutants with reduced epiphytic fitness. *Appl. Environ. Microbiol.* **59:**1586–1592.

Lindow, S. E., G. Andersen, and G. Beattie. 1993. Characteristics of insertional mutants of *Pseudomonas syringae* with reduced epiphytic fitness. *Appl. Environ. Microbiol.* **59:**1593–1601.

Lindow, S. E., D. C. Arny, W. R. Barchet, and C. D. Upper. 1978a. The role of bacterial ice nuclei in frost injury to sensitive plants, p. 249–263. *In* P. Li (ed.), *Plant Cold Hardiness and Freezing Stress.* Academic Press, New York.

Lindow, S. E., D. C. Arny, and C. D. Upper. 1978b. Distribution of ice nucleation active bacteria on plants in nature. *Appl. Environ. Microbiol.* **36:**831–838.

Lindow, S. E., D. C. Arny, and C. D. Upper. 1982. Bacterial ice nucleation: a factor in frost injury to plants. *Plant Physiol.* **70:**1084–1089.

Lindow, S. E., E. Lahue, A. G. Govindarajan, N. J. Panopoulos, and D. Gies. 1989. Localization of ice nucleation activity and the *iceC* gene product in *Pseudomonas syringae* and *Escherichia coli. Mol. Plant-Microbe Interact.* **2:**262–272.

Loper, J. E., and S. E. Lindow. 1987. Lack of evidence for *in situ* fluorescent pigment production by *Pseudomonas syringae* pv. *syringae* on bean leaf surfaces. *Phytopathology* **77:**1449–1454.

Loper, J. E., and S. E. Lindow. 1994. A biological sensor for iron available to bacteria in their habitats on plant surfaces. *Appl. Environ. Microbiol.* **60:**1934–1941.

Morgan, J. V., and H. B. Tukey. 1964. Characterization of leachate from plant foliage. *Plant Physiol.* **39:**590–593.

Morris, C. E., and D. I. Rouse. 1985. Role of nutrients in regulating epiphytic bacterial populations, p. 63–82. *In* C. E. Windels and S. E. Lindow (ed.), *Biological Control on the Phylloplane.* American Phytopathological Society, St. Paul, Minn.

Rahme, L. G., M. N. Mindrinos, and N. J. Panopoulos. 1992. Plant and environmental sensory signals control the expression of *hrp* genes in *Pseudomonas syringae* pv. *phaseolicola. J. Bacteriol.* **174:**3499–3507.

Rouse, D. I., E. V. Nordheim, S. S. Hirano, and C. D. Upper. 1985. A model relating the probability of foliar disease incidence to the population frequencies of bacterial plant pathogens. *Phytopathology* **75:**505–509.

Silverstone, S. E., D. G. Gilchrist, R. M. Bostock, and T. Kosuge. 1993. The 73-kb pIAA plasmid increases competitive fitness of *Pseudomonas syringae* subspecies *savastanoi* in oleander. *Can. J. Microbiol.* **39:**659–664.

Tukey, H. B. J. 1970. The leaching of substances from plants. *Annu. Rev. Plant Physiol.* **21:**305–324.

Warren, G., and L. Corotto. 1989. The consensus sequence of ice nucleation proteins from *Erwinia herbicola, Pseudomonas fluorescens* and *Pseudomonas syringae. Gene* **85:**239–242.

Warren, G., and P. Wolber. 1991. Molecular aspects of microbial ice nucleation. *Mol. Microbiol.* **5:**239–243.

Wilson, M., and S. E. Lindow. 1993. Effect of phenotypic plasticity on epiphytic survival and colonization by *Pseudomonas syringae. Appl. Environ. Microbiol.* **59:**410–416.

Wilson, M., and S. E. Lindow. 1994a. Ecological differentiation and coexistence between epiphytic Ice$^+$ *Pseudomonas syringae* strains and an Ice$^-$ biological control agent. *Appl. Environ. Microbiol.* **60:**3128–3137.

Wilson, M., and S. E. Lindow. 1994b. Coexistence among epiphytic bacterial populations mediated through nutritional resource partitioning. *Appl. Environ. Microbiol.* **60:**4468–4477.

Wolber, P., and G. Warren. 1989. Bacterial ice-nucleation proteins. *Trends Biochem. Sci.* **14:**179–182.

Wolber, P. K. 1992. Bacterial ice nucleation. *Adv. Microb. Physiol.* **34:**205–237.

Molecular Biology of Pseudomonads
Edited by T. Nakazawa et al.

Chapter 44

Iron Regulation in Plant-Associated *Pseudomonas fluorescens* M114: Implications for Biological Control

D. N. Dowling, R. Sexton, A. Fenton, I. Delany, S. Fedi, B. McHugh, M. Callanan, Y. Moenne-Loccoz, and F. O'Gara

THE IRON UPTAKE REGULON IN PLANT-ASSOCIATED PSEUDOMONADS

Fluorescent *Pseudomonas* species produce a range of metabolites that are inhibitory to other microorganisms, some of which are implicated as playing a role in the biological control of plant pathogens (Dowling and O'Gara, 1994). For example, iron-chelating compounds (siderophores) have both fungistatic and bacteriostatic effects in the laboratory under low-iron conditions. Under field conditions, these iron chelators are thought to contribute directly to the suppression of plant disease by the biocontrol agent. Indirectly, siderophores may play an important role in the general persistence and survival of biocontrol *Pseudomonas* strains by facilitating iron uptake to support metabolism in iron-limiting environments.

Siderophores are produced by many microorganisms for taking up iron which is not readily available because of the poor solubility of iron oxides and hydroxides formed in the environment. Pseudomonads produce a range of iron-chelating compounds, including salicylic acid, pyochelins, and fluorescent pseudobactins and pyoverdines. Fluorescent siderophores such as pseudobactins have a very high affinity for ferric ions. These molecules consist of a fluorescent chromophore, i.e., a quinoline moiety with two hydroxyl groups that are involved in binding iron in conjunction with hydroxamate, hydroxyl, or carboxyl, groups from the peptide backbone (Leong, 1986). Pseudobactins can be often strain specific as a result of variation in this peptide. Uptake of the fluorescent iron-siderophore complex requires a specific outer membrane receptor. Although an individual *Pseudomonas* strain usually produces only one type of pseudobactin, it is possible to isolate strains that can utilize a range of different pseudobactins by harboring a number of different outer membrane siderophore receptors (Morris et al., 1992; Koster et al., 1993). Under iron-limiting conditions, *Pseudomonas fluorescens* M114 produces

D. N. Dowling, R. Sexton, A. Fenton, I. Delany, S. Fedi, B. McHugh, M. Callanan, Y. Moenne-Loccoz, and F. O'Gara • Department of Microbiology, University College Cork, Cork, Ireland.

a fluorescent siderophore, termed pseudobactin M114, and its cognate receptor PbuA, a casein protease, and demonstrates antifungal properties under iron limitation in laboratory conditions (O'Gara et al., 1986). The structure of pseudobactin M114 was determined and shown to be the same as that of pseudobactin B10 (Ruangviriyachal, 1991).

Siderophore Biosynthetic Genes in *P. fluorescens* M114

Pseudobactin biosynthesis requires numerous genes, and many are clustered; e.g., the *pvd* (pyoverdine) cluster of *P. aeruginosa* PAO maps within a 103-kb region located at 47 min on the genetic map of strain PAO (Tsuda et al., 1995). *P. aeruginosa* encodes two characterized pyoverdine biosynthetic genes, *pvdA*, encoding an L-ornithine N^5-oxygenase which catalyzes ornithine hydroxylation, an early step in hydroxamate synthesis (Visca et al., 1994), and a peptide synthetase gene, *pvdD* (Merriman et al., 1995). At the DNA level, there is considerable homology between the siderophore biosynthetic genes of *P. aeruginosa* and species of *P. fluorescens, P. syringae, P. putida*, and *Pseudomonas* sp. strain B10, yet few *Pseudomonas* biosynthetic genes have been fully characterized (Rombel and Lamont, 1992).

Complementation studies of Tn*5*-induced siderophore-minus mutants of *P. fluorescens* M114 indicated that at least five genetic loci are required for the synthesis of pseudobactin M114 (O'Sullivan et al., 1990). Adams et al. (1994) characterized the *P. fluorescens* M114 *pbsC* gene, which is similar to *pvdD* and exhibits significant homology to the AMP-binding siderophore biosynthetic gene products of *angR* and *entF* from *Vibrio anguillarum* and *Escherichia coli*, respectively. Recently two more biosynthetic genes from strain M114, *pbsD* and *pbsE*, have been isolated and characterized. The deduced gene products of *pbsD* and *pbsE* exhibit homology to the products of the previously characterized siderophore biosynthetic genes, M114 *pbsC* and *E. coli iucB*, respectively (R. Sexton, D. Dowling, and F. O'Gara, unpublished results).

Pseudobactin Uptake by *P. fluorescens* M114

Under iron stress conditions, *P. fluorescens* M114 secretes pseudobactin M114 into the environment to chelate ferric ions. The iron-bound siderophore complex is reassimilated into the host cell via the specific outer membrane receptor, PbuA (Morris et al., 1992). PbuA is similar to other pseudobactin-type receptors which require the inner membrane TonB protein in association with the ExbB and ExbD proteins to generate the necessary energy for active transport (Bitter et al., 1992). The *pbuA* gene has been cloned and confers the ability to transport pseudobactin M114 when expressed in heterologous pseudomonads. The finding shows that although ferric-pseudobactin transport across the outer membrane is siderophore specific, the pseudobactin-dependent iron transport through the inner membrane is conserved among pseudomonads (Morris et al., 1994).

P. fluorescens M114, like *E. coli* and *P. aeruginosa*, has the capacity to utilize heterologous siderophores, and the outer membrane receptor specific for *Pseudomonas* sp. strain B24 pseudobactin has been identified in M114 (O'Sullivan et al., 1990; Morris et al., 1992). Siderophore production and uptake may provide the producing strain with a competitive advantage under low-iron conditions, which would contribute directly or indirectly to antagonizing the establishment of pathogens with less potent iron uptake systems in the rhizosphere. Indeed, the introduction of an additional siderophore receptor gene may improve the performance of the host strain in laboratory experiments (Dowling et al., 1992; Y. Moenne-Loccoz and F. O'Gara, unpublished results).

Wild-type strains with multiple pseudobactin receptors also exist in nature, and the genes encoding these receptors may contribute to the organisms' ecological fitness. *P. putida* WCS358 encodes numerous receptors for heterologous pseudobactins, some of which are inducible by specific pseudobactins; for example, strain WCS358 is capable of utilizing its own pseudobactin via PupA and the siderophores of strains BN7 and BN8 via the PupB receptor (Bitter et al., 1991; Koster et al., 1993).

Regulation of Iron Assimilation in *P. fluorescens* M114

In *E. coli*, the iron regulon is negatively regulated at the transcriptional level by a repressor, Fur, and the cofactor Fe^{2+} (for a review see Neilands, 1990). A *fur*-like gene from *P. aeruginosa* has been characterized (Prince et al., 1993), and homologs of the gene have been found in the pseudomonads, including strain M114 (M. Callanan, D. N. Dowling, and F. O'Gara, unpublished results). Also, an iron-regulated promoter from *P. fluorescens* M114 (O'Sullivan and O'Gara, 1991) was shown to be deregulated in an *E. coli fur* mutant and to bind purified *E. coli* Fur in vitro (O'Sullivan et al., 1994).

There is also a requirement for positive effectors of iron-regulated transcription in pseudomonads (Venturi et al., 1993; Dowling et al., 1994). A Tn*5lacZ*-induced mutant (M114FA1) that exhibits a pleiotropic phenotype and lacks the ability to express iron-regulated genes was isolated (Sexton et al., 1995). A cosmid clone which complements this mutation was identified. This clone was capable of activating a number of iron-regulated promoter fusion constructs from *P. fluorescens* M114 and *P. putida* WCS358 and could also promote expression of these fusions in *E. coli*. DNA sequence analysis of the complementing region identified an open reading frame termed *pbrA* (for pseudobactin regulation activation). Two recently identified genes, *pfrI* (Venturi et al., 1995) and *pvdS* (Cunliffe et al., 1995), which regulate pseudobactin production in *P. putida* WCS358 and *P. aeruginosa*, respectively, show 80% identity with *pbrA*, indicating the requirement of a PbrA regulator for pseudobactin production in all pseudomonads.

The deduced amino acid sequence of the *pbrA* gene product also shows domains with significant homology to a number of ECF (extracytoplasmic function) transcriptional regulators of the σ^{70} sigma factor family, including FecI, which is required for expression of the ferric dicitrate outer membrane receptor protein of *E. coli* (Sexton et al., 1995) (Fig. 1). The ECF family of alternative sigma factors represents a novel group proposed by Lonetto et al. (1994), who observed that not only do these proteins maintain the sequence characteristics and/or biochemical functions of group III σ^{70} sigma factors, but each controls a regulon in response to a specific environmental stimulus. The ECF sigma factors usually regulate a small regulon which often includes a cognate regulator modulating the ability of the sigma factor to activate transcription in response to the specific environmental stimulus. Some new regulators which are proposed as sigma factors within the ECF family were previously characterized as transcriptional activators. Along with FecI and AlgU, Lonetto et al. (1994) include five other regulators in the

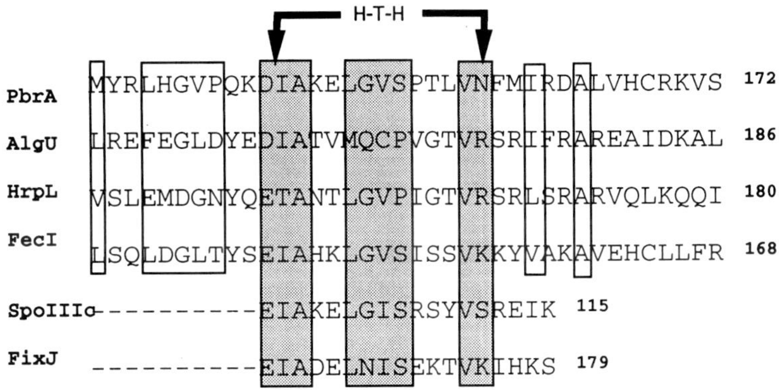

Figure 1. Homology of the amino acid sequence of PbrA to sequences of members of the subgroup of ECF sigma factors, AlgU, HrpL, and FecI, over functional region 4.2. The most-conserved sequences are boxed and numbered with respect to the complete amino acid sequence. The homology among PbrA, SpoIIIc, and FixJ at the α-helix–turn–helix motif is shown as shaded boxes.

family: σ^E of *Streptomyces coelicolor*, σ^E of *E. coli*, CarQ of *Myxococcus xanthus*, HrpL of *P. syringae*, and CnrH of *Alcaligenes eutrophus*. Members of the ECF family are not readily recognizable as sigma factors, but each member shows homology to the four specific functional regions of group III σ^{70} factors (Helmann and Chamberlain, 1988). One of the conserved regions, region 4.2, contains an α-helix–turn–helix DNA binding motif (Fig. 1).

Regulatory studies of *pbrA* expression using promoter-*lacZ* transcriptional fusions demonstrate that expression of *pbrA* dictates the cellular response to iron. *pbrA* is transcribed at all phases of iron-limited growth but maximally at late logarithmic to stationary phase. *pbrA* expression is independent of autoregulatory control but is strictly repressed in iron-rich conditions in a Fur-dependent fashion. Constitutive expression of *pbrA* from an inducible *tac* promoter permits the induction of PbrA-dependent transcription and pseudobactin M114 biosynthesis in high-iron conditions (Sexton et al., 1996).

ANTIFUNGAL METABOLITES PRODUCED BY FLUORESCENT PSEUDOMONADS

In addition to producing fluorescent siderophores, *Pseudomonas* spp. produce an array of low-molecular-weight metabolites, some of which are potent antifungal agents. Important metabolites include phenazines (Thomashow and Weller, 1992) and the c-acetylphloroglucinols (Keel et al., 1992; Shanahan et al., 1992). 2,4-Diacetylphloroglucinol (Phl) (Fig. 2) has been shown to be largely responsible for the prevention of damping off (caused by *Pythium ultimum*) of sugar beets (Shanahan et al., 1992) and responsible for the control of black root rot of tobacco (caused by *Thielabiopsis basicola*) by *P. fluorescens* CHA0, although in the latter case hydrogen cyanide (HCN) also contributes to biocontrol (Voisard et al., 1989; Keel et al., 1992).

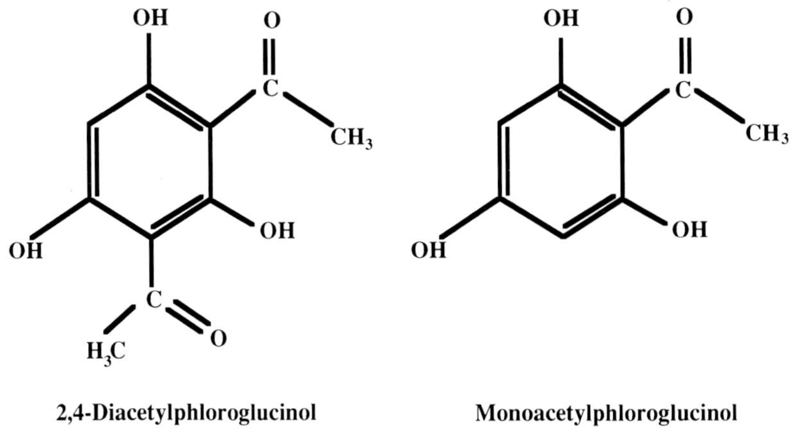

Figure 2. Chemical structures of the antifungal metabolites monoacetylphloroglucinol and 2,4-diacetylphloroglucinol (Phl).

Factors Affecting Antifungal Metabolite Production

Adequate production of secondary metabolites by the producing strain in laboratory media requires a suitable carbon and nutrient source. In the field, these nutrients may be supplied in the form of root or seed exudates. Carbon sources usually have a major influence on the types and levels of antibiotics produced (James and Gutterson, 1986). Laboratory studies on the production of the antifungal metabolite Phl by the biocontrol strain *P. fluorescens* F113 are yielding interesting results.

Key factors influencing Phl production by strain F113 include temperature, a suitable carbon source (e.g., succinate reduces the detectable level of Phl whereas sucrose permits production), and micronutrients (e.g., iron stimulates Phl production) (A. Fenton, D. Dowling, and F. O'Gara, unpublished results). With knowledge of the relative amounts and types of sugars, amino acids, etc., present in the rhizosphere, it may be possible to exploit this information for field use in order to predict whether metabolites will be produced in situ.

Genetic Approaches to Improving Phl Production in Fluorescent Pseudomonads

The ability to genetically improve nutrient uptake may be an approach to enhance the production of useful metabolites, particularly with respect to micronutrients. In the laboratory, production of Phl by strain F113 requires high levels of soluble iron (100 μM). However, if the P_{tac}-regulated *pbrA* sigma factor gene from M114 is introduced into this strain, Phl synthesis can be achieved upon induction with isopropylthiogalactopyranoside (IPTG) under low-iron conditions (Fenton et al., unpublished results). The precise explanation for this observation is unknown; however, it is possible that the presence of the construct increases the ability of the strain to assimilate iron as a result of increased production of fluorescent siderophore.

Genes involved in the biosynthesis of Phl have been cloned from different strains (Bangera et al., 1994; Fenton et al., 1992), including F113. The structural genes have been partially characterized and reveal sequence homology with plant chalcone synthesis genes (Bangera et al., 1994; I. Delany, A. Fenton, D. Dowling, and F. O'Gara, unpublished results). In the case of strain F113, the final step in the putative biochemical pathway, a monoacetylphloroglucinol acetyltransferase activity, is encoded by a 6-kb DNA fragment (Fenton et al., 1992). This fragment was cloned in the multicopy cloning vector pSUP106 to create plasmid pFO1, which was introduced into a wild-type strain (M114) that is unable to synthesize Phl. The engineered strain expresses the enzyme activity that apparently converts monoacetylphloroglucinol to Phl and is able to synthesize Phl at 0.37 μM. The presence of this new trait has enhanced the biocontrol ability of strain M114 against *Pythrum ultimum*, both in the laboratory and in greenhouse experiments (Fenton et al., 1992). Introduction of the fragment into other pseudomonads or *E. coli* does not lead to Phl production, which suggests that these organisms may lack other components necessary for production of the antifungal metabolite. The introduction of pFO1 into the wild-type producer F113 (producing 0.34 μM Phl) confers a significantly higher level of Phl (0.72 μM), presumably as a result of increased gene dosage. These strategies may offer a practical solution to construct strains that produce additional bioactive metabolites.

Global Regulation of Antibiotic Production

The GacA protein acts as a response regulator of many traits, including the production of Phl, pyoluteorin, and HCN in *P. fluorescens* CHA0 (Laville et al., 1992), disease lesion formation of *P. syringae* in bean plants (Rich et al., 1994), and the production of chitinase, HCN, and pyrrolnitrin in *P. fluorescens* BL915 (Gaffney et al., 1994). The GacA protein contains the conserved aspartate and lysine residues of the response regulator domains of two-component regulatory systems, and Rich et al. (1994) have obtained genetic evidence that the sensor component which couples to GacA in *P. syringae* is LemA.

There is also physiological and genetic evidence that a cell density-dependent autoinduction mechanism analogous to the prototype *luxR/I* system of *Vibrio fischeri* may be involved in regulation of antifungal antibiotics. Recently, the *phzR* gene of *P. aureofaciens* was shown to be required for the regulation of phenazine biosynthesis and to be a homolog of *luxR*. Production of phenazines is enhanced by the presence of a putative autoinducer in culture supernatants of the producing strain (Pierson et al., 1994). It is also of interest that an autoinducer-like activity has been detected in supernatants of the biocontrol strain *P. fluorescens* CHA0 (Voisard et al., 1994). In our laboratory, we have shown that Phl production may also be regulated by such a factor. Phl can be produced earlier in batch culture and in higher amounts if the producing culture is supplemented with an extract of the cell-free supernatant from the spent medium of a stationary-phase culture (Fig. 3).

PSEUDOMONAS SPP. AS BIOLOGICAL CONTROL AGENTS: ECOLOGICAL IMPLICATIONS

Microbial compounds such as siderophores and metabolites with antimicrobial properties are considered to play a major role in disease suppression by fluorescent pseudomonads. Direct killing or inhibition of the pathogen by the metabolite is observed

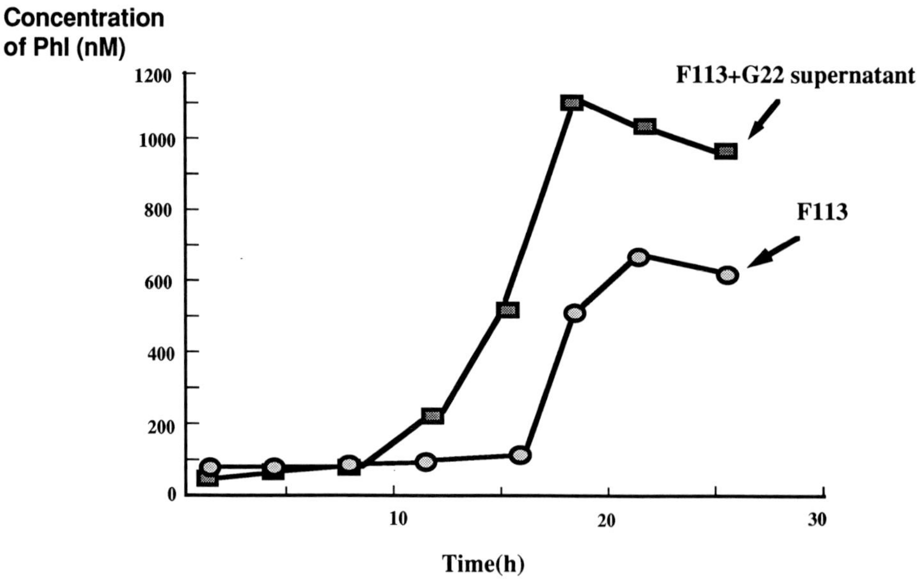

Figure 3. Phl production of wild-type F113 as a function of time and addition of sterile culture supernatant containing a putative auto-inducing compound. Addition of supernatant harvested from stationary-phase cells of a batch culture of the Phl biosynthetic mutant of strain F113, G22 (F113+G22), leads to earlier and increased production of Phl compared with the wild-type strain grown without the supernatant (F113).

in laboratory experiments, and there are a number of studies indicating a direct effect of antimicrobial metabolites on pathogen numbers in soil (Kloepper et al., 1981; Bull et al., 1991). It is important that the large-scale introduction of antifungal metabolite-producing strains into the environment for agricultural purposes affects only the target pathogen and presents little risk to the beneficial microflora. There is evidence that the production of the antifungal compound phenazine by *P. aureofaciens* contributes to the ecological fitness of the producing strain in wheat rhizosphere microcosm experiments (Mazzola et al., 1992). By contrast, in experiments with near-isogenic strains of *P. fluorescens* F113, Phl producers were compared with nonproducers following coinoculation of sugar beet rhizosphere microcosms. It was found that even after 10 simulated cropping and resowing cycles over a total of 270 days, there was no significant advantage to the Phl producer under the experimental conditions (Carroll et al., 1995). These data suggest that the long-term impact on the target ecosystem following introduction of Phl producers is likely to be minimal.

The potential interaction between the target pathogen and the biocontrol agent is also of relevance to biological control. Fungal pathogens produce metabolites (elicitors) that interact with plants to produce a variety of reactions. Recent work from our laboratory indicates that the fungal pathogen *Pythium ultimum* and its crude supernatant extracts can alter gene expression in the biocontrol strain *P. fluorescens* F113 in that F113 cells grown in the presence of *Pythium* extracts show a significant reduction in both fluorescent siderophore and Phl production. The effect on Phl production is also observed in in vitro bioassays in which pretreating the biocontrol strain with *Pythium* extract reduces the ability of the strain to control the pathogen on agar plates. We are currently characterizing the fungal supernatants for putative elicitors and the bacterial genes that respond to them.

Acknowledgments. We thank Pat Higgins for technical support. This work was supported in part from grants from the European Commission (BIOTECH-BIO2-CT92-0084, BIO2-CT93-0196, BIO2-CT93-0053, and BIO2-CT94-300).

REFERENCES

Adams, C., D. N. Dowling, D. J. O'Sullivan, and F. O'Gara. 1994. Isolation of a gene (*pbsC*) required for siderophore biosynthesis in fluorescent *Pseudomonas* sp. strain M114. *Mol. Gen. Genet.* **243:**515–524.

Bangera, M. G., D. M. Weller, and L. S. Thomashow. 1994. Genetic analysis of the 2,4-diacetylphloroglucinol biosynthetic locus from *Pseudomonas fluorescens* Q2-87. *Adv. Mol. Genet. Plant-Microbe Interact.* **3:**383–386.

Bitter, W., J. D. Marugg, L. A. deWeger, J. Tommassen, and P. J. Weisbeek. 1991. The ferric-pseudobactin receptor PupA of *Pseudomonas putida* WCS358: homology to TonB-dependent *Escherichia coli* receptors and specificity of the protein. *Mol. Microbiol.* **5:**647–655.

Bitter, W., J. Tommassen, and P. J. Weisbeek. 1992. Identification and characterization of the *exbB, exbD,* and *tonB* genes of *Pseudomonas putida* WCS358: their involvement in ferric-pseudobactin transport. *Mol. Microbiol.* **7:**117–130.

Bull, C. T., D. M. Weller, and L. S. Thomashow. 1991. Relationship between root colonization and suppression of *Gaeumannomyces graminis* var. *tritici* by *Pseudomonas fluorescens* strain 2-79. *Phytopathology* **81:**954–959.

Carroll, H., Y. Moenne-Loccoz, D. N. Dowling, and F. O'Gara. 1995. Mutational disruption of the biosynthesis genes coding for the antifungal metabolite 2,4-diacetylphloroglucinol does not influence the ecological fitness of *Pseudomonas fluorescens* F113 in the rhizosphere of sugarbeet. *Appl. Environ. Microbiol.* **61:**3002–3007.

Cunliffe, H. E., T. R. Merriman, and I. Lamont. 1995. Cloning and characterization of *pvdS*, a gene required for pyoverdine synthesis in *Pseudomonas aeruginosa*: PvdS is probably an alternative sigma factor. *J. Bacteriol.* **177:**2744–2750.

Dowling, D. N., B. Boesten, P. R. Gill, Jr., and F. O'Gara. 1994. Developing concepts in biological control: a molecular ecology approach, p. 57–65. *In* F. O'Gara, D.N. Dowling, and B. Boesten (ed.), *Molecular Ecology of Rhizosphere Bacteria.* VCH, Weinheim, Germany.

Dowling, D. N., B. Boesten, D. J. O'Sullivan, P. Stevens, J. Morris, and F. O'Gara. 1992. Genetically modified plant-microbe interacting strains for potential release into the rhizosphere, p. 408–414. *In* E. Galli, S. Silver, and B. Witholt (ed.), *Pseudomonas: Molecular Biology and Biotechnology.* American Society for Microbiology, Washington, D.C.

Dowling, D. N., and F. O'Gara. 1994. Metabolites of *Pseudomonas* involved in the biocontrol of plant disease. *Trends Biotechnol.* **12:**133–141.

Fenton, A. M., P. M. Stephens, J. Crowley, M. O'Callaghan, and F. O'Gara. 1992. Exploiting gene(s) involved in 2,4-diacetylphloroglucinol biosynthesis to improve the biocontrol ability of a pseudomonad strain. *Appl. Environ. Microbiol.* **58:**3873–3878.

Gaffney, T. D., S. T. Lam, J. Ligon, K. Gates, A. Frazelle, J. Di Maio, S. Hill, S. Goodwin, N. Torkewitz, A. M. Allshouse, H. J. Kempf, and J. O. Becker. 1994. Global regulation of expression of antifungal factors by a *Pseudomonas fluorescens* biological control strain. *Mol. Plant-Microbe Interact.* **7:**455–463.

Helmann, J. D., and M. J. Chamberlain. 1988. Structure and function of bacterial sigma factors. *Annu. Rev. Biochem.* **57:**839–872.

James, D. W., and N. I. Gutterson. 1986. Multiple antibiotics produced by *Pseudomonas fluorescens* HV37A and their differential regulation by glucose. *Appl. Environ. Microbiol.* **52:**1183–1189.

Keel, C., U. Schnider, M. Maurhofer, C. Voisard, J. Laville, U. Burger, P. Withner, D. Haas, and G. Defago. 1992. Suppression of root diseases by *Pseudomonas fluorescens* CHA0: importance of the bacterial secondary metabolite 2,4-diacetylphloroglucinol. *Mol. Plant-Microbe. Interact.* **5:**4–13.

Kloepper, J. W., and M. N. Schroth. 1981. Relationship of in vitro antibiosis of plant growth promoting rhizobacteria to plant growth and the displacement of root microflora. *Phytopathology.* **71:**1020–1024.

Koster, M., J. van der Vossenberg, J. Leong, and P. J. Weisbeek. 1993. Identification and characterisation of the *pupB* gene encoding an inducible ferric-pseudobactin receptor of *Pseudomonas putida* WCS358. *Mol. Microbiol.* **8:**591–601.

Laville, J., C. Voisard, C. Keel, M. Maurhofer, G. Defago, and D. Haas. 1992. Global control in *Pseudomonas fluorescens* mediating antibiotic synthesis and suppression of black root rot of tobacco. *Proc. Natl. Acad. Sci. USA* **89:**1562–1566.

Leong, J. 1986. Siderophores: their biochemistry and possible role in the biocontrol of plant pathogens. *Annu. Rev. Phytopathol.* **24:**187–209.

Lonetto, M. A., K. L. Brown, K. E. Rudd, and M. J. Buttner. 1994. Analysis of the *Streptomyces coelicolor sigE* gene reveals the existence of a subfamily of eubacterial RNA polymerase s factors involved in the regulation of extracytoplasmic functions. *Proc. Natl. Acad. Sci. USA* **91:**7573–7577.

Mazzola, M., R. J. Cook, L. S. Thomashow, D. M. Weller, and L. S. Pierson III. 1992. Contribution of phenazine antibiotic biosynthesis to the ecological competence of fluorescent pseudomonads in soil habitats. *Appl. Environ. Microbiol.* **58:**2616–2624.

Merriman, T. R., M. E. Merriman, and I. L. Lamont. 1995. Nucleotide sequence of *pvdD,* a pyoverdine biosynthetic gene from *Pseudomonas aeruginosa*: PvdD has similarity to peptide synthetases. *J. Bacteriol.* **177:**252–258.

Morris, J., D. F. Donnelly, E. O'Neill, F. McConnell, and F. O'Gara. 1994. Nucleotide sequence analysis and potential environmental distribution of a ferric pseudobactin receptor gene of *Pseudomonas* sp. strain M114. *Mol. Gen. Genet.* **242:**9–16.

Morris, J., D. J. O'Sullivan, M. Koster, J. Leong. P. Weisbeek, and F. O'Gara. 1992. Characterization of fluorescent ferric siderophore mediated uptake in *Pseudomonas* sp. strain M114: evidence for the existence of an additional ferric siderophore receptor. *Appl. Environ. Microbiol.* **58:**630–635.

Neilands, J. B. 1990. Ferric uptake regulation (Fur) repressor: facts and fantasies, p. 382–395. *In* S. Silver, A. M. Chakrabarty, B. Iglewski, and S. Kaplan (ed.), *Pseudomonas: Biotransformations, Pathogenesis, and Evolving Biotechnology.* American Society for Microbiology, Washington, D.C.

O'Gara, F., P. Treacy, D. O'Sullivan, M. O'Sullivan, and P. Higgins. 1986. Biological control of phytopathogens by *Pseudomonas* spp: genetic aspects of siderophore production and root colonization, p. 331–339. *In* T. R. Swinburne (ed.), *Iron, Siderophores and Plant Diseases.* Plenum Press, New York.

O'Sullivan, D. J., D. N. Dowling, V. deLorenzo, and F. O'Gara. 1994. *Escherichia coli* ferric uptake regulator (Fur) can mediate regulation of a pseudomonad iron regulated promoter. *FEMS Microbiol. Lett.* **117:**327–332.

O'Sullivan, D. J., J. Morris, and F. O'Gara. 1990. Identification of an additional ferric siderophore uptake gene clustered with receptor, biosynthesis, and *fur*-like regulatory genes in fluorescent *Pseudomonas* sp. M114. *Appl. Environ. Microbiol.* **56:**2056–2064.

O'Sullivan, D. J., and F. O'Gara. 1991. Regulation of iron assimilation: nucleotide sequence analysis of an iron-regulated promoter from a fluorescent pseudomonad. *Mol. Gen. Genet.* **228:**1–8.

Pierson, L. S., III, D. D. Keppenne, and D. W. Wood. 1994. Phenazine antibiotic biosynthesis in *Pseudomonas aureofaciens* 30-84 is regulated by PhzR in response to cell density. *J. Bacteriol.* **176:**3966–3974.

Prince, R. W., C. D. Cox, and M. L. Vasil. 1993. Coordinate regulation of siderophore and exotoxin A production: molecular cloning and sequencing of the *Pseudomonas aeruginosa fur* gene. *J. Bacteriol.* **175:**2589–2598.

Rich, J. J., T. G. Kinscherf, T. Kitten, and D. K. Willis. 1994. Genetic evidence that the *gacA* gene encodes the cognate response regulator for the *lemA* sensor in *Pseudomonas syringae. J. Bacteriol.* **176:**7468–7475.

Rombel, R. T., and I. L. Lamont. 1992. DNA homology between siderophore genes from fluorescent pseudomonads. *J. Gen. Microbiol.* **138:**181–187.

Ruangviriyachal, C. 1991. Liquid chromatographic and complexation analysis of natural and synthetic chelating agents. Ph.D. thesis. University College Cork, Cork, Ireland.

Sexton, R., P. R. Gill, Jr., M. J. Callanan, D. J. O'Sullivan, D. N. Dowling, and F. O'Gara. 1995. Iron-responsive gene expression in *Pseudomonas fluorescens* M114: cloning and characterization of a transcription-activating factor, PbrA. *Mol. Microbiol.* **15:**297–306.

Sexton, R., P. R. Gill, Jr., D. N. Dowling, and F. O'Gara. 1996. Transcriptional regulation of the non-responsive sigma factor gene *pbrA. Mol. Gen. Genet.* **250:**50–58.

Shanahan, P., D. O'Sullivan, P. Simpson, J. D. Glennon, and F. O'Gara. 1992. Isolation and characterization of an antibiotic-like compound from a fluorescent pseudomonad and investigation of physiological parameters influencing its production. *Appl. Environ. Microbiol.* **58:**353–358.

Thomashow, L. S., and D. M. Weller. 1992. Role of phenazine antibiotic from *Pseudomonas fluorescens* in biological control of *Gaeumannomyces graminis* var. *tritici*. *J. Bacteriol.* **170:**3499–3508.

Tsuda, M., H. Miyazaki, and T. Nakazawa. 1995. Genetic and physical mapping of genes involved in pyoverdin production in *Pseudomonas aeruginosa* PAO. *J. Bacteriol.* **177:**423–431.

Venturi, V., C. Ottevanger, M. Bracke, and P. J. Weisbeek. 1995. Iron regulation of siderophore biosynthesis and transport in *Pseudomonas putida* WCS358: involvement of a transcriptional activator and of the Fur protein. *Mol. Microbiol.* **15:**1081–1093.

Venturi, V., C. Ottevanger, J. Leong, and P. J. Weisbeek. 1993. Identification and characterization of a siderophore regulatory gene (*pfrA*) of *Pseudomonas putida* WCS358: homology to the alginate regulatory gene *algQ* of *Pseudomonas aeruginosa*. *Mol. Microbiol.* **10:**63–73.

Visca, P., A. Ciervo, and N. Orsi. 1994. Cloning and nucleotide sequence of the *pvdA* gene encoding the pyoverdin biosynthetic enzyme L-orntithine N^5-oxygenase in *Pseudomonas aeruginosa*. *J. Bacteriol.* **176:**1128–1140.

Voisard, C., C. T. Bull, C. Keel, J. Laville, M. Maurhofer, U. Schnider, G. Defago, and D. Haas. 1994. Biocontrol of root diseases by *Pseudomonas fluorescens* CHA0: current concepts and experimental approaches, p. 67–89. *In* F. O'Gara, D. N. Dowling, and B. Boesten (ed.), *Molecular Ecology of Rhizosphere Bacteria*. VCH, Weinheim, Germany.

Voisard, C., C. Keel, D. Haas, and G. Defago. 1989. Cyanide production by *Pseudomonas fluorescens* helps suppress black root rot of tobacco under gnotobiotic conditions. *EMBO J.* **8:**351–358.

Molecular Biology of Pseudomonads
Edited by T. Nakazawa et al.

Chapter 45

Function and Regulation of *Pseudomonas syringae hrp* Genes

Steven W. Hutcheson, Sunggi Heu, Songmu Jin, Michael C. Lidell, Minna U. Pirhonen, and Daniel L. Rowley

Many strains of *Pseudomonas syringae* have the capacity to cause disease in several economically important plant species (Agrios, 1988). Most commonly, this bacterium is found growing asymptomatically on plant surfaces. Disease occurs when bacteria are introduced into tissue of a susceptible plant species and begin to multiply in the intercellular spaces. Tissue necroses, called leaf blights, commonly develop following colonization of tissue, but some strains have the capacity to induce tissue hyperplasias. Extracellular polysaccharides, peptide toxins, and phytohormones appear to be the major virulence factors for this bacterium (Long and Staskawicz, 1993).

Individual strains of *P. syringae* usually cause disease in only one or a few plant species and in some cases are limited to specific variants (cultivars or ecotypes) of a plant species (Keen, 1992). The ability of a strain to cause disease thus is the exception rather than the rule. In most other plants, a *P. syringae* strain elicits a set of inducible cellular defense responses, which restricts further multiplication of the bacteria and invasion of tissue. The plant's defense mechanisms include the production of active oxygen species, secondary metabolites with antimicrobial activity, and hydrolytic enzymes with lysozymal activity as well as alteration of plant cell wall structure (Keen, 1992). A laboratory manifestation of the initiation of these defense mechanisms is the hypersensitive response (HR), a rapid localized necrosis induced in response to a bacterial inoculum sufficient to cause 50% or more of the cells in the tissue to respond (Klement, 1982). It is the elicitation of these HR-associated defenses which appears to be a primary factor in limiting the host range of a *P. syringae* strain (Keen, 1992). Recognition of the invading pathogen by the resistant plant differs from mammalian paradigms for host-pathogen recognition. No stable

---

Steven W. Hutcheson, Songmu Jin, Michael C. Lidell, and Daniel L. Rowley • Department of Plant Biology, University of Maryland at College Park, College Park, Maryland 20742. ***Sunggi Heu*** • Plant Molecular Biology Laboratory, Agricultural Research Service, U.S. Department of Agriculture, Beltsville, Maryland 20705. ***Minna U. Pirhonen*** • Department of Molecular Genetics, Swedish University of Agricultural Sciences, Box 7010, 75007 Uppsala, Sweden.

surface feature of *P. syringae* strains is correlated with host range, indicating that other factors control the host range of *P. syringae* strains.

Two classes of genes which affect the ability of *P. syringae* strains to elicit the HR and thus affect the host range have been identified. The *hrp* genes control the basic pathogenicity of a *P. syringae* strain in susceptible plant hosts and are also essential for the elicitation of the HR in nonhost plant species (Bonas, 1994; Willis et al., 1991). Most *P. syringae hrp*::Tn mutants lose both pathogenicity in the susceptible plant species and the ability to elicit the HR in other nonhost plant species (Huang et al., 1991; Lindgren et al., 1986). A *hrp* cluster cloned from *P. syringae* pv. syringae Pss61 enables nonpathogenic bacteria such as *Escherichia coli* to elicit the HR in tobacco (Huang et al., 1988). In addition to carrying the *hrp* genes, many *P. syringae* strains also carry avirulence (*avr*) genes which function to restrict the host range of the strain to those variants of the susceptible plant species which lack a corresponding resistance (R) gene product (Dangl, 1994, 1995; Staskawicz et al., 1995).

ORGANIZATION AND BIOCHEMICAL FUNCTION OF THE *P. SYRINGAE hrp* GENE CLUSTER

Mutational analyses have shown that most *hrp* genes cluster in a 25-kb region of the chromosome and are conserved among *P. syringae* strains (Lindgren et al., 1988). The complete nucleotide sequence of the *hrp* gene cluster isolated from *P. syringae* pv. syringae Pss61 has recently been assembled through the efforts of several laboratories (He et al., 1993; Heu and Hutcheson, 1993; Huang et al., 1992; Huang et al., 1995; Huang et al., 1993; Lidell and Hutcheson, 1994; Xiao et al., 1994). The deduced organization of the cluster indicates the presence of 26 genes organized as at least eight transcriptional units (Fig. 1) (Huang et al., 1995; Hutcheson et al., 1994; Xiao and Hutcheson, 1994). Extensive similarities exist between the deduced gene products of the *hrp* cluster and virulence determinants of enteric bacteria pathogenic to mammals, such as the *ysc* genes of *Yersinia* spp., the *spa* and *mxi* genes of *Salmonella* and *Shigella* spp., and the *sep* genes of enteropathogenic *E. coli* strains, that are required for the secretion of virulence proteins (Huang et al., 1995). Similarities are also observed with the *fli* genes of *Bacillus* and *Salmonella* spp., which function in flagellar biosynthesis (Huang et al., 1995; Hutcheson et al., 1994; Lidell and Hutcheson, 1994). The sequence similarities are detected both at the translational level (deduced protein sequences) and at the transcriptional level (gene organization). In general, the highest level of similarity is observed with the *ysc* genes of *Yersinia* spp. Several other species of plant-pathogenic bacteria also carry partially homologous genes, some of which are also termed *hrp* genes (Fenselau et al., 1992; VanGijsegem et al., 1994). The relatively low sequence similarities, differences in transcriptional organization and regulation, and the products secreted in these other phytopathogens suggest that these genes form analogous systems in their host bacteria.

Most of the gene products exhibiting similarities to the *P. syringae hrp* gene products appear to function in the recently described type III protein secretion pathway (Salmond and Reeves, 1993; VanGijsegem et al., 1994). Proteins secreted by this mechanism lack an obvious N-terminal signal sequence and do not appear to be processed during the secretion process. In *Yersinia* strains, each secreted Yop protein also has a dedicated

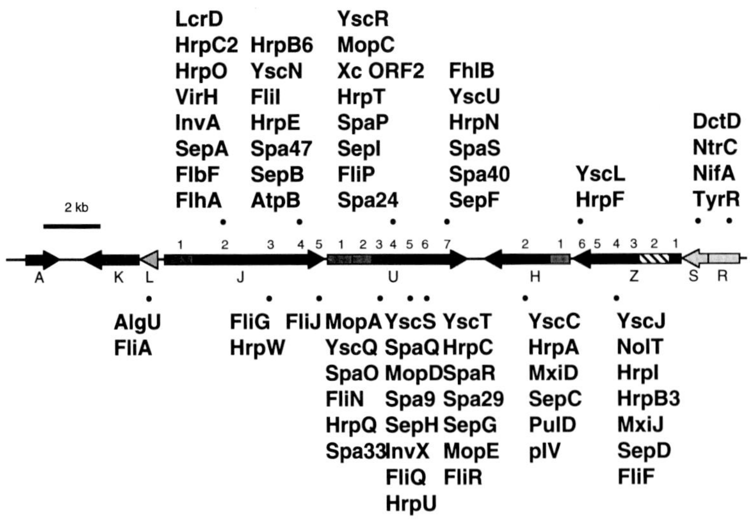

Figure 1. Organization of the *P. syringae* Pss61 *hrp* cluster and sequence similarities with related proteins. Genes identified within the *P. syringae* Pss61 *hrp* cluster are shown. The genetic nomenclature used is that of Xiao and Hutcheson (1994), which employs letters to indicate deduced operons and numbers to indicate genes within an operon. An alternative nomenclature for the *hrp* cluster has been proposed by Huang et al. (1995). Direction of transcription is indicated by the arrowheads. Operons are designated by capital letters, and genes are indicated by numbers. Darkly shaded boxes indicate *hrp* gene products functioning in protein translocation; lightly shaded boxes indicate gene products with regulatory activity; the hatched box indicates the gene producing harpin$_{Pss}$. Gene products exhibiting sequence similarities are indicated. Source organisms: Ysc, *Yersinia* sp.; Spa and Mxi, *Salmonella* and *Shigella* spp.; Sep, enteropathogenic *E. coli*; Mop, *Erwinia carotovora;* Fli and Fih, *Salmonella* and *Bacillus* spp.; Xc, *Xanthomonas campestris;* Hrp, *X. campestris* or *Burkholderia solanacearum;* Alg, *P. aeruginosa.*

chaperone to facilitate the secretion process (Cornelis, 1994). The mechanism for protein secretion by the Hrp pathway has not been fully elucidated. An indication of the organization of the *hrp* gene products in the membrane may be indicated by the similarities with the gene products of many of the late genes involved in flagellar biosynthesis. These genes form the secretion system for flagellar proteins, and the physical relationships of several gene products have been established (MacNab, 1992; Shapiro, 1995). FliF is thought to form the mounting plate for the secretion system. Attached to the mounting plate is a switch complex which includes FliG and FliN. Built upon this complex is the export apparatus formed from FlhA and FliI together with other proteins (possibly FliJ, FliP, FliQ, FliR, and FlhB). FlhB has been postulated to function as a gatekeeper for the secretion apparatus (Shapiro, 1995). Since homologs to these proteins are present in the *P. syringae hrp* cluster, it is tempting to speculate that the *hrp* gene products may form similar structures in the inner membrane. Consistent with this hypothesis, HrpJ2, HrpU4, HrpU5, HrpU6, and HrpU7 (also known as HrpI, HrpW, HrpO, HrpX, and HrpY, respectively) contain regions of hydrophobic residues typical of transmembrane domains (Huang et al., 1992; Huang et al., 1995) and suggestive of an inner membrane location. HrpH2 (also known as HrpH) has properties of an outer membrane protein (Huang et al., 1992). HrpJ4 appears to be an ATPase and is predicted to be associated with the cytoplasmic face of the inner membrane (Lidell and Hutcheson, 1994).

At least one protein, termed harpin$_{Pss}$, has been shown to be secreted by the Hrp secretion system and to function as an elicitor of the HR in some plants, such as tobacco (He et al., 1993). Harpin$_{Pss}$ is the product of the second gene of the *hrpZ* operon (*hrpZ2*) (Huang et al., 1995; Xiao and Hutcheson, 1994). It is a 35-kDa protein which is relatively glycine rich and heat stable. Deletion derivatives of *hrpZ2* carrying either the N or C portion of the protein retain at least partial elicitor activity, suggesting that at least two domains in the protein carry HR-eliciting activity (Collmer et al., 1994). Specific deletion of the *hrpZ2* gene in several strains of *P. syringae,* however, had little or no effect on the pathogenicity of the mutant or its ability to elicit the HR. Since inactivation of the genes encoding components of the secretion system causes a loss of pathogenicity and ability to elicit the HR, this observation suggests other proteins necessary for pathogenesis are secreted by the *hrp* secretion system. Recently, several other proteins have been identified which may also be secreted by the *hrp* secretion system in *P. syringae* pv. tomato DC3000 (Collmer et al., 1994). It has not yet been established whether any of these secreted proteins function as an elicitor of the HR or are required for pathogenicity. The specific biochemical functions of these proteins have not been elucidated. The earliest effects of harpin detected in plant cells responding hypersensitively include production of active oxygen and leakage of K^+ from plant cells (Baker et al., 1993). The involvement of receptors in the harpin-mediated initiation of the HR has not been established.

REGULATION OF *hrp* GENES

The expression of *hrp* genes is affected by growth conditions, including amino source, carbon source, osmotic conditions, and pH (Huynh et al., 1989; Rahme et al., 1992; Xiao et al., 1992). Thus far several positive-acting transcriptional factors that mediate the environmental regulation of *hrp* genes have been identified in the *hrp* cluster. HrpR and HrpS show sequence similarity with members of a large protein family that usually function in two-component regulatory systems and activate σ^{54}-dependent promoters (Felley et al., 1991; Grimm et al., 1995; Grimm and Panopoulos, 1989; Xiao et al., 1994). While the domains deduced to interact with σ^{54}-RNA polymerase holoenzyme and a helix-turn-helix involved in DNA binding (Morett and Segovia, 1993) are detected in both HrpR and HrpS, the N-terminal domains thought to function in the modulation of the regulatory activity are absent in both proteins. The *hrpR* gene appears to be expressed from a σ^{70}-dependent promoter located about 100 bp upstream of the initiation codon. The Pss61 *hrpR* and *hrpS* open reading frames are separated by a 50-bp intergenic region which lacks an obvious terminator or sequences similar to known promoter consensus sequences, suggesting that these genes may be part of a single transcriptional unit.

By using plasmid-borne constructs to express the Pss61 *hrpR* and/or *hrpS* in an *E. coli* strain singly or in combination, HrpR and HrpS were shown to be positive activators of the *hrpL* promoter (Xiao et al., 1994). Both HrpR and HrpS were required to activate the *hrpL* promoter in *E. coli.* A dissection of the *hrpL* promoter revealed the presence of a strong candidate σ^{54} promoter, as predicted from the deduced structural features of HrpR and HrpS

(Hutcheson et al., 1994; Zhang and Jones, 1995). The transcriptional start site was consistent with the functionality of the σ^{54} promoter consensus sequence, and the HrpR/S-dependent activity of the *hrpL* promoter was lost in an *rpoN* mutant of *E. coli* (S. Heu, S. Jin, and S. W. Hutcheson, unpublished results). Proteins similar to HrpR and HrpS frequently bind to enhancer-like elements located 100 to 500 bp upstream of a σ^{54} promoter (Morett and Segovia, 1993). Approximately 100 bp upstream of the σ^{54} promoter consensus sequence in the *hrpL* promoter is a region of dyad symmetry similar to an enhancer-like element (Hutcheson et al., 1994). Deletion analysis showed this region to be essential to *hrpRS*-dependent activation of the *hrpL* promoter (Heu et al., unpublished results).

The HrpL gene product has properties which suggest that it functions as an alternative sigma factor controlling transcription of *hrp* and *avr* genes (Xiao et al., 1994). It is a required positive-acting transcriptional factor for the *hrpK, hrpJ, hrpU, hrpH,* and *hrpZ* operons as well as for several *avr* genes and *hrmA* (Felley et al., 1991; Heu and Hutcheson, 1993; Huynh et al., 1989; Innes et al., 1993; Xiao et al., 1994). The deduced gene product shows sequence similarity with several alternative sigma factors such as AlgU and CnrA (Xiao et al., 1994), which are members of the extracytoplasmic function family of sigma factors (Lonetto et al., 1994). A conserved bipartite sequence motif, originally identified in the promoter-active regions of several *avr* genes (GGAACCNAN$_{14}$CCACNNA) (Innes et al., 1993; Salmeron and Staskawicz, 1993; Shen and Keen, 1993), has been shown to function as an HrpL-dependent promoter (Xiao and Hutcheson, 1994). This putative promoter motif has in common with the promoters recognized by related sigma factors (Lonetto et al., 1994) a conserved −35 region, but only weak similarity is observed in the −10 region. Transcription initiated by HrpL begins six to eight nucleotides downstream of this motif (Innes et al., 1993; Salmeron and Staskawicz, 1993; Shen and Keen, 1993).

These results indicate that the expression of the *hrp* cluster is controlled by a regulatory cascade involving σ^{70} (*hrpR* promoter), σ^{54} (*hrpL* promoter), and σ^{L} (various HrpL-dependent promoters). An alternative model for the action of HrpR and HrpS which suggests that HrpS alone functions to regulate expression of the *hrp* genes in *P. syringae* strains has been proposed (Grimm et al., 1995). Since our data are presently inconsistent with some features of this model, we are examining both models more closely. Recent evidence suggests that at least one additional regulatory factor modulates the activity of HrpR and HrpS, a second unidentified factor functions to repress *hrpL* promoter activity, and a third postulated component appears to act as a positive activator of HrpL to mediate the environmental regulation of *hrp* genes (D. Rowley and S. W. Hutcheson, unpublished results). An overview of the apparent *hrp* regulatory network is shown in Fig. 2.

INTERACTION OF *hrp* AND *avr* GENES

A long-standing quandary in plant-microbe interactions has been the function of *avr* genes. *avr* genes have been cloned from a number of *P. syringae* strains and demonstrated to control race-specific interactions with the susceptible plant species (Dangl, 1994; Keen, 1990; Staskawicz et al., 1995). *P. syringae* strains carrying an *avr* gene elicit the HR in cultivars of the susceptible plant species that express the corresponding R gene. Current models to describe these interactions invoke race-specific elicitors produced directly or indirectly by *avr* genes which are recognized by receptors in the plant

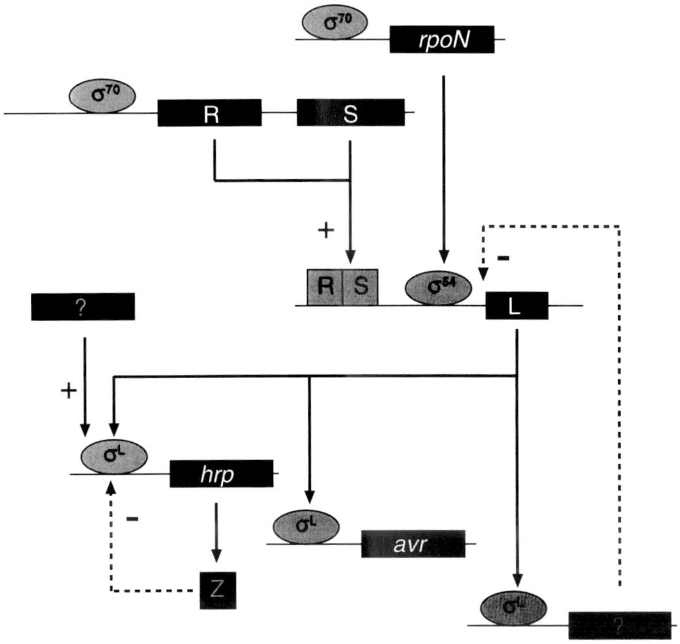

Figure 2. Transcriptional factors controlling expression of *hrp* and *avr* genes in *P. syringae* Pss61. Sigma factors are indicated by ovals, promoters are represented by lines, genes are represented by black rectangles, and regulatory components are shown as boxes. Arrows indicate target promoters for regulatory factors, and dashed lines indicate negative-acting regulatory components. The *hrpR* promoter appears to be constitutively expressed, whereas promoters below are conditional. Current analyses suggest that a presently unidentified positive activator and a negative-acting component linked to HrpZ2 mediate the activity of HrpL (D. Rowley, V. Kotraiah, and S. W. Hutcheson, unpublished results). Other data suggest that the activity of the *hrpL* promoter is negatively regulated by a third component acting as a negative repressor (Rowley and Hutcheson, unpublished results).

cell that are encoded by R genes to initiate the HR (Keen, 1992). With the exception of *avrD* (Midlands et al., 1993), however, the identity of the postulated race-specific elicitor has been elusive. Cell-free fractions of bacteria carrying constitutively expressed *avr* genes (other than *avrD*) have failed to exhibit elicitor activity. The deduced gene products thus far lack features indicative of a biochemical activity. Indications that Hrp and Avr gene products may interact to control the host range of *P. syringae* strains come from a largely overlooked observation that in one strain of *P. syringae hrp* mutations suppressed the phenotype of an *avr* gene (Huynh et al., 1989) and the above-mentioned findings that *avr* genes are regulated by the same mechanism as the *hrp* operons in *P. syringae* strains.

Experimental evidence demonstrating that the *hrp* gene cluster mediates the phenotypic expression of *avr* genes came from studies using the heterologous expression of *hrp* genes in *E. coli* (Pirhonen et al., 1996). *E. coli* is not a plant pathogen and thus fails to elicit a response when inoculated into tobacco or any other plant. Both the *hrp*-linked secretion system and the *hrp* regulatory system have been shown to be active in *E. coli* (Heu and Hutcheson, 1993; Lidell and Hutcheson, 1994; Xiao et al., 1994). *E. coli* strains carrying the Pss61 *hrp* cluster are capable of eliciting the HR in tobacco, but a relatively high inoculum level is required even when expression of the cluster is increased by the presence of a constitutively expressed *hrpL* construct. In other plants, such as soybean cultivars or ecotypes of *Arabidopsis thaliana,* a null response is consistently observed. In collaboration with N. Keen, we showed that *E. coli* transformants carrying a constitutively expressed *hrpL* construct, the cloned *P. syringae* Pss61 *hrp* cluster, and *avrB* expressed from vector *lac*UV5 promoters elicit the HR specifically in soybean cultivars that carry the reactive *Rpg1* resistance gene (Pirhonen et al., 1996). Similarly, in *A. thaliana* an HR was observed in ecotype Col-0, which carries the reactive *RPM1* resistance gene, but not in the Col-0 (*rps*3-1) mutant, which carries an *rpm1* mutation, or in five ecotypes of *A. thaliana* which lack the *RPM1* gene. These results are consistent with phenotypic expression of *avrB* in *E. coli.* Similar experiments demonstrated that phenotypic expression of *avrA, avrC, avrPto, avrRpt2, avrRpm1,* and *avrPph3* in *E. coli* also requires an activity of the *hrp* cluster. *E. coli* transformants carrying each of these *avr* genes and the induced Pss61 *hrp* cluster elicited the HR in soybean cultivars that carry a reactive R gene. Therefore, for at least seven *avr* genes isolated from *P. syringae* strains, phenotypic expression in an *E. coli* strain is dependent directly upon the *hrp* genes.

Subsequent experiments showed that two activities associated with the *P. syringae hrp* cluster are required for phenotypic expression of *avr* genes. As discussed above, transcription of *avr* genes is controlled by the HrpL-dependent regulatory system. Mutational analyses showed that the *hrp*-linked secretion system is also necessary for phenotypic expression of *avr* genes. These observations provide an indication of a mechanism by which the Avr phenotype is generated. One possibility could be that the complete *hrp* cluster is needed for the presentation of the *avr* gene product to the plant cell. Alternatively, harpin and the *avr* gene product could serve as coelicitors in a dual-stimulus model. Experiments are in progress to test these hypotheses.

CONCLUDING REMARKS

It is now apparent that the *hrp* genes play a central role in the pathogenicity of *P. syringae* strains, controlling both virulence and host range. Thus in phytopathogenic bacteria and in several enteric bacteria pathogenic to mammals, a conserved type III protein secretion system is a necessary component for virulence. The similarity in organization and components of the *hrp*-related secretion systems found in the *P. syringae* strains and the enteric bacteria, such as *Yersinia* strains, suggests a common origin. Because *P. syringae* strains are common epiphytes of many plants and are capable of conjugal transfer of DNA to heterologous bacteria, lateral transfer of a functional secretion system between bacteria could have occurred. Alternatively, the similarity with the late genes of flagellar biosynthesis could suggest that these secretion systems evolved from a duplication and adaptation of these genes. Further analysis will be necessary to determine if either of these models is correct.

In the mammalian pathogens, the virulence factors secreted by this system facilitate attachment and, in some cases, invasion of target cells. Pathogenesis of *P. syringae* strains differs from that of most mammalian pathogens: strains remain external to the cell wall of living plant cells in colonized tissue. To exert their pathogenic effects, however, both types of pathogens require contact with the host cell before a response is initiated. In view of the similarity with the flagellar biosynthesis systems, it may be that type III protein secretion systems form structures that inject secreted proteins into the parasitized cell (Rosqvist et al., 1994). Since R-gene products are apparently cytoplasmic (Dangl, 1995), the function of *hrp* genes in *P. syringae* strains might be to introduce an *avr*-linked elicitor or the *avr* gene products directly into plant cells.

Acknowledgments. The experiments on the interaction of *hrp* and *avr* genes were done in collaboration with N. Keen (University of California, Riverside). This work was supported in part by grants to S.W.H. from the National Science Foundation (DMB 92221670), the U.S. Department of Agriculture (PPW9501170), and the Maryland Agricultural Experiment Station. M.U.P. was supported by a grant from the Swedish Council for Forestry and Agricultural Research.

REFERENCES

Agrios, G. N. 1988. *Plant Pathology*, 3rd ed. Academic Press, New York.

Baker, C. J., E. W. Orlandi, and N. M. Mock. 1993. Harpin, an elicitor of the hypersensitive response in tobacco caused by *Erwinia amylovora,* elicits active oxygen production in suspension cells. *Plant Physiol.* **102:**1341–1344.

Bonas, U. 1994. *hrp* genes of phytopathogenc bacteria. *Curr. Top. Microbiol. Immunol.* **192:**79–98.

Collmer, A., D. W. Bauer, J. R. Alfano, G. Preston, A. O. Loniello, H. C. Huang, and S. Y. He. 1994. The role of *Pseudomonas syringae* and *Erwinia chrysanthemi hrp* gene products in plant interactions. *Adv. Mol. Genet. Plant-Microbe Interact.* **3:**49–56.

Cornelis, G. R. 1994. *Yersinia* pathogenicity factors. *Curr. Top. Microbiol. Immunol.* **192:**243–263.

Dangl, J. L. 1994. The enigmatic avirulence genes of phytopathogenic bacteria. *Curr. Top. Microbiol. Immunol.* **192:**99–118.

Dangl, J. L. 1995. Piece de resistance: novel classes of plant disease resistance genes. *Cell* **80:**363–366.

Felley, R., L. G. Rahme, M. N. Mindrinos, R. D. Frederick, A. Pisi, and N. J. Panopoulos. 1991. Genes and signals controlling the *Pseudomonas syringae* pv. *phaseolicola*-plant interaction. *Adv. Mol. Genet. Plant-Microbe Interact.* **1:**45–52.

Fenselau, S., I. Balbo, and U. Bonas. 1992. Determinants of pathogenicity in *Xanthomonas campestris* pv. vesicatoria are related to proteins involved in secretion in bacterial pathogens of animals. *Mol. Plant-Microbe Interact.* **5:**390–396.

Grimm, C., W. Aufsatz, and N. J. Panopoulos. 1995. The *hrp*RS locus of *Pseudomonas syringae* pv. phaseolicola constitutes a complex regulatory unit. *Mol. Microbiol.* **15:**155–165.

Grimm, C., and N. J. Panopoulos. 1989. The predicted protein product of a pathogenicity locus from *Pseudomonas syringae* pv. phaseolicola is homologous to a highly conserved domain of several prokaryotic regulatory proteins. *J. Bacteriol.* **171:**5031–5038.

He, S. Y., H. C. Huang, and A. Collmer. 1993. *Pseudomonas syringae* pv. syringae harpin$_{Pss}$: a protein that is secreted via the Hrp pathway and elicits the hypersensitive response in plants. *Cell* **73:**1255–1266.

Heu, S., and S. W. Hutcheson. 1993. Nucleotide sequence and properties of the *hrm*A locus associated with the *P. syringae* pv. syringae 61 *hrp* gene cluster. *Mol. Plant-Microbe Interact.* **6:**553–564.

Huang, H. C., S. Y. He, D. W. Bauer, and A. Collmer. 1992. The *Pseudomonas syringae* pv. syringae 61 *hrpH* product: an envelope protein required for elicitation of the hypersensitive response in plants. *J. Bacteriol.* **174:**6878–6885.

Huang, H. C., S. W. Hutcheson, and A. Collmer. 1991. Characterization of the *hrp* cluster from *Pseudomonas syringae* pv. syringae 61 and Tn*pho*A tagging of exported or membrane-spanning Hrp proteins. *Mol. Plant-Microbe Interact.* **4:**469–476.

Huang, H. C., R. H. Lin, C. J. Chang, A. Collmer, and W. L. Deng. 1995. The complete *hrp* gene cluster of *Pseudomonas syringae* pv. syringae 61 includes two blocks of genes required for harpinPss secretion that are arranged colinearly with *Yersinia ysc* homologs. *Mol. Plant-Microbe Interact.* **8:**733–746.

Huang, H. C., R. Schuurink, T. P. Denny, M. M. Atkinson, C. J. Baker, I. Yucel, S. W. Hutcheson, and A. Collmer. 1988. Molecular cloning of a *Pseudomonas syringae* pv. *syringae* gene cluster that enables *Pseudomonas fluorescens* to elicit the hypersensitive response in tobacco. *J. Bacteriol.* **170:**4748–4756.

Huang, H. C., Y. Xiao, R.-H. Lin, Y. Lu, S. W. Hutcheson, and A. Collmer. 1993. Characterization of the *Pseudomonas syringae* pv. syringae 61 *hrpJ* and *hrpI* genes: homology of HrpI to a superfamily of proteins associated with protein translocation. *Mol. Plant-Microbe Interact.* **6:**515–520.

Hutcheson, S. W., S. Heu, and Y. Xiao. 1994. Mechanism for environmental regulation of *Pseudomonas syringae* pathogenicity and host range determinants. *Adv. Mol. Genet. Plant-Microbe Interact.* **3:**33–36.

Huynh, T., D. Dahlbeck, and B. J. Staskawicz. 1989. Bacterial blight of soybean: regulation of a pathogen gene determining host cultivar specificity. *Science* **245:**1374–1377.

Innes, R. W., A. F. Bent, B. N. Kunkel, S. R. Bisgrove, and B. J. Staskawicz. 1993. Molecular analysis of avirulence gene *avrRpt2* and identification of a putative regulatory sequence common to all known *Pseudomonas syringae* avirulence genes. *J. Bacteriol.* **175:**4859–4869.

Keen, N. 1990. Gene-for-gene complementarity in plant-pathogen interactions. *Annu. Rev. Genet.* **24:**447–463.

Keen, N. T. 1992. The molecular biology of disease resistance. *Plant Mol. Biol.* **19:**109–122.

Klement, Z. 1982. Hypersensitivity, p. 149–177. *In* M. S. Mount and G. H. Lacy (ed.), *Phytopathogenic Prokaryotes,* vol. 2. Academic Press, New York.

Lidell, M., and S. W. Hutcheson. 1994. Characterization of the *hrpJ* and *U* operons of *Pseudomonas syringae* pv. syringae Pss61: similarity with components of enteric bacteria involved in flagellar biogenesis and demonstration of their role in harpin$_{Pss}$ translocation. *Mol. Plant-Microbe Interact.* **7:**488–497.

Lindgren, P. B., N. J. Panopoulos, B. J. Staskawicz, and D. Dahlbeck. 1988. Genes required for pathogenicity and hypersensitivity are conserved and interchangeable among pathovars of *Pseudomonas syringae. Mol. Gen. Genet.* **21:**499–506.

Lindgren, P. B., R. C. Peet, and N. J. Panopoulos. 1986. Gene cluster of *Pseudomonas syringae* pv. phaseolicola controls pathogenicity on bean plants and hypersensitivity on nonhost plants. *J. Bacteriol.* **168:**512–522.

Lonetto, M. A., K. L. Brown, K. E. Rudd, and M. J. Bittner. 1994. Analysis of the *Streptomyces coelicolor sigE* gene reveals the existence of a subfamily of eubacterial RNA polymerase σ factors involved in the regulation of extracytoplasmic functions. *Proc. Natl. Acad. Sci. USA* **91:**7573–7577.

Long, S. R., and B. J. Staskawicz. 1993. Prokaryotic plant pathogens. *Cell* **73:**921–935.

MacNab, R. M. 1992. Genetics and biogenesis of bacterial flagella. *Annu. Rev. Genet.* **26:**131–158.

Midlands, S. L., N. T. Keen, J. J. Sims, M. M. Midland, M. M. Stayton, V. Burton, M. J. Smith, E. P. Mazzola, K. J. Graham, and J. Clardy. 1993. The structure of syringolides 1 and 2, novel C-glycosidic elicitors from *Pseudomonas syringae* pv. tomato. *J. Org. Chem.* **58:**2940–2945.

Morett, E., and L. Segovia. 1993. The sigma 54 bacterial enhancer-binding protein family: mechanism of action and phylogenetic relationship of their functional domains. *J. Bacteriol.* **175:**6067–6074.

Pirhonen, M. U., D. Rowley, M. C. Lidell, S. W. Lee, S. Silverstone, Y. Liang, N. T. Keen, and S. W. Hutcheson. 1996. Phenotypic expression of *Pseudomonas syringae avr* genes in *Escherichia coli* is linked to the activities of the *hrp*-encoded secretion system. *Mol. Plant Microbe Interact.* **9:**252–260.

Rahme, L. G., M. N. Mindronos, and N. J. Panopoulos. 1992. Plant and environmental sensory signals control the expression of *hrp* genes in *Pseudomonas syringae* pv. phaseolicola. *J. Bacteriol.* **174:**3499–3507.

Rosqvist, R., K. E. Magnusson, and H. Wolf-Waltz. 1994. Target cell contact triggers expression and polarized transfer of *Yersinia* YopE cytotoxin into mammalian cells. *EMBO J.* **13:**964–972.

Salmeron, J. M., and B. J. Staskawicz. 1993. Molecular characterization and *hrp*-dependence of the avirulence gene *avr*Pto from *Pseudomonas syringae* pv. tomato. *Mol. Gen. Genet.* **239:**6–10.

Salmond, G. P. C., and P. J. Reeves. 1993. Membrane traffic wardens and protein secretion in gram-negative bacteria. *Trends Biochem. Sci.* **18:**7–12.

Shapiro, L. 1995. The bacterial flagellum: from genetic network to complex architecture. *Cell* **80:**525–527.

Shen, H., and N. T. Keen. 1993. Characterization of the promoter of avirulence gene D from *Pseudomonas syringae* pv. tomato. *J. Bacteriol.* **175:**5916–5924.

Staskawicz, B. J., F. M. Ausubel, B. J. Baker, J. G. Ellis, and J. D. G. Jones. 1995. Molecular genetics of plant disease resistance. *Science* **268:**661–667.

VanGijsegem, F., S. Genin, and C. Boucher. 1994. Conservation of secretion pathways for pathogenicity determinants of plant and animal bacteria. *Trends Microbiol.* **1:**175–180.

Willis, D. K., J. J. Rich, and E. M. Hrabak. 1991. The *hrp* genes of phytopathogenic bacteria. *Mol. Plant-Microbe Interact.* **4:**132–138.

Xiao, Y., S. Heu, J. Yi, Y. Lu, and S. W. Hutcheson. 1994. Identification of a putative alternate sigma factor and characterization of a multicomponent regulatory cascade controlling the expression of *Pseudomonas syringae* pv. *syringae* Pss61 *hrp* and *hrmA* genes. *J. Bacteriol.* **176:**1025–1036.

Xiao, Y., and S. W. Hutcheson. 1994. A single promoter sequence recognized by a newly identified alternate sigma factor directs expression of pathogenicity and host range determinants in *Pseudomonas syringae*. *J. Bacteriol.* **176:**3089–3091.

Xiao, Y., Y. Lu, S. Heu, and S. W. Hutcheson. 1992. Organization and environmental regulation of the *Pseudomonas syringae* pv. syringae 61 *hrp* cluster. *J. Bacteriol.* **174:**1734–1741.

Zhang, L. Z., and A. L. Jones. 1995. Organization of the *hrp* gene cluster and nucleotide sequence of the *hrp*L gene from *Pseudomonas syringae* pv. morspurorum. *Phytopathology* **85:**118–123.

INDEX